CARDIAC OUTPUT AND REGIONAL FLOW IN HEALTH AND DISEASE

Developments in
Cardiovascular Medicine

VOLUME 138

The titles published in this series are listed at the end of this volume.

Cardiac Output and Regional Flow in Health and Disease

edited by

ABDUL-MAJEED SALMASI

Department of Cardiology, Central Middlesex Hospital, London, UK

and

ABDULMASSIH S. ISKANDRIAN

Philadelphia Heart Institute, Presbyterian Medical Center, Philadelphia, Pennsylvania, USA

KLUWER ACADEMIC PUBLISHERS

DORDRECHT / BOSTON / LONDON

Library of Congress Cataloging-in-Publication Data


```
Cardiac output and regional flow in health and disease / edited by
  Abdul-Majeed Salmasi and Abdulmassih S. Iskandrian.
       p.   cm. -- (Developments in cardiovascular medicine ; v. 138)
    Includes bibliographical references and index.
    ISBN 0-7923-1911-7 (alk. paper)
    1. Cardiac output.  2. Regional blood flow.  I. Salmasi, Abdul
  -Majeed.  II. Iskandrian, Abdulmassih S., 1941-   . III. Series.
    [DNLM: 1. Cardiac Output--drug effects.  2. Cardiac Output-
  -physiology.  3. Regional Blood Flow--drug effects.  4. Regional
  Blood Flow--physiology.   W1 DE997VME v. 138 / WG 106 C2665]
  QP113.C369  1993
  612.1'71--dc20
  DNLM/DLC
  for Library of Congress                             92-49733
```


ISBN 0-7923-1911-7

Published by Kluwer Academic Publishers,
P.O. Box 17, 3300 AA Dordrecht, The Netherlands.

Kluwer Academic Publishers incorporates
the publishing programmes of
D. Reidel, Martinus Nijhoff, Dr W. Junk and MTP Press.

Sold and distributed in the U.S.A. and Canada
by Kluwer Academic Publishers,
101 Philip Drive, Norwell, MA 02061, U.S.A.

In all other countries, sold and distributed
by Kluwer Academic Publishers Group,
P.O. Box 322, 3300 AH Dordrecht, The Netherlands.

Printed on acid-free paper

Table of contents

List of contributors

RALPH ABRAHAM MA, PhD, BMBCh, MRCP
London Diabetes and Lipid Centre
London
UK

MUNTHER I. ALDOORI PhD, FRCS
Consultant Transplant Surgeon, Clinical Lecturer
St. James' University Hospital
Leeds
UK

JONATHAN D. BEARD, ChM, FRCS
Consultant Vascular Surgeon
The Royal Hallamshire Hospital
Sheffield
UK

LOUIS J. BRISSON MD
Presbyterian Medical Center
Philadelphia Heart Institute
Philadelphia
Pennsylvania 19104
USA

JOHN G.F. CLELAND MD, MRCP
Senior Lecturer and Consultant Cardiologist
Division of Clinical Cardiology
Department of Medicine
Royal Postgraduate Medical School
Hammersmith Hospital
London
UK

WILLIAM J. CORIN MD
Philadelphia Heart Institute
Presbyterian Medical Center
Philadelphia
Pennsylvania 19104
USA

MARK R. DRAYTON MR3P
Consultant Neonatal Paediatrician
University Hospital of Wales
Cardiff
UK

FAWZI HABBOUSHE MD, FACS
Clinical Assistant Professor of Surgery
University of Pennsylvania
Attending Thoracic and General Surgeon
The Graduate Hospital
Philadelphia Pennsylvania 19104
USA

HOPE BETH HELFELD DO
Philadelphia Heart Institute
Presbyterian Medical Center
Philadelphia
Pennsylvania 19104
USA

JAEKYEONG HEO MD
Philadelphia Heart Institute
Philadelphia
Pennsylvania 19104
USA

WALTER R. HEPP MD
Philadelphia Heart Institute
Presbyterian Medical Center
Philadelphia
Pennsylvania 19104
USA

LEONARD N. HOROWITZ MD
Philadelphia Heart Institute
Presbyterian Medical Center
Philadelphia
Pennsylvania 19104
USA

ABDULMASSIH S. ISKANDRIAN MD, FACP, FCCP, FACC
Clinical Professor of Medicine
Co-Director
Philadelphia Heart Institute
Presbyterian Medical Center
Philadelphia
Pennsylvania 19104
USA

MARIELL JESSUP MD
Director, Heart Failure Unit
Philadelphia Heart Institute
Presbyterian Medical Center
Philadelphia
Pennsylvania 19104
USA

STUART D. KATZ MD
Division of Cardiology
Albert Einstein College of Medicine
New York
New York 10461
USA

RICHARD E. LEE ChM, FRCS
Church House
Drayton, Somerset
UK

THIERRY H. LEJEMTEL MD
Division of Cardiology
Albert Einstein College of Medicine
New York
New York 10461
USA

PAUL L. MARINO MD, PhD, FCCM
Associate Clinical Professor
University of Pennsylvania
Director, Critical Care
Presbyterian Medical Center
Philadelphia
Pennsylvania 19104
USA

DAVID P. MOORE MB, MRCPI
Division of Clinical Cardiology
Department of Medicine
Royal Postgraduate Medical School
Hammersmith Hospital
London
UK

KYPROS H. NICOLAIDES MRCOG
Consultant Obstetrician and Gynaecologist
Harris Birthright Research Centre for Fetal Medicine
King's College Hospital Medical School
London
UK

PETROS NIHOYANNOPOULOS MD, FACA
Senior Lecturer and Consultant Caradiologist
Director of Echocardiography Laboratory
Royal Postgraduate Medical School
Hammersmith Hospital
London
UK

THACH N. NGUYEN MD
Philadelphia Heart Institute
Presbyterian Medical Center
Philadelphia
Pennsylvania 19104
USA

J. DAVID OGILBY MD
Clinical Assistant Professor of Medicine
Associate Director, Cardiac Catheterization Laboratory
Philadelphia Heart Institute
Presbyterian Medical Center
Philadelphia
Pennsylvania 19104
USA

MIKE W. RAMPLING BSc, PhD
Reader
Departmerlt of Physiology and Biophysics
St. Mary's Hospital Medical School
London
UK

ABDUL-MAJEED SALMASI MD, PhD, FACA, FICA
Department of Cardiology
Central Middlesex Hospital
London
UK

WILLIAM P. SANTAMORE PhD
Philadelphia Heart Institute
Presbyterian Medical Center
Philadelphia
Pennsylvania 19104
USA

JEFFREY J. SCHWARTZ MD
Assistant Professor
Department of Anesthesiology
Yale University School of Medicine
New Haven
Connecticut 06510-8068
USA

BERNARD L. SEGAL MD, FACC
Clinical Professor of Medicine
University of Pennsylvania School of Medicine
Director, Philadelphia Heart Institute
Presbyterian Medical Center
Philadelphia
Pennsylvania 19104
USA

NANCY M. SHERWIN
Lankenau Hospital
Philadelphia
Pennsylvania 19104
USA

JAMES D. SINK MD
Associate Clinical Professor
University of Pennsylvania
Chief, Division of Cardiothoracic Surgery
Presbyterian Medical Center
Philadelphia
Pennsylvania 19104
USA

IBRAHIM SUKKAR BSc, MSc, PhD
Irvine Laboratory for Cardiovascular Investigation and Research
Department of Surgery
St. Mary's Hospital Medical School
London
UK

J. GUY THORPE-BEESTON MRCOG
Department of Obstetrics and Gynaecology
St. Mary's Hospital Medical School
London
UK

GARY J. VIGILANTE MD, FACP, FACC
Philadelphia Heart Institute
Presbyterian Medical Center
Philadelphia
Pennsylvania 19104
USA

HARRY G. ZEGAL MD
Presbyterian Medical Center
Philadelphia Heart Institute
Philadelphia
Pennsylvania 19104
USA

Preface

Although cardiac output has received much attention throughout this century, the last decade has been rather rich in major developments in, and a better understanding of, the clinical aspects of "cardiac output" and its application in different branches of medicine. Much of these advances have been made as a result of the introduction of the innovative non-invasive techniques to measure cardiac output which have also made it easier to study changes in the heart or other organs as a result of variation in cardiac output.

Because of the popularity of the cardiac output to the understanding of the hemodynamic adaptation in health and disease and its critical role in managing acutely ill patients, it seemed appropriate to compose a book that assembles all aspects of "cardiac output". We are fortunate to have a distinguished group of authors who have written what we believe to be state-of-the-art chapters. We hope that this book will stand out as a reference on the subject and that the readers will find it both stimulating and useful. Because of the relevance of cardiac output in cardiac and non-cardiac diseases, we hope this book will be useful not only to cardiologists, but also to physicians in other fields of medicine and surgery, and to their trainees.

Finally we are greatful to the help and support of the Kluwer Academic Publishing Company.

Abdul-Majeed Salmasi   Abdulmassih S. Iskandrian
London, U.K.   *Philadelphia, PA, U.S.A.*

PART ONE

Technical considerations

1. Determination of cardiac output by invasive methods

WILLIAM J. CORIN and WILLIAM P. SANTAMORE

The fundamental role of the heart within the circulatory system is to pump blood. This blood flow supplies oxygen and nutrients to all of the tissues in the body, and removes metabolic waste products. Cardiac output is the term used to represent the quantity of blood flowing through the systemic circulation per unit time, and is expressed in the units liters/minute. To account for differences in patients' body height and weight, the cardiac output is related to the body surface area and termed the cardiac index; it is expressed in the units liters/minute/m^2.

At present, there are four fundamental methods to invasively measure cardiac output: the Fick oxygen method; the indicator dilution method, including the thermodilution and indocyanine green dye techniques; the angiographic approach; and the conductance method. These methods are complementary and each approach provides the accuracy and responsiveness most applicable to certain clinical situations. Advances in technology permit more rapid and accurate determination of cardiac output than was previously possible; measurement and computation were previously performed by hand. Computers presently calculate oxygen consumption, measure hemoglobin saturation, determine indicator concentrations, and perform integration and multiple computations. Microprocessor systems will often provide a result despite incorrect or inconsistent input data. As these systems become increasingly sophisticated, certain algorithms have been incorporated to evaluate the quality and consistency of the data. However, to insure consistent accuracy of cardiac output determinations, continued operator attention is essential.

The Fick oxygen technique

In 1870, Adolf Fick described a method to determine cardiac output: "The total uptake or release of a substance by an organ is the product of the blood flow to the organ and of the arteriovenous concentration of the substance" [1]. The Fick oxygen technique applies this principle to the specific substance oxygen, which is infused at a constant rate (at steady state) into the circulatory system via the lungs. This method is accurate to within 10%, and remains the standard for steady-state measurements of systemic cardiac output [2]. By measuring the oxygen uptake from the lungs and the difference in oxygen

A.-M. Salmasi and A.S. Iskandrian (eds): Cardiac output and regional flow in health and disease, 3–29.

content of blood across the pulmonary circulation, the Fick technique actually determines pulmonary blood flow. In the absence of an intracardiac shunt, pulmonary and systemic blood flow are equal and this method provides the systemic blood flow. The systemic cardiac output (CO, liters/minute) is computed as the quotient of the systemic oxygen consumption, (VO_2, ml/minute) and the difference between the arterial and venous oxygen content of blood (A-V O_2 difference, ml/dl, multiplied by 10 to convert to liters), and is expressed as:

$$CO = \frac{VO_2}{\text{A-V } O_2 \text{ difference} \cdot 10}.$$

Thus, in order to determine cardiac output by the Fick oxygen method, both the oxygen consumption and arteriovenous oxygen difference must be assessed.

Oxygen consumption

Oxygen consumption is presently determined in two ways: by collecting the exhaled air in a Tissot or Douglas bag, and by the polarographic method.

Tissot/Douglas bag method. This approach measures the volume and oxygen content of the air expired by the patient to compute oxygen consumption. The patient breathes room air and exhales into a Tissot gasometer (or a collecting Douglas bag) for a predetermined period of time (Figure 1.1). To calculate the difference in oxygen content, the proportion of oxygen in the inhaled and exhaled air is measured using an oxygen analyzer (for room air the inhaled oxygen fraction equals 0.209). The absolute volume of exhaled gas in the Tissot or Douglas bag is measured and then corrected, using the barometric pressure and temperature of the ambient air obtained from a barometer and thermometer, and applied to standard tables (e.g. Documenta Geigy-Scientific Tables). Oxygen consumption is determined as the corrected volume of ventilation multiplied by the difference in oxygen between inspired and expired air. When corrected for the period of collection, the oxygen consumption per minute is obtained; this result divided by body surface area, yields the oxygen consumption index.

Polarographic oxygen method. This instrument contains an oxygen sensor, face hood or mask, and a variable-speed blower which maintains a flow directing room air into the hood, through a connecting hose to the oxygen sensor (Figure 1.2). The rate of air volume blown (V_M, ml/min) is controlled by a negative feedback system that maintains the content of oxygen passing the detector at a constant level. The oxygen content of air flowing through the hose to the sensor is a function of the rate of air entering the hood (V_R, ml/min), and the patient's ventilatory rate (V_I, air inhaled ml/min; V_E, air exhaled ml/min); V_M will vary with oxygen consumption. At steady state, the

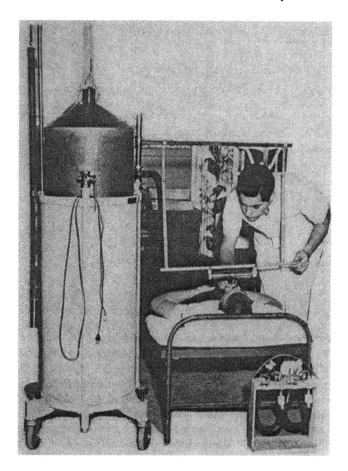

Figure 1.1. The Tissot spirometer. The patient (supine) is assisted in breathing into a mouthpiece connected via tubing to the Tissot bell. With permission.

patient's oxygen consumption is determined by measuring the volume rate V_M, and the proportion of oxygen in the air passing the polarographic sensor.

Arteriovenous oxygen difference

Computation of the difference in the oxygen content of blood across the pulmonary circulation is central to the Fick oxygen method. To perform this technique most accurately, blood should be obtained from both the pulmonary artery and pulmonary vein during the period of oxygen consumption measurement. In the absence of a left to right intracardiac shunt, the pulmonary artery is the most reliable location to obtain mixed venous blood; right

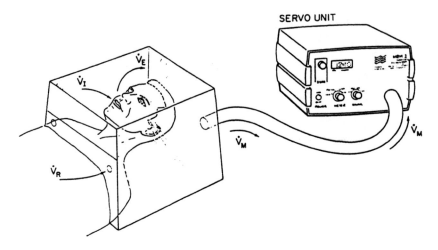

SERVO UNIT

Figure 1.2. The metabolic rate meter (Waters instruments) employs the polarographic cell to measure oxygen consumption. In this schematic, air enters the transparent hood, that fits over the patients head at the flow rate V_R. V_M is the air flow rate leaving the hood and entering the servo-unit which contains the oxygen sensor. V_M is equal to V_R plus the difference between the inspired V_I and expired air V_E. The flow rate V_M is determined by a blower that, via a negative feedback system with the oxygen sensor, maintains the oxygen content of the air reaching the polarographic cell at a constant level. With permission.

ventricular or atrial blood may be substituted if necessary. In the absence of a right to left shunt, systemic arterial blood may be sampled in place of pulmonary venous blood, and assumed to have a similar oxygen content. (Due to the drainage of thesbian and bronchial veins into the left atrium, systemic blood has a 1–2% lower oxygen content than pulmonary venous blood.) Systemic arterial blood may be acquired via a catheter positioned in any convenient location in the systemic circulation: central aorta or a peripheral artery. While for the majority of patients the sample location is not critical, an aortic sample is preferred in patients with diminished peripheral flow.

The oxygen saturation of the sampled blood is presently determined in one of two ways. Most modern cardiac catheterization laboratories are equipped with a co-oximeter that measures the oxygen saturation and content of a blood sample. These instruments measure the proportion of hemoglobin and oxyhemoglobin present in the blood sample using the principle that light absorption by these substances varies at different wavelengths (Figure 1.3). The relative transmission of multiple narrow wavelength bands of light through the blood to a photodetector is measured, permitting the relative proportions of hemoglobin and oxyhemoglobin to be determined (Figure 1.4).

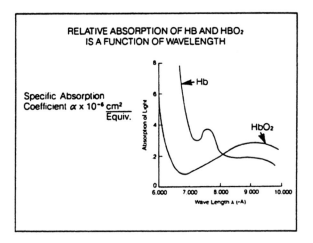

Figure 1.3. The different light absorption characteristics of hemoglobin (Hb) and oxyhemoglobin (HbO$_2$) are shown across a range of light wavelengths. Transmission and reflectance oximetry utilizes these differences to measure the oxygen saturation of blood. With permission.

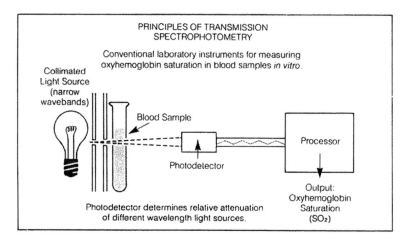

Figure 1.4. The principles of transmission spectrophotometry are presented in schematic. The transmission of multiple narrow wavelength bands of light through a blood sample is measured by a photodetector. These signals are provided to a processor that computes the relative proportions of hemoglobin and oxyhemoglobin in the sample. With permission.

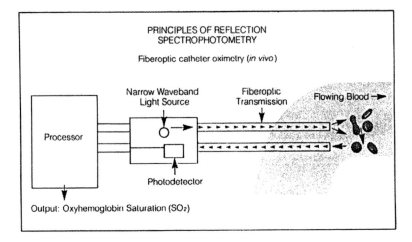

Figure 1.5. The principles of reflection spectrophotometry are presented in schematic. An optical module transmits light of different wavelength via the fiberoptic filament to the flowing blood and the reflected light is returned by a separate monofilament. The photodetector measures the reflected light and sends this electrical signal to the processor. After filtering these signals, the processor computes blood oxygen concentration. With permission.

Central venous oxygen saturation can be continuously monitored and cardiac output calculated, using an intravascular oximetry catheter. This catheter transmits a beam of light from a variable wavelength light source via a fiberoptic monofilament to the bloodstream, and returns the reflected signal to a photodetector via a separate monofilament (Figure 1.5). This catheter is used primarily in the post-operative and intensive care setting, where it permits continuous *in vivo* measurement of blood oxygen saturation. While right heart 'pullback' oximetry can also be performed using these catheters, reservations concerning cost, accuracy and sensitivity to manipulation have limited their use in the cardiac catheterization laboratory.

Oxygen is transported in the blood bound almost exclusively to hemoglobin. The oxygen carrying capacity of hemoglobin is approximately 1.36 ml O_2/gm Hb [3]. This value may be significantly altered in smokers in whom quantities of carboxyhemoglobin are present, and in patients with hemoglobinopathies. Changes in the oxygen carrying capacity of hemoglobin reduce the accuracy of the arteriovenous calculation.

The relationship of the partial pressure of oxygen in blood to the hemoglobin saturation (and content) is represented by the oxygen dissociation curve (Figure 1.6). The oxygen affinity of hemoglobin is enhanced by an increase in blood pH, or a decrease in blood temperature, 2,3 DPG level, pCO_2. There is also a quantity of oxygen dissolved in the plasma, though it contributes minimally to oxygen content in the patient breathing room air (approxi-

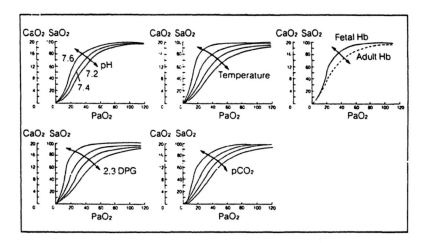

Figure 1.6. The oxygen dissociation curve relates the partial pressure of oxygen in blood (PaO_2) to oxygen saturation (SaO_2). Oxygen saturation is a non-linear function of oxygen pressure, and is also affected by blood pH, temperature, type of hemloglobin, 2,3 DPG level and pCO_2. With permission.

mately 1% of the total). However in the anemic patient receiving supplemental oxygen, the dissolved oxygen may comprise a significant proportion of the total blood oxygen content (up to 8%) and introduce a significant error into the calculation of the arteriovenous oxygen difference.

The arteriovenous oxygen difference is calculated as (Table 1.1):

Arteriovenous oxygen difference =
systemic oxygen content − PA oxygen content.

The oxygen consumption and arteriovenous oxygen difference are used to calculate the cardiac output.

Clinical utility and advantage

The Fick oxygen technique remains the standard to which all other methods are compared. The error in determining the arteriovenous oxygen difference and oxygen consumption are approximately 5% [4–6]; the total error using this method is about 10% [2].

The Fick oxygen method is most accurate in patients with a *reduced* cardiac output, in whom the arteriovenous oxygen difference is large [7]. This method is the most accurate approach in atrial fibrillation: the longer period required to determine the Fick output eliminates the effect of the beat to beat variation.

This technique may be used in the setting of an intracardiac shunt. To

Table 1.1. Calculation of cardiac output by Fick principle.

Cardiac output (liters/minute)	O$_2$ consumption (ml O$_2$/minute)	A-V O$_2$ difference (ml O$_2$/L blood)

Arteriovenous oxygen difference (ml O$_2$/dl blood) = systemic oxygen content/dl blood − PA oxygen content/dl blood

(a)   Systemic O$_2$ content   =   Hemoglobin (gm/dl)   ×   Systemic   O$_2$ saturation × 1.36[a]

(b)   (Venous O$_2$ content   =   Hemoglobin (gm/dl)   ×   PA O$_2$ saturation × 1.36[a]

(c)   A-V O$_2$ difference   =   Systemic O$_2$ content   −   Venous O$_2$ content
(ml O$_2$/dl blood)   (equation a)   (equation b)

A-V O$_2$ difference
(ml O$_2$/L blood)   =   A-V O$_2$ difference × 10[b]
(ml O$_2$/dl blood)

[a]The theoretic oxygen carrying capacity of blood, 1.36 ml O$_2$/gm Hb, is used for these calculations. Use of this theoretic factor provides the theoretic blood oxygen content, a close approximation to the actual blood oxygen content.
[b]The arteriovenous oxygen difference is usually expressed as the difference per 100 ml of blood, but must be expressed as the difference per liter of blood to calculate the cardiac output in liters/minute.

maximize accuracy in the presence of a left to right shunt, multiple samples must be obtained (and averaged) from the chamber just proximal to the level of the shunt. For example, in the patient with a ventricular septal defect, right atrial blood is sampled. In the patient with an atrial septal defect, the mixed venous oxygen saturation is a weighted average of the results obtained from sampling the superior (SVC) and inferior (IVC) vena cavae:

Mixed venous O$_2$ saturation = (3 · SVC saturation
+ 1 · IVC saturation)/4 [7].

Accurate computation of cardiac output requires determination of both the oxygen consumption and arteriovenous oxygen difference. When the metabolic rate and hemoglobin remain stable, changes in the arteriovenous oxygen difference sensitively reflect alterations in cardiac output. The oximetry catheter is designed to detect these changes and thereby monitor the cardiac output. The use of an assumed oxygen consumption to calculate cardiac output may introduce a large error into the calculation [8].

Limitations and sources of error

The method assumes that the patient is in a metabolic steady state, and that oxygen consumption and cardiac output remain stable during the measurement period. Dynamic changes in either during the period of measurement can lead to large errors.

This technique requires more time and calculation than other methods: several minutes are required to accurately assess oxygen consumption.

An arterial puncture is necessary to obtain the systemic hemoglobin saturation.

Inaccuracies in determining cardiac output using the Fick oxygen method are due mainly to errors in measuring the oxygen consumption. The specific causes include:

- an incomplete collection of expired air. One of the main sources of inaccuracy is due to the loss of expired air from leaks around the mouthpiece, through the nose (despite the use of noseclips), around the mask, and in the tubing system [9].
- variations in the volume of lung air during the collection period. Although the calculation utilizes the quantity of air entering the bloodstream, this volume is approximated by the volume of expired air. The lung can act as an air reservoir, and changes in lung volume can significantly alter the volume of air collected and the calculation of oxygen consumption [10].
- the difference between inspired and expired air volume. This method assumes that the inspiratory and expiratory volumes are equivalent, which will only be correct when the respiratory quotient = 1.0. In the majority of patients the respiratory quotient < 1, and the expired air volurne is slightly smaller than the inspiratory volume. This causes an underestimation of oxygen consumption and of cardiac output. Neglecting this factor introduces only a minimal error.
- uncertainty in the inspiratory oxygen fraction. It is very difficult to determine the net oxygen fraction provided by face mask or nasal cannulae. The oxygen delivery and alarm systems found in modern ventilators also interfere with the accurate measurement of oxygen consumption.

Indicator dilution techniques

The indicator dilution methods are a specific application of Fick's general principle, using an injected solution as the indicator in place of oxygen. Stewart in 1897 was the first to measure cardiac output using indocyanine green [11]. The technique of rapid green dye injection was developed in the early part of this century [12] and remained the most widely used indicator method until development of the thermodilution method. Determination of cardiac output by thermodilution was initially introduced by Fegler in 1954

[13], and adapted clinically by Branthwaite [14] and Ganz [15]. Ganz and associates [15] were the first to report these measurements using a single pulmonary venous catheter.

Thermodilution technique

The thermodilution technique represents an application of the indicator-dilution method, the measured indicator is the change in blood temperature due to the mixing of circulating blood with a cold injectate. It has been validated by comparison to *in vitro* flow [16] and to the Fick and indocyanine green methods [17, 18]. It is presently the most widely used method because of its high accuracy, technical simplicity, and the ability to obtain multiple outputs at frequent intervals.

To determine cardiac output by thermodilution, cold injectate is rapidly introduced via the right atrial port of a catheter that has a thermistor located at its distal end, situated in a pulmonary artery. The thermistor is coupled to a computer that samples pulmonary artery blood temperature. Introduction of a specific quantity of cold indicator (I), is followed by measurement of its concentration (C) in the pulmonary artery over time (t). Since (in an ideal system) all of the indicator passes downstream:

$$I = Q \int C(t)dt;$$

where Q is the volume of blood flow. This may be rearranged to calculate the cardiac output:

$$Q = \frac{I}{\int C(t)dt}$$

The quantity of cold indicator introduced into the right atrium is calculated as a function of the injectate volume and temperature, and the specific heat and density of the injectate and of blood:

$$I = Vi \times \frac{(Di \times Si)}{(Db \times Sb)} \times (Tb - Ti).$$

The average pulmonary artery blood temperature change and its duration are calculated by the computer. The computational approach to obtain the cardiac output (liter/minute) is:

$$\text{Cardiac output} = Vi \times \frac{(Di \times Si)}{(Db \times Sb)} \times F \times \frac{(Tb - Ti)}{(\Delta T \times t)} \times CF,$$

  Vi = volume of injected solution (minus the dead space in the injecting catheter, ml);
  Di = the specific gravity of the injected solution; Si = the specific heat of the injected solution; Db = specific gravity of blood (1.055); Sb =

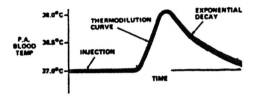

Figure 1.7. The thermodilution temperature-time curve of pulmonary artery blood after a rapid injection of cooled injectate into the right atrium. The curve is characterized by a rapid change in temperature to a maximum, followed by a slower exponential return to the baseline. With permission.

specific heat of blood (0.887). The term $(Di \times Si)/(Db \times Sb)$ is equal to 1.08 when the indicator solution is 5% dextrose;

F = is an electronic scaling factor determined by the material and dimensions of the injection catheter;

Tb = baseline temperature of pulmonary artery blood, (°C);

Ti = temperature of the injected solution, (°C);

ΔT = average change in pulmonary artery blood temperature, (°C);

t = duration of the temperature change, (seconds);

CF = correction factor. Unless the temperature of the injectate is measured directly using a cossette thermistor, the cardiac output calculated by this formula is multiplied by an empiric factor (usually 0.825) to correct for the warming of the injectate as it is handled.

In practice following a rapid injection, there is an initial temperature decline of the pulmonary artery blood from 0.1 to 1.8°C [19]. This is followed by a slow return of the blood temperature to the baseline as an exponential function (Figure 1.7). Cardiac output is inversely proportional to the area under the thermodilution curve, and it also determines the shape of the curve (Figure 1.8). During the first injection of cold solution there is increased warming of the injectate by the catheter, and this output calculation may be unreliable. The initial result is usually disregarded and three to five subsequent measurements within a 10% variation are used to confirm an accurate determination.

More sophisticated microprocessor and thermodilution catheter systems to determine right ventricular volume and ejection fraction are being developed [20, 21]. More frequent measurement of pulmonary artery temperature is required to obtain diastolic 'plateau' temperatures that are used for these computations (Figure 1.9). The values obtained using this method correlate well with measurements derived from other techniques, although end diastolic volume is generally overestimated and ejection fraction is underestimated [20, 22]. To obtain reliable results, it is essential to position the thermistor in the pulmonary artery close to the pulmonic valve [22]. At present, use

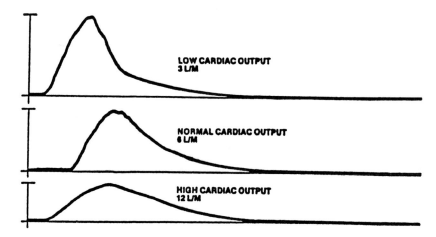

Figure 1.8. Cardiac output is inversely proportional to the area under the thermodilution temperature-time curve. The level of cardiac output determines the shape of the curve: there is a large maximum temperature change, broad peak and slow return to baseline with a low cardiac output, and a small temperature change and rapid return to baseline with a high output. With permission.

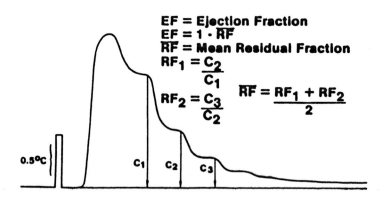

Figure 1.9. An idealized thermodilution curve demonstrating the diastolic temperature plateaus obtained with more frequent measurement of the pulmonary artery temperature. The method is a more sophisticated application of the thermodilution technique, requiring specifically designed catheters and complex processing to calculate right ventricular volume and ejection fraction. With permission.

of the rapid thermodilution approach is limited to patients in normal sinus rhythm who have no tricuspid regurgitation.

Clinical utility and advantages

The thermodilution cardiac output is highly accurate and reproducible, with an approximate error of 5 to 10 percent [7]. The results obtained by this method correlate closely with those from the Fick oxygen and green dye methods [18, 19].

Since withdrawal of blood is not necessary, it does not require an arterial puncture.

The accuracy of this method is not affected by supplemental oxygen. This approach is preferred to the Fick technique when additional oxygen is provided to the patient.

In the absence of an intracardiac shunt, there is virtually no recirculation of the indicator. The blood is warmed during its course through the systemic circulation and returns to the central venous system at ambient body temperature.

The indicator used is inexpensive, inert, and easily available.

Limitations and sources of error

Since the indicator using this method is a temperature change in pulmonary artery blood, factors that interfere with the accurate measurement of temperature changes introduce errors in the determination of cardiac output.

In low flow states due to a reduced cardiac output or with significant tricuspid regurgitation [18], a greater time is required for the cold injection solution to traverse the heart and reach the thermistor located in the pulmonary artery. During this prolonged period, the solution is warmed not only by the circulating blood, but also by the myocardium and surrounding structures. The result is a reduction in the measured temperature deflection. Cardiac output is overestimated in patients with a cardiac output < 3.5 liters/minute [23], an error that may approach 35% in patient with a cardiac output <2.5 liters/minute.

Pulmonary artery flow increases with inspiration and decreases with expiration; the proper timing of injection has not been established.

Fluctuations may occur in the temperature of blood within the pulmonary artery due to the respiratory or cardiac cycle. This may occur with the onset of exercise, deep respiratory efforts, and Cheyne-Stokes respiration. The temperature variations due to these physiologic processes may approach those due to the injection of the cold solution, and significantly alter the computation of cardiac output.

To exclude a poor quality signal, the microprocessor compares the shape of the detected curve to a 'normal' thermodilution curve. Common causes of an irregular curve message include incorrect catheter position, an uneven or irregular injection, and kinking of the catheter (Figure 1.10). The range of curves accepted by the microprocessor includes irregular signals: it cannot detect all invalid curves. When the cardiac output is computed without reviewing the thermodilution temperature-time curve, the absence of an error message can provide false security about the accuracy of the output determination.

Indocyanine green dye

When used to measure cardiac output, the indocyanine dye is injected rapidly into the pulmonary artery while blood is sampled from a peripheral systemic artery. The appearance and concentration of the indocyanine dye in systemic arterial blood is measured and used to calculate the cardiac output. The concentration-time curve recorded from the measurement of dye concentration is normally characterized by a rapid rise to a maximum followed by a gradual decline (Figure 1.11). During the latter portion of concentration decline, a second increase in dye concentration is observed: this secondary rise is due to the recirculation of the indocyanine green in the systemic arterial system. To accurately compute cardiac output, it is necessary to separate the first pass dye concentration from that due to recirculation. The method of Kinsman [12] and subsequently validated [24], or the Bradley triangulation method [25] are the approaches usually used.

Cardiac output is computed as:

Cardiac output (liters/minute) = $I/(c \cdot t) \cdot 60$,

in which I = the quantity of green dye injected into the pulmonary artery (mg); c = the mean concentration during the first pass (mg/l); t = the total duration of the concentration-time curve (seconds). In order to compute the mean concentration of dye, the area of the concentration-time curve is determined either by planimetry or numeric integration, and divided by the duration of the analyzed curve. Since the injected quantity of indocyanine green is known, cardiac output may be computed.

Clinical utility and advantages

The indocyanine green method generates an accurate calculation of cardiac output without the need to determine oxygen consumption, often a tedious task.

Cardiac output can be determined without the need to measure hemoglobin or saturations.

The shape of the concentration-time curve provides information concerning the presence of intracardiac shunts.

Indocyanine provides an accurate cardiac output in the presence of tricuspid regurgitation, a situation in which the thermodilution output may be inaccurate.

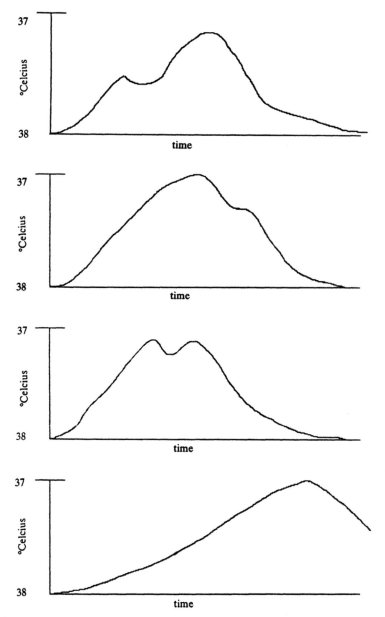

Figure 1.10. The cardiac output computer utilizes several algorithms to detect aberrant thermo-dilution curves. Curves such as these will result in an error message and the processor will not calculate a cardiac output.

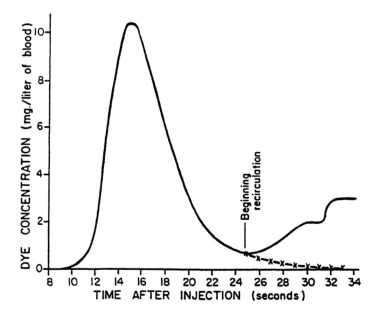

Figure 1.11. A typical indocyanine green dye concentration curve after pulmonary artery injection, illustrating a rapid increase and an exponential decline. The curve requires correction by the semilog replot method because of the recirculation that begins (in this example) at 25 seconds. With permission.

Limitations and sources of error

The accuracy of the dye-dilution method depends mainly upon the ability to separate the first pass dye concentration from the additional concentration due to recirculation. This is compromised in the presence of intracardiac and arterial-venous shunts which cause premature recirculation, and with a low cardiac output or severe mitral regurgitation, which prolong the downslope the dye-dilution curve.

Indocyanine green causes inaccuracies in the determination of blood oxygen saturation and affects the computation of cardiac output by the Fick-oxygen technique.

This method requires an arterial puncture to obtain the systemic concentration of green dye.

Indocyanine green is unstable with exposure to light and over time.

Repeated output determinations result in an accumulation of the indicator within the circulation, and require multiple blood withdrawals.

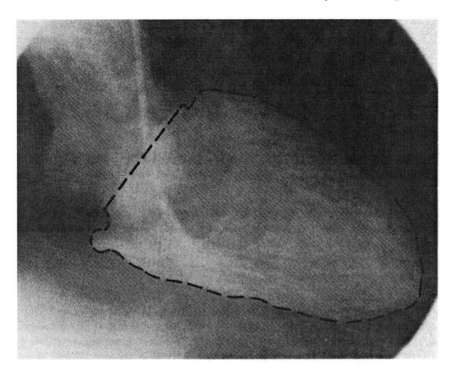

Figure 1.12. The right anterior oblique projection of the left ventriculogram. The broken line indicates the margins of the left ventricular silhouette, which is used to calculate ventricular volume. With permission.

Angiographic technique

Injection of iodinated contrast material directly into the left ventricle permits direct fluoroscopic and cineangiographic visualization of the ventricular silhouette (Figure 1.12). Ventriculography is performed primarily to assess regional and global left ventricular wall motion. Given the difficulty in employing the technique to determine cardiac output, this approach is not often used as a primary method.

In the process of calculating the ejection fraction, the left ventricular end-diastolic and end-systolic volumes are often obtained. The angiographic cardiac output is calculated as the product of stroke volume and heart rate, and is represented by:

Cardiac Output = (end diastolic volume – end systolic volume) · heart rate.

To obtain the left ventricular silhouette, ventriculography may be performed in either monoplane (right anterior oblique 30°, RAO) or biplane (RAO and left anterior oblique 60°, LAO) projections. For each laboratory the calculated ventricular volumes should be validated against other techniques and a regression equation developed [7]. Previous studies have compared angiographically calculated left ventricular volume with postmortem measurement of the same ventricles and provide regression equations to correct for the inherent errors of ventriculography. The most commonly used regression equations are:

Volume = 0.81 V_A + 1.9 (adults, RAO monoplane imaging) [26]
Volume = 0.938 V_A − 5.7 (adults, RAO monoplane imaging) [27]
Volume = 0.989 V_A − 8.1 (adults, biplane imaging) [27].

To compute left ventricle volume, the chamber is approximated by an ellipse of rotation, with one long and two short axes [28]. The volume of the left ventricle is mathematically represented as:

$$\text{Volume} = \frac{4\pi}{3}\frac{L}{2}\frac{D_1}{2}\frac{D_2}{2}, \tag{1.1}$$

where L = long axis, D_1 = the short axis in the RAO projection and D_2 = the short axis in the LAO projection. Ventricular volume may be calculated by directly measuring the long and short axes. If only monoplane ventriculography is performed, the ventricle is assumed to be a prolate ellipse of rotation, that is, the two short axes are assumed to be equal.

An alternate approach developed by Sandler and Dodge, permits computation of left ventricular volume using the planimetered ventricular area and the longest chords of the ventricle (aortic valve plane to the apex) from the RAO and LAO projections [28]. The *area length method* utilizes the following geometric formulae:

$$\text{Area (RAO)} = \pi\frac{L_{RAO}}{2}\frac{D_1}{2} \quad \text{Area (LAO)} = \pi\frac{L_{RAO}}{2}\frac{D_2}{2} \tag{1.2}$$

$$D_1 = \frac{4\,\text{Area(RAO)}}{\pi L_{RAO}} \qquad D_2 = \frac{4\,\text{Area(RAO)}}{\pi L_{RAO}}$$

Combining equation (1.1) and equations (1.2):

$$\text{Volume} = \frac{\pi\,L_{max}}{6}\left(\frac{4\,\text{Area(RAO)}}{\pi\,L_{RAO}}\right)\left(\frac{4\,\text{Area(LAO)}}{\pi\,L_{LAO}}\right) \tag{1.3}$$

$$= \frac{8}{3\pi}\frac{\text{Area(RAO)}\,\text{Area(LAO)}}{L_{min}}.$$

The areas from both projections are used. Since L_{RAO} is usually greater than L_{LAO} the latter will usually be used as L_{min}. In the case of monoplane ventriculography, Equation (1.3) simplifies to the following:

$$\text{Volume} = \frac{8(\text{Area}_{\text{RAO}})^2}{3\pi L_{\text{RAO}}}. \tag{1.4}$$

The volume obtained must be corrected to the actual volume by taking into account the manipulation of ventricular size by the cineangiographic imaging system. When performing angiography, the ventricle is magnified onto the surface of the image intensifier by the dispersion of the x-rays, and then reduced by the use of lenses onto the 35 mm film. Imaging either a grid or a sphere at the midchest or 'zero' pressure level with the image intensifier in the same angle and distance as during ventriculography, reproduces the magnification process. Correcting the dimensions of the analyzed ventricular silhouette permits accurate calculation of ventricular volume. This process must be repeated for each patient to correctly calculate left ventricular volume. Newer cineangiographic systems that permit the positioning of the left ventricle in the isocenter eliminate the need to image a grid for each patient, since image manipulation is the same for all objects at the isocenter. The one dimensional correction factor is represented by:

$$CF = \frac{L_{\text{measured}}}{L_{\text{actual}}}.$$

This factor must be corrected in each dimension, and is cubed for the volume of the left ventricular chamber. Equations (1.3) and (1.4) are further modified to:

$$\text{Volume} = \frac{8}{3\pi CF^3} \frac{\text{Area(RAO) Area(LAO)}}{L_{\text{LAO}}} \qquad (1.3a) \quad \text{(biplane imaging)}$$

$$= \frac{8}{3\pi L_{\text{RAO}}CF^3}(\text{Area}_{\text{RAO}})^2. \qquad (1.4a) \quad \text{(monoplane imaging)}$$

Advantages and clinical utility

Ventriculographic beat-to-beat data provides a sensitive method to detect rapid changes in cardiac output, due for example to exercise or pharmacologic intervention.

In the setting of valvular regurgitation, calculation of ventricular volumes permits determination of the total quantity of blood ejected by the left ventricle; this value cannot be assessed by the Fick oxygen or indicator dilution methods. This is particularly important with combined regurgitation and stenosis, a situation in which total transvalvular flow is required to calculate valve area.

Limitations and sources of error

Ventricular arrhythrnias occur frequently during contrast injection. Calculations using premature ventricular and post-PVC beats will lead to large errors in computing cardiac output. Similarly in the setting of atrial fibrillation, beat to beat variation requires that several beats be analyzed and averaged to obtain an accurate cardiac output.

The cardiac output determined by angiography is usually somewhat greater than when determined by the Fick or thermodilution techniques because:

– The left ventricular volume is directly overestimated: the papillary muscle and trabeculae are included within the traced ventricular silhouette but do not contribute to intraventricular blood volume.
– The geometric approximation of the left ventricle is imperfect. The left ventricle is not ellipsoid, and it deviates further from this shape in both disease states and at end systole.
– Stroke volume probably increases slightly due to the increased preload effect of injecting contrast into the left ventricle. The increase in preload enhances the contractile performance via the Starling mechanism.

With repeated contrast injections, there is an accumulation of contrast within the circulation and an increase in intravascular volume. Ionic contrast material has a negative inotropic effect and may directly depress the cardiac output

Ventriculography is more tedious and time consuming (e.g. film must be developed, images reviewed, traced, and analyzed) than the other invasive techniques, and is therefore infrequently used as a primary method.

Conductance catheters

The conductance catheter is a multielectrode electronic device that both produces an electric field within the left (or right) ventricle and measures the time-varying voltage of blood within the chamber. Efforts to validate the accuracy and reproducibility of the volumes obtained with this catheter require simplification of an otherwise complex electrical field technique [29]. At present, the conductance catheter remains primarily a investigational tool to measure ventricular volumes and cardiac output. The technical difficulties in accurately placing a correctly sized catheter in the ventricle and the need to validate the results against a reference volume [30], continue to limit its clinical utility.

To measure cardiac output by the conductance method, the catheter (with eight platinum electrodes) is placed within the ventricle with the distal electrode (number 1) near the apex and the proximal electrode (number 8) at

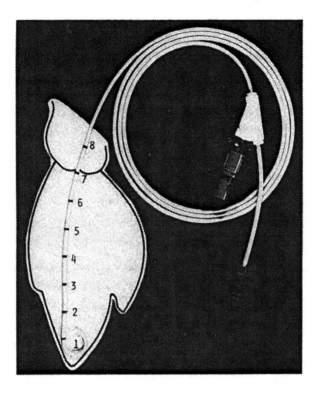

Figure 1.13. A pigtail conductance catheter is schematically positioned in the left ventricle along the long axis. Electrode number 1 is placed near the apex and number 8 is located at the level of the aortic valve, with an equal distance between each of the electrodes. An electric current is emitted from electrode 1 to 8 and the intraventricular voltage is measured by electrodes 2 through 7. With permission.

the level of the aortic valve (Figure 1.13). The conductance catheter emits an electric current from electrode 1 to electrode 8, and continuously measures the voltages generated between each pair of electrodes 2–7 (i.e. between electrode pairs 2–3, 3–4, 4–5, 5–6, 6–7). Dividing the emitted electric current by the five measured potentials, provides five conductances. Summing these conductance values provides a signal that is (theoretically) linearly related to ventricular volume. Results from this method (Volume$_{cath}$) have been shown to correlate with ventricular volume (Volume$_{stand}$) determined by thermodilution [29], angiography [31], an intraventricular volume servosystem [32] and endocardial crystals [33]:

$$\text{Volume}_{cath} = m\ \text{Volume}_{stand} + b.$$

The slope and intercept of this relationship varies between patients and becomes non-linear with large changes in ventricular volume [30].

Cardiac output is calculated from the end diastolic and end systolic volumes, and heart rate:

Cardiac output = (end diastolic volume − end systolic volume) · heart rate.

Clinical utility and advantages

The primary advantage of this method is that it provides continuous volume data without the need to directly expose the heart (closed chest) or tediously calculate ventricular volume.

The conductance method provides physiological information concerning left ventricular and stroke volume over the range of volumes usually observed during the cardiac cycle.

The conductance catheter is able to accurately assess relative changes in ventricular volume and significantly simplifies determination of left ventricular function. This catheter has been used to measure contractility using ventricular elastance [34].

Limitations and sources of error

The main limitation of the conductance method is that the relationship between the impedance signal and ventricular volume is complex. While the output signal is (usually) linearly related to volume, the slope of this relationship is less than unity and there is a large offset volume. There is no simple way to determine the slope of this relationship and the absolute volume is difficult to obtain [30].

The conductive activity of the structures that surround the left ventricular chamber (e.g. lung, right ventricle, ventricular myocardium) enhance the conductance signal and increase the apparent volume.

The electric field theory underlying this method is complex. One simplifying assumption is the presence of parallel conductance within the ventricle. The lines of electric current within the chamber are not exactly parallel, and contributes to the error in volume computation.

When ventricular volume is varied over a wide range [35], it has been shown that the relation between left ventricular volume and conductance becomes *non-linear*. At extremes of volume, this method may become very inaccurate.

Exercise and cardiac output

During exercise there is an increase in dynamic exertion due to the force generated by activated skeletal muscle. The contraction of these muscles is translated into motion, and enables the individual to perform external work. During exercise, there is an increase in the oxygen consumption and carbon dioxide production of striated muscle, which necessitates an increase in oxygen and carbon dioxide transport by the circulatory system. At rest, oxygen consumption is approximately 110–150 ml O_2/minute/m^2 body surface area [10]. At maximal exercise, an individual increases basal oxygen consumption by a factor of 12 to 18. Since the normal reserve for oxygen extraction is 3 [10], cardiac output must increase to a level 4 to 6 times the baseline to provide for this increased demand.

There is a strong correlation between the increase in cardiac output and oxygen consumption. Dexter [36] found that for every 100 ml/min/m^2 increase in oxygen consumption, the cardiac index increased by 590 ml/min/m^2. The relationship between these two factors is expressed as:

cardiac index (lit/min/m^2) = 0.0059 (O_2 consumption, ml/min/m^2) + 2.99,

and may be used to assess the the adequacy of a patient's response to exercise. During exercise, the patient's measured cardiac index is compared to the predicted index based upon oxygen consumption. A normal cardiac output response is defined as a measured/predicted index ≥ 0.8. Donald. *et al.* [37] found an increase in cardiac output of ≥ 600 ml/minute for each increase of 100 ml/minute of oxygen consumed. These ratios termed by Grossman [7] as the 'exercise index', permit evaluation of the heart's ability to respond to exercise.

The preferred invasive method to determine cardiac output during exercise depends upon the form of exercise, the need for multiple determinations and their frequency, and the desire for measurements during steady state vs. dynamic changes in cardiac output. The Fick oxygen technique provides accurate determinations, but requires that the patient exercise at a constant level for a period of minutes, to allow oxygen consumption and blood oxygen saturations to equilibrate. Both arterial and venous access are necessary, and with large increases in the arteriovenous oxygen difference near the anaerobic threshold, oxygen saturation measurements may become inaccurate.

The thermodilution technique requires only one central venous catheter, no withdrawal of blood, and the cardiac output can be repeated frequently with minimal hemodynamic or systemic interference. At present this is the most frequently used method to determine cardiac output during exercise. However, thermodilution cannot provide beat-to-beat dynamic changes in cardiac output, as during an acute change in work load. The indocyanine green dye approach requires both arterial and venous access, and since reproducible arterial blood withdrawal is necessary, the arterial source must be nearly stationary. The need to reinject green dye for each output measurement causes systemic accumulation of this substance. The dye technique is infrequently used to measure cardiac output during exercise.

Angiography may be used to advantage during acute changes in cardiac output or when a limited number of determinations are required. This technique requires placement of an intraventricular catheter and injection of contrast material during exercise, and must be performed in a cardiac catheterization laboratory. The frequency of ventricular arrhythmias, the potential negative inotropic and other hemodynamic effects of contrast agents, limit this technique. The conductance catheter is designed to provide both beat-to-beat data during dynamic changes in work load, and continuous cardiac output information during steady state. However, this method requires the placement of a stable intraventricular catheter in the catheterization laboratory. The validity of the conductance catheter over a wide range of ventricular volumes has not been established.

Summary

Advantages and disadvantages of variouus invasive techniques to measure cardiac output.

Method	Advantages	Disadvantages
Fick oxygen	–The Fick oxygen method is most accurate in patients with a reduced cardiac output. –May be used in the setting of intracardiac shunts; with a left to right shunt, multiple samples must be obtained from the chamber just proximal to the shunt. –When the metabolic rate and hemoglobin remain stable, the arteriovenous oxygen difference sensitively reflects changes in cardiac output.	–Assumes that the patient is in a metabolic steady state, and that oxygen consumption and cardiac output remain stable. –This technique requires more time and calculation than thermodilution. –An arterial puncture is necessary to obtain the systemic oxygen saturation.
Thermodilution	–Thermodilution is highly accurate and reproducible; results are closely correlated with the Fick cardiac output. –It does not require an arterial puncture. –There is virtually no recirculation of the indicator in the absence of an intracardiac shunt. –The indicator used is inexpensive, inert, and easily available.	–The accuracy decreases in low flow states (cardiac output (<3.5 l/m) or with significant tricuspid regurgitation. –Fluctuations may occur in the temperature of pulmonary artery blood during the respiratory or cardiac cycles. –The temperature-time curve is often unavailable to validate the injection and calculation.

Method	Advantages	Disadvantages
Indocyanine dye	–The indocyanine green method generates an accurate cardiac output without the need to determine oxygen consumption. –Cardiac output can be determined without measuring hemoglobin or oxygen saturation. –The shape of the concentration-time curve provides information concerning the presence of intracardiac shunts.	–The accuracy depends upon the ability to separate the dye concentration due to the first pass and recirculation. –Indocyanine green affects the oxymetric blood oxygen saturation. –With repeated injections, there is an accumulation of the indicator within the circulation
Angiogaphy	–Ventriculography provides beat-to-beat data to detect rapid changes in cardiac output. –With combined valvular regurgitation and stenosis, this method provides transvalvular flow data necessary to calculate valve area.	–Ventricular arrhythmias occur frequently during contrast injection, and affect the cardiac output calculation. –The cardiac output determination is usually greater than Fick or thermodilution. –Repeated contrast injections cause a large increase in intravascular volume.
Conductance	–Provides continuous volume data. –Relative changes in ventricular volume are accurately assessed in the physiologic range of ventricular volume.	–The relationship between conductance and ventricular volume may be complex. –It is difficult to obtain absolute ventricular volume and cardiac output –Large changes in ventricular volume may cause significant inaccuracy.

References

1. Fick A. Über die Messung des Blutquantums in den Herzventrikeln. Sitz der Physik-Med ges Wurtzberg 1870, 16.
2. Visscher MB, Johnson JA. The Fick principle: analysis of potential errors in its conventional application. J Appl Physiol 1953;5:635–8.
3. Bernhart FW, Skeggs L. The iron content of crystalline human hemoglobin. Biol Chem 1943;147:19–22.
4. Seltzer A, Sudrann RB. Reliability of the determination of cardiac output in man by means of the Fick principle. Circ Research 1958;6:485–90.
5. Barrat-Boyes BG, Wood EH. The oxygen saturation of blood in the venae cavae, right heart chambers, and pulmonary vessels of healthy subjects. J Lab Clin Med 1957;50:93–106.
6. Thomassen B. Cardiac output in normal subjects under standard conditions. The repeatability of mesurements by the Fick method. Scand J Clin Lab Invest 1957;9:365–76.

7. Grossman W. Blood flow measurement: the cardiac output. In: Cardiac Catheterization and Angiography, 3rd Ed. Philadelphia: Lea and Febiger, 1986:101–17.

8. Dehmer G, Firth BG, Hillis LD. Oxygen consumption in adult patients during cardiac catheterization. Clin Cardiol 1982;5:436–40.

9. Bursztein S, Elwin DH, Askanazi J. *et al.* Methods of measurement and interpretation of indirect calorimetry. In: Energy metabolism, indirect calorimetry and nutrition. Baltimore: Williams and Wilkins, 1989:173–209.

10. Guyton AC, Jones CE, Coleman TG. Circulatory physiology: cardiac output and its regulation. Philadelphia: WB Saunders, 1973:4–80.

11. Stewart GN. Researches on the circulation time and on the influences which affect it. IV: the output of the heart. J Physiol 1897;22:159–83.

12. Kinsman JM, Moore JW, Hamilton WF. Injection method: physical and mathematical considerations. Am. J Physiol 1929;89:322–31.

13. Fegler G. Measurement of cardiac output in anesthetized animals by a thermodilution method. Q J Exp Physiol 1954;39:153–64.

14. Branthwaite MA, Bradley RD. Measurement of cardiac output by thermal dilution in man. J Appl Physiol 1968;24:434–8.

15. Ganz W, Donosco R, Marcus HS *et al.* A new technique for measurement of cardiac output by thermodilution in man. Am. J Cardiol 1971;27:392–6.

16. Forrester JS, Ganz W, Diamond G. *et al.* Thermodilution cardiac output determination with a single flow-directed catheter. Am Heart J 1972;83:306–11.

17. Weisel RD, Berger RL, Hechtman HB. Measurement of cardiac output by thermodilution. N Engl J. Med 1975;292:682–4.

18. Levett JM, Replogle RL. Thermodilution cardiac output: a critical analysis and review of the literature. J Surg Res 1979;27:392–404.

19. Shaw TI. The Swann Ganz pulmonary artery catheter. Anesth 1979;34:651–6.

20. Dhainut JF, Brunet F, Monsallier JF *et al.* Bedside evaluation of right ventricular performance using a rapid computerized thermodilution method. Crit Care Med 1987;15:148–52.

21. Mukherjee R, Spinale FG, von Recum AF, Crawford FA. Rapid response thermistors to measure ventricular ejection fraction: *in vitro* validation. Presented at the 12th Annual International Conference of the IEEE-EMBS, Philadelphia, 1990.

22. Spinale FG, Smith AC, Carabello BA, Crawford FA. Right ventricular function computed by thermodilution and ventriculography. J Thorac Cardiovasc Surg 1990;99:141–52.

23. van Grondelle A, Ditchey RV, Groves BM *et al.* Thermodilution method overestimates low cardiac output in humans. Am J Physiol (Heart Circ Physiol) 1983;14:H690–H692.

24. Hamilton WF, Riley RL, Atayah AM *et al.* Comparison of the Fick and dye injection methods of measuring the cardiac output in man. Am J Physiol 1948;153:309–321.

25. Bradley EC, Barr JW. Fore-n-aft triangle formula for rapid estimation of curves. Am Heart J 1969;78:643–8.

26. Kennedy JW, Trenholme SE, Kasser IS. Left ventricular volume and mass from single-plane cineangiogram. A comparison of anteroposterior and right anterior oblique methods. Am Heart J 1970;80:343–52.

27. Wynne J, Green LH, Mann T *et al.* Estimation of left ventricular volumes in man from biplane cineangiograms filmed in oblique projections. Am J Cardiol 1978;41:726–32.

28. Dodge HT, Sandler H, Baxley WA *et al.* Usefulness and limitations of radiographic methods for determining left ventricular volume. Am J Cardiol 1966;18:10–24.

29. Baan J, Aouw Jong TT, Kerkhof PLM *et al.* Continuous stroke volume and cardiac output from intraventricular dimensions obtained with impendance catheter. Cardiovasc Res 1981;15:328–34.

30. Burkhoff D. The conductance method of left ventricular volume estimation: Methodological limitations put into perspective. Circulation 1990;81:703–6.

31. Tjon-A-Meeuw L, Hess OM, Nonogi H *et al.* Left ventricular volume determination in dogs: a comparison between conductance technique and angiocardiography. Eur Heart J 1988;9:1018–26.

32. Burkhoff D, Van der Velde ET, Kass D *et al*. Accuracy of volume measurement by conductance catheter in isolated, ejecting canine hearts. Circulation 1985;72:440–7.

33. Applegate RJ, Cheng CP, Little WC. Simultaneous conductance catheter and dimension assessment of left ventricular volume in the intact animal. Circulation 1990;81:638–48.

34. Kass DA, Beyar R, Lankford E *et al*. Influence of contractile state on curvilinearity of in situ end-systolic pressure-volume relations. Circulation 1989;79:167–78.

35. Boltwood CM, Appleyard RF, Glantz SA. Left ventricular volume measurement by conductance catheter in intact dogs. Circulation 1989;80:1360–77.

36. Dexter L, Whittenberger JL, Haynes FW *et al*. Effect of exercise on circulatory dynamics of normal individuals. J Appl Physiol 1951;3:439–53.

37. Donald KW, Bishop JM, Cumming G *et al*. The effect of exercise on the cardiac output and circulatory dynamics of normal subjects. Clin Sci 1955;14:37–73.

2. The use of echo-Doppler cardiography in measuring cardiac output

PETROS NIHOYANNOPOULOS

Repeated determinations of systemic haemodynamics are often necessary for effective follow-up of patients. Both short-term and long-term follow-up of patients with cardiovascular disease require sequential evaluation of stroke volume and cardiac output, blood volume distribution, as well as indices of cardiac performance. These indices may be altered positively or negatively by the natural history of the disease and/or by therapeutic interventions.

An ideal method to calculate stroke volume and cardiac output should be inexpensive, non-invasive and radiation-free, it should provide accurate and reproducible measurements and be easily tolerated by the patient for serial determinations.

Echocardiography has become a well established, reliable and readily available non-invasive cardiac imaging modality. These properties have made it an attractive diagnostic tool in a large number of patients with known or suspected heart disease. A much wider application of this technique however would be in the assessment of left ventricular function and today there is no comprehensive echocardiographic study without the necessity for assessing left ventricular function. Estimation of left ventricular function can be based upon an eye-ball subjective evaluation of myocardial contraction, to the most sophisticated and complex calculations of left ventricular volumes.

Historically, the first reported use of cardiac Doppler was for the assessment of aortic flow velocity, a measure of left ventricular systolic function. In 1969, Light [1] demonstrated that aortic velocity could be obtained easily and non-invasively from the suprasternal notch with Doppler echocardiography. Six years later Huntsman [2] demonstrated the reliability of determining aortic blood flow velocity using transcutaneous Doppler ultrasound and Boughner *et al.* [3] showed that the aortic flow pattern was different in patients with hypertrophic cardiomyopathy from normal subjects. During the ensuing five years the emphasis shifted to the use of Doppler ultrasound for evaluating valvular heart disease. Only recently has there been a resurgence of interest in aortic flow patterns in a variety of diseases.

A.-M. Salmasi and A.S. Iskandrian (eds): Cardiac output and regional flow in health and disease, 31–45.
© 1993 *Kluwer Academic Publishers. Printed in the Netherlands.*

Echocardiographic measurement of ventricular volumes

M-mode echocardiography

Cubing the left ventricular dimensions was the earliest and perhaps one of the most widely used methods for calculating left ventricular volume and excelled by its simplicity, using the formula: volume = diameter cubed. This was based on the fact that the left ventricle resembles a prolate ellipsoid with a long axis twice the length of the short axis [4, 5]. Left ventricular stroke volume was then determined by subtracting the end-systolic from the end-diastolic volume and good correlation between the ultrasound and angiographic stroke volume were found [4, 5]. However, the shape of the left ventricle varies with heart size so that the geometrical assumptions necessary for these calculations can not be valid for all ventricles. For example, when the ventricle dilates it becomes more spherical and the ratio of long-axis to short-axis dimensions decreases. Conversely, when the left ventricle is underfilled becomes a more exaggerated ellipse. As a result, the simple cube function method tends to overestimate the volume of enlarged ventricles and to underestimate that of small chambers.

Teichholz *et al.* [6], modified the diameter cube formula for calculating volume by correcting the relation between minor and major left ventricular axis from a wide range of volume and subsequently this has become the most widely used formula. However, these measurements can only be applied when the left ventricular contraction is uniform and symmetrical. In many patients with coronary artery disease, congenital heart disease or pulmonary hypertension, segmental wall motion abnormalities may exist which render M-mode measurements of the length and shortening of a single axis unrepresentative of the overall left ventricular size and function. Finally, extrapolating from a single linear dimension to three-dimensional measurements of stroke volumes and cardiac outputs means that any error in primary measurements will be cubed in these volume calculations.

Two-dimensional echocardiography

With the development of two-dimensional echocardiography it was expected that the advantages of more complete spatial information would improve the accuracy of measurements of cardiac chamber volumes. Many of the echocardiographic tomographic sections of the left ventricle contain dimensions and areas that appear similar to those found in angiographic projections of the left ventricle. As a result, a number of the angiographic ellipsoid volume formulas have been applied to echocardiographic volume calculations. In addition other left ventricular volume calculations have been based upon mathematic models.

Methods based on simple geometric models

The ellipsoid model contains two orthogonal angiographic images of the left ventricle both of which contain a long axis and a minor axis perpendicular to each other. The assumptions required for the application of this formula are that the ventricle must be orientated parallel to at least one of the angiographic planes, so that the true long axis is projected and secondly, the ventricle must be a true ellipse. The echocardiographic application of these formulas is a little more complex since it provides a number of additional short axis planes.

There are two basic echocardiographic approaches based on the ellipsoid model; the length – diameter method and the area – length method [7].

1. *Length – diameter method.* The long axis dimension is usually taken from the apical four-chamber view (occasionally from apical long axis). The minor axes (D1 and D2) may be directly measured or a common minor axis may be derived as the mean radius from measured cavity dimension in the short axis parasternal view. The equation for volume (V) of a length-diameter prolate ellipsoid is:

$$V = 4/3\pi(L/2)(D1/2)(D2/2).$$

2. *Area – length method.* A slight modification of the above is the prolate ellipsoid area-length method. The inherent irregularities of left ventricular shape should have less effect on measurements if ventricular areas are calculated instead of the ventricular radii. There are two variations of this method depending of the echocardiographic windows used. The first variation utilises one of the apical planes, usually the four chamber view, from which the left ventricular length is measured (planimetered) and one of the parasternal short axis projections, usually at the tips of the mitral valve, for measuring the short axis area. Alternatively, both, short axis and longitudinal areas are obtained from two orthogonal to each other apical projections, the apical four and two chamber views. A simple internal check of the accuracy of measurements used by this second method is provided by the fact that the two longitudinal axes should be similar. This is particularly important because the true left ventricular apex is commonly missed in the four-chamber view, resulting in underestimation of chamber length and area.

The Simpson's rule method

According to Simpson's rule, the volume of a large figure can be calculated from the sum of the volumes of a series of smaller similar figures which, when put together, reproduce the larger figure. In practice, a sequence of three short axis cross-sectional scans of the ventricle are taken at mitral, papillary muscle level and cardiac apex, each one of which is planimetered.

From apical long axis projection, the ventricle is planimetered in its long axis. The major advantage of the Simpson's rule method is that it can readily be adapted to gross distortion in ventricular shape and therefore be used to calculate volume in patients with coronary artery disease or in patients with hypertrophic cardiomyopathy.

Combined geometrical models

The final geometric models to estimate left ventricular volume employ a number of short axis imaging planes to divide the ventricle into segments of different shape. The volume of each segment is measured separately and then summed to provide the total left ventricular volume. The geometric figures commonly used for the various ventricular components are the cylinder, the cone, the truncated cone and the ellipsoid segment. In each of these models, the long axis length is measured from the apical two or four chamber view and the short-axis dimensions are measured at the level of the mitral valve and the papillary muscles. It is assumed that these two planes divide the left ventricular long axis into three equal segments so that the height of each segment is equal to one third of the long axis.

Doppler ultrasound estimation of ventricular volumes

Over the past few years, Doppler ultrasound methods combined with echocardiography have been widely used for the evaluation of stroke volume and cardiac output in man. From the study of aortic velocity curves (Figure 2.1), it has been possible to evaluate and validate maximal (time from onset of systolic flow to the peak velocity) and mean aortic acceleration, ejection time and pre-ejection period and to calculate stroke distance (area under the time velocity curve). All these measurements have been suggested to be valid indices of cardiac contractility and performance.

More recently, a number of reports have validated the use of Doppler echocardiography to calculate stroke volume and cardiac output [8–19]. With Fick and thermodilution output used as gold standards, these studies have shown that Doppler measurements from a variety of sites throughout the heart and great veins can be used to calculate cardiac output non-invasively.

However, although Doppler ultrasound estimates of cardiac output compared favourably with hemodynamically derived peak estimates, there were several limitations to the Doppler approach:

1. Potential for error due to the excessive angle of the Doppler ultrasound beam with respect to the vector representing flow velocity.
2. Potential error when measuring the diameter of the vessel.
3. Potential of a non-uniform flow profile at the Doppler ultrasound sample site.

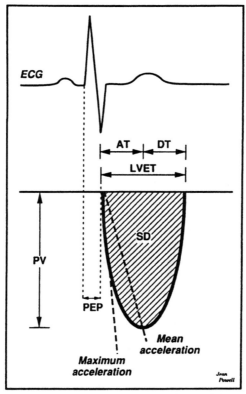

$$\text{Mean acceleration:} = \frac{\text{Peak velocity}}{\text{Acceleration time}}$$

$$\text{Cross sectional area } (cm^2): = \pi \times \left(\frac{d}{2}\right)^2$$

Stroke volume (ml): = CSA x SD
Cardiac output (ml/min): = SV x HR

Figure 2.1. Schematic representation of the various Doppler measurements of left ventricular function derived from the systolic waveform obtained at the left ventricular outflow tract. The peak velocity (cm/sec), left ventricular ejection time (msec), Stroke distance (cm), acceleration time (m/sec) are demonstrated. Peak acceleration (m/sec^2) is the maximal slope from onset to peak of the systolic waveform, while the mean acceleration (m/sec^2) is the peak velocity divided by the acceleration time.

Theoretical considerations

The physical principles underlying the use of the Doppler ultrasound frequency shift to measure blood flow velocity have been well described [1]. When an ultrasonic wave meets a moving object, any reflected wave so produced will have a frequency shift proportional to the reflecting object's velocity vector in the direction of the incident wave. Thus the measurement of the frequency shift produced by ultrasound reflecting off a moving column of blood can be used to measure the velocity vector of the blood parallel to the ultrasound beam.

While flow velocity is a linear measurement representing both speed and direction, flow is a measurement of volume versus time. Flow measurements using Doppler ultrasound techniques are based upon the fluid hydraulic principle citing that flow volume in a straight and non-expandable tube is related to the cross-sectional area at one point and the velocity of flow at that particular point: Flow = velocity × cross-sectional area. If velocity is defined in cm/sec and the cross-sectional area in cm^2, the resulting flow is calculated in cm^3/sec. Thus in theory, blood flow can be measured at any one point along a tubular structure which can clearly be defined, so that the cross-sectional area at that particular point can accurately be measured. There are a number of assumptions to be met in order for this hydraulic formula to be applied; these are: (i) the tube must be filled with incompressible fluid; (ii) the tube size does not change; and (iii) all the fluid at that point of measurement is laminar with uniform flow profile.

Measurements of stroke volume and cardiac output have been made at many points in the circulation, including left ventricular outflow tract, ascending aorta, aortic arch, descending thoracic aorta, pulmonary artery, mitral valve and tricuspid valve. Each site has some advantages and disadvantages taking into account factors such as (i) the ability to align the ultrasonic beam parallel to the flow direction; (ii) the profile of the blood velocity distribution; (iii) the proportion of the total cardiac output traversing the vessel or valve; (iv) the velocity signal-to-noise ratio; and (v) the quality of echocardiographic imaging of the diameter of the vessel for cross-sectional area measurements.

Blood flow profile

The calculation of blood flow from flow velocity integral multiplied by cross-sectional area depends on the assumption that the velocity profile at the measurement site is uniform across a vessel or chamber. This is reasonable for sites that approximate to inlet conditions where blood flow is accelerating through a narrowing. These conditions exist at most valve inlets and immediately downstream of a valve, but are lost as the blood moves further down the vessel.

In a large blood vessel such as the aorta, two major patterns of flow occur. At the left ventricular outflow tract (subaortic) area and immediately above the aortic valve most of the blood cells are travelling at similar speed, describing a flat flow profile. Further up at the ascending aorta and aortic arch, a parabolic flow profile develops, that is flow in the central area of the vessel is relatively fast with progressive slowing of the blood cell velocity towards the walls. Measurement of only the central velocities create the possibility of overestimation of flow, while using an off-centre sampling position may cause a significant underestimation of the average velocity in the vessel. During high flow states, the differences are exaggerated and make accurate measurement even more difficult. In addition, the ascending aorta is curved and has side branches, both of which contribute to skewing of the velocity profile [8–12].

As the Doppler ultrasound method measures blood flow velocity at one particular point in the circulation, it only measures volume flow at that point and hence only measures cardiac output if that point receives the full cardiac output. The term "cardiac output" usually refers to left ventricular output which enters and stays in the arterial system. Some measurement sites receive only a proportion of the total output. A measurement taken several centimetres down the aorta from the valve will not include coronary blood flow and hence will be approximately 5% less than total cardiac output.

Similarly, in the presence of intracardiac communication between left and right heart chambers there may be discrepancy between right and left ventricular outputs. This discrepancy is commonly used to calculate the magnitude of shunt (*vide infra*).

Tube diameter

The other major assumption of the hydraulic formula is that the tube size remains constant during the period of velocity measurement. In reality, none of the specific areas measured echocardiographically has a constant size during the cardiac cycle. When M-mode echocardiography of the aortic root is performed on the normal aorta, a systolic expansion of up to 14% of resting diameter can be seen. Furthermore, if the tube is one of the veins (superior vena cava, inferior vena cava, pulmonary veins), this systolic expansion may reach 50% so that volume measurements from the venous system may seriously be questioned.

It therefore becomes apparent that to improve the accuracy of volume measurements one should choose a cross-sectional area that has solid internal reference points, so that it can be found easily and in which the blood volume can be repetitively sampled.

Measurements of cross-sectional area

The cross-sectional area of the vessel, valve annulus, or heart chamber must be measurable accurately at the level blood velocity measurements are taken. Poor image quality often limits measurements of pulmonary artery and tricuspid annulus cross-sectional area because the whole circumference of these areas may not be imaged. Any assumption of the geometrical shape of the valve annulus may also be very important in calculating cross-sectional area from two-dimensional measurements.

The best and perhaps the most reproducible measurements of cross-sectional area in conjunction with the most accurate sampling (practical and theoretical) of blood flow velocity are just under the aortic valve (aortic root). The cross-sectional area of the aortic root is commonly measured from inner wall to leading edge, anteriorly at the point where the aortic root joins the membranous septum and posteriorly at the point where the posterior aortic wall becomes anterior mitral leaflet (Figure 2.2, top). The aortic root area is then treated as a circular structure and the area calculated by the formula for the area of a circle is given by: area = 3.14 × diameter half, all squared.

Flow calculation

Aortic blood flow velocity may be recorded with a hand-held transducer from the cardiac apex or the suprasternal notch using pulsed or continuous wave Doppler. Numerous studies have resulted in a wide variety of validated methods for calculating stroke volume and cardiac output. However, the best method uses aortic flow and measures the aortic root dimensions from inner wall to inner wall. Integrating aortic velocity over one cardiac cycle gives a value proportional to the blood volume passing through the sample volume during the cardiac cycle.

Calculation of stroke volume and cardiac output by Doppler ultrasound remains controversial despite the apparently good results. The two main controversies involve determination of the cross-sectional area, as it may markedly vary independently from patient to patient and the use of thermo-dilution as a gold standard since the reproducibility of cardiac output measurements by thermodilution vary greatly. Consequently, the isolated Doppler ultrasound determination of cardiac output often provides little useful information about cardiac function in cross-sectional studies. The good reproducibility of these measurements however may be very useful indeed during follow-up studies on individual patients.

The angle of incidence between blood flow and ultrasonic beam is an important determinant of the accuracy of Doppler ultrasound measurements of blood flow velocity and ideally it should either be zero or well known. In practice, this angle cannot be measured precisely from a two-dimensional image for two basic reasons: First, because the total flow within the vessel or through an orifice is not seen and therefore to measure an angle it has to be assumed that flow is directly parallel to an apparent anatomic landmark. Second, in a given two-dimensional plane the angle may be significantly underestimated due to the orientation of the sound waves with flow on the orthogonal plane. For these reasons, angle correction should not be used as it may lead to false calculations of blood flow velocities and decrease reproducibility. Fortunately, the angle Θ can vary by as much as 20 degrees with an error in under-estimating flow velocity of no more than 6%. Use of the apical window has the advantage of providing a shallow (<20°) angle between the ultrasonic beam and left ventricular outflow. The audio signal from the Doppler or the colour Doppler display can also be used to find the

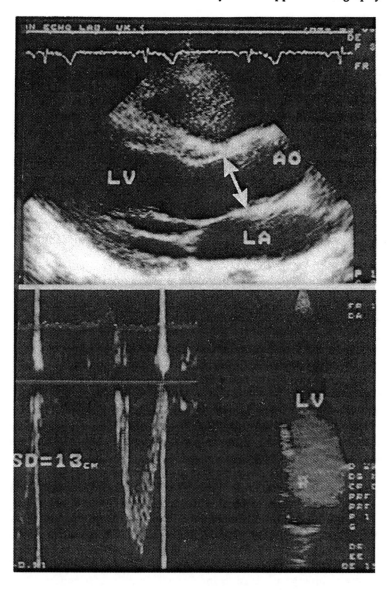

Figure 2.2. Calculation of stroke volume and cardiac output. The diameter of the left ventricular outflow tract is demonstrated in the parasternal long axis view (top panel). The area under the velocity curve obtained from the apical five-chamber view (stroke distance) is illustrated in the bottom panel. Stroke Volume (mls) = Stroke Distance × Cross Sectional Area. Cardiac Output (mls/min) = Stroke Volume × Heart Rate. Ao = Aorta, LA = Left Atrium, LV = Left ventricle, SD = Stroke Distance.

highest frequency shift that can be obtained (i.e. the smallest angle to the flow direction) (Figure 2.2, bottom).

The advantage of measuring flow velocity from the suprasternal notch using continuous wave Doppler is that the technique is easy and can be performed by non-experts. The major disadvantage however, is that the flow velocity measurements are a summation of blood flow velocities from the left ventricular outflow tract up to the ascending aorta and aortic arch, along the line of the ultrasound beam. The diameter of these assumed tubular structures is by far non-uniform and greatly changes from the outflow tract to the aortic arch, a necessary assumption for flow calculation. Another problem is that the flow velocity is not uniform along the assumed tubular structure and closer to the aortic arch the flow profile assumes a parabolic profile. Because of the uneven flow velocity distribution and the non-uniform tubular structure, small changes in preload may lead to over or under estimation of flow volumes.

The use of pulse wave Doppler ultrasound

The two main methods to calculate blood flow velocity are continuous wave with no limits to detectable velocity but no range resolution, and pulsed wave with range resolution but with a limited maximal detectable velocity. Although similar results have been reported on accuracy using both these Doppler modalities, there are theoretical advantages in favour of pulsed wave Doppler, that is the position of the sample volume is known and can be fixed, so that repeat measurements will always be taken at approximately the same point in the circulation.

There is no doubt that sampling a small volume of blood flow at a specific site can best be performed with pulsed wave Doppler ultrasound. It is however of great importance to be able to sample the flow volume at the same site easily with sufficient reproducibility. The success rate will depend upon the internal reference point of the sample area. The ascending aorta lacks specific internal reference points, while the cross-sectional area greatly differs from sinuses to arch. The direct consequence is that small changes in the site of flow sampling may lead to incorrect volume measurement.

The site that can be sampled easily is the left ventricular outflow tract as seen from apical projections and the cross-sectional area of the aortic annulus can easily be measured from long axis parasternal views (Figure 2.3). Furthermore, the aortic annulus changes little with time and the loading conditions.

The limitations on peak velocities detected by pulsed wave Doppler ultrasound is not a major draw-back in adults because blood velocities above 150 cm/sec are rare in the absence of valvular disease or shunts, so the velocity limit is rarely reached.

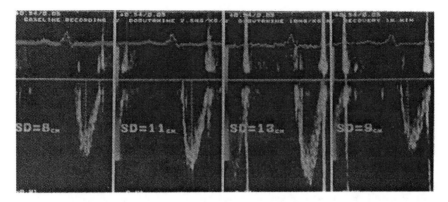

Figure 2.3. Serial pulsed wave Doppler recordings of the ejection systolic blood flow from the left ventricular outflow tract (apical 5-chamber view) at baseline and during incremental doses of dobutamine infusion at 1, 2.5 and 10 μg/kg/min, in a patient with severe heart failure. Note the progressive increase of the stroke distance (SD) from 8 cm to a maximum of 13 cm at maximal dose. This is followed by re-normalisation of the stroke distance 18 minutes after cessation of the infusion.

Calculations

Although early studies only used maximal velocities for calculations, the wider variations of instantaneous velocities are seen particularly during the deceleration phase. It therefore became important to use an estimate of the entire systolic flow velocity during the time objection. The area under the systolic velocity curve (flow velocity integral) of the Doppler signal is now commonly calculated. Today, this is automatically calculated by either a built-in or an off-line computer after tracing the velocity profile manually with a track-ball. Thus, the tracing is automatically broken up into a series of rectangles, the areas of which are summoned to provide an estimate of the area under the curve Doppler tracing. The area under the Doppler flow velocity curve (flow velocity integral) is directly proportional to the stroke volume. The integrated mean velocity over a distance is termed "stroke distance" and represents the distance covered by a column of blood through the aortic root during one cardiac cycle. Stroke distance (SD) is then related to stroke volume by the equation:

SD = Stroke Volume/Cross Sectional Area.

Stroke Distance is dimensionally a distance and has units of length (centimetres). The stroke volume is then calculated by multiplying the stroke distance by the cross- sectional area at the same level where the blood flow velocity is sampled. The product of the stroke volume and heart rate is the cardiac output.

Stroke distance is usually unrelated to patients morphologic characteristics such as body surface area and aortic valve cross-sectional area so that it may be considered as a more sensitive index of cardiac performance than stroke volume which depends on the cross-sectional area.

It is interesting that Doppler ultrasound measurements of flow volumes have yielded good correlations with invasive cardiac output in several studies using a variety of techniques (continuous wave, pulsed wave, ascending aortic flow, etc.). It must be remembered however that correlation is a comparison of the amount of change measured by one technique to a proportionate amount of change of another technique and not a measurement of accuracy of the tested measurement. It would therefore be surprising for any of the studies not to show a good correlation between invasive and non-invasive measurements. Nevertheless, it wouldn't really matter provided that one laboratory always uses the same technique but where it would matter is in longitudinal studies in patients in whom loading conditions may change, the percent of change of volume changes measured by Doppler ultrasound will greatly depend upon the method used.

Mitral inflow method

Another way of calculating blood volume is by using the mitral inflow volume from apical four chamber view. The mitral inflow is calculated by multiplying the area and the diastolic inflow curve (time velocity integral) by the cross-sectional area of the mitral annulus assumed to be a circle. The problem here is that the flow velocity greatly varies with respiration and the position of the sample volume and for serial measurements of blood flow sampling exactly the same point at the mitral inflow may be very difficult. The assumption that the mitral ring is a circle may not be true and furthermore, the annular area change averages 12% from early to end-diastole.

During exercise and drug-induced changes in cardiac output cross-sectional area seems to change substantially at the mitral valve level in contrast with the aortic annulus were there is little or no change in cross-sectional area.

Tricuspid and pulmonic valves

Blood flow volume measurements have also been performed using the right ventricular inflow and outflow tract. The area of the tricuspid valve is probably the most difficult to measure from any echocardiographic projection as this cannot be obtained from a single echocardiographic projection.

Similarly, measurements of the area of the right ventricular outflow tract or pulmonary annulus, although easy in children and young adults, is difficult in older people. This measurement however, is useful in calculating shunts in patients with congenital heart disease. Measurements of pulmonary artery flow profiles can be performed from the left parasternal window with the patient in the left lateral decubitus position. After visualisation of the short axis view of the aorta the transducer is then rotated to the left and superiorly, "opened-out" the main pulmonary artery and right ventricular outflow tract. Flow recording is performed in the right ventricular outflow tract immediately below the pulmonic valve. This measurement of pulmonary flow is particularly useful in patients suspected to have an intracardiac shunt so that the ratio between pulmonary to systemic blood flow can be calculated.

Clinical applications

Regurgitant fractions and shunts

The methodology that allows us to measure by Doppler echocardiography can also be used to measure differences in volume in certain pathologic states. These including assessment of intracardiac shunts and valvular regurgitant lesions.

Mitral regurgitation

As it is possible to measure Doppler ultrasound derived blood flow at several points in the circulation, it is possible to compare the flows across two valves and hence to estimate the regurgitant fractions. The stroke volume across the mitral valve is calculated as the product of the mitral velocity integral and the cross-sectional area of the mitral annulus. The volume of flow across the aortic valve will be calculated at the left ventricular outflow tract and cross-sectional area at this level. The difference between the mitral and aortic volume will be the mitral regurgitant volume. Dividing this value by the calculated mitral stroke volume will provide an estimate of mitral regurgitant fraction.

Shunt calculations

The ratio of pulmonary to systemic blood flow (QP:QS) can also be determined by measuring the right ventricular stroke volume at the sub-pulmonic area and the left ventricular stroke volume at the aorta [13]. The pulmonary to systemic flow ratio is abnormal in patients with atrial septal defects and correlated well with oximetric estimates suggesting the usefulness of this method. This can be used to determine the size of the shunt. However, the calculation of volume flow in the two vessels is not accurate enough to diagnose or to exclude small shunts, but the method has been proven useful to differentiate between small, moderate and larger shunts.

Monitoring effects of drug administration

ElKayam et al. [14] examined the effect of vasodilators and Doppler aortic blood flow measurements. Thirteen patients underwent a total of 18 drug interventions. Peak flow velocity left ventricular ejection time and flow velocity integral were determined with each intervention. There was good overall correlation between thermodilution and Doppler derived flow velocity integral. The flow velocity integral accurately reflected changes in stroke volume and the inverse relationship between vascular resistant and peak flow velocity. Therefore, changes in aortic flow caused by vasodilators can be measured accurately and non-invasively by Doppler echocardiography.

Although Doppler measurements of stroke volume and cardiac output are affected by changes in vascular resistance, they are altered even more dramatically by changes in the inotropic state. Wallmeyer *et al.* [20] studied the effects of positive and negative inotropes in an animal model. With pre-load and after-load held constant, a positive inotrope (dobutamine) increased the peak aortic flow velocity and mean acceleration. Both were decreased when a negative inotrope (beta-blocker) was administered.

A substantial number of data now exist regarding the effect of inotropes, daily variations in Doppler ultrasound measurements and observer variability of these measurements. Consequently, we can define as significant a change >15% in peak flow velocity or flow velocity integral occurring after an intervention. Figure 2.3 shows a progressive increase of the time velocity integral (stroke distance) and consequently of stroke volume and cardiac output following incremental doses of intravenous infusion of dobutamine in a patient with severe heart failure (class III of the New York Heart Association classification).

Conclusions

Systolic cardiac function can be analysed using a variety of invasive and non-invasive techniques. Stroke volume and cardiac output can be reliably calculated using Doppler echocardiography. This technique can particularly be used in the serial determination of the effects of therapy on the individual patient, as well as in the non-invasive measurement of regurgitant fractions and shunts. The aortic root method (cross-sectional area of the aortic root and left ventricular outflow tract flow velocity) is simpler and less influenced by variations in cross-sectional area measurement and has been more extensively validated.

References

1. Light LH. Noninvasive ultrasonic technique for observing flow in the human aorta. Nature 1969;224:1119.
2. Huntsman LL, Gams E, Johnson CC *et al*. Transcutaneous determination of aortic blood flow velocities in man. Am Heart J 1975;89:605.
3. Boughner DR, Schnild RL, Persaud JA. Hypertrophic obstructive cardiomyopathy: assess-

ment by echocardiographic and Doppler ultrasound techniques. Br Heart J 1975;37:917–23.

4. Popp RL, Harrison DC. Ultrasonic cardiac echography for determining stroke volume and valvular regurgitation. Circulation 1970;41:493–502.
5. Pombo JF, Troy BL, Russel RO. Left ventricular volumes and ejection fraction by echocardiography. Circulation 1971;43:480–90.
6. Teichholz LE, Kreulen T, Herman MV *et al*. Problems in echocardiographic determinations: echocardiographic-angiographic correlations in the presence or absence of asynergy. Am J Cardiol 1976;37:7–11.
7. Gehrke J, Leeman S, Raphael M *et al*. Non-invasive left ventricular volume determination by two-dimensional echocardiography. Br Heart J 1975;37:911–6.
8. Seed WA, Wood NB. Velocity patterns in the aorta. Cardiovasc Res 1971;5:319.
9. Nerem RM, Seed WA, Wood NB. An experimental study of the velocity distribution and transition to turbulance in the aorta. Cardiovasc Fluid Mech 1972;52:137.
10. Clark C, Schultz DL. Velocity distribution in aortic flow. Cardiovasc Res 1973;7:601.
11. Nerem RM, Rumberger JA, Gross DR *et al*. Hot film anemometer velocity measurements of arterial blood flow in horses. Circ Res 1974;34:193.
12. Farthing S, Peronneau P. Flow in the thoracic aorta. Cardiovasc Res 1979; 13:607.
13. Kitabatake A, Inone M, Asad M *et al*. Non-invasive evaluation of the ratio of pulmonary to systemic blood flow in atrial septal defect by duplex Doppler echocardiography. Circulation 1984;69:73.
14. Elkayam U, Gondin JM, Berkley R *et al*. The use of Doppler flow velocity measurement to assess the haemodynamic response to vasodilators in patients with heart failure. Circulation 1983;67:377–83.
15. Brubakk AO, Givold SE. Pulsed Doppler ultrasound for measuring blood flow in the human aorta. In: Hatle I, Angelsen B (eds), Doppler ultrasound in cardiology. Philadelphia: Lea & Febiger, 1982;185–93.
16. Feigenbaum H. Echocardiography. 3rd ed. Philadelphia: Lea & Febiger, 1981:110–5.
17. Steingart RM, Meller J, Barovick *et al*. Pulsed Doppler echocardiographic measurement of beat to beat changes in stroke volume in dogs. Circllation 1980;62:542–8.
18. Greenfield JC Jr, Patel DJ. Relation between pressure and diameter in the ascending aorta of man. Circ Res 1962;10:778–81.
19. Magnin PA, Stewart JA, Myers S *et al*. Combined Doppler and phased-array echocardiographic estimation of cardiac output. Circulation 1981;63:388–92.
20. Wallmeyer K, Wann LS, Sagar KB *et al*. The influence of preload and heart rate on Doppler echocardiographic indexes of left ventricular performance: comparison with invasive indexes in an experimental preparation. Circulation 1986;74:181–6.

3. Measurement of cardiac output by magnetic resonance imaging

HARRY G. ZEGEL, LOUIS J. BRISSON and
NANCY M. SHERWIN[1]

The application of the principles of nuclear magnetic resonance, or, as it is more commonly referred to, magnetic resonance imaging (MRI), to the study of cardiac function and morphology dates back to the mid-1980s [1–6]. Since that time, many improvements in image quality, data acquisition time, and scanning techniques have contributed to make cardiac MRI and important and practical tool in the investigation and treatment of heart disease.

In this chapter, we will present the fundamental principles of magnetic resonance imaging, the various methods of determining the parameters of left ventricular function by MRI, and the potential applications of this relatively new modality in the vast realm of cardiac imaging.

The basic principles of magnetic resonance imaging

Magnetic resonance is an imaging modality which takes advantage of the principle that certain atomic nuclei, primarily hydrogen in the human body, possess a small magnetic field, by virtue of their intrinsic charge and spin, which can be stimulated by the application of external radio waves of specific frequency, causing them to induce a signal when placed within a strong, uniform magnetic field. This emitted radio signal is then processed and refined via computer to create the clear and impressive images characteristic of MRI.

In a strong, uniform magnetic field such as exists within present super-conducting MRI units (0.35–1.5T; 1 Tesla (T) = 10,000 Gauss), the hydrogen nuclei align themselves in either high or low energy states with respect to the principal magnetic field, i.e. along the z-axis. When external radio waves of the appropriate resonant frequency (Larmor frequency) are presented to the hydrogen ion, a small number of these nuclei (6 per 10^6) become stimulated with a resultant displacement of their magnetization vector from the z-axis to the x-y plane. When this brief radio frequency stimulation is no longer applied, the hydrogen nuclei tend to return to their initial low energy state.

1. We wish to express our thanks to MRI Diagnostics Inc. for their assistance in providing images for this manuscript.

A.-M. Salmasi and A.S. Iskandrian (eds): Cardiac output and regional flow in health and disease, 47–61.

Table 3.1. Signal appearance of principle tissue components in MRI with T_1 weighted and T_2 weighted images.

	T_1 weighted $= \dfrac{\text{Short TR}}{\text{Short TE}}$ e.g. 600 ms/20 ms	T_2 weighted $= \dfrac{\text{longTR}}{\text{long TR}}$ e.g. 2000 ms/100 ms
Water	Dark	Bright
Fat	Bright	Slightly less bright
Soft Tissue	Intermediate	Intermediate

TR = time to repetition; TE = time to echo.

In doing so, they induce an electrical signal which is computer reconstructed into an MRI image.

Briefly, this hydrogen ion relaxation occurs in two ways. The longitudinal (spin lattice) relaxation rate is referred to as T_1 and the transverse (spin-spin) relaxation rate is referred to as T_2. T_1 and T_2 are intrinsic tissue characteristics.

The most common form of MRI is spin-echo utilizing 2D Fourier transformation. The signal intensities with this method are approximated by the formula:

$$SI = N(H) \times F(V) \times (1 - E^{-TR/T}1) \times E^{-TE/T}2,$$

where SI represents signal intensity, T_1 and T_2 are intrinsic tissue relaxation rates, TR (time to repetition) and TE (time to echo) are variable instrument settings, N(H) is the number of hydrogen nuclei, and F(V) is function of velocity of flow. By varying TR and TE we can "weight" the signal intensity formula to produce T_1 or T_2 weighted images and, thus, emphasize signal characteristics between adjacent tissues (Table 3.1).

Spatial resolution is acheived by encoding positional information into the MRI signal. Additional small magnetic field gradients are applied in the z, y, and x axes, known as slice selection, phase encoding, and frequency encoding, respectively. These gradients alter the signal to allow spatial information to be encoded [7–9].

In magnetic resonance imaging, a tomographic plane of tissue can be represented in either the standard x, y, or z axis orientation or any intermediate plane or obliquity. Within each tomographic plane, the tissue is divided into multiple volume elements called voxels. Each voxel is represented by a solitary pixel in the computer image. In cardiac MRI scanning, the pixel matrix is usually 256 × 256 which results in approximately 1.25 mm of resolution, depending on the size of the field of view. Flowing blood generally does not produce a signal with standard spin-echo MRI [10]; and "artificial signal intensity" within vessels can be selectively eliminated by the application of pre-saturation gradients which are available on more current equipment. With respect to cardiac MRI, this phenomenon is advantageous as it

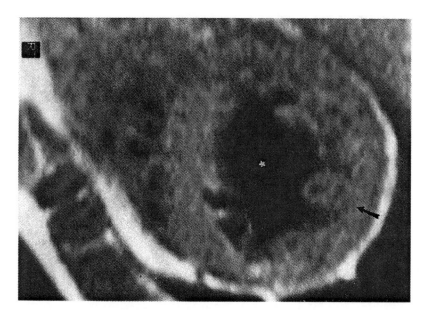

Figure 3.1. Spin-echo cardiac MR image of left ventricle (black arrow) in systole (short axis cross-section of the heart) demonstrating flowing intracavitary blood as a region of signal void (white asterisk).

creates a natural contrast between flowing blood within the chambers of the heart and great vessels, depicted as an area of signal void, and the surrounding myocardium (Figure 3.1). Thus, the need for intravenous or intraarterial contrast material to opacify blood is obviated.

The initial cardiac gated MRI studies were plagued by long scanning and data acquisition times which brought the total time to complete the study in the range of 60 to 90 mintues. Clearly, this was impractical both in its application to a non-academic setting, and for patients as well, when compared to ventriculography and, especially, 2-D echocardiography. The development of fast echo "gradient echo imaging" (GRE) [11–15] allowed the acquisition of up to 32 images per cardiac cycle at up to four levels within a few minutes time. Since GRE rather than spin-echo sequences are utilized, flowing blood demonstrates increased signal in relation to the surrounding myocardium (Figure 3.2).

This facilitates the detection of the endocardial border for the purpose of calculating left ventricular end-systolic volume (LVESV) and left ventricular end-diastolic volume (LVEDV). When the information is presented in a cine format, movie-like images display the heart in a dynamic fashion which simplifies evaluation of regional left ventricular motion by accurately out-

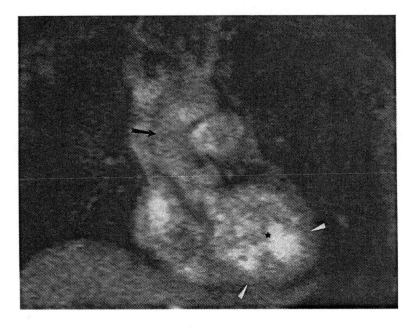

Figure 3.2. Gradient echo (GRE) MR image of the heart in coronal projection demonstrating intracavitary left ventricular blood as an area of increased signal intensity (black asterisk) with respect to the surrounding myocardium (white arrowheads). The ascending aorta is indicated (black arrow).

lining the intraventricular blood pool, as well as the actual heart wall, in the appropriate systolic and diastolic images.

Recent developments include single gradient echo tomographic slices which can be obtained in the subsecond (50–150 msec) range, thus allowing cardiac motion to be frozen in time.

The measurement of heart wall motion is a sensitive method for the evaluation of myocardial function. Heart motion, however, is a complex combination of translation, rotation, and concentric contraction [16]. Recently, a new pulse sequence technique has been developed which "tags" myocardium with a cross-hatched, lattice-like pattern. The true complex motion of the heart can be precisely analyzed by the way in which this superimposed "grid pattern" geometrically deforms during the cardiac cycle [16, 17].

MRI assessment of left ventricular function

The prerequisite for the use of MRI in determining the basic parameters of left ventricular (LV) function (i.e. left ventricular end-diastolic volume

(LVEDV), left ventricular end-systolic volume (LVESV), and ejection fraction (EF)) are two-fold: first, that there must exist standardized techniques to obtain such measurements; and, second, that those same measurements must be reproducible in the same patient when no significant interval change in cardiac function has occurred between studies [18].

With regard to the standardized techniques of measurement, two important features of MR imaging are particularly salient. As previously mentioned, the natural contrast between flowing blood and myocardium is equivalent to that obtained in ventriculography as part of a cardiac catheterization procedure. Consequently, the endocardial margins are clearly defined, hence, facilitating the measurement of LVEDV and LVESV (Figure 3.3). In addition, the ability of an MRI unit to obtain and reproduce a tomographic slice of tissue in transverse, coronal, sagittal, and, most important, any oblique plane is a necessary component in assessing its utility *vis-à-vis* ventriculography, 2-D echocardiography (2-D echo), and gates blood-pool scintigraphy [19, 21].

The standard projections used in cardiac MRI are the same as the cardiac axes for angiography and 2-D echo: (a) the long axis of the LV, parallel to the interventricular septum: (b) the long axis of the LV, perpendicular to the septum; and (c) the short axis of the LV at multiple levels including outflow, papillary muscle, and apex (Figures 3.3 and 3.4). The first two axes correspond to the 30° right anterior oblique view and the 60° left anterior oblique positions, respectively, in ventriculography.

Although the optimal planes for performing cardiac MR imaging are well-established, there remains some controversy as to the best reference points for the definition of the longitudinal LV axis. Various proposals included portions of the mitral valve and apex, a "line of symmetry" [22] within the LV, and an axis through the apex and the aortic valve. We concur with the position held by Dinsmore [23] who states that the apex/aortic valve is the most appropriate choice because: (a) it is usually the longest plane in the LV; (b) parts of the ventricular outflow tract can be excluded in measuring LVEDV and LVESV when other axes are used; (c) the aortic valve can be reliably identified in most MRI studies of the heart; and (d) the aortic valve and apex are the reference points in the area-length calculation of LVEDV and LVESV in contrast ventriculography.

The original static ECG-gated MRI studies calculated LVEDV, LVESV, and, hence, EF from a single image for each of end-diastole and end-systole located in a single optimal plane, i.e. the long axis of the LV parallel to the interventricular septum. The area of the intra-cavitary portion of the ventricle is determined by scanner software which sums the size of the individual pixels (i.e. representing voxels of tissue) outlined within the endocardial border which is marked manually with a planimeter or more recently with automatic edge-detecting software. The long axis of the ventricle is then measured directly (Figure 3.5). The volumes are calculated by a modification of the area-length formula, which assumes the LV cavity is a ellipsoid, used in ventriculography:

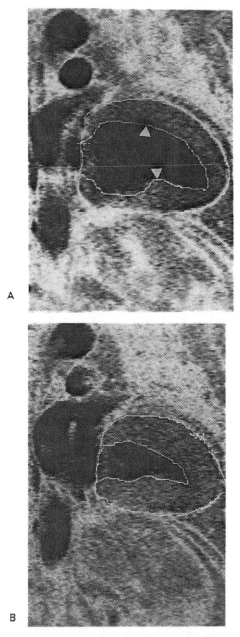

A

B

Figure 3.3. (a) Long axis view of the left ventricle parallel to the interventricular septum during end-diastole. The delineation of the endocardial borders (inner hatched line/white arrowheads) is facilitated by the natural contrast between flowing intracavitary blood (signal void) and myocardium in this spin-echo technique. (b) Same projection and technique as in (a) but left ventricle is now in end-systole.

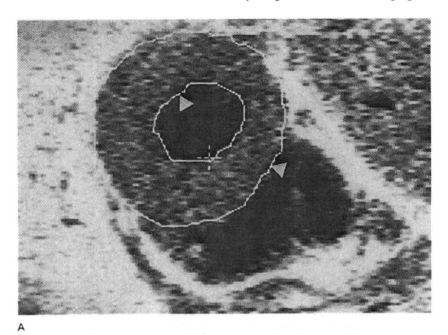

A

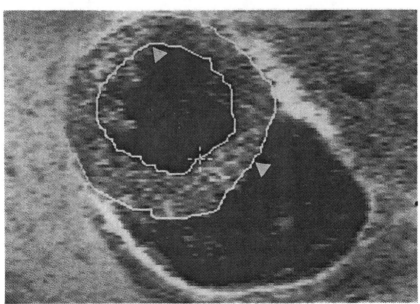

B

Figure 3.4. Spin-echo MR images of the left ventricle (short-axis view) during end-systole (a) and end-systole (b). White arrowheads indicate epicardial and endocardial borders of the left ventricle.

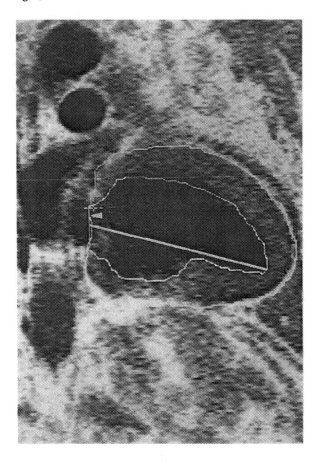

Figure 3.5. Long axis view of left ventricle for purpose of measuring distance (white line) between apex (black arrowhead) and aortic valve (white arrowhead) which is then used for calculated LVEDV by area/length method.

Volume = $0.849 \times$ (area)^2/length [24],

where area is the total area in the region of interest in cm; length represents the length of the long axis of the LV in cm; and volume is either LVEDV or LVESV in cm. Ejection fraction and cardiac output are then calculated in the usual manner.

The fast echo pulse sequence measures LVEDV and LVESV from multiple images obtained at different levels of the LV in the appropriate short axis plane during end-diastole and end-systole, i.e. after tracing the endocardial borders. Volume is calculated by a modification of Simpson's rule which assumes the ventricle to be cylindrical and divides the LV into 1 cm slices where the volume of each slice equals h(A × B)/4 (h = slice thickness, A = axis in one view, B = axis in second view at same level). The total volume of LV is the sum of the individual slice volumes corrected for image distortion:

$$\text{Volume} = 1.047h'\left(A_i'B_i' + \Sigma 1/2A_j'B_j'\right) [25],$$

where h' is segment height corrected for image distortion, A'B' represent the respective AP and lateral measured axes, i denotes the odd-numbered slices, and j denotes the even-numbered slices.

Both the modified area-length and Simpson's rule methods of calculating LVEDV and LVESV contain inherent inaccuracies stemming from the geometric assumptions made in these formulae. However, the cine MRI technique of measuring LVEDV and LVESV, by computer-assisted calculation of the LV intra-cavitary area within the endocardial borders in contiguous 1 cm slices through the short axis plane and subsequent summation of the volume within each 1 cm slice, provides the most accurate, though somewhat tedious, assessment of the true LVEDV and LVESV. Besides eschewing any geometric assumptions or corrections for image distortion, this technique excludes the papillary muscles from the intracavitary portion of the LV which further enhances the veracity of the volume measurements.

The second prerequisite to the consideration of MRI as being equal or superior to the other modalites is the reproducibility of measurements between studies in the same patient. In this regard, we refer the reader to the recent work of Semelka *et al.* [18] which examined interstudy variability of measurements of ventricular dimensions and LV function obtained with cardiac cine MRI. Their work indeed proved that "anatomic and functional measurement from the cine MRI images are reproducible". The parameters of LV function not only included LVESV, LVEDV, and EF, but also LV mass (end-diastolic and end-systolic) and LV end-systolic wall stress.

Table 3.2 summarizes and compares LV function indices for various imaging modalities. A recurrent issue when examining these values is the consistent finding that cardiac MRI LVEDV and LVESV are smaller than those obtained in angiography. This is likely attributable to a variety of factors including an overestimation of volume in ventriculography secondary to the inclusion of the papillary muscles, manual errors in tracing endocardial borders in cardiac MRI, and the combination of the chronotopic effects of contrast agents and the angiographic procedure itself. However, ejection fraction is logically more accurate between various modalities as it measures the relative change from diastole to systole.

A recent method for determining ejection fraction involves the detection of the velocity of blood flowing in the aortic root (Figures 3.6 and 3.7). By anatomically measuring the cross-sectional area of the aortic root and identifying the velocity of a given volume of blood that traverses this region.

Table 3.2. Comparison of left ventricular end-diastolic volume (LVEDV), left ventricular endsystolic volume (LVESV), and left ventricular ejection fraction (LVEF) of various cardiac imaging modalities.[a]

Modality	LVEDV (ml)	LVESV (ml)	LVEF (%)
Cine MR			
Semelka [18]	113.3	39.6	65.1
Sechtem [11]	101.0	31.0	69.3
2-D echo			
Gordon [39]	95.5	38.6	60.0
Michaelson [40]	****	****	70.0
Angiography			
Wynne [20]	*****	****	72.0
Kennedy [21]	*****	****	67.0

[a] Adapted from Semelka *et al.* [18] in reference guide.

An accurate estimation of cardiac output can be made [26]. The velocity mapping technique (Figure 3.8), although still experimental, is based on either phase shifts proportional to flow velocity or to the "time-of-flight" of a tagged volume of blood [27]. This same technique can also be applied to the pulmonary artery to give an accurate estimation of right ventricular output, or to the pulmonary veins to assess blood return to the left atrium.

Advantages and disadvantages of cardiac MRI

Each of the major cardiac imaging modalities, including MRI, have inherent advantages and restrictive features. The benefits of MRI with respect to ventriculography are that it is completely non-invasive, does not require the use of contrast agents, involves no risk of radiation exposure, and is potentially a superior marker of the parameters of LV function by its greater spatial resolution and almost equivalent temporal resolution. Moreover, with the advent of cine GRE MRI, the geometric assumptions which distort the measurement of LVEDV and LVESV by other means are avoided.

The pitfalls of cardiac MRI are highlighted when it is compared to gated blood-pool scintigraphy and 2-D echo. Although the latter two modalities do not approach the image quality of MRI, they are more versatile in several respects. Cardiac MRI is not helpful in the assessment of a bed-ridden or moderately ill patient whereas both 2-D echo and gated blood-pool scintigraphy are portable examinations which can be performed at the bedside in unstable persons requiring extensive cardiac monitoring. In addition, the requirement of stable rhythms for the acquisition of cardiac MRI images precludes the use of this modality in persons who are afflicted with relatively common arrhythmias, e.g. atrial fibrillation. Finally, cardiac MRI is presently limited by numerous intrinsic contraindications. Absolute contraindications

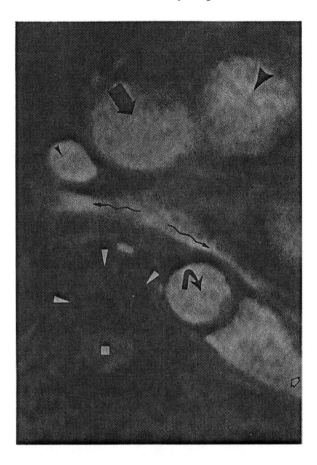

Figure 3.6. Transverse gradient-echo (GRE) MR image of the great vessels, used for detection of ejection fraction by measuring velocity of flowing blood in the aortic root, landmarked as follows: ascending aorta (large black arrow), descending aorta (curved black arrow), superior vena cava (small black arrowhead), pulmonary outflow tract (large black arrowhead), main pulmonary arteries (wavy black arrows), thoracic vertebral body (white arrowheads), and spinal canal (white square). Incidental note is made of a left pleural effusion (open arrowhead).

to MRI are the presence of: (1) a cardiac pacemaker; (2) certain brands of ferromagnetic intracerebral aneurysm clips; (3) metallic intraocular foreign bodies (metal workers should be screened with CT scanning of the orbits prior to any MRI study); (4) cochlear implants; (5) neurostimulators; and (6) certain early generation prosthetic heart valves. Relative contraindications include pregnancy and claustrophobia. Patients with malleable surgical clips, orthopedic implants, and most prosthetic heart valves may undergo MRI imaging. Life-supporting ventilators and intravenous pumps are now avail-

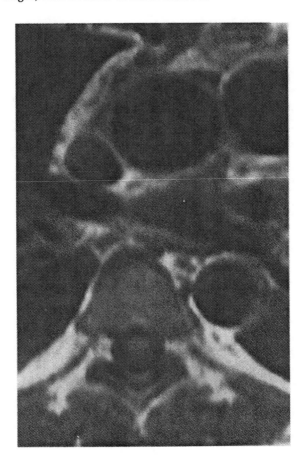

Figure 3.7. Identical image of great vessels in transverse plane as seen in Figure 3.6 but performed with spin-echo technique. See legend of Figure 3.6 for identification of particular great vessels and supporting structures.

able in non-ferromagnetic versions which allow the imaging of critically-ill patients, but the logistics involved in producing a study on such individuals make the use of MRI limited in these situations.

Other present and future applications of cardiac MRI

Beyond the previously discussed role of MR imaging in the assessment of left ventricular function, cardiac MRI has established roles in the preoperative investigation of congenital heart disease involving complex morphologic anomalies [28], the evaluation of intracardiac and pericardial masses, as well as

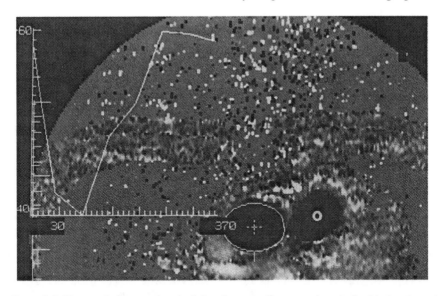

Figure 3.8. Phase velocity mapping depicting the ascending aorta (+ sign) with demarcated phase velocity shifts (on graph) allowing calculation of cardiac output. The pulmonary outflow tract is marked by the white circle.

the characterization of primary myocardial abnormalities of infectious and ischemic origin.

There are also potential roles for dynamic cardiac MR imaging of the proximal coronary arteries and coronary bypass grafts [29–31]. Future applications will include quantification of cardiac, aortic, and pulmonary vascular flow rates. Tissue characterization either by T_2 weighting or Gadolinium-DTPA enhancement has shown to be highly accurate in depicting the area and extent of myocardial infarction [32–35].

Recently, pharmacologic stress testing [36–38] has been used in conjunction with MRI ventricular wall motion studies. This appears to be a clinically useful investigative procedure and yields more diagnostic information than merely scanning the patient in a non-physiologic state [39, 40].

The ultimate goal of cardiac MRI is to incorporate, in one study, the ability to detect cardiac anatomy, wall motion, blood flow through chambers and vessels, as well as to depict the signal characteristics of normal, ischemic, and infarcted myocardium. In the not-too-distant future, it is hoped that a single MRI examination will quickly and accurately render the above anatomic and physiologic information and, thus, eliminate the need for multiple alternative, or more invasive, studies.

In summary, this promising modality has earned a position on the same stage with the other principal forms of cardiac imaging. Magnetic resonance imaging has enormous untapped potential only limited by today's existing technology.

References

1. Dinsmore RE, Wismer GL, Levine RA *et al*. Magnetic resonance imaging of the heart: positioning and gradient angle selection for optimal imaging planes. Am J. Radiol 1984;143:1135–42.
2. Ehman RL, Julsrud PR. Magnetic resonance of the heart: current status. Mayo Clin Proc 1989;64:1134–46.
3. Byrd BF, Schiller NB, Botvinick EH *et al*. Normal cardiac dimensions by magnetic resonance imaging. Am J Cardiol 1985;55:1440–2
4. Sechtem U, Somnerhoff BA, Markiewicz W *et al*. Regional left ventricular wall thickening by magnetic resonance imaging: evaluation in normal persons and patients with global and regional dysfunction. Am J Cardiol 1987;59:145–51.
5. Higgins CB. MR of the heart: anatomy, physiology, and metabolism. Am J Radiol 1988;151:239–48.
6. Akins EW, Hill JA, Fitzsimmons JR *et al*. Importance of imaging plane for magnetic resonance imaging of the normal left ventricle. Am J. Cardiol 1985;56:366–72.
7. Longmore DB. The principles of magnetic resonance. Br Med Bull 1989;45:948–67.
8. Sprawls P. Physical principles of medical imaging. Rockville: Aspen Publishers Inc, 1987.
9. Underwood R, Firman D. An introduction to magnetic resonance of the cardiovascular system. London: Current Medical Literature Ltd, 1987.
10. Mirowitz SA, Lee JK, Guiterrez FR *et al*..
11. Sechtem U, Pflugfelder PW, Gould RG *et al*. Measurement of right and left ventricular volumes in healthy individuals with cine MR imaging. Radiology 1987;163:697–702.
12. Pflugfelder PW, Sechtem UP, White RD *et al*. Quantification of regional myocardial function by rapid cine MR imaging. Am J Radiol 1988;150:523–9.
13. Underwood ST. Cine magnetic resonance imaging and flow measurements in the cardiovascular system. Br Med Bull 1989;45:848–80.
14. Lotan CS, Cranney GB, Bouchard A. *et al*. The value of cine MR for assessing regional ventricular function. J Am Coll Cardiol 1989;14:1721–9.
15. Pettigrew RI. Dynamic cardiac MR imaging: techniques and applications. Radiol Clin North Am 1989;27:1183–203.
16. Thomsen C, Mogelvana J, Peng Q *et al*. Chess-pattern spatial modulation of MR image intensity: assessment of myocardial function. Appeared in Book of Abstracts, Vol. 1, of the Society of Magnetic Resonance in Medicine–9th annual meeting & exhibition, New York City, USA, August 1990.
17. Axel L, Dougherty L. Heart wall motion: improved method of spatial modulation of magnetization for MR imaging. Radiology 1989;172:349–50.
18. Semelka RC, Tomei E, Wagner S *et al*. Normal left ventricular dimensions and function: interdstudy reproducibility of measurements with cine MR imaging. Radiology 1990;174:763–8.
19. Stratemeier EJ, Thompson R, Brady TJ *et al*. Ejection fraction determination by MR imaging: comparison with left ventricular angiography. Radiology 1986;158:775–7.
20. Wynne J, Greene LH, Mann T *et al*. Estimation of left ventricular volumes in man from biplane cineangiograms filmed in oblique projections. Am J Cardiol 1978;41:726–32.
21. Kennedy JW, Baxley WA, Figley MM *et al*. Quantitative angiocardiography: i. the normal left ventricle in man. Circulation 1966;34:272–8.
22. Bernstein MA, Perman WH, Besozzi MC *et al*. Pulse sequence generated oblique magnetic resonance imaging: applications to cardiac imaging. Med Phys 1986;13:648–57.

23. Dinsmore RE. Quantitation of cardiac dimensions from ECG-synchronized MRI studies. Cardiovasc Intervent Radiol 1987;10:356–64.
24. Buckwalter KA, Aisen AM, Dilworth LR *et al*. Gated cardiac MRI: ejection fraction determination using the right anterior oblique view. Am J Radiol 1986;147:33–7.
25. Utz JA, Hefkens RJ, Heinsimer JA *et al*. Cine MR determination of left ventricular ejection fraction. AJ Radiol 1987;148:839–43.
26. Bogren HG, Klipstein RH, Firmin DN *et al*. Quantitation of antegrade and retrograde blood flow in the human aorta by MR velocity mapping. Am Heart J 1989;117:1214–22.
27. Firmin DN, Nayler GL, Klipstein RH *et al*. *In vivo* validation of MR velocity imaging. J Comput Assist Tomogr 1987;11:751–6.
28. Soulen RL, Donner RM, Capitanio M. Postoperative evaluation of complex congenital heart disease by magnetic resonance imaging. Radiographics 1987;9:975–1000.
29. Rubinstein RI, Askenase AD, Thickman D *et al*. Magnetic resonance imaging to evaluate patency of aortocoronary bypass grafts. Circulation 1987;76:786–91.
30. White RD, Pflugfelder PW, Lipton MJ *et al*. Coronary artery bypass grafts: evaluation of patency with cine MR imaging. Am J Radiol 1988;150:1271–4.
31. White RD, Caputo GR, Mark AS *et al*. Coronary artery bypass graft patency: non-invasive evaluation with MR imaging. Radiology 1987;164:681–6.
32. Saeed M, Wendland MF, Takehara Y *et al*. Reversible and irreversible injury in the reperfused myocardium: differentiation with contrast material-enhanced MR imaging. Radiology 1990;175:633–7.
33. De Roos A, Van Rossum AC, Van der Wall EE *et al*. Reperfused and non-reperfused myocardial infarction: diagnostic potential of Gd-DTPA-enhanced MR imaging. Radiology 1989;172:717–20.
34. Brown JJ, Higgins CB. Myocardial paramagnetic contrast agents for MR imaging. Am J Radiol 1988;151:865–72.
35. Rozeman Y, Zou X, Kantor HL. Cardiovascular MR imaging with iron oxide particles: utility of a superparamagnetic contrast agent and the role of diffusion in signal loss. Radiology 1990;175:655–9.
36. Pennell DJ, Underwood SR, Longmore DB. Detection of coronary artery disease using MR imaging with dipyridamole infusion. J Comput Assist Tomogr 1990;14:167–70.
37. Beer S, Zegel HG, Feldman *et al*. The efficacy of oral dipyridamole cine-magnetic resonance imaging in detecting coronary artery disease. American College of Cardiology 40th Annual Scientific Session, Atlanta, Georgia, March 1991.
38. Pennell DJ, Underwood SR, Manzara CC, *et al*. Magnetic resonance imaging of reversible myocardial ischaemia during dobutamine stress. Proceedings of the Society of Magnetic Resonance in Medicine–9th lnnual meeting & exhibition, New York City, USA, August 1990.
39. Gordon EP, Schnittger I, Fitzgerald PJ *et al*. Reproducibility of left ventricular volumes by two-dimensional echocardiography. J Am Coll Cardiol 1983;2:506–13.
40. Michaelson JK, Byrd BF, Bouchard A *et al*. Left ventricular dimension and mechanics in distance runners. Am Heart J 1986;112:1251–6.

4. Measurement of cardiac output by nuclear techniques

JAEKYEONG HEO and ABDULMASSIH S. ISKANDRIAN

Cardiac output measurement using radionuclide angiographic (RNA) techniques is feasible, accurate and reproducible. Since it is non-invasive, it may be repeated as necessary for serial follow-up changes or to evaluate effect of therapeutic interventions [1–7]. Most nuclear techniques (except for the indicator dilution method) rely on measurement of end-diastolic (EDV) and end-systolic volume (ESV). The nuclear techniques will be discussed in four broad categories (Tables 4.1 and 4.2):

1. indicator dilution;
2. geometric method;
3. nongeometric method;
4. newer approaches.

Indicator dilution method using Tc-99m labeled RBC

This method is based on the same principle as the indocyanine dye dilution method used in the hemodynamic laboratory (see chapter 1). A 20 mCi bolus of Tc-99m labeled RBC is injected into the antecubital vein or jugular vein and images of the heart are obtained during the first transit [8, 9]. A multi-crystal camera is prefered due to its high count rate capability. A framing rate of 40 frames/sec is adequate for this purpose.

Images are reformatted to give 2 frames/sec and left ventricular (LV) region of interest is drawn to generate time activity curve. A typical time activity curve is shown in Figure 4.1 and is presented mathematically in Equation (4.1).

$$I = Q \times \int C(t)\, dt. \tag{4.1}$$

Where, I is the total amount of radioactivity injected, Q is the flow rate or cardiac output, C(t) is the concentration of radioactivity at time t, thus $\int C(t)\, dt$ represents the primary curve (area under the broken line) after elimination of the recirculation portion of the original curve either by gamma variate function or exponential curve fitting method. Approximately 10 min post injection or at equilibrium, the radioactivity will be diluted in the total

A.-M. Salmasi and A.S. Iskandrian (eds): Cardiac output and regional flow in health and disease, 63–76.
© 1993 Kluwer Academic Publishers. Printed in the Netherlands.

Table 4.1. Nuclear technique measuring cardiac output.

A) Indicator dilution method
   1) gamma variate function
   2) exponential function
B) Geometric method
   1) gated RNA[a]
   2) first pass RNA[a]
C) Nongeometric method
   1) regression equation method
   2) surface marker technique
   3) balloon tipped catheter
   4) esophageal transmission measurement
D) Newer approaches
   1) SPECT technique
   2) Count-proportional method
   3) Ambulatory nuclear monitoring

[a]RNA = Radionuclide angiography.

blood volume, which may be estimated using sex, weight, height, etc. or directly measured using I-125 labeled human serum albumin.

A static image of the heart is obtained without changing the patient position to generate LV counts at equilibrium (C_{eq}). Thus, the total activity injected (I) is expressed in equation (4.2).

$$I = \text{Total blood volume} \times C_{eq}. \tag{4.2}$$

Table 4.2. Radionuclide angiographic volume measurements.

Author	RNA	Vol	Attn	Reference	Camera	#	Corr	SEM
Anderson	G	EDV	−	sonomicrometer	MC	6 dogs	0.98	1.1
Caputo	S	EDV/ESV	−	contrast angio	SC	30 pts	0.89	24
Dehmer	C	EDV	−	contrast angio	SC	15 pts	0.91	10
Gill	S	EDV	−	contrast angio	SC	12pts	0.94	20
Harpen	I	EDV	−	contrast angio	SC	12 pts	0.99	17
Iskandrian	G	EDV	−	contrast angio	MC	30 pts	0.94	46
Kronenberg	C	EDV	+	contrast angio	SC	7 dogs	0.96	−
Links	C	EDV	+	contrast angio	SC	35 pts	0.95	36
Massardo	R	EDV	−	contrast angio	SC	25 pts	0.95	23
Maurer	C	EDV	+	contrast angio	SC	36 pts	0.96	21
Petru	G	CO	+	contrast angio	SC	28 pts	0.91	1.3
Rerych	G	EDV	−	Fick CO	MC	23 pts	0.98	23
Slutsky	C	EDV	+	contrast angio	SC	52 pts	0.98	7.3
Starling	C	EDV	+	contrast angio	SC	27 pts	0.98	25

Abbreviations: +, yes; −, no; Attn, attenuation correction; C, count based nongeometric method; I, indicator dilution; G, geometric method; pts, patients; R, count-based ratio method; S, SPECT technique; MC, multi-crystal camera; SC,single-crystal; Corr, correlation; SEM, standard error of mean; vol, measured volume.

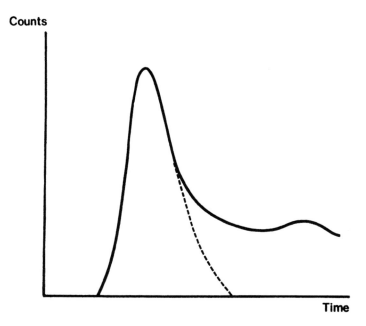

Figure 4.1. Time activity curve with indicator dilution method. The primary curve is represented by the initial solid line and the subsequent broken line.

From Equations (4.1) and (4.2)

$$Q = \frac{C_{eq} \times \text{Total blood volume}}{\int C(t)\, dt} \qquad (4.3)$$

or

$$CO = \frac{\text{Counts at equilibrium} \times \text{Total blood volume}}{\text{Area under primary curve}}. \qquad (4.4)$$

The two types of curve fitting used to exclude the recirculation are briefly summarized below.

Exponential method

If washout of the tracer is a mono-exponential function, one can use semi-logarithmic paper (activity on logarithmic scale and time on regular scale) to plot this time activity curve from the region of interest. However, a computer program using curve fitting method will identify primary curve to eliminate recirculation component.

Gamma variate function

Curve fitting method by gamma variate function is expressed in Equation (4.5).

$$C(t) = k(t - AT)^\alpha \cdot e^{-(t-AT)/\beta},\tag{4.5}$$

where C(t) is concentration of radioactivity at time t, AT = appearance time of the bolus activity; k, α, β = coefficients variables for curve fitting. Gamma variate function also is included in the software package of nuclear computers. In general, the exponential method slightly overestimates the primary curve, thus underestimates cardiac output than gamma variate extrapolation method. Although this method is simple and provides good correlation with conventional methods, several precautions are necessary.

The *in vitro* labeling of RBC with Tc-99m should be carefully observed to reach high labeling efficiency. The injection of the bolus should be compact without tracer hangup elsewhere. The assumption of adequate mixing of the tracer in the proximal chamber is important. Lastly, unlike thermodilution technique, serial measurements during a short time period are not feasible because of buildup of background activity due to previous studies.

Geometric method

Ventricular volumes can be determined by applying the similar principle and geometric assumptions used in the catherization laboratory using contrast ventriculography [10–12]. With the first-pass technique with a multi-crystal gamma camera a modification of area-length method is used for the anterior projection using the Equation (4.6) (Figure 4.2).

$$LV\ EDV = 0.85\ A^2/L.\tag{4.6}$$

Where A is the end-diastolic area and L is the long axis of the left ventricle. These parameters are derived automatically by the computer using the built-in software packages. Thus, the stroke volume and cardiac output are calculated by the formula:

$$Stroke\ volume = EDV \times ejection\ fraction\ (EF).\tag{4.7}$$

$$Cardiac\ output = Stroke\ volume \times heart\ rate.\tag{4.8}$$

An important difference between contrast ventriculography and first-pass RNA is that in the former both the EDV and ESV are measured by the geometric method while the ESV by the RNA method is a derived measurement from the EDV which is geometrically derived and the EF which is based on count differences independent upon geometric assumptions. The same method maybe also be applied to the gated RNA technique; however, the long axis of the heart is foreshortened in the left anterior oblique projec-

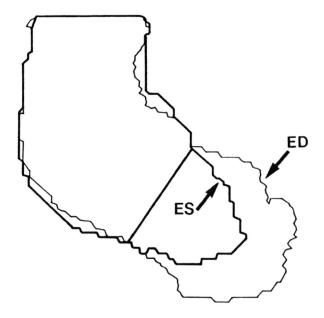

Figure 4.2. An example of end-diastolic (ED) and end-systolic (ES) perimeters in a first-pass study.

tion which is the only way to separate LV from RV [13]. Therefore, LV volumes may be underestimated.

The above described geometric methods have some problems related to the resolution limitation of the gamma camera system, inaccurate region of interest definition and valve plane identification. In addition, geometric assumption of an ellipsoidal shape may not apply in patients with segmental wall motion abnormalities and abnormal configuration of LV cavity.

Non-geometric method (count-based method)

This method is based on the fact that the radioactive count is proportional to the volume at equilibrium. End-diastolic counts are obtained from LV ROI and 2–5 ml of blood sample is withdrawn for counting (Figure 4.3). The LV EDV is measured with Equation (4.9).

$$EDV = \frac{\text{Count rate from LV at ED}}{\text{Count rate*/ml of blood sample}}. \tag{4.9}$$

The count rate from the sample should be corrected for decay and attenuation. Several techniques are used for attenuation correction.

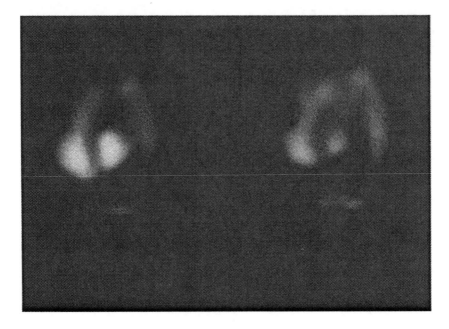

Figure 4.3. A gated radionuclide angiogram. Region-of-interests are drawn at end-diastole (right panel) and end-systole (left panel) to generate counts from either LV or RV.

A. *Regression equation method*

A linear relationship between LV end-diastolic count rate and LV volume is established from experimental studies either by phantom or contrast ventriculograms in men, producing coefficients for slope and intercept (Volume by cath = a + b × volume by RNA) [14–16]. From these coefficients, the true volume can be calculated. However, this method is based on the assumption that all attenuations are uniform from patient to patient and does not take into consideration the individual variation in the position of the heart, and the size of the thorax.

B. *Acquisition of 30° RAO*

To determine the distance between the LV center and the skin surface of the patient's chest, a static acquisition during the first-pass study in 30° right anterior oblique projection is obtained with a marker on the skin surface [17]. The distance is calculated afterwards using the computer technique. The attenuation is addressed using the Equation (4.10).

$$A_1 = A_0 e^{-\mu l}. \tag{4.10}$$

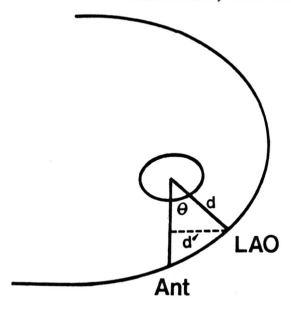

Figure 4.4. Schematic presentation of two images (anterior and left anterior oblique projections). The distance (d') (between LV centers of two projections and angle (θ) are determined to calculate the distance (d) between the LV center and the skin surface using sine function.

Where A_1 is activity after distance 1, A_0 is the true original activity, μ is attenuation coefficients and 1 is the distance between the chest surface and center of the LV cavity. A conventional gated RNA is acquired after the first-pass study. The EDV is calculated using Equation (4.11).

$$\text{EDV} = \frac{\text{End-diastolic counts}}{\text{Frame duration} \times \# \text{ of cycles} \times \text{blood counts} \times e^{-\mu l}}, \qquad (4.11)$$

where end-diastolic counts is obtained from LV ROI and corrected for background activity. Frame duration and # of cardiac cycles are determined from computer parameters during processing of the study. Two milliliters of blood sample is drawn, counted and decay corrected. This blood count is corrected for attenuation using the factor $e^{-\mu l}$.

C. *Distance calculation by anterior and LAO projection images*

Links *et al.* and others used combination of anterior projection and left anterior oblique projection from gated RNA to calculate the distance between the chest surface and the center of the LV cavity [18–20]. This technique is explained in Figure 4.4. From the LAO projection, the angle is determined and a point source is placed to indicate the center of the LV cavity. Then d' is determined from the anterior projection. The distance in the LAO projection is easily obtained using the Equation (4.12).

$$d = \frac{d'}{\sin \theta}.$$

(4.12)

The other important parameter, attenuation coefficient μ is evaluated using phantom studies, where μ measured $0.14 - 0.15$/cm for 50–250 ml flasks in water 4–13 cm from the collimator. In studies with patients, this coefficient was proved to be accurate in providing good correlation with contrast angiography without systematic under- or over-estimation. LV EDV was calculated from Equations (4.13) and (4.14).

$$LV\ EDV = \frac{\text{Count rate from LV in ED}/e^{-\mu d}}{\text{Count rate/ml from blood sample}}$$

(4.13)

$$\text{Count rate from LV at ED} = \frac{\text{Total LV counts in ED frame}}{\text{Time per frame} \times \#\ \text{of cycles acquired}}.$$

(4.14)

D. *Direct attenuation measurement using a balloon tipped catheter*

The intrathoracic attenuation of radioactivity was measured in the catherization laboratory in seven mongrel dogs [21, 22]. A dose of Tc-99m was injected into a balloon-tipped catheter that was placed on the skin surface of the chest and imaged in the LAO projection. The balloon was then aspirated and catheter was advanced to the right atrial-inferior vena cava junction. The Tc-99m was reinjected, and an image obtained maintaining the same angle of view. The attenuation factor (AF) was calculated using Equation (4.15).

$$AF = \frac{\text{Count rate outside thorax}}{\text{Count rate inside thorax}}.$$

(4.15)

The dog was then positioned for contrast ventriculography by moving the imaging table. The reproducibility of nuclear volume determinations was excellent. This method was especially accurate for estimating changes in LV volumes.

E. *Esophageal transmission measurement*

Maurer et al. determined attenuation factor using gated RNA and esophageal transmission measurement [23]. Patients swallowed a small capsule containing a calibrated dose of Tc-99m sulfur colloid, which is tied to a sewing thread. To determine the capsule count rate behind the LV cavity, a region of interest was drawn from the 40° LAO gated RNA study. For background subtraction, another ROI was selected that did not include an area of increased activity from adjacent vascular structures (aorta or spleen) or decreased activity from an area such as fluid or gas-filled stomach. The individual transmission factors measured in this study ranged from 0.11 to 0.35. There was no significant difference between scintigraphic and angiographic end-diastolic volumes in this study in 36 patients. In general a counts-based method using gated RNA is more reproducible and accurate than geometric methods, which assume ellipsoid configuration of the LV cavity [7, 24]. The ROI for the LV cavity and background may be drawn manually, however automated programs for drawing are more reproducible without significant inter- or intra-observer variability.

Since the volume is dependent on the radioactivity concentration, measurements of cardiac output and LV volumes may be affected by the changes in concentration. Studies that examined changes in blood activity, RBC count and splenic activity show an increase in hemoglobin concentration during exercise secondary to splenic contraction [25, 26]. They reported that the cardiac output and LV volumes may be overestimated in the range of 7–14%. Thus additional blood sampling during exercise is required to circumvent this radio-activity concentration change. In the absense of valvular regurgitation or intra cardiac shunts, the LV stroke volume and right ventricular stroke volumes are equal and hence the right ventricular volumes can be calculated from LV stroke volume and right ventricular ejection fraction. Alternatively, the above count methods can also be adopted to measure right ventricular volumes and right ventricular stroke volume and output from right ventricular ROI.

Newer approaches

SPECT technique

Single photon emission computed tomography (SPECT) is gaining popularity in myocardial perfusion imaging to eliminate overlap and superimposition problems. However, its use in gated RNA is limited due to time consuming processing and too many images with problems of display and storage.

Recently, Gill and associates (1986) used multigated SPECT in blood pool imaging to measure LV volumes and assessing regional wall motion [27]. The patients' RBC were labeled with 25 mCi of Tc-99m by the modified *in vivo* technique. Data were collected at 60 views over a 360° rotation using a 1.4 zoom mode for 25 sec/view. Each cardiac cycle was divided into 16 frames with fixed interval gating using 90% of the R-R interval and rejecting all beats that did not fall within a timing window of 20% of the average of the preceding four beats. For analysis, short axis slices were selected to extend from the apex to the base of LV ROI. The total number of counts and number of pixels within the LV ROI with counts above the threshold value were determined for each slice.

The LV volume can be expressed by Equation (4.16).

$$\Sigma \frac{\text{count density of LV slice (i)}}{\text{count of LV slice with max count density}}$$

$$\cdot \text{\# pixels in slice(i)} \cdot \text{voxel volume.} \tag{4.16}$$

The correlation between measured LV volumes using this SPECT technique and actual volumes in a phantom study and volumes by contrast angiogram was excellent. This technique represents a SPECT equivalent of geometric RNA volume measurement.

Count based method by SPECT

Caputo *et al.* applied a count-based method using ungated SPECT. After the gated planar study, 128 ten second nongated tomographic images were acquired over 360° with a total acquisition time of 22 min using 64 × 64 matrix [28]. After reconstruction, tomographic slices were used to determine the counts per milliliter in the mid-LV chamber slice and total LV counts which were used to derive mean LV volume. The EDV and ESV were calculated from the mean volume using the LV time activity curve from planar gated blood pool images. The EDV is the mean tomographic LV ratio of the end-diastolic counts to mean counts of time activity curve. The clinical application of this technique in 30 patients showed good correlation with cineangiography ($r = 0.89$, standard error of mean = 24).

Count-proportional non geometric method

The count-proportional method is based on the fact that the radioactivity recorded from a chamber at equilibrium is proportional to the volume of the chamber. Massardo and associates studied 25 patients using this RNA technique and compared with contrast angiographic volumes [29]. The total count (C_t) is proportional to the total volume of the sphere (V_t), k is constant and D is its diameter hence:

$$C_t = kV_t = k\frac{\pi}{6}D^3 \tag{4.17}$$

$$V_t = \frac{\pi}{6}D^3. \tag{4.18}$$

The pixel with maximum count (N_m) is proportional to the volume M^2D where M is pixel dimension and D is the diameter:

$$N_m = kM^2D. \tag{4.19}$$

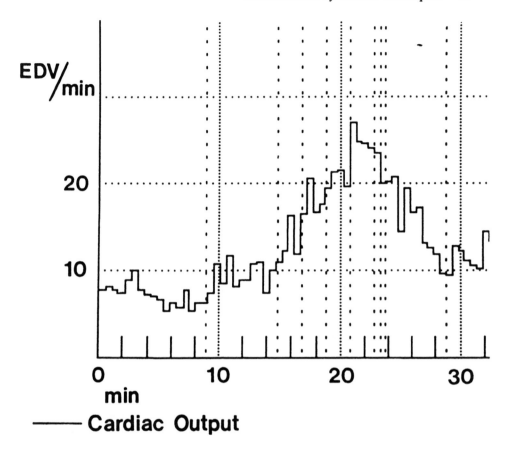

Figure 4.5. Continuous recording of cardiac output from a VEST study. Broken vertical lines represent event markers indicating different stages of exercise.

The constant, k, is eliminated by taking the ratio $R = C_t/N_m$ resulting following equation:

$$R = \frac{C_t}{N_m} = \frac{k\pi D^3/6}{kM^2D} = \frac{\pi D^2}{6M^2}. \tag{4.20}$$

Equation (4.20) may be solved from D as follows:

$$D^2 = 6M^2R/\pi. \tag{4.21}$$

From Equations (4.18) and (4.21), the volume of the sphere is solved:

$$V_t = \pi/6 \cdot D^3 \tag{4.22}$$

$$V_t = 1.38\,M^3R^{3/2}. \tag{4.23}$$

This method appears to be reproducible and requires no additional procedures such as attenuation correction or blood sampling.

Ambulatory nuclear monitoring

Recent advance in technology in a nuclear detector and computer hardware/software made it possible to monitor left ventricular function on ambulatory basis. C-VEST™ is such a unit and consists of a sodium iodide crystal detector and a parallel hole collinator weighing approximately 1.5 lbs [30]. The detector is mounted on a plastic garment, which is worn like a vest, thus named VEST.

In addition there are two leads that constantly record two channel electrocardiogram. These nuclear and ECG signals are sent by wire to a tape recorder that may be carried over the shoulder or wheeled along side the patient. An event marker is available for recording any special events. This tape is fed into the computer for data processing. After acquisition of gated RNA, the detector is positioned to cover the center of the LV cavity with the use of different sizes of collimators. The average recording time is 3–4 hours during which time various measurements are obtained such as heart rate, ECG changes, systolic and diastolic LV function (EF, PFR, etc.) and volumes (EDV, SV, CO, etc.). Figure 4.5 shows a recording of cardiac output up to 30 minutes, where the vertical broken lines represent events indicating different stages of exercise. Thus, ambulatory monitoring of cardiac output during daily activities, physiologic or pharmacologic interventions is feasible during extended periods of time. These volume measurements are relative in that the unit is in EDV/min. However, if the absolute baseline EDV or cadiac output is known with other technique such as RNA, echo and angiographic method etc, these relative volumes may be converted easily to absolute volumes.

References

1. Huff RL, Feller DD, Oliver JJ et al. Cardiac output of men and dogs measured by *in vivo* analysis of iodinated (I-131) human serum albumin. Circ Res 1955;3:564–9.
2. Mack RE, Herschel JW, Pollack R. An *in vivo* method for the determination of cardiac output. Radiology 1957;68:245–48.
3. Zipf RE, McGuire TF, Webber JM et al. Determination of cardiac output by means of external monitoring of radioisotope injected intravenously. Clin Path 1957;28:134–44.
4. Shackman R. Radioactive isotope measurements of cardiac output. Clin Sci 1958;17:317–29.
5. Pritchard WH, MacIntyre WJ, Moir TW. The determination of cardiac output by the dilution method without arterial sampling. II. Validation of precordial counting. Circulation 1958;18:1147–55.
6. Schreiner BF, Lovejoy FW, Yu PN. Estimation of cardiac output from precordial dilution curves in patients with cardiopulmonary disease. Circ Res 1959;595–601.
7. Iskandrian AS. Thallium-201 myocardial imaging andradionuclide ventriculogram. In: Nu-

clear cardiac imaging: principles and applications. Philadelphia: F.A. Davis Co, 1986;137–43.

8. Harpen MD, Dubuisson RL, Mead GB *et al*. Determination of left-ventricular volume from first-pass kinetics of labeled red cells. J Nucl Med 1983;4:98–103.

9. Glass EC, Rahimian J, Hines HH. Effect of region of interest selection on first-pass radionuclide cardiac output determination. J Nucl Med 1986;27:1282–92.

10. Rerych SK, Scholz PM, Newman GE *et al*. Cardiac function at rest and during exercise in normals and in patients with coronary heart disease: evaluation by radionuclide angiography. Ann Surg 1978;187:449.

11. Iskandrian AS, Hakki A-H, Kane SA *et al*. Quantitative radionuclide angiography in the assessment of hemodynamic changes during upright exercise = observations in normal subjects, patients with coronary artery disease and patients with aortic regurgitation. Am J Cardiol 1981;48:239.

12. Anderson PAW, Rerych SK, Moore TE *et al*. Accuracy of left ventricular end-diastolic dimension determinations obtained by radionuclide angiocardiography. J Nucl Med 1981;22:500–5.

13. Strauss, H, Zaret B, Hurlley P *et al*. A scintiphotographic method for measuring left ventricular ejection fraction in man without cardiac catheterization. Am J Cardiol 1971;28:575.

14. Dehmer GJ, Lewis SE, Hillis DL *et al*. Nongeometric determination of left ventricular volumes from equilibrium blood pool scans. Am J Cardiol 1980;45:293–300.

15. Kronenberg MW, Parrish MD, Jenkins DW *et al*. Accuracy of radionuclide ventriculography for estimation of left ventricular volume changes and end-systolic pressure-volume relations. J Am Coll Cardiol 1985;6:1064–72.

16. Slutsky R, Karliner J, Ricci *et al*. Left ventricular volumes by gated equilibrium radionuclide angiography a new method. Circulation 1979;60:556–64.

17. Parrish MD, Graham TP, Born ML *et al*. Radionuclide ventriculography for assessment of absolute right and left ventricular volumes in children. Circulation 1982;66:811–9.

18. Links JM, Becker LC, Shindledecker JG *et al*. Measurement of absolute left ventricular volume from gated blood pool studies. Circulation 1982;65:82–91.

19. Starling MR, Dell Italia LJ, Walsh RA *et al*. Accurate estimates of absolute left ventricular volumes from equilibrium radionuclide angiographic count data using a simple geometric attenuation correction. J Am Coll Cardiol 1984;3:789–98.

20. Petru MA, Sorensen SG, Chaudhuri TK *et al*. Attenuation correction of equilibrium radionuclide angiography for noninvasive quantitation of cardiac output and ventricular volumes. Am Heart J 1984;107:1221.

21. Keller AM, Simon TR, Smitherman TC *et al*. Direct determination of the attenuation coefficient for radionuclide volume measurements. J Nucl Med 1987;28:102–7.

22. Burow RD, Wilson MF, Heath PW *et al*. Influence of attenuation on radionuclide stroke volume determinations. J Nucl Med 1982;23:781–5.

23. Maurer AH, Siegel JA, Denenberg BS *et al*. Absolute left ventricular volume from gated blood pool imaging with use of esophageal transmission measurement. Am J Cardiol 1983;51:853–8.

24. Massie BM, Kramer BL, Gertz EW *et al*. Radionuclide measurement of left ventricular volume: comparison of geometric and count based methods. Circulation 1982;65:725.

25. Sandler MP, Kronenberg MW, Foreman MB *et al*. Dynamic fluctuations in blood and spleen radioactivity: splenic contraction and relation to clinical radionuclide volume calculations. J Am Coll Cardiol 1984;3:1205–11.

26. Konstam MA, Tu'meh S, Wynne J *et al*. Effect of exercise on erythrocyte count and blood activity concentration after technetium-99m *in vivo* red cell labeling. Circulation 1982;66:638–42.

27. Gill JB, Moore RH, Tamaki N *et al*. Multigated blood-pool tomography: new method for the assessment of left ventricular function. J Nucl Med 1986;27:1916–24.

28. Caputo GR, Graham MM, Brust KD *et al*. Measurement of left ventricular volume using single photon emission computed tomography. Am J Cardiol 1985;56:781–6.
29. Massardo T, Gal RA, Grenier RP *et al*. Left ventricular volume calculation using a count-based ratio method applied to multigated radionuclide angiography. J Nucl Med 1990;31:450–6.
30. Iskandrian AS, Heo J. Ambulatory nuclear monitoring of left ventricular function. J Myo Ischemia 1989;1:82–95.

5. Comparison between the invasive and noninvasive methods

ABDULMASSIH S. ISKANDRIAN

The previous chapters (Chapters 1 to 4) discussed the various methods of measuring the cardiac output invasively and noninvasively. Some of the methods are geometrically dependent, others are not. The geometrically independent methods are preferred because in diseased states, assumptions made on a prolate ellipse may not be valid.

In my opinion, the best method for measuring the cardiac output in the catheterization laboratory is the thermodilution technique. This is a convenient method which can be repeated many times and does not require blood sampling. It is accurate and geometrically independent. Furthermore, the Swan-Ganz catheter permits simultaneous assessment of pulmonary artery wedge and the right heart pressures. There are obviously some pitfalls and these are nicely summarized by Drs. Koren and Santamore in Chapter 1. For example, the method is not reliable in patients with low cardiac output, intracardiac shunts or right-sided valvular regurgitation.

For research purposes, the thermodilution method can be used in the exercise laboratory but for routine clinical use, the method is not practical because of the inherent risk, inconvenience and the cost associated with the method. Hence, the choice between invasive and noninvasive methods should take into consideration the circumstances in which the test is being used; in the catheterization laboratory invasive tests are appropriate while for out-patients, noninvasive tests are mandatory. Any comparison between the two methods is done merely to determine the accuracy of a newer technique. Some methods may be reproducible though not quite accurate; these are acceptable if directional changes are being examined e.g. what happens to the cardiac output during exercise or during other interventions?

Furthermore, for purposes of comparison it should be mentioned that biological variability may be significant in absolute measurements. For example, changes in preload, afterload, contractility, heart rate, body position, relaxation and filing characteristics of the left ventricle may all affect the cardiac output. Therefore, when independent methods are compared to each other, they should be done in very close temporal relation to each other. Studies done on separate days are probably not acceptable.

The non-geometric method for measuring the left ventricular volume by the gated-equilibrium radionuclide angiographic technique is the most suitable for out-patients. This method permits assessment discussed by Heo

A.-M. Salmasi and A.S. Iskandrian (eds): Cardiac output and regional flow in health and disease, 77–78.

and Iskandrian, left ventricular end-diastolic volume, end-systolic volume, ejection fraction as well as relaxation and filing characteristics of the left ventricle. It is geometrically independent. It does not require blood sampling and can be repeated serially. It can be studied with the patient in the supine, semi-erect, or even the erect position. It can be obtained with commercially available gamma cameras and can be done at rest and during exercise. It should, however, be recognized that the cardiac output measured by this method reflects the total cardiac output. Hence, in patients with mitral regurgitation or aortic regurgitation this method tends to overestimate the true (net) cardiac output. The first-pass method though reliable, requires for optimum results, the use of a multi-crystal gamma camera which is not routinely available in most laboratories. The correlation between the nuclear techniques and the invasive techniques were summarized in in Chapter 4. The magnetic resonance imaging method is not well suited for routine use because of cost and inconvenience of obtaining such measurements in acutely ill patients or during exercise.

The two dimensional echocardiographic method and possibly also the doppler technique are increasingly being used during pharmocologic interventions and exercise to detect wall motion abnormality reflective of ischemia. It is possible to use the methods also to generate volume and output data. The echocardiographic technique is inherently geometrically dependent but the doppler technique can provide information on flow velocity or flow that is geometrically independent.

In summary, both invasive and non-invasive techniques permit cardiac output measurements. The invasive techniques will remain as the "Gold Standard" to validate newer non-invasive techniques which may have more of an impact on patient management and clinical utility than the invasive techniques.

6. Linear cardiac output

ABDUL-MAJEED SALMASI

The main or perhaps the only function of the heart is to maintain an adequate cardiac output and hence regional flow and within the physiological limits. In physiological conditions, subject to the effect of various reflex stimuli and mechanisms the cardiac output can vary widely. Similarly in pathological conditions cardiac output and/or regional flow may be subject to a wide range of variation (see other chapters). It has been, therefore, a prime objective in clinical practice to measure cardiac output hence representing myocardial performance. From previous chapters one can realise that measurement of cardiac output varies widely depending upon the technique used. In addition and from the practical point of view it is not feasible to measure cardiac output repeatedly using an invasive method in order, for example, to assess the response to an intervention or therapy. Therefore cardiac output in its "volumetric" term may not be so easy to use for clinical purposes.

The concept of linear cardiac output

One of the methods used to measure cardiac output is the combination of echocardiographic measurement of aortic cross-sectional area and the Doppler ultrasound measurement of the aortic blood velocity deriving the distance travelled by the blood at a point where the Doppler ultrasound beam is in line with the direction of flow. By placing the Doppler ultrasound transducer in the suprasternal notch, it is possible to have an access to a wide area and alternative direction of the transducer will make the measurement obtained either in the aortic root or in the aortic arch. Figures obtained from both these sites were similar. For this reason the term "stroke distance" is introduced to denote the distance travelled by the blood in the aortic arch per beat or the systolic velocity time integral [1]. Similarly "minute distance" represents stroke distance times heart rate [1]. The main parameter missing from both the stroke distance and the minute distance is the aortic cross-sectional area. Measurement of the aortic blood velocity is highly reproducible, simple and safe [2] while measurement of the aortic cross-sectional area is the least reproducible and technically difficult [4]. For serial measurements on the same subject in order to assess effect of therapy or surgical intervention it is more appropriate and practical to use stroke distance and

A.-M. Salmasi and A.S. Iskandrian (eds): Cardiac output and regional flow in health and disease, 79–81.
© 1993 *Kluwer Academic Publishers. Printed in the Netherlands.*

minute distance or "linear" stroke volume and cardiac output than the volumetric.

There have been several reports to correlate cardiac output measured by Doppler ultrasound and echocardiography and that measured by invasive techniques (for further detail see Chapter 2). In order to have an accurate method of measuring the stroke distance the whole flow within the aorta should be measured and insonated. Such a signal should contain a wide range of frequencies to cover nearly all velocities from the stationary vessel wall to the fastest midstream blood flow. This can be achieved practically via using a wide bore transducer [2].

The maximal velocity of the aortic blood flow is seen in the midstream [3] where under physiological condition it is not disturbed. Although it is assumed that blood velocity is the same within the aorta, measuring this velocity is better made at the aortic arch rather than the root. Another challenge to trying to make accurate measurement of cardiac output from the echo/ Doppler cardiography is the correct measurement of the aortic cross-sectional area. The various reporters who used this technique made the measurement of the aortic cross-sectional area at different levels, namely at the aortic valve orifice, at the sinus of Valsalva and the narrowest point of the sinotubular junction. There is a substantial difference between these levels of measurements hence giving differences in the measurements of the cardiac output made. The other observation made with regards to obtaining a correct measurement of the aortic cross-sectional area was the poor correlation made between the echocardiographic measurement and that made during aortic valve replacement surgery [4].

There have been reports on a good correlation between body surface area and aortic cross sectional area. A correlation coefficient of 0.84 was reported by Feigenbaum (1976) between the aortic root diameter and the square root of the body surface area [5]. Since the cardiac index is the cardiac output divided by the body surface area, it is appropriate to use the minute distance as being proportional to the cardiac output divided by the aortic cross sectional area. Towfiq and associates reported that aortic cross-sectional area increased with advancing age in 200 patients [6]. Thus, this is one of the causes why minute distance declines with age (see Chapter 10). This is further supported by the observation of Rawles that the stroke distance is not related to body surface area but declines with advancing age [3].

References

1. Mowat DHR, Haites NE, Rawles JM. Aortic blood velocity measurement in healthy adults using a simple ultrasound technique. Cardiovasc Res 1983;17:75.
2. Salmasi SN. Electrocardiographic chest wall mapping and transcutaneous aortovelography [M Phil thesis]. Univ of London, 1989.

3. Rawles JM. Measurement of linear cardiac output. In: Salmasi AM, Nicolaides AN, (eds), Cardiovascular applications of Doppler ultrasound. London: Churchill-Livingstone, 1989:85.
4. Mackay A, Been M, Rodrigues A et al. Preoperative of prosthesis size using cross-sectional echocardiography in patients requiring aortic valve replacement. Brit Heart J 1985;53:507.
5. Feigenbaum H. Echocardiography. 2nd ed. Philadelphia: Lea & Febiger, 1976:471.
6. Towfiq BA, Weir J, Rawles JM. Effect of age and blood pressure on aortic size and stroke distance. Brit Heart J 1986;55:560.

PART TWO

Cardiac output: physiological considerations. Cardiac output in normal subjects at rest and during exercise

7. Cardiac output: physiological concepts

ABDUL-MAJEED SALMASI

The main function of the heart is to maintain an adequate cardiac output. The physiological regulation of cardiac output is complicated and is beyond the scope of this book. However, under normal physiological conditions cardiac output is maintained equal to the perfusion needs of various tissues. Various mechanisms interact to achieve such a control. Cardiac output varies widely according to physiological and/or environmental factors.

As cardiac output is the product of heart rate and stroke volume, it is anticipated that factors which affect either of these two components would in turn affect the cardiac output. However, human cardiac output varies according to differences in age, size or sex of the subjects. Changes in the posture or in the enviromental temperature can also affect measurements of cardiac output.

Because there are different techniques of measuring cardiac output there have been, as a result, wide variations in the results obtained from such techniques. However, in a young healthy adult male, cardiac output averages approximately 5.6 litres per minute. In general, cardiac output in females is 10% lower than that of a male subject of the same age and body size [1].

The basic phenomena that control the regulation of cardiac output is the venous return, the total peripheral resistance and the myocardial contractility.

The rate of venous return plays the major role in the regulation of cardiac output and under normal physiological circumstances it is the main determinant of cardiac output. This mechanism follows the Frank-Starling law of the heart. However, it should be remembered that during normal physiological circumstances there is a limit beyond which the pumping action of the heart does not increase in parallel with the increase in the venous return. This permissive level of the heart action is estimated to be upto 13–15 litres per minute. Increase in the permissive level of heart pumping action under normal physiological circumstances occurs in autonomic stimulation of the heart. Athletes are another example of individuals who have high level of permissive heart pumping action under physiological conditions. Whereas the increase in the permissive level of the pumping action of the heart is physiological in the majority of circumstances, a reduction is always pathological and occurs when the heart fails. Such a situation is encountered in congenital valvular and myocardial heart disease. It also occurs after my-

A.-M. Salmasi and A.S. Iskandrian (eds): Cardiac output and regional flow in health and disease, 85–88.

ocardial infarction. Under these pathological circumstances the heart fails to cope with the rate of the venous return and the cardiac output may fall to below 3 or even 2 litres per minute at rest.

Myocardial contractility

One of the characteristics of ventricular contraction is that the myocardial fibres contract sequentially. This means that the strength of contraction of myocardial fibre depends on the rate, strength and sequence of contraction of the fibres that have contracted earlier [2–6].

Sympathetic stimulation increases ventricular contractility directly and indirectly by increasing heart rate, while parasympathetic stimulation produces an opposite effect. Myocardial contractility is affected by drugs and hormones. Most beta-adrenergic blocking agents, calcium-channel blockers, lignocaine, disopyramide, procainamide and quinidine decrease contractility. Hypoxia and acidosis decrease myocardial contractility too. However, contractility increases by catecholamine, thyroxine and serotonin.

Afterload (or the total peripheral resistance)

Cardiac output increases when there is a decrease in the vascular resistance such as in anaemia, arteriovenous fistula and pregnancy. Also total peripheral resistance decreases when cardiac output increases; this has particularly been noticed during exercise.

Body size

Although changes in cardiac output in obesity will be discussed in Chapter 28, a consideration of physiological changes in accordance to body size will be discussed here.

It is well recognised that cardiac output varies markedly with body size; a reason why and for comparative purposes cardiac output has been normalised for body surface area thus introducing the term "cardiac index", which is cardiac output per square metre of body surface area. For a normal man under normal physiological conditions the cardiac index is 3.3 l/minute/sq. metre [6].

Gender

While there has been no concrete evidence to indicate that cardiac output in females is different from that in males there have been controversial reports on the subject. A report by Buonanno and associates [7] suggested the presence of a hyperdynamic condition of the left ventricle in females under normal physiological conditions as compared to males. However, the population used in their study were patients presenting with chest pain and though their coronary arteriography was normal, 59% of the female population had resting S-T segment changes and 17% had positive stress ECG testing. None of the male subjects had positive stress ECG testing but yet 22% of them had resting S-T segment abnormalities.

Posture

It is well documented that changing the posture while at rest is accompanied by changes in cardiac output. This was well shown in the report of Donald *et al.* [8] that changing the posture was associated by a small, though significant, change in the cardiac output. This was further confirmed by the work of Wang and associates [9] who in 4 normal subjects reported a decrease in cardiac output from 6.9 l/minute in the supine position to 5.4 l/minute in the standing position [10]. In a study using dye dilution method to determine cardiac output in men ranging in age between 32 and 58 years, a change in cardiac output from 6.6 l/minute in the supine position to 5.3 l/minute in the sitting position was reported [11].

Excitement

Our knowledge of the effect of excitement on cardiac output goes back to the work of Linhard in 1915 [12] who reported that cardiac output increased at rest when individuals were subjected to excitement.

No doubt that cardiac output increases when the subject is excited, an effect which may persist if the individual is subjected to exercise. Various circumstances have been attempted such as anxiety, apprehension, tests and academic examination and in all a significant increase in cardiac output was noted [13].

High altitude

Hypoxia as a result of high altitudes stimulates the sympathetic nervous system. This in combination with a decrease in the parasympathetic activity will lead to increased cardiac output [14]. This response reaches its peak within one hour of the ascent to high altitudes but within a day or two it reaches the sea level value and within 10 days it plateaus to about 20% below the cardiac output at sea level [15]. This value applies both at rest and during exercise. The main mechanism responsible for this process is an increase in heart rate which also reaches its maximum within an hour of ascent to the high altitude then decreases within a day or two but plateaus at a level above that at the sea level. The stroke volume on the other hand remains unchanged upon ascent to high altitude but starts to decrease after that till it levels up to a plateau on the tenth day to 25% below the sea level value.

References

1. Guyton AC. Human physiology and mechanisms of disease. 3rd ed. Philadelphia: WB Saunders, 1982.
2. Hawthorne EW. Instantaneous dimensional changes of the left ventricle in dogs. Circ Res 1961;9:110.
3. Schlant RC, Dixon F, Elson SH et al. Modification of the law of the heart: influence of early contracting areas. Circulation 1964;30 (Suppl 3):153.
4. Schlant RC, Rawls WJ, Dixon F et al. Intraventricular kick: an additional determinant of ventricular performance. Clin Res 1965;13:62.
5. Schlant RC. Idioventricular kick. Circulation 1966;34(Suppl 3):209.
6. Lentner C. Geigy scientific tables. Volume 5, heart and circulation. Ciba-Geigy 1990:47.
7. Buonanno C, Arbustini E, Rossi B et al. Left ventricular function in men and women. Another difference between sexes. Eur Heart J 1982;3:525.
8. Donald KW, Bishop JM, Wade OL. Effect of nursing positions on cardiac output in man with a note on the repeatability of measurements of cardiac output by the direct Fick method and with data on subjects with normal cardiovascular system. Clin Sci 1953;12:199.
9. Wang Y, Marshall RJ, Shepherd JT. The effect of changes in posture and of graded exercise on stroke volume in man. J Clin Invest 1960;39:1051.
10. Holmgren A, Ovenfors CO. Heart volume at rest and during muscular work in the supine and in the sitting position. Acta Med Scand 1960;167:267.
11. Thadani U, West RO, Mathew TM et al. Hemodynamics at rest and during supine and sitting bicycle exercise in patients with coronary artery disease. Am J Cardiol 1977;39:776.
12. Lindhard J. Über das minutenvolumen des Herzens bei Ruhe und bei Muskelarbeit. Pflug Arch Ges Physiol 1915;161:233.
13. Wade OL, Bishop JM. Cardiac output and regional flow. Oxford: Blackwell, 1961:43.
14. Hammill SC, Wagner WW Jr., Latham LP et al. Autonomic cardiovascular control during hypoxia in the dog. Circ Res 1979;44:569.
15. Alexander JK, Hartley LH, Modelski M et al. Reduction of stroke volume during exercise in man following ascent to 3100m altitude. J Appl Physiol 1967;23:849.

8. Cardiac output in athletes and the effect of training

ABDUL-MAJEED SALMASI

Both from the scientific and the clinical points of views, the changes observed in the cardiac output during athletic activity is an acute one. Athletic training increases maximal oxygen uptake, and the subject involved will have a reduced heart rate but compensated for by an increase in the stroke volume. Peak heart rate is not altered by training but there is an increase in both the stroke volume and the arteriovenous oxygen difference; the latter together with an increased cardiac output will be the reason for increased oxygen uptake.

In athletes or in continuous athletic training there are histological changes which take place in the myocardium. Macroscopically cardiac size, mass and the volume all increase; the latter may increase up to 60–80% of that of a non-athletic individual.

Mitchell and Blomqvist pointed out that during acute exercise there is a huge increase in blood flow to active muscle; this increase is from an average of 650 ml per minute to 20,850 ml per minute during maximal exercise [1]. Opening up of capillary beds which are not open at rest is the main reason for the increase in the blood flow to active muscles. It is important to remember that blood flow to the brain during acute exercise shall remain unchanged. As a result of acute exercise heat is liberated by the exercising muscles and body temperature increases. Heat loss occurs entirely throughout the skin via opening up of skin capillaries and increasing the cutaneous flow.

Augmentation of the heart rate and stroke volume during acute exercise is mainly brought up via sympathetic stimulation. This is attenuated by 20–40% after blocking the beta-adrenergic receptor of the heart by pharmacological agents [2].

Systolic blood pressure increases during acute dynamic exercise while the diastolic blood pressure remains unchanged or show a slight decrease. This, in the presence of a huge increase in cardiac output, reflects a decrease in the total peripheral resistance.

Sympathetic overactivity during acute exercise also leads to vasoconstriction of resistant vessels which occurs in all areas except in the exercising muscles.

After prolonged exercise programmes there is a progressive increase in stroke volume, which in endurance athletes may be up to 50–75% higher

A.-M. Salmasi and A.S. Iskandrian (eds): Cardiac output and regional flow in health and disease, 89–90.

than that of sedentary men [3]. In terms of myocardial oxygen consumption, increasing volume load is the most efficient method of increasing the cardiac output. This can be achieved via various methods of sports. However, it should be remembered that weight lifting produces no significant change in heart volume as it is an isometric type of exercise.

Another factor that mediates increased blood volume in the heart is the increase in the venous return brought about by increasing venous tone mediated by sympathetic reflex. With a very minute rise in intraventricular pressure, the right ventricle can accept a huge volume of blood during diastole, thus cardiac output increases immediately.

A considerable influence on the stroke volume at rest comes from the position of the body during acute exercise. Venous return is higher during supine exercise and hence cardiac output increases during exercise in such a position such as swimming. This is further assisted by a drop in the peripheral resistance which is encountered during acute exercise.

References

1. Mitchell JH, Blomqvist G. Maximal oxygen uptake. N Eng J Med 1971;284:1018.
2. Wallace AG. The heart in athletes. In: Hurst JW, (ed), The Heart. New York: McGraw-Hill Book Company, 1985:1398.
3. Bates DV. Commentary on cardiorespiratory determinants of cardiovascular fitness. Can Med Assoc J 1967;96:704.

9. Cardiac output during exercise

ABDUL-MAJEED SALMASI

Being on organ which only function is to pump blood to various tissues of the body including itself, the heart must increase its function and capacity during exercise thus resulting in an increase in the cardiac output in order to cope with the extra demand.

In normal individuals and under physiological conditions exercise will result in an increase in sympathetic tone and thus causing a rise in the heart rate and contractility. This together with the decrease in total peripheral resistance and simultaneous increase in venous return result in an increase in the cardiac output and stroke volume [1]. Sharma and associates (1976) using angiographic techniques have confirmed these physiological observations [2]. In normal subjects the increase in the cardiac output during exercise is the result of combination of increased heart rate and stroke volume; the latter being mainly due to enhanced contractility. An increase in the left ventricular end-diastolic pressure combined with a simultaneous decrease in the left ventricular end-systolic pressure results in an increase in stroke volume. This enhanced Starling effect during exercise has been the subject of study by many investigators and acted as the basis for studying changes in cardiac output with exercise in various clinical cardiac conditions.

There has been no evidence by radiological studies to suggest any remarkable increase of heart size during exercise. Brynjolf and associates by using multiple gated blood pool imaging of left ventricular volumes at rest and during upright submaximal exercise in 22 normal subjects, they reported an increase of 14% in the left ventricular ejection fraction with exercise as a result of an increase of 14% in the left ventricular end-diastolic volume offset by a decrease of 14% in the left ventricular end-systolic volume [3]. These results confirmed previously reported similar findings [4–6]. The disparity in the resting cardiac output and the stroke volume between the supine and the upright positions remains also during exercise. Thadani and Parker [7] carried out a study on healthy volunteers in the age range of 32 and 58 years and reported that cardiac output, which was determined by dye dilution, increased from a resting value of 6.6 l/minute to 14.3 l/minute during exercise in the supine position. However in the upright position, cardiac output increased from 5.3 l/minute at rest to 13.8 l/minute during exercise.

In clinical situations assessment of left ventricular function is best carried out during exercise as dysfunction is often unvailed during physical stress.

A.-M. Salmasi and A.S. Iskandrian (eds): Cardiac output and regional flow in health and disease, 91–96.
© 1993 *Kluwer Academic Publishers. Printed in the Netherlands.*

Also it is well established in exercise physiology that data derived from exercise are better indices of the individual's tolerance and fitness than the measurements carried out at rest. Since cardiac output is the best measure of global left ventricular function its assessment during exercise bears the same importance. However, from the clinical and practical points of views, assessment of cardiac output during physical exercise is not without difficulties. This arises especially if such measurements are required for following up patients or assessing a clinical situation or study the response to therapy or a surgical procedure or interference. For these reasons emphasis in the past decade has been put on non-invasive methods of measuring cardiac output which can be repeated safely and without inconvenience to the patient. Various approaches have been introduced which were discussed in details in the previous part of this book. For some time, and until now, assessment of left ventricular function using radionucleides has been carried out. This approach has unvailed lots of pathophysiological situations and established effects of different therapeutic measures and substances on the myocardium.

More recently echo/Doppler cardiographic techniques have been widely used as being simple, safe and probably the easiest available method of assessing left ventricular function noninvasively. This is specially the case when compared to the currently available techniques of measuring cardiac output and stroke volume during exercise thus offering a major potential advantage technically and clinically.

As explained in the previous part of this book the term "linear cardiac output" was used in Doppler ultrasound measurement of cardiac output during exercise assuming the aortic diameter remains unchanged during exercise hence the systolic velocity time integral (which is the distance travelled by the aortic blood per beat) denoted the stroke distance or a measure of the stroke volume. Similarly cardiac output is expressed by the minute distance and it is equal to the stroke distance times the heart rate.

Doppler ultrasound measurement of the aortic blood velocity during exercise

It was in 1982 when the first report was published by Salmasi and associates [7] on characterising left ventricular performance during exercise in normal subjects and in patients with coronary artery disease using Doppler ultrasound. Further reports by the same authors were published from 1983–1985 [8–10]. In a preliminary study the stroke distance and the minute distance were measured in 10 normal subjects every minute during an upgraded supine exercise to their voluntary maximum manifested by exhaustion (Figure 9.1). Aortic blood velocity was insonated via the suprasternal notch using the transcutaneous aortovelography (TAV) [11]. For the first three minutes the stroke distance and the minute distance (hence the stroke volume and the cardiac output, respectively) rose progressively and significantly until a pla-

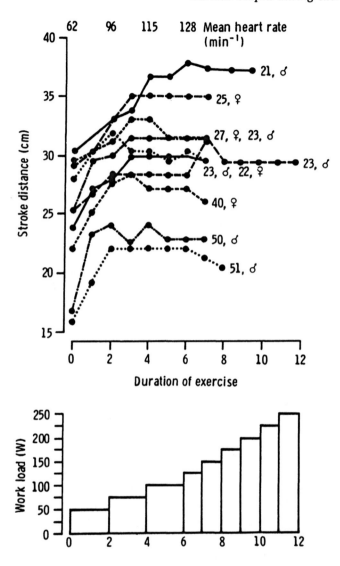

Figure 9.1. Change in the stroke distance (the systolic velocity-time integral) with exercise duration in ten healthy subjects throughout the step-wise increasing workload protocol shown in the bottom figure. Mean heart rate is shown at 2-minute intervals. Subject's ages and gender are indicated against the individual's curves. The minute distance (stroke distance × heart rate) increased during exercise mainly as a result of increasing heart rate. (Salmasi AM. In Cardiovascular Applications of Doppler ultrasound. Edited by A.M. Salmasi and A.N. Nicolaides, 1989. Churchill-Livingstone. Edinburgh. p. 131. Reproduced with permission from the publisher.)

teau was reached and maintained for the rest of the exercise period. For the stroke distance the plateau was on average 24% above the resting baseline. The plateau value was attained at low workload levels (125 Watts at 60 revolution per minute) of exercise and decreased only slightly, but non-significantly at the highest levels reached. This, therefore, shows that the stroke distance in normal subjects is robust against variations in exercise level provided a certain minimum is exceeded. The increase in the minute distance (hence in the cardiac output) in the first three minutes of exercise is therefore due to the increase in both the stroke volume and the heart rate while later during exercise the increase in the cardiac output is mainly the result of the increase in the heart rate.

To establish the response during exercise in a wider population of normal subjects, a study was carried out by Salmasi and associates in 1987 [12]. The authors studied 66 normal volunteers (43 males and 23 females) who were clinically free from any cardiovascular or other illnesses. The stroke distance increased from 21.9 cm per beat at rest to 27 cm per beat at maximal exercise. The minute distance, on the other hand, increased from a resting value of 1.57 metre per minute to a maximal exercise value of 3.34 metre per minute. The increase in the minute distance was mainly due to the increase in the heart rate.

Physiological background

The rise in systolic blood pressure which occurs during dynamic exercise results in some dilatation of the aorta, so that the actual flow changes will be somewhat greater than the observed velocity changes. In the 1987 study of Salmasi and associates [12] the systolic blood pressure rose progressively with increasing work load; the maximum change ranged from 15 mm Hg (2 kPa) to 50 mm Hg (6.8 kPa). Representative measurements of the *in situ* diameter changes of the human thoracic aorta, from which the resultant dilatation might be deduced, exist only for the pressure range between normal systolic and normal diastolic; a pressure range has shown that pulsa-tile diameter changes in the descending aorta average 2.6% and in another report [13] 10% for the thoracic aorta. A study carried by Wilkins and Light (Light, personal communication) on normal subjects with normal cardiac output and without local vascular disease in the distal part of the aortic arch (the site of the TAV insonation) suggests that pulsatile changes exceeding 6% are uncommon. Because of the non-linear compliance of arterial walls, the corresponding diameter change resulting from the maximum observed systolic pressure increase of 50 mm Hg should be less than proportionate (say 5%). Underestimation of flow changes, which depends on diameter squared, should thus rarely exceed 10% at maximal exercise level, and be less at intermediate workloads.

Although potential errors in the derivation of cardiac output and stroke distance measurements are greater under the conditions of the studies of Salmasi and associates [12] than in many other applications, they are not excessive. They are of the same order as errors in comparable techniques of proven utility. The findings in this study [12] are indeed in general accord with previous studies on the effect of supine exercise under similar conditions. Investigators who used invasive or gas exchange techniques found that stroke volume increased on average by 10–35% already at low levels of exercise [1, 14–18]. Most series also showed only relatively small further changes with increased workload. The divergence that exists between these reports is attributed to the effect on baseline readings of apprehension [19], which is minimum in the study of Salmasi and associates [12], and the position of the subject's legs during the baseline readings prior to pedaling [20]. Quantitative and qualitative agreement between the stroke distance and the stroke volume and between minute distance and cardiac output during exercise are thus satisfactory.

References

1. Topham WS, Warner HR. The control of cardiac output during exercise. In: Reeve EB, Guyton AC (ed), Physical bases of circulatory transport: regulation and exchange. Philadelphia: Saunders, 1967.
2. Sharma B, Goodwin JF, Raphael MJ *et al.* Left ventricular angiography on exercise, a new method of assessing left ventricular function in ischaemic heart disease. Br Heart J 1976;38:59.
3. Brynjolf I, Kelbaek H, Munck O *et al.* Right and left ventricular ejection fraction and left ventricular volume changes at rest and during exercise in normal subjects. Eur Heart J 1984;5:756.
4. Upton MT, Rerych SK, Newman GE *et al.* The reproducibility of radionuclide angiographic measurement of left ventricular function in normal subjects at rest and during exercise. Circulation 1982;62:126.
5. Poliner LR, Dehmer GJ, Lewis SE *et al.* Left ventricular performance in normal subjects: a comparison of the responses to exercise in the upright and supine positions. Circulation 1980;62:528.
6. Iskandrian AS, Hakki AH, Kane SA *et al.* Quantitative radionuclide angiography in assessment of haemodynamic changes during upright exercise: observations in normal subjects, patients with coronary artery disease and patients with aortic regurgitation. Am J Cardiol 1981;48:239.
7. Salmasi SN, Salmasi AM, Hendry WG *et al.* Exercise-induced changes in stroke volume measured noninvasively in coronary artery disease. Ultrasound Med Biol 1982;8:170.
8. Salmasi AM, Salmasi S, Light LH *et al.* Assessment of left ventricular function in coronary artery disease by continuous-wave Doppler during exercise. Proceedings of the First International Cardiac Coppler Symposium; 1983 Jan; Florida.
9. Salmasi SN, Salmasi AM, Hendry WG *et al.* Exercise-induced changes in stroke volume measured noninvasively in coronary artery disease. Acta Cardiol 1983;6:337.
10. Salmasi AM, Salmasi SN, Light LH *et al.* Exercise-induced changes in the aortic blood velocity and its derivatives in the assessment of coronary artery bypass grafting. Proceedings of the Second International Symposium of Cardiac Doppler Diagnosis; 1984 May; Florida.
11. Salmasi AM. Doppler stress testing. In: Salmasi A-M, Nicolaides AN. Cardiovascular applications of Doppler ultrasound (eds). Edinburgh: Churchill-Livingstone, 1989:127.

12. Salmasi AM, Salmasi S, Dore C *et al*. Non-invasive assessment of changes in aortic blood velocity and its derivatives with exercise in normal subjects by Doppler ultrasound. J Cardiovasc Surg 1987;28:321.
13. Gonza ER, Shaw AJ, Marble AE *et al*. Distention and the geometric taper of the thoracic aorta. Can J. Surg 1972;15:113.
14. Bevegard BS, Sheperd JT. Regulation of the circulation during exercise in man. Physiol Rev 1967;47:178.
15. Wang Y, Marshall RJ, Sheperd JT. Effect of changes in posture and of graded exercise in man. J. Clin Invest 1980;39:1051.
16. Asmussen E, Neilsen M. Cardiac output during muscular work and its regulation. Physiol Rev 1955;35:778.
17. Bevegard S, Freyschuss U, Strandell T. Circulatory adaptation to arm and leg exercise in supine and sitting position. J. Appl Physiol 1967;22:61.
18. Stenberg J, Astrand P, Bjorn E *et al* Haemodynamic response to work with different muscle groups, sitting and supine. J Appl Physiol 1967;22:61.
19. Donald KW, Bishop JM, Cumming G *et al*. The effect of exercise on cardiac output and circulatory dynamic of normal subjects. Clin Sci 1955;14:37.
20. Frick MH, Somer T. Base-line effects on response of stroke volume to leg exercise in the supine position. J Appl Physiol 1964;19:639.

10. Effect of age on cardiac output

ABDUL-MAJEED SALMASI

The effect of advancing age on cardiovascular parameters has been the subject of considerable study for many years. Age changes in the cardiovascular functional parameters are more pronounced during stress. However several parameters measured at rest do show changes with age. Amongst these parameters and probably the most important of all are the stroke volume and cardiac output.

The original work of Brandfonbrener and associates showed a decline in both stroke volume and cardiac output with age [1]. Using indicator dilution technique they studied 67 male subjects between ages 19 and 86 years. They found that cardiac output fell by an average of 1% per year from a mean of 6.49 l/minute at age 20 years to 3.87 l/minute in the ninth decade. Within the same period stroke volume fell from an average of 85.6 ml to 60.1 ml. In another study by Gerstenblith and associates, cardiac output was estimated and found to be 7.89 l/minute in ten young healthy subjects, while in 17 other healthy male subjects aged 60–83 years, cardiac output was found to be 5.85 l/minute [2]. As no change with age in the heart rate was detected, the decline in the cardiac output can only be explained as a result of the decrease in the stroke volume.

Evidence from Doppler ultrasound study of aortic blood velocity

Reporters who used Doppler ultrasound to assess aortic blood velocity at rest have shown that the normal range in blood velocity and derived variables for resting adults varies with age but not with other anthropometric variables [3–5]. In a report by Salmasi and Dore who studied changes in the aortic blood Doppler ultrasound signals, they found that the reason for the decline in stroke distance with age was the decline in the peak velocity against a fixed flow time [6]. The results obtained from studying 66 normal volunteers showed that the peak velocity decreased with age both at rest and at maximal exercise. Between ages 20 and 70 years the peak velocity declined by 1.11% at rest and by 1.05% at peak exercise. Similarly the stroke distance declined with advancing age at an annual rate of 1.13% at rest and 1.1% at peak exercise. The minute distance, on the other hand, decreased by 1.01% per

A.-M. Salmasi and A.S. Iskandrian (eds): Cardiac output and regional flow in health and disease, 97–105.
© 1993 *Kluwer Academic Publishers. Printed in the Netherlands.*

Table 10.1. Age regression relationship for the peak velocity, stroke distance and minute distance at pre- and peak maximal tolerated supine exercise in 66 normal subjects aged 18–67 years.

Measure	Exercise	Intercept	Slope	Residual SD	Slope p-value
Peak velocity	Pre	184.04	− 1.6727	10.70	<0.0001
	Peak	232.59	− 2.0198	15.05	<0.0001
Stroke distance	Pre-	33.45	− 0.3082	2.47	<0.0001
	Peak	40.92	− 0.3698	3.07	<0.0001
Minute distance	Pre-	2380.00	−19.3970	212.20	<0.0001
	Peak	5084.40	−46.4350	518.80	<0.0001

year at rest and by 1.11% at peak exercise. Table 10.1 demonstrates the age regression relationship for the peak velocity, stroke distance and the minute distance. The regression slope of the peak exercise data for the minute distance is more than twice the slope of the resting data ($p < 0.001$). Comparison of the residual standard deviations about the regression line with the standard deviation of each variable indicates that about half the variability can be explained by the age dependence.

Evidence from patients with coronary artery disease

Fifty consecutive patients with documented coronary artery disease were studied by Salmasi and associates [6]. In contrast to the normal subjects there was no age relation with the stroke distance either at rest or at peak exercise. However there was a slight age dependence of the minute distance at rest ($p < 0.05$) and the slope was not significantly different from that of the normal subjects. On the other hand, the minute distance did not show age dependence at peak exercise. These age relations are demonstrated in Figures 10.1–10.3. In these figures the age relations in the normal subjects were taken as reference ranges.

Pathophysiological mechanisms

The fall in the stroke distance and the minute distance throughout adult life has been attributed to the normal progressive dilatation of the aorta [3, 7] and falling cardiac output with advancing age [1, 2]. The decline in cardiac output is mainly due to the reduction in the stroke volume. The relatively small spread around the age regression lines supports the suggestion that blood velocity is not the result of random interaction between the aortic cross-sectional area and cardiac output but that a control mechanism correlates these two variables throughout the individual's life so as to bring velocities under basal conditions close to a "set-point" value [5, 8].

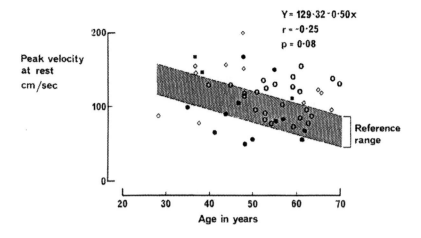

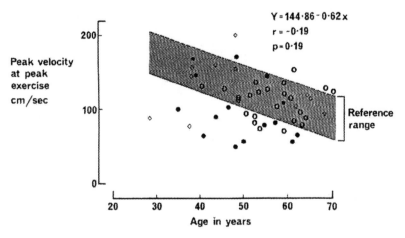

Figure 10.1. Decline with advancing age in the peak velocity of aortic blood recorded from the suprasternal notch by TAV at rest (top figure) and at maximal tolerated supine exercise (bottom figure) in 50 patients with proven coronary artery disease who are not taking beta-adrenergic blockades. Shaded area represents reference range (based on values + 2 RSD) for peak velocity in 66 normal subjects. (Salmasi AM, Dore C. In: Cardiovascular applications of Doppler ultrasound. Edited by Salmasi and Nicolaides. 1989. Churchill-Livingstone. Edinburgh. p. 145. Reproduced with permission from the publisher.)

The decline in the resting minute distance by a factor of 1.01% per annum relative to the predicted value at age 20, is almost identical to the findings of Brandfonbrener [1] who reported a fall of 1% per annum in the resting cardiac output between ages 20 and 80 using invasive techniques. Similarly, other groups found that the resting minute distance diminished by 0.87%

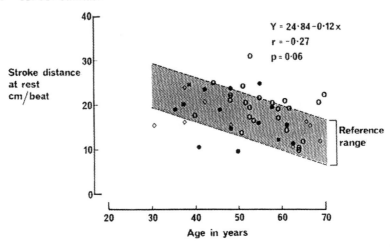

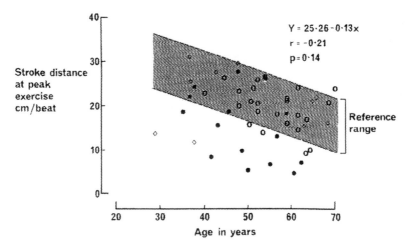

Figure 10.2. Variation of the stroke distance (systolic velocity-time integral) with advancing age in 50 consecutive patients with proven coronary artery disease who were not taking beta-adrenergic blockades both at rest (top figure) and at maximal tolerated exercise (bottom figure). Shaded area represents reference range (based on values + 2 RSD) for stroke distance in 66 normal subjects. (Salmasi AM, Dore C. In: Cardiovascular applications of Doppler ultrasound. Edited by Salmasi & Nicolaides. 1989. Churchill-Livingstone. Edinburgh. p. 145. Reproduced with permission.)

per annum between the ages of 20 and 70, while the resting stroke distance declines by 0.86% per annum and the resting peak velocity by 0.82% per annum [9]. As the stroke distance is mainly a function of the peak velocity and to much lesser extent the flow time [9, 10], both the stroke distance and the peak velocity (but not flow time) are age-dependent and both decline

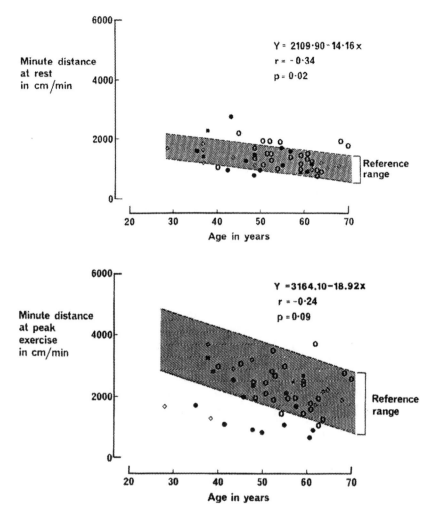

Figure 10.3. Decline in the minute distance (stroke distance × heart rate) with advancing age in 50 consecutive patients with proven coronary artery disease and who are not receiving beta-adrenergic blockades at rest (top figure) and at maximal tolerated supine exercise (bottom figure). Reference range (based on values + 2 RSD) obtained from 66 normal subjects is represented by shaded area. (Salmasi AM, Dore C. In: Cardiovascular applications of Doppler ultrasound. Edited by Salmasi & Nicolaides. 1989. Churchill-Livingstone. Edinburgh. p. 145. Reproduced with permission.)

with age at a similar rate. Also the minute distance is a function of the stroke distance rather than the heart rate. Therefore the main factors responsible for the decline in the minute distance are the reduction in the peak velocity haemodynamically and an increase in the aortic cross-sectional area anatomically. The peak velocity was reported to be a functional representative of the status of left ventricular performance [11]. Jewitt and associates measured the blood velocity in the ascending aorta invasively using a catheter tip velocity probe [11]. They reported a lower peak velocity in patients with coronary artery disease than in normal subjects and much lower in patients with lower ejection fraction. The authors also found that the peak velocity decreased from the resting value with increasing heart rate by pacing until the onset of angina.

Effect of exercise on the age relation of cardiac output

Using direct Fick principle to measure cardiac output both at rest and during exercise, Hossack and associates studied the variation of cardiac output and stroke volume according to different age groups in 99 normal sedentary men [12]. They used the age relation in the normal subjects as reference range to study the relation to age of the stroke volume and cardiac output in 77 patients with coronary artery disease. While a significant age relation existed in the normal subjects it did not exist in the patient group.

In the study of Salmasi and associates on 66 normal subjects whose age ranged between 20 and 70 years it was reported that similar to the resting conditions, both the stroke volume and the minute distance declined with advancing age [6]. The decline in the minute distance was mainly due to the decline in the stroke distance; the latter fell mainly due to the decline in the peak velocity. How much does the change in the minute distance relate to changes in the cardiac output and how much does the change in the stroke distance relate to changes in the stroke volume? To answer these questions it is important to mention that the aorta, and particularly, the thoracic aorta is an elastic tube which will change its diameter with the change in the blood pressure; the latter increases with exercise in normal subjects. Changes in aortic cross-sectional area as a result of changing blood pressure (say due to exercise) depend upon the age of the subject and the part of the aorta from which the aortic signal is recorded [7]. In young adults, elasticity of the aorta causes a considerable dampening of the changes in the aortic blood velocity that results from increasing cardiac output and a concomitant increase in the mean blood pressure [7]. The rigidity of the aorta increases with advancing age, hence the cross-sectional area is less vulnerable to change in blood pressure produced by exercise. Therefore there is more departure from exact linearity between stroke distance and stroke volume during exercise in lower age groups than at more advanced age.

In aged individuals, at maximal work loads, oxygen uptake and heart rate are lower while the pulmonary wedge pressure is higher when compared to those in younger age group [13]. These observations, beside lower cardiac output and stroke volume may indicate an increased impedance to ejection in older individuals, limitations of intrinsic myocardial contractility, increased ventricular stiffness or prolonged myocardial relaxation and decreased inotropic responsiveness to catecholamine stimulation [13, 14]. hence the reduced cardiac output at maximal exercise in the elderly is due to lower maximum heart rate and increased impedance to ejection. Iskandrian and Hakki studied the effect of age on left ventricular function during upright exercise in patients who underwent myocardial revascularization (thus free of myocardial ischaemia) [14]. They studied 90 subjects ranging in age between 36 and 75 years. The authors found no age relation in the resting level of the heart rate, stroke volume index, cardiac index and ejection fraction. However the cardiac index, ejection fraction and the heart rate during exercise decreased with advancing age. The exercise duration was highly age dependant being higher in younger age group and some residual coronary artery disease has thus been suggested to be a possible explanation. Age was reported not to influence resting ejection fraction while a significant decline with advancing age was observed at peak exercise.

Effect of coronary artery disease on the age trend of cardiac output

In the presence of coronary artery disease the age trend of the Doppler ultrasound-derived peak velocity, stroke distance and minute distance no longer exists both at rest and at maximal exercise. The possible explanations for this observation include heterogeneity in the distribution of (1) both numbers of significantly diseased coronary arteries and the severity of the coronary lesion itself; and (2) the presence of a history of myocardial infarction amongst individuals at different age groups. There is a tendency for the 15 patients with a history of myocardial infarction to be younger (mean age 49.1 years, S.D. 8.9) than the 35 patients without such a history (mean age 53.9 years, S.D. 9.8) although this difference failed to reach significance ($p = 0.11$). All these causes may, amongst patients with various ages, have resulted in heterogeneity of myocardial performance and hence stroke volume and cardiac output with exercise. The age relation of the stroke distance and the minute distance was the same in patients who were receiving beta-adrenergic blockades and those who were not receiving them.

Hossack and associates (1980) measured cardiac output noninvasively by dividing oxygen uptake by the difference in oxygen concentration between arterial and venous blood in normal subjects and in patients with coronary artery disease both at rest and during upright exercise. They reported a decline in the exercise values for the stroke volume and the cardiac output with age in normal subjects but not in patients with coronary artery disease [12].

Effect of coronary artery bypass graft surgery on the age relation of cardiac output

The evidence on the effect of the operation of coronary artery bypass grafting comes from the study of Salmasi and associates [15] which was carried out on 30 patients with proven coronary artery disease who underwent coronary artery bypass graft surgery (CABG). There was no significant change in the slope of the age relation of either the stroke distance, the minute distance, or the peak velocity with age after CABG. This was noticed despite the improvement in the intercept of the age relation of the peak velocity, stroke distance and the minute distance both at rest and during exercise.

Conclusion

Cardiac output and stroke volume decline with advancing age both at rest and during exercise. The decline in the former is due to combination of decline in both the heart rate and the stroke volume while the decline with advancing age in the stroke volume is due to the reduction in the contractility of the left ventricle. Decreased inotropic responsiveness to the effect of catecholamine during exercise with advancing age was said to be the reason for the reduced stroke volume. This however may also be the reason for the reduction in the aortic blood velocity which is measured noninvasively by Doppler ultrasound.

References

1. Brandfonbrener M, Landowne M, Shock NW. Changes in cardiac output with age. Circulation 1955;12:557.
2. Strandell T. Circulatory changes on healthy old men. Acta Med Scand 1964;175 (Suppl 414):1.
3. Light LH, Sequeira RF, Cross G et al. Flow orientated circulatory patients assessment and management using transcutaneous aortovelography, a noninvasive Doppler technique. J Nucl Med ALL Sci 1979;23:137.
4. Mowat DHR, Haites NE, Rawles JM. Aortic blood velocity measurement in healthy adults using a simple ultrasound technique. Cardiovasc Res 1983;17:75.
5. Light LH, Cross G. Convenient monitoring of cardiac output and global left ventricular function by transcutaneous aortovelography an effective alternative to cardiac output measurement. In: Spencer MP (ed). Cardiac Doppler diagnosis. The Hague: Martinus Nijhoff, 1983:69.
6. Salmasi AM, Dore C. Variation of linear cardiac output with age. In: Salmasi AM, Nicolaides AN (eds), Cardiovascular applications of Doppler ultrasound. Churchill-Livingstone, Edinburgh: 1989:145.
7. Towfiq BA, Weir J, Rawles JM. Effect of age and blood pressure on aortic size and stroke distance. Br Heart J 1986;55:560.
8. Light LH. Implications of aortic blood velocity measurements in children. J Physiol 1978;285:17.

9. Haites N, McLennan F, Mowat DHR *et al.* Assessment of cardiac output by the Doppler ultrasound technique alone. Br Heart J 1985;53:13.
10. Salmasi AM. Doppler stress testing. In: Salmasi AM, Nicolaides AN (eds), Cardiovascular application of Doppler ultrasound. edinburgh: Churchill-Livingstone, 1989:127.
11. Jewitt D, Gabe I, Mills C *et al.* Aortic velocity and acceleration measurements in the assessment of coronary heart disease. Eur J Cardiol 1974;13:299.
12. Hossack KF, Bruce RA, Green B *et al.* Maximal cardiac output during upright exercise: Approximate normal standards and variations with coronary heart disease. Am J Cardiol 1980;46:204.
13. Gerstenblith G, Lakatta EG, Weisfeldt ML. Age changes in myocardial function and exercise response. Prog Cardiovasc Dis 1976;19:1.
14. Iskandrian AS, Hakki AH. The effect of aging after arterial bypass grafting on the regulation of cardiac output during upright exercise. Int J Cardiol 1985;7:347.
15. Salmasi AM, Salmasi S, Nicolaides AN *et al.* Assessment of the effect of coronary artery bypass grafting on left ventricular performance by Doppler measurement of the aortic blood velocity during exercise. J Cardiovasc Surg 1988;29:89.

11. Effect of blood rheology on cardiac output

MICHAEL W. RAMPLING

The cardiovascular system consists essentially of a double, reasonably synchronised, pumping system each side of which feeds the other through a peripheral circulation made up of a vast number of series and parallel circuits. Two overall factors determine finally the rate of flow or, to put this another way, the cardiac output. The first is the time-averaged pressure generated in the aorta by the heart (for the purpose of this discussion it will be assumed that the corresponding pressure of the blood returning to the heart is zero). It in turn depends on the heart rate and the contractility of the heart muscle, which are under a variety of physiological controls and are discussed elsewhere in this book. This is the drive to maintain blood flow, but what it is actually allowed to achieve by way of flow is determined by the second factor, i.e. the flow resistance. The relationship between these two factors and the cardiac output is:

$$\text{cardiac output} = \frac{\text{time-averaged blood pressure}}{\text{flow resistance}}. \tag{11.1}$$

The variables that determine the flow resistance are external to the heart, and are geometrical terms related to the dimensions of the conducting vessels and rheological terms related to the flow properties of the blood.

In order to give an idea of how blood rheology relates to flow resistance, a simple model of the circulation will be considered. The first simplification is the assumption that blood is a Newtonian fluid, i.e. that it has a constant viscosity η. The second is that the blood vessels are rigid tubes connected in series or parallel, each having a constant radius but, generally, differing in size from one another. The other assumptions are that the flow is streamlined and constant rather than turbulent and pulsatile.

Under these assumptions it can be shown (see the next section in this chapter) that the flow resistance, R_1, of any one tube of radius r_1 and length l_1 is given by:

$$R_1 = \frac{K \cdot \eta \cdot l_1}{r_1^4}, \tag{11.2}$$

where K is a constant. When several of these tubes are connected in series

A.-M. Salmasi and A.S. Iskandrian (eds): Cardiac output and regional flow in health and disease, 107–124.
© 1993 Kluwer Academic Publishers. Printed in the Netherlands.

the resistance, R_{series}, is given by:

$$R_{series} = R_1 + R_2 + R_3 + \cdots \tag{11.3}$$

$$R_{series} = \frac{K \cdot \eta \cdot l_1}{r_1^4} + \frac{K \cdot \eta \cdot l_2}{r_2^4} + \frac{K \cdot \eta \cdot l_3}{r_3^4} + \cdots \tag{11.4}$$

$$R_{series} = K \cdot \eta \left(\frac{l_1}{r_1^4} + \frac{l_2}{r_2^4} + \frac{l_3}{r_3^4} + \cdots \right) \tag{11.5}$$

$$R_{series} = K \cdot \eta \left[\sum_{i=1}^{n} \frac{l_i}{r_i^4} \right]. \tag{11.6}$$

When such tubes are connected in parallel the corresponding resistance, $R_{parallel}$, is given by:

$$\frac{1}{R_{parallel}} = \frac{1}{R_1} + \frac{1}{R_2} + \frac{1}{R_3} + \cdots \tag{11.7}$$

$$\frac{1}{R_{parallel}} = \frac{r_1^4}{K \cdot \eta \cdot l_1} + \frac{r_2^4}{K \cdot \eta \cdot l_2} + \frac{r_3^4}{K \cdot \eta \cdot l_3} + \cdots \tag{11.8}$$

or

$$R_{parallel} = K\eta \left\{ \frac{1}{\dfrac{r_1^4}{l_1} + \dfrac{r_2^4}{l_2} + \dfrac{r_3^4}{l_3} + \cdots} \right\} \tag{11.9}$$

$$R_{parallel} = \frac{K\eta}{\left\{ \displaystyle\sum_{i=1}^{n} \frac{r_i^4}{l_i} \right\}}. \tag{11.10}$$

Hence it can be seen that in either case the resistance term is a product of the viscosity and a composite geometrical term, and thus that resistance is directly and significantly affected by the rheological properties of the blood.

The simplifications of the above model are considerable. First, the viscosity of blood is not constant but varies according to prevailing conditions of flow. Second, the vessels are not rigid but variously distensible. Third, the flow is pulsatile at least on the arterial side, though the assumption of non-turbulence is not unreasonable as little turbulence actually occurs in the healthy circulation. A further complication is the fact that in a substantial proportion of the circulation the vessels are of similar radius to the cells that are passing through them. The consequence is that in this part of the circulation the concept of whole blood viscosity then has limited value, and it is more usual to deal in terms of factors such as cellular deformability and adhesion. Needless to say, more realistic models than the one used here are more complex and difficult to analyse, but the essential principles of Equations (6)

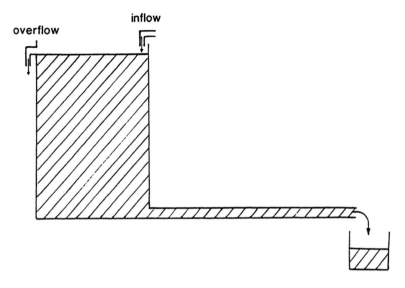

Figure 11.1. The inflow and overflow produce a constant head of liquid maintaining a constant driving pressure forcing liquid through the horizontal tube. Dynamic equilibrium obtains.

and (10) still obtain [1], i.e. that flow resistance is directly related to a rheological term and to a geometric one, and that both have a significant role to play in determining the resistance of the system.

In what follows the relevant haemorheological factors will be discussed.

Viscosity

This is a cornerstone concept to the current chapter. At a qualitative level it is not difficult to understand; thus, under identical conditions a thick liquid such as treacle will flow slower than a thinner one such as water because it has a higher viscosity. However, it is important to be able to quantitate viscosity and so a rigorous definition is required, but first two new concepts must be introduced.

Consider a simple liquid such as water in a cylindrical tube with a constant pressure applied across it, say from a reservoir as in Figure 11.1. The system quickly comes to equilibrium such that the volume flow rate through the tube is constant. What actually happens is that as the liquid first enters the tube it quickly accelerates (this is called the entrance effect) until an effectively steady rate of flow is achieved. Thus, in spite of a continuous pressure difference across the tube there is no overall change of flow rate. The reason, of course, is that there is a frictional force opposing the pressure effect – in other words we see here the retarding effect of viscosity.

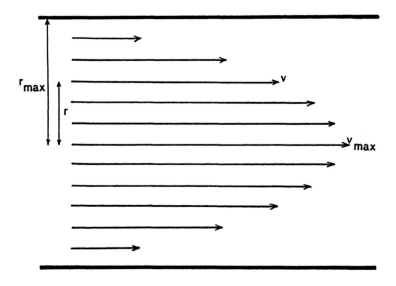

Figure 11.2. The velocity profile across the horizontal tube of Figure 11.1. The flow rate is maximum at the centre and minimum at the wall. For a Newtonian liquid the equation of the profile is:

$$\frac{V}{V_{max}} = 1 - \left(\frac{r}{r_{max}}\right)^2.$$

If now a cross-section were cut across the tube at any point beyond the initial 'entrance effect' region, the velocity profile would look like that shown in Figure 11.2. It can be seen that there is a continuous variation in velocity across the tube, from a minimum (of zero) at the wall, to a maximum in the centre of the tube. Consider now two adjacent planes, A and B, in the tube shown in enlargement in Figure 11.3. The first plane has a greater velocity than the second, by an amount dv, and the planes are separated by a small distance dr. This allows an important rheological parameter to be introduced, i.e. the shear rate. At the point in the system illustrated in Figure 11.3 it is given by:

$$\text{shear rate} = \frac{dv}{dr}. \tag{11.11}$$

To put this in general terms, the shear rate is the difference in velocity of two adjacent planes of flowing liquid divided by the distance separating them. This parameter gives a measure of the rate at which the planes of liquid are separating from one another. Thus, referring back to the Figure 11.2 it should be clear that the shear rate at the vessel wall is high, indeed it is

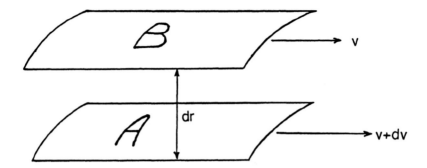

Figure 11.3. Two adjacent planes of liquid in the tube of Figure 11.2 with velocities that differ by dv and separted by a distance dr.

maximal, and it falls progressively to become zero at the very centre of flow. Because this parameter is the ratio of a speed to a length it has the units of reciprocal time, usually expressed as reciprocal seconds or s^{-1}.

Returning again to the two planes of Figure 11.3, some of the molecules of plane A will inevitably diffuse to and interact with those of plane B and because they have, on average, a higher speed than those of plane B they will tend to speed up that plane. Correspondingly, molecules from B will diffuse to and interact with those of plane A tending to slow it down. This phenomenon manifests itself as a tangential frictional or, better, viscous force acting between the planes. The magnitude of the force per unit area of the planes is called the shear stress and has the units of pressure, usually Pascal or Pa. This principle, of course, applies to any such planes possessing different speeds.

With this information it is possible to define viscosity in an absolute fashion. It is simply the shear stress divided by the shear rate operating between the planes i.e.:

$$\text{viscosity} = \frac{\text{shear stress}}{\text{shear rate}}. \tag{11.12}$$

The units are Pa.s.

If the liquid in question has a constant viscosity (such liquids are usually referred to as Newtonian) it can be shown theoretically [2] that when flowing in a cylindrical tube under constant pressure the velocity profile is parabolic in shape. The equation of this velocity profile is:

$$\frac{V}{V_{max}} = 1 - \left\{ \frac{r}{r_{max}} \right\}^2, \tag{11.13}$$

where v is the velocity at any radius r in the flowing liquid, r_{max} is the radius of the tube and the maximum velocity (at the centre of the tube) is V_{max} (see Figure 11.2).

A more important theoretical derivation [2] that can be made for such a liquid is an expression for the volume rate of flow, Q/t, through the tube:

$$\frac{Q}{t} = \frac{\pi P r_{max}^4}{8\eta l},$$ (11.14)

where P is the driving pressure across the tube of length l and the viscosity of the liquid is η. This is the famous Poiseuille-Hagen equation. It is useful not only because it allows flow rates to be determined if P, r_{max}, l and η are known, but it also provides a simple basis for a viscometer because if the volume flow rate, pressure and tube dimensions are known then η can be derived. A large number of simple liquids such as water, alcohol, glycerol etc. are strictly Newtonian, in the sense that their viscosities are constant at a given temperature, and so their viscosities can be measured using this principle. Blood plasma is also simple in this sense, i.e. a given sample has a constant viscosity at a given temperature. A number of commercial plasma viscometers are now available based on the use of the Poiseuille-Hagen equation and on apparatus similar in principle to that shown in Figure 11.1 [3]. Such an apparatus is called a capillary viscometer.

Plasma viscosity

The normal range for plasma viscosity is usually taken as 1.25 ± 0.1 mPa.s at 37° C, with no sex difference and little if any increase with age in healthy individuals [4]. The viscosity of plasma is considerably greater than that of water, which is about 0.7 mPa.s at the same temperature. The difference is due to the proteins in the plasma. Of these the large asymmetric ones, especially fibrinogen and some of the immunoglobulins, have a much greater molar effect than the smaller more symmetric ones, such as albumin. Thus, plasma viscosity is very sensitive to the concentrations of the large proteins, and because their concentrations vary in sympathy with a variety of clinical conditions, so does the plasma viscosity. For example, most reports find it elevated in association with some specific conditions such as chronic is-chaemic heart disease [5], and diabetes [6] and also with more generalised ones such as those associated with the acute phase reaction [7]. In some situations it can achieve amazingly high values, particularly in paraproteinae-mias where it can reach as high as 5 mPa.s or more [8]. Indeed, the sensitivity of plasma viscosity to a wide variety of clinical conditions has resulted in its being proposed as a non-specific index of pathology to replace the older erythrocyte sedimentation rate test [9].

Blood viscosity

Unfortunately, blood is not a simple viscometric liquid in the sense used above. Thus, when its viscosity is estimated using a capillary viscometer it is found to vary with the rate of flow of the sample, to be sensitive to its recent history of deformation and to depend on the size of vessel in which the determination is being made. In other words blood is a non-Newtonian liquid and as such does not rigorously obey the Poiseuille-Hagen equation. Hence, there follows a section considering the complex, non-Newtonian characteristics of blood viscosity and the responsible factors.

Shear rate

Perhaps the most interesting of the non-Newtonian characteristics of blood is the variation of its viscosity with shear rate. This is ultimately the reason that the capillary viscometer is inadequate for the estimation of blood viscosity. The problem for a non-Newtonian liquid is that the shear rate varies continuously, but in an unknown way, across the bore of the capillary, so only a shear-rate-averaged viscosity over an undefined shear rate profile is obtained. If the size of the capillary or the rate of flow is altered the shear rate profile also changes (again in an unknown way) and so does the measured averaged-viscosity. The obvious way to overcome the problem is to devise a viscometer in which the blood is subjected to a single, known shear rate during the measurement. The shear rate may be changed to a different value for the next measurement and so on, in order to cover a range of shear rates, but no averaging over unknown shear rate profiles is involved. The newer generation of viscometers based on cone-on-plate or bob-in-cup configurations are designed to do just this [3].

Using these newer viscometers it is possible to obtain the variation of the viscosity of a blood sample as a function of shear rate, and Figure 11.4a shows the results for a typical sample of normal blood. It can be seen that at low shear rates the viscosity is very high, but that it falls rapidly as the shear rate rises – indeed, over the range of shear rate shown in the figure, there is a fall of an order of magnitude. It is often preferable to plot the data on log:log axes since then, to a good approximation, a double linear plot is obtained as shown in Figure 11.4b. This has the advantage of simplifying the picture, but it also suggests that there are different factors causing the rapid fall at low shear rates and the slower fall at higher shear rates. These factors are illustrated in Figure 11.5 [10]. It shows that at very low shear rates large, weakly bonded red cell aggregates (known as rouleaux) form in normal blood leading to a high viscometric drag, as the shear rate increases the increasing shear stress causes progressive break up of these aggregates and the viscous drag steadily declines until the cells become monodispersed. After this a slower but continuing fall in viscosity occurs because of the inherent deformability of the erythrocytes; as the shear rate

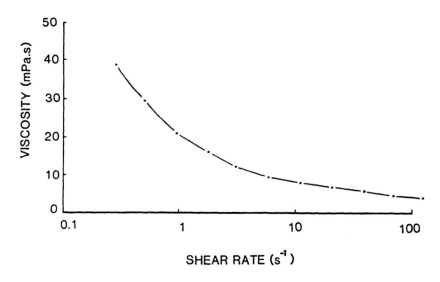

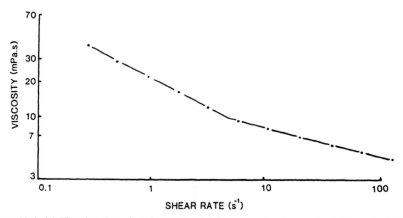

Figure 11.4. (a) The viscosity *v* log shear rate plot for a sample of normal adult blood of 45% haematocrit. (b) The same data plotted on double logarithmic axes, showing the bilinearity so generated.

increases so the cells progressively deform and their viscous drag steadily declines.

Thus, overall it can be seen that the viscosity of blood is very shear rate dependent, but the question that then arises is what shear rates are relevant to the circulation *in vivo*? This however depends on the position in the circulation. The highest values are found at the arterial walls where they can be $1000 \, s^{-1}$ or more in magnitude. Generally, they are lower in the venous circulation, of the order of $200 \, s^{-1}$, but in the smallest veins they may be an

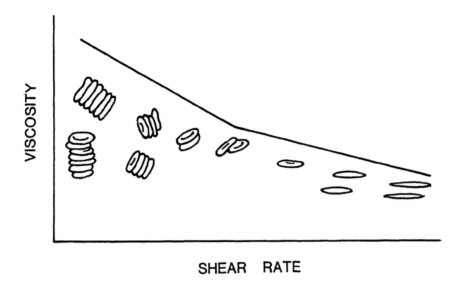

Figure 11.5. This illustrates the major factors causing the shear dependence of blood viscosity, i.e. rouleaux formation at low shear rates and red cell deformation at high.

order of magnitude less than this [1]. However, it must be remembered that across every vessel the shear rate falls progressively from that at the wall to ZERO at the centre of flow (see Figure 11.2). Thus, it can be seen that the whole viscosity:shear rate profile of Figures 11.4a and 11.4b is relevant to the situation *in vivo* and the effective viscosity of the blood increases in moving from the wall towards the centre of the vessel.

Consideration will next be given to the two factors which are largely responsible for the Non-Newtonianism of blood, i.e. rouleaux formation and red cell deformability.

Rouleaux formation

The ultimate cause of rouleaux formation is the presence in the plasma of a number of large asymmetric proteins of which fibrinogen is the most important, but of which IgG, IgM and α_2-macroglobulin are also known to be effective [11–13]. It was originally thought that the mechanism by which rouleaux formed was a cross-bridging one, in which these large proteins adhered to adjacent cells to produce intercellular links holding the rouleaux together [11]. However, a new hypothesis based on steric exclusion of these proteins from the inter-membrane region has recently been proposed [14]. It is not yet clear which of these is the more acceptable, but the actual mechanism is of no great importance to the current discussion. What is

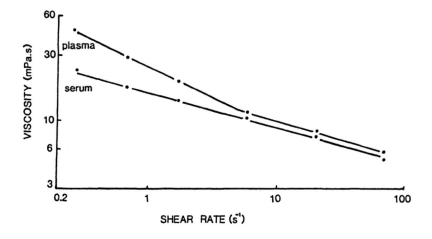

Figure 11.6. The viscosity:shear rate relationship of a suspension of erythrocytes at 45% haematocrit in autologous plasma or serum.

important and clear is that as the concentrations of these proteins increase so their effects on low shear rate viscosity become more prominent. To give an illustrative example for the case of fibrinogen, Figure 11.6 shows the viscosity:shear rate curves for erythrocytes suspended in plasma or autologous serum (i.e. with only fibrinogen missing). It can be seen that there is a striking change in the slope of the line at low shear rates but very little difference at high shear rates. Figure 11.7 shows the situation for erythrocytes suspended in buffered saline containing increasing concentrations of fibrinogen. Again it can be seen that there are only small differences between the lines at high shear rates, while at low shear rates there are dramatic variations with fibrinogen concentration. The same sort of phenomena can be elicited by changing the concentrations of the other proteins mentioned above [12].

Because fibrinogen is an acute phase protein and because the others play a role in defence against infection and are also frequently affected by malignancy, their concentrations are very variable in association with a wide variety of clinical conditions [7]. The consequence is that the degree of rouleaux formation is altered in these conditions and this is reflected in the viscosity characteristics of the blood.

Red cell deformability

The normal red cell is highly deformable and when subjected to increasing shear stresses it is increasingly stretched until it achieves an elongated cigar shape. This progressive deformation steadily reduces the viscometric drag of the cell and is responsible for the decline in viscosity with increasing shear

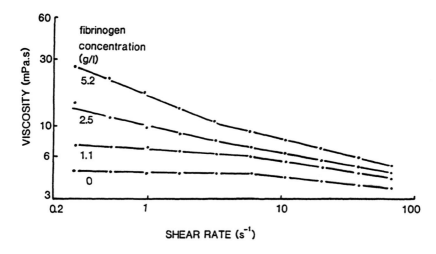

Figure 11.7. The viscosity:shear rate relationship of a suspension of erythrocytes at 45% haematocrit in phosphate-buffered saline containing different concentrations of fibrinogen.

rate that occurs at the high shear rate end of the viscosity:shear rate curve. Chien *et al.* [15] showed that this phenomenon is abolished if the cells are made rigid by fixing them with glutaraldehyde. They showed that as the red cells stiffen so the high shear rate fall in blood viscosity becomes less pronounced, the blood becomes increasingly Newtonian and the overall blood viscosity rises. However, apart from a few specific clinical conditions where erythrocytes are very inflexible, such as sickle cell anaemia [16], the other naturally occurring alterations in the deformability of the red cell are rarely sufficient to cause substantial effects on blood viscosity.

Haematocrit

It was explained previously that plasma is a Newtonian liquid while blood is not–this indicating one importance of the cellular compartment to the viscometric properties of blood. Furthermore, the viscosity of plasma is about 1.25 mPa.s while that of normal blood varies from about 4 to 40 in the shear rate range from about 100 to $0.3 \, s^{-1}$. This illustrates the importance of the cells in determining the magnitude of blood viscosity. However, in the vast majority of blood samples, the leukocyte and platelet volume concentrations are so small that they can generally be ignored and it is only the red cell volume concentration, or haematocrit, that is relevant. Indeed, it is the major determinant of blood viscosity, e.g. increasing haematocrit from 35 to 55% causes an increase of almost 100% in blood viscosity at $100 \, s^{-1}$, while at low shear rate of about $0.3 \, s^{-1}$ the increase is about 500%. In practice it is found that over a limited range the following relationship holds to a good approximation:

$$\ln \eta = A + BH, \qquad (11.15)$$

where A and B are shear-rate-dependent constants and η and H are respectively the viscosity and haematocrit. Furthermore, at high shear rates this relationship becomes:

$$\ln \eta = \ln \eta_p + BH, \qquad (11.16)$$

where η_p is the plasma viscosity.

One result of these considerations is that anaemia almost inevitably leads to enhanced blood fluidity. On the other hand polycythaemia leads to elevated blood viscosity, and at haematocrits of 60% or more the elevation is massive, especially at low shear rates. This frequently leads to symptoms in the subjects which have been interpreted as due to the hyperviscosity [17, 18].

Leukocrit

It was stated above that generally the leukocytes have little or no effect on blood viscosity, the reason being their normally low volume concentration compared to that of the erythrocytes. However, when the white cells become massively elevated in number their effect can become noticeable and can also lead to the hyperviscosity syndrome [19]. The number concentration necessary for these effects to become manifest is of the order of $200.10^9/1$ or more for myeloid leukaemia, while for lymphocytic leukaemia it needs to exceed about $400.10^9/1$ [19]. The reason for this difference may relate to the differing cellular deformabilities of the various white cell lines involved [20].

Plasma viscosity

Since about half of the volume of blood is the plasma, it is to be expected that this too will have an effect on the viscosity of whole blood. In general the effect is, to a reasonable approximation, a simple proportional one in the sense that an increase in plasma viscosity by, say, 10% will lead to a similar increase in the viscosity of blood at high shear rate. The effect at low shear rate, however, is less easy to predict because any increase in plasma viscosity is usually due to an increase in the plasma protein concentration. The influence on blood viscosity at low shear rate will then depend on whether the rouleaugenic protein concentrations change as well as on the change in plasma viscosity itself.

In general the variations induced in plasma viscosity by clinical conditions are fairly small, of the order of a few tens of percent. Thus, under most circumstances these effects on the viscosity of whole blood are not great. However, in cases of Waldenstrom's macroglobulinaemia, where plasma viscosity can reach in excess of four times the normal value, the blood viscosity is elevated by similar amounts at high shear rates and by even more at low [8], and can lead to severe hyperviscosity syndrome.

Temperature

In general, the effect of temperature on blood viscosity is fairly small and simple in the sense that, to a good approximation, high shear rate blood viscosity exhibits a similar temperature coefficient to that of water, i.e. it increases by about 2.4% for each °C drop in temperature [4]. However, at low shear the changes can be more pronounced and depend on the plasma protein composition [21].

Microvascular flow

The overall rheological resistance of the circulation is, of course, a combination of that from the large and the small vessels. Large in this sense means that the vessels are sufficiently bigger than the blood cells that the blood can be treated as effectively homogeneous, and so blood viscosity can be used as the composite rheological determinant. The situation in the small vessels is, however, fundamentally different for reasons discussed below.

In the microcirculation the dimensions of the vessels and the cells become of similar magnitude, and under these circumstances the concept of blood viscosity becomes of less use because the flowing blood is clearly multiphasic. Here the determining parameters are plasma viscosity, red cell aggregation, red and white cell deformability and number concentrations and white cell adhesiveness to the vessel wall. These factors are, of course, similar to those that affect blood viscosity, but their relative importance changes in this small vessel area.

Red cell deformability

It is obvious from the dimensions of the capillaries that the red cells have to deform in order to enter them. Studies using micropore filters as models of the microcirculation have shown that this requirement for the red cell to deform in order to enter small vessels, and their viscous properties while flowing, produce a significant hindrance to flow [22]. Thus, for example, a 10% volume suspension of normal red cells in buffer will flow through 5 μm filters at about half the speed of the buffer alone. However, the sensitivity of the microfiltration technique is such that a number of conditions, apart from the extreme cases of sickle cell anaemia and spherocytosis, have been documented where erythrocyte deformability is sufficiently reduced to affect filtration rates and consequently, it is assumed, to hinder microcirculatory flow as well [5, 6, 23]. Thus, while naturally occurring alterations in red cell deformability are relatively unimportant in large vessel flow, they are considered to be significant determinants of flow in the microcirculation.

White blood cell deformability

Similar considerations also apply to the white cells. The deformabilities of these vary amongst their subclasses, but it is a reasonable generalisation to say that they are some three orders of magnitude less deformable than erythrocytes [24]. The result is that although leukocytes are normally present in numbers some three orders of magnitude less than the red cells their contribution to microvascular resistance is probably of a similar magnitude. This is compounded by the stickiness of these cells which causes them frequently to adhere to the endothelium and further impede flow [24]. Clearly in conditions where their numbers are elevated they will cause even greater effects.

Red cell aggregation

The shear rates present in the microcirculation are extremely variable. Thus, those at the walls of the capillaries are probably amongst the highest in the whole circulation, while those at the walls of the draining venules are probably the lowest [1]. This variation is further accentuated on a temporal scale because of the effects of vasomotion. This is the result of rhythmic contraction and relaxation of the feeding arterioles leading to variations in flow in the dependent capillaries and venules. The contraction can be sufficient to stop flow in the dependent vessels completely. During the closed period the shear rate will fall to something of the order of zero. Under these conditions rouleaux can develop in the blood. They are then thought to act like a log jam, such that a considerable force is required to break them down before flow can restart. This is manifest as a yield stress [11] and will contribute to flow resistance. Clearly, in any condition where rouleagenic proteins are in high concentration, so that rouleaux formation is enhanced, the effects will be magnified.

Plasma viscosity

When erythrocytes flow in small capillaries it is believed that a layer of plasma exists between them and the vessel wall. There are also good reasons for believing that in the gaps between cells in this region the plasma undergoes lateral circulation. Dissipation of energy must therefore take place governed by the viscosity of the plasma, hence this is another factor determining resistance in the microcirculation. Indeed, Tooke et al. [25] showed directly by capillaroscopic methods that alterations in plasma viscosity can influence capillary flow to a significant degree.

Haematocrit

It would be reasonable to suppose that haematocrit has a significant affect on flow rate and resistance in the microcirculation. However, there is a problem here in that the haematocrit in these small vessels is not the same as the systemic value. The phenomenon is known as the Fahreaus Effect [26], and what it amounts to is that in a capillary fed by a larger reservoir the capillary haematocrit is less than that in the feed. However, the difference only becomes significant for tubes with diameters less than about 300 μm, but is the more pronounced the smaller the tube. The result is that in the smallest vessels *in vivo* the haematocrit may be as little as 20% of the feed value [1]. Thus, the dependence of microcirculatory resistance on haematocrit is less significant than would be expected from measurements of venous haematocrit.

Measurements *in vivo*

The essential argument that leads to the expectation of a significant rheological component to flow resistance *in vivo* was presented in the earlier part of this chapter. It was followed by a detailed discussion of the various factors that can affect blood rheology and which can be expected, therefore, to have an effect on circulatory flow resistance. This was somewhat theoretical but now a summary will be given of evidence obtained *in vivo*.

One of the earliest studies was that of Whittaker and Winton [27], who altered the viscosity of blood in the isolated hindlimb of a dog by changing its haematocrit and measured the effect on its flow. They found an inverse relation between flow rate and haematocrit, but the calculated apparent viscosity determined from the data obtained *in vivo* did not alter with haematocrit as much as did the viscosity measured *in vitro* using a viscometer. Similar studies by other workers [28, 29] confirmed these results showing that there was a significant affect of blood viscosity on flow resistance, but that this was less than would be interpreted from *in vitro* measurements of blood viscosity. This difference may be explained as due to the influences of the Fahraeus Effect in the microcirculation and of vascular distensibility.

Other organs in the dog have been studied, where again haematocrit was varied in order to alter viscosity and the effect on flow rate determined. These organs include the lungs [30, 31] and the coronary circulation [31]. Once more a clear inverse relation was found between flow and viscosity, which was prominent above a haematocrit of 40%. Thus in the dog, at least, evidence is available for a significant effect on blood flow of viscosity changes.

Dormandy [32] performed one of the earliest of such studies in the human. He estimated blood flow in the leg using plethysmography and altered blood viscosity by haemodilution with dextran or Hartmann's infusions. He found that flow rate changed by three times as much, and in the opposite direction, as the change in blood viscosity (determined *in vitro*), concluding that a clear rheological component was evident.

An area where considerable study has taken place in man has been in relation to cerebral blood flow, this being triggered largely by the finding that subjects suffering from polycythaemia exhibit reduced flow rates. Thomas *et al.* [33] showed a substantial inverse relation between haematocrit and flow rate in polycythaemics who had been venesected to reduce their haematocrits. Thus, reducing haematocrit from an average of 54% to 45% led to an increase in cerebral blood flow of 73% and a fall in viscosity by 20 to 30%. A study comparing anaemic patients with normal plasma viscosity to those with high plasma viscosity due to paraproteinaemia, showed that autoregulatory effects resultant on the altered oxygen-carrying capacity of the diluted blood could only partly explain the changes observed, and that blood viscosity changes also had a significant role to play [34]. Incidentally, this study indicated that elevated plasma viscosity could also affect flow resistance to a significant degree. A more recent paper by Grotta *et al.* [35] shows an inverse relation between cerebral blood flow and fibrinogen concentration, which is again interpreted in terms of the effect of fibrinogen on plasma viscosity and on low shear rate blood viscosity.

These studies all point to the conclusion that blood viscosity has a significant role to play in determining flow resistance in particular organs *in vivo*. This being the case it is to be expected that such resistance summed over the whole system should be reflected in an effect on cardiac output. A number of studies have provided evidence in this direction. One of the earliest was that of Murray *et al.* [36] who used dextran infusions in dogs to reduce haematocrit normovolaemically, but also altered blood viscosity by using solutions of dextrans of differing molecular weights to dilute the blood. They concluded that peripheral resistance was significantly changed by the rheological alterations and that this had a direct effect on cardiac output. Similar studies in the human by Schmidt Schonbein and Reiger [37] showed that, in spite of no change in arterial pressure or heart rate, cardiac output increased by 24% when the haematocrit was reduced from 44 to 31%, and concluded that this was predominantly rheologically caused. Other human studies have produced broadly similar results [31, 33, 39]. However, one of the most interesting was that of Murray and Escobar [40] who induced anaemia with or without accompanying methaemoglobinaemia and were able to show directly that irrespective of oxygen-carrying capacity of the blood substantial cardiac output changes occurred, and so had to be due to rheological causes.

Results of the sort discussed above seem to make it clear that individual organ blood flow and cardiac output are influenced by blood viscosity. Most of the studies have relied upon haematocrit changes to induce the changes in viscosity. There is clearly a need for much more study in this area in particular looking at other methods of varying blood viscosity and investigating other rheologically important factors.

References

1. Chien S. Physiological and pathophysiological significance of hemorheology. In: Chien S, Dormandy J, Ernst E (eds), Clinical haemorheology. Dordrecht: Martinus Nijhoff, 1987:125–64.
2. Caro CG, Pedley TJ, Schroter RC *et al*. The mechanics of the circulation. Oxford: Oxford University Press, 1978:44–50.
3. Matrai A, Whittington RB, Skalak R. Biophysics. In: Chien S, Dormandy J, Ernst E (eds), Clinical hemorheology. Doredrecht: Martinus Nijhoff, 1987:9–72.
4. Lowe GDO, Barbenel JC. Plasma and blood viscosity. In: Lowe GDO (ed), Clinical blood rheology Vol I. Boca Raton: CRC Press, 1988:11–43.
5. Lowe GDO, Forbes CD. Rheology of cardiovascular disease. In: Lowe GDO (ed), Clinical blood rheology Vol. II. Boca Raton: CRC Press, 1988:113–39.
6. Barnes AJ. Rheology of diabetes mellitus. In: Lowe GDO (ed), Clinical blood rheology Vol II. Boca Raton: CRC Press, 1988:63–187.
7. Lowe GDO. Rheology of disease. In: Lowe GDO (ed), Clinical blood rheology Vol II. Boca Raton: CRC Press; 1988:89–111.
8. Lowe GDO. Rheology of paraproteinemias and leukemias. In: Lowe GDO (ed), Clinical blood rheology Vol II. Boca Raton: CRC Press, 1988:67–87.
9. International Committee for Standardization in Haematology. Guidelines on selection of laboratory tests for monitoring the acute phase response. J Clin Pathol 1988;41:1203–12.
10. Meiselman HJ. Measures of blood rheology and erythrocyte mechanics. In: Cokelet GR, Meiselman HJ, Brooks DE (eds), Erythrocyte mechanics and blood flow. New York: Alan R Liss, 1980:75–117.
11. Rampling MW. Red cell aggregation and yield stress. In: Lowe GDO (ed), Clinical blood rheology Vol I. Boca Raton: CRC Press, 1988:45–64.
12. Schmid Schonbein H, Gallasch G, Volger E *et al*. Microrheology and protein chemistry of pathological red cell aggregation (blood sludge) studied *in vitro*. Biorheology 1988;10:213–27.
13. Rovel A, Vigneron C, Streiff F. Comparison of *in vitro* effects of normal IgG and of monoclonal IgG on the rheological behaviour of erythrocytes. Br J Haematol 1979:41:509–13.
14. Janzen J, Brooks DE. Do plasma proteins adsorb to red cells? Clin Hemorheol 1989;9:695–714.
15. Chien S, Usami S, Dellenbeck RJ *et al*. Blood viscosity: influence of erythrocyte deformation. Science 1967;157:825–31.
16. Stuart J, Kenny MW. Sickle-cell disease and vascular occlusion. In: Lowe GDO, Barbenel JC, Forbes CD (eds), Clinical aspects of blood viscosity and cell deformability. Berlin: Springer-Verlag, 1981:109–22.
17. Pearson TC. Rheology of polycythaemias. In: Lowe GDO (ed), Clinical blood rheology Vol II. Boca Raton: CRC Press, 1988:23–41.
18. Walker CHM. Rheology of the newborn and their disorders. In: Lowe GDO (ed), Clinical blood rheology Vol II. Boca Raton: CRC Press, 1988:213–31.
19. Preston FE. Circulatory complications of leukaemia and paraproteinaemia. In: Lowe GDO, Barbenel JC, Forbes CD (eds), Clinical aspects of blood viscosity and cell deformability. Berlin: Springer-Verlag, 1981:123–32.
20. Nash GB, Jones JG, Mikita J *et al*. Methods and theory for analysis of flow of white cell subpopulations through micropore filters. Br J Haematol 1988;70:165–70.
21. Rampling MW, Whittingstall P. The effect of temperature on the viscosity characteristics of erythrocyte suspensions. Clin Hemorheol 1987;7:745–55.
22. Stuart J. Erythrocyte deformability. In: Lowe GDO (ed), Clinical blood rheology Vol I. Boca Raton: CRC Press, 1988:65–85.
23. Stuart J. Rheology of the hemolytic anemias. In: Lowe GDO (ed), Clinical blood rheology Vol II. Boca Raton: CRC Press, 1988:43–65.

24. Chien S. White blood cell rheology. In: Lowe GDO (ed), Clinical blood rheology Vol I. Boca Raton CRC Press, 1988:43–65.

25. Tooke JE, Milligan DW. Capillary blood flow in haematological disorders; the role of the red cell, white cell and plasma viscosity. Clin Hemorheol 1987;7:311–9.

26. Gaehtgens P, Pries AR, Ley K. Structural, hemodynamic and rheological characteristics of blood flow in the circulation. In: Chien S, Dormandy J, Ernst E *et al*. (eds), Clinical hemorheology. Dordrecht: Martinus Nijhoff, 1987:99–124.

27. Whittaker SRF, Winton FR. The apparent viscosity of blood flowing in the isolated hind limb of the dog: and its variation with corpuscular concentration. J Physiol 1933;78:339–69.

28. Levy MN, Share L. The influence of erythrocyte concentration upon pressure-flow relationships in the dog's hind limb. Circ Res. 1953;1:247–55.

29. Benis AM, Usami S, Chien S. Effect of hematocrit and inertial losses in pressure-flow relations in the isolated hind-paw of the dog. Circ Res 1970;27:1047–68.

30. Murray JF, Karp RP, Nadel JA. Viscosity effects on pressure-flow relations and vascular resistance of dog's lungs. J App Physiol 1969;27:336–41.

31. Jan KM, Chien S. Effect of hematocrit variation on coronary hemodynamics and oxygen utilization. Am J Physiol 1977;233:H106–H113.

32. Dormandy JA. Influence of blood viscosity on blood flow and the effect of low molecular weight dextran. Br Med J 1971;4:716–9.

33. Thomas DS, du Boulay GH, Marshall J *et al*. Cerebral blood-flow in polycythaemia. Lancet 1977;ii:161–3.

34. Pearson TC, Humphrey PRD, Thomas DJ *et al*. Haematocrit, blood viscosity, cerebral blood flow and vascular occlusion. In: Lowe GDO, Barbanel JC, Forbes, CD (eds), Clinical aspects of blood viscosity and cell deformability. Berlin: Springer-Verlag, 1980:97–108.

35. Grotta J, Ackerman R, Correia J. Whole blood viscosity parameters and cerebral blood flow. Stroke 1982;13:296–301.

36. Murray JF, Escobar E, Rapaport E. Effect of blood viscosity on hemodynamic responses in acute normovolemic anaemia. Am J Physiol 1969;216:638–40.

37. Schmid-Schonbein H, Reiger H. Isovolaemic haemodilution. In: Lowe GDO, Barbenel JC, Forbes CD (eds), Clinical aspects of blood viscosity and cell deformability. Berlin: Springer-Verlag, 1980:211–27.

38. Weisse AB, Maschos CB, Frank MJ *et al*. Hemodynamic effects of staged haematocrit reduction in patients with stable Cor Pulonale and severely elevated haematocrit levels. Am J Med 1975;58:92–8.

39. Rosenthal A, Nathan DG, Marty AT *et al*. Acute hemodynamic effects of red cell volume reduction in polycythaemia of cynotic congenital heart disease. Circulation 1970;42:297–307.

40. Murray J, Escobar E. Circulatory effects of blood viscosity in comparison of methemoglobinaemia and anaemia. J App Physiol 1968;25:594–9.

PART THREE

Cardiac output in cardiac disease

12. Cardiac output in coronary artery disease

ABDUL-MAJEED SALMASI

Stroke volume and cardiac output are haemodynamic variables of global left ventricular function which are of great clinical importance specially in assessing patient with coronary artery disease. Their importance lies in parallel with that of the anatomical distribution of the coronary arterial lesion. In an individual with coronary artery disease it is not uncommon to find normal cardiac output and stroke volume at rest. However the tendency to increase stroke volume and cardiac output which is encountered in normal subjects is not altered in patients with coronary artery disease if the degree of coronary artery stenosis is not too severe and their left ventricle is relatively preserved; hence the resting cardiac output and stroke volume may be normal or near normal for their age. With the progress in the coronary artery stenosis or in the presence of previous infarction there is an increase in the scar tissue of the left ventricle resulting in poor response to exercise with a drop in the stroke volume or even cardiac output during physical stress.

One of the commonly used invasive ways of hemodynamic determination of myocardial oxygen consumption has been the measurement of left ventricular end-diastolic pressure (LVEDP). Unfortunately LVEDP may not necessarily reflect changes in left ventricular end-diastolic volume (LVEDV) [1] and thus it was regarded as a poor substitute for the LVEDV which is the core measure in constructing Frank-Starling ventricular function curve in man. Using left ventriculography during exercise, Sharma and associates (1976) were able for the first time to measure stroke volume and cardiac output at rest and during physical stress and thus classify left ventricular performance in patients with ischaemic heart disease according to the presence or absence of chest pain during the time of the study. The authors measured stroke volume and cardiac output at rest and during supine leg exercise in a homogeneous group of 17 patients with ischaemic heart disease, of whom 5 did not develop angina during leg exercise while the rest (n =12) developed angina. Prior to exercise there was no significant difference between the two groups in the heart rate, stroke volume and cardiac output. However during exercise the stroke volume and cardiac output decreased significantly in the 17 patients as a whole but without any significant difference between those who developed angina and those who did not develop angina during exercise.

In the last decade there have been various reports on using non-invasive

A.-M. Salmasi and A.S. Iskandrian (eds): Cardiac output and regional flow in health and disease, 127–135.

approaches to study left ventricular function. With the advent of Doppler ultrasound and radionuclide angiography a new era has emerged with better studies of left ventricular function mainly via determination of stroke volume and cardiac output non-invasively. This was specially the case with understanding the relationship between cardiac output and stroke volume and the extent of the coronary pathology and the presence of a myocardial infarct scar. These methods also allowed for a better approach to understand the mechanism of the effect of various therapeutic intervention.

By using radionucleide techniques Kirshenbaum and associates found that the left ventricular ejection fraction decreased during exercise in patients with ischaemic heart disease [3]. However much of the work in the application of nuclear angiographic techniques in studying changes in cardiac output and ejection fraction in coronary artery disease have been generated by the group of Iskandrian from Pennsylvania. In one of their reports they studied 69 patients with myocardial ischaemia [4] and found the ejection fraction decreased during exercise in 11 of the patients with restion ejecting fraction below 50% and in 13 of 16 patients with resting ejection fraction over 50% who had reversible thallium defects. However, the ejection fraction increased as a response to exercise in 13 of the 16 patients with resting ejection fraction <50% and in 20 of 26 patients with resting ejection fraction >50% with no reversible thallium defects. Also using radionuceide angiography, Nestico and associates [5] discussed the effect of various therapeutic agents on cardiac output and left ventricular function.

Doppler ultrasound assessment of stroke distance and minute distance in coronary artery disease

In series of studies by Salmasi and associates [6–8] using the continuous wave Doppler ultrasound technique of transcutaneous aortovelography (TAV), the aortic blood velocity was measured via the suprasternal notch (see Chapters 2 and 9 for more details on the technique). The main aim of the study was to characterise left ventricular performance in coronary artery disease and establish the relationship of the changes of the stroke volume and cardiac output as a result of exercise with the anatomical distribution of the coronary lesion and the presence of an old myocardial infarct. Fifty consecutive normotensive patients (40 males and 10 females) were studied. Their age was 52.4 (S.D. 10.1) years (range 27-70 years). They presented with chest pain suggestive of angina pectoris. They were not receiving beta-adrenergic blocking agents and calcium antagonists and nitrates were discontinued one week prior to the TAV recording. Doppler ultrasound recordings were carried out at rest and at maximal tolerated supine exercise limited by the development of >3 mm S-T segment depression or if the patients themselves stopped exercising as a result of the development of chest pain, shortness of breath or fatigue. None of the patients developed serious arrhythmia. Coronary

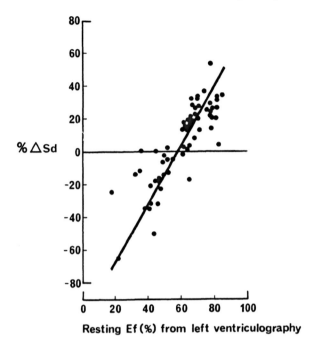

Figure 12.1. Distribution of the percentage change in the stroke distance (%ΔSd) as measured noninvasively by transcutaneous aortovelography (TAV) plotted against resting injection fraction measured invasively by left ventriculography in 62 patients presenting with chest pain. None of the patients with ejection fraction below 60% had %Sd of more than 6. (Salmasi A.M. In: Cardiovascular applications of Doppler ultrasound. Edited by Salmasi and Nicolaides. 1989. Churchill-Livingstone. Edinburgh. p. 132. Reproduced with permission).

arteriography confirmed the presence of significant (>50%) lesion in 1, 2 or 3 coronary arteries in 50 patients. The systolic velocity-time integral (or the stroke distance) and the minute distance were all derived and the results were compared to these obtained from the recordings carried out on 66 normal individuals described in Chapter 9. It was found that the response of the stroke distance to exercise was very much related to the global left ventricular function. In the presence of abnormally low ejection fraction the stroke distance decreased with exercise and the increase in the minute distance was due mainly to the increase in the heart rate (Figure 12.1). The response of the stoke distance and the minute distance in 12 patients in whom no significant lesion was detected on coronary arteriography was very much similar to that in the normal subjects (Figures 12.2, 12.3). Analysis of variance demonstrated the presence of linear trend in the response of stroke distance and minute distance to exercise according to the presence of number of coronary arteries with significant stenoses and history of myocardial infarc-

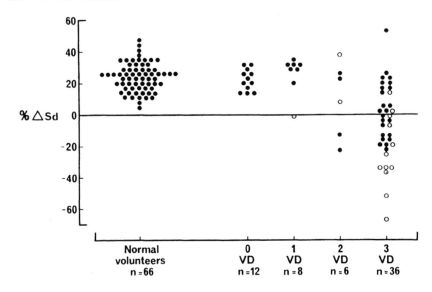

Figure 12.2. Distribution of the %ΔSd (the percentage change in the stroke distance) in 62 subjects presenting with chest pain (12 patients with normal coronary arteriogram and 50 patients with significant coronary artery lesion) and 66 normal asymptomatic subjects. (VD: number of diseased coronary vessels; (○) patients with history of myocardial infarction; (●) patients without history of myocardial infarction.).

tion. Interestingly both the stroke distance and the minute distance did not vary according to the number of the diseased coronary arteries or the presence of history of myocardial infarction [8]. The results were compared to those obtained from 66 normal volunteers in whom the stroke distance increased by 6–48% during exercise [9]. However, 23 of the 50 patients with coronary artery disease showed stroke distance increase below this normal range. In the majority of these patients the stroke distance actually decrease with exercise thus opposing the effect of the increased heart rate on cardiac output.

Inability to respond to the normal physiological stress of dynamic exercise by appropriate increase of cardiac output constitutes direct evidence of impaired pump performance. A variety of measurement techniques have shown that the increase in cardiac output with supine exercise results principally from increased heart rate with a lesser but positive contribution coming from a modest (10–35%) increase in stroke volume [10].

Effect of myocardial revascularization

Because preserving normal cardiac output is the only function of the heart, the effect of coronary artery bypass grafting on cardiac output has received

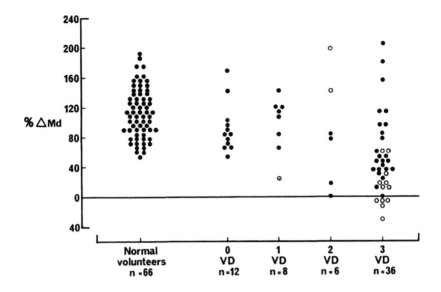

Figure 12.3. Distribution of the percentage change in the minute distance (%ΔMd) in 66 normal healthy asymptomatic subjects and 62 patients presenting with chest pain (12 patients had normal coronary arteriogram and 50 patients had significant (>50%) stenosis in 1, 2 or 3 coronary arteries). Number of diseased coronary arteries is indicated by VD. ((○) Patients with history of myocardial infarction; (●) patients without history of myocardial infarction.)

much attention. The discrepancies observed in the various reports on the effect of this operation on left ventricular function have emerged mainly because these studies were made either too soon after surgery or they were carried out at rest and not during exercise. Some of these reports indicated improvement [10, 11] while others [12, 13] showed deterioration in left ventricular function.

It remains certain that improvement of left ventricular performance during exercise is the best indicator of the effectiveness of the operation of CABG. Certainly a non-invasive approach is an ideal method of assessment as it may be necessary to repeat the technique frequently in certain cases. Exercise ECG testing per se has its own limitations in assessing the effect of the operation. The disappearance of chest pain after the operation does not always imply improved coronary blood flow as intraoperative infarcts or even placebo effect may be responsible for the relief of pain [14]. Despite the improvement in exercise tolerance and disappearance of symptoms following CABG reversal of ischaemic S-T segment changes during exercise following CABG was noted in only 50% of patients [15]. Another mechanism which may influence the result of exercise testing is the training programme which may produce improvement in exercise tolerance following CABG [16].

Effect of CABG on left ventricular performance has been evaluated using Doppler ultrasound technique of transcutaneous aortovelography to derive the stroke distance and minute distance [17]. For this purpose 30 consecutive patients (all male) were studied. Their mean age was 55.4 years (S.D. 7.9) and all had significant coronary arterial lesion confirmed by coronary arteriography. The Doppler TAV study was carried out prior to surgery and sex weeks follow the operation. None of the patients developed perioperative myocardial infarction. Prior to CABG the stroke distance in 19 patients; 10 of whom had history of myocardial infarction. In 16 of these 19 patients the resting ejection fraction was abnormal. Following CABG, a significant increase in the exercise values for the stoke distance and the minute distance was noted. However the resting values for the stroke distance did not change whereas the minute distance increased significantly following CABG. The latter may well be due to discontinuation of the beta-adrenergic blocking agents after CABG. These results indicate, therefore, that left ventricular stroke volume and cardiac output improve following CABG and that this improvement is noted during exercise rather than at rest.

Another important observation in this study was that patients with a history of myocardial infarction, who had a significantly lower response of the stroke distance to exercise that patients without history of myocardial infarction, continued to have weaker response following CABG though their stroke distance response to exercise had improved after CABG (Figure 12.4). The explanation for this observation is that revascularization has only improved the function in the ischaemic myocardium but not in the dead (infarcted) area of the myocardium which remained non-functioning following CABG.

Left ventricular function in patients with intermittent claudication

The majority of the 2–5% of perioperative mortality and the 30–40% of the 3-year mortality encountered in patients undergoing peripheral vascular reconstruction are the result of myocardial infarction and stroke [18–22]. It is therefore important to ensure a good myocardial blood supply and well preserved cardiac output and stroke volume prior to peripheral vascular reconstruction. In the Cleveland Clinic, Hertzer and associates (1984) studied a series of 1000 consecutive patients with peripheral arterial disease [23]. In these patients coronary artery disease was clinically suspected in 52% of 263 patients presenting with abdominal aortic aneurysm and 56% of 381 with lower limb ischaemia. However when routine angiography was performed in all 1000 patients only 18% were found to have normal coronary arteries indicating the presence of occult coronary artery disease in a very large number of patients. Severe but correctable disease in three coronary artery territories was found in 25%, while severe but correctable disease in three coronary artery territories was found in 25%, while severe but inoperable

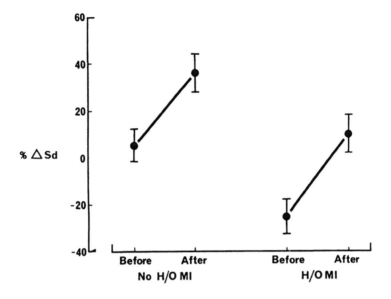

Figure 12.4. Comparison of the (mean ± S.D.) of the %ΔSd (percentage change in the stroke distance) before and after coronary artery bypass graft surgery (CABG) in patients with and without history of myocardial infarction (H/O MI). No significant (p = 0.7) difference was found in the increase of the %ΔSd after CABG between patients with H/O MI (mean 36.0, se 6.0) and patients without H/O MI (mean 32.0, se 4.6). Patients with H/O MI tended to have a lower %ΔSd than patients without H/O MI both before and after CABG.

disease because of diffuse distal coronary disease or impaired left ventricular function was present in only 6%.

It has been found that patients who underwent myocardial revascularization for concomitant severe coronary artery disease prior to peripheral vascular reconstruction had a lower rate of perioperative mortality than similar patients who had not undergone coronary artery bypass grafting [24]. Assessment of left ventricular function prior to peripheral vascular reconstruction is therefore necessary and a simple non-invasive approach during exercise to achieve that is appropriate. The cause of any left ventricular dysfunction must be determined and accordingly treated especially if it was due to coronary artery disease.

Another benefit of evaluating the stroke volume and cardiac output in patients with peripheral vascular disease is haemodynamic which will also help in assessing the pathophysiology of the condition. It was over three decades ago when Donald and associates established the relationship between the drop in the cardiac output and the impairment in the circulation to the lower limbs. The blood flow to the legs and the cardiac output were measured invasively and simultaneously at rest and during bicycle ergometer in the supine position in 11 normal subjects and 11 patients with rheumatic valve disease. In normal subjects whose cardiac output increased during exercise the femoral blood flow also increased in paralled. On the other hand patients with poor response of the cardiac output to exercise had lower leg blood flow than patients with normal response.

The Continuous-wave Doppler ultrasound technique of TAV was used to measure the stroke distance and the minute distance at rest and at maximal-tolerated supine exercise in 100 consecutive patients who presented with intermittent claudication [25]. The ankle/brachial systolic pressure index in response to exercise was also determined. Left ventricular dysfunction (as demonstrated by a decrease in the stroke distance by more than 9% in response to exercise) was observed in 44 of the 47 patients with positive stress ECG testing. On the other hand an increase of more than 6% in the response of the stroke distance to exercise was observed in the 52 of the 53 patients with negative stress ECG test. A good correlation was obtained between the percentage change in the stroke distance with exercise and the response of the ankle/brachial systolic blood pressure index with exercise hence indicating that inability of the heart to maintain an adequate stroke volume during physical exercise, which is the outcome of coronary arterial lesion, is partially responsible for the drop in the ankle systolic blood pressure and therefore resulting in intermittent claudication which is observed in subjects with combined atherosclerotic lesions in two or more sites.

References

1. Sharma B, Goodwin JF, Raphael MJ et al. Left ventricular angiography on exercise: a new method of assessing left ventricular function in ischaemic heart disease. Br Heart J. 1976;38:59.
2. Kirshenbaum HD, Okada RD, Boucher CA et al. Relationship of thallium-201 myocardial perfusion pattern to regional and global left ventricular function with exercise. Am Heart J. 1981;101:734.
3. Iskandrian AS, Hakki A, Newman BS. The relationship between myocardial ischaemia and the ejection fraction response to exercise in patients with normal or abnormal resting left ventricular function. Am Heart J 1985;109:1253.
4. Nestico PF, Hakki AH, Iskandrian AS. Effect of cardiac medication on ventricular performance: emphasis on evaluation with radionuclide angiography. Am Heart J 1985; 109: 1070.
5. Salmasi SN, Salmasi A-M, Hendry WG et al. Exercise-induced changes in stroke volume measured noninvasively in coronary artery disease. Ultrasound Med Biol 1982;8:170.
6. Salmasi S, Salmasi A-M, Hendry WG, et al. Exercise-induced changes in stroke volume measured noninvasively in coronary artery disease. Acta Cardiol 1983;6:337.
7. Salmasi AM, Salmasi S, Nicolaides AN et al. Noninvasive assessment of left ventricular function in coronary artery disease by Doppler stress testing. J Cardiovasc Surg 1987;28:313.
8. Salmasi AM, Salmasi SN, Dore C et al. Noninvasive assessment of changes in aortic blood velocity and its derivative with exercise in normal subjects by Doppler ultrasound. J Cardiovasc Surg 1987;28:321.
9. Salmasi AM. Doppler stress testing. In:Salmasi A-M, Nicolaides AN (eds.) Cardiovascular application of Doppler ultrasound. London:1989: Churchill-Livingstone, 127.
10. Taylor NC, barber RW, Crossland P et al. Effects of coronary artery bypass grafting on

left ventricular function assessed by multiple gated ventricular scintigraphy. Br Heart J 1983;50:149.

11. Roberts AJ, Lichtenthal PR, Spies SM *et al*. Perioperative myocardial damage in coronary artery bypass graft surgery: analysis of multifactorial aetiology and evaluation of diagnostic techniques. In: Moran JM, Michaelis LL (eds.), Surgery for the complications of myocardial infarction. New York: Grune and Stratton Inc, 1980:79.

12. Wolf NM, Kreulen oF, Bove AA *et al*. Left ventricular function following coronary artery bypass surgery. Circulation 1978;58:63.

13. Hammermeister KE, Kennedy JW, Hamilton GW. Aorto-coronary saphenous vein bypass. Failure of successful grafting to improve resting left ventricular function in chronic angina. N Eng J Med 1974;290:186.

14. Hossack KF. Bruce RA, Ivey TD *et al*. Changes in cardiac functional capacity after coronary artery bypass surgery in relation to adequacy of revascularization. J Am Coll Cardiol 1984;3:47.

15. Laptin ES, Murray JA, Bruce RA *et al*. Changes in maximal exercise performance in the evaluation of saphenous vein bypass surgery. Circulation 1973;47:1164.

16. Boudoulas H, Lewis RP, Vasco JS, *et al*. Left ventricular function and adrenergic hyperactivity before and after saphenous vein bypass. Circulation 1976;53:802.

17. Salmasi A-M, Salmasi S, Nicolaides AN *et al*. Assessment of the effect of coronary artery bypass grafting on left ventricular performance by Doppler measurement of the aortic blood velocity during exercise. J Cardiovasc Surg 1988;29:89.

18. Cooley DA, Wakasch DC. Techniques in vascular surgery. Philadelphia: Saunders & Co., 1979: 261.

19. Jameison WRE, Jancesz TM, Miaygishima RT *et al*. Influence of ischaemic heart disease on early and late mortality after surgery for peripheral occlusive disease. Circulation 1982;66:92.

20. Crawford ES, Bomberger RA, Glaeser DH, *et al*. Aortoiliac occlusive disease: factors influencing survival and function following reconstructive operation over a twenty-five-year period. Surgery 1981;90:1055.

21. Burnham NR, Johnson G, Gurri JA. Mortality risks for survivors of vascular reconstructive procedures. Surgery 1982;92:1072.

23. Hertzer NR, Beven EG, Young JR. Coronary artery disease in peripheral vascular patients. A classification of 1000 coronary angiograms and results of surgical management. Ann Surg 1984;199:223.

22. Hertzer NR. Fatal myocardial infarction following lower extremity revascularization. Two-hundred seventy-three patients followed 6 to 11 postoperative years. Ann Surg 1981;193:492.

24. Hertzer NR, Beven EG, *et al*. Late results of coronary bypass in patients with peripheral vascular disease. I. Five-year survival according to age and clinical cardiac status. Clev Clin Quart 1986;53:133.

25. Donald KW, Wormald PN, Taylor SH *et al*. Changes in the oxygen content of femoral venous blood and leg blood flow during leg exercise in relation to cardiac output response. Clin Sci 1957;16:567.

13. Cardiac output in valvular heart disease

J. DAVID OGILBY and ABDULMASSIH S. ISKANDRIAN[1]

The emphasis of this paper will be on changes in cardiac output in patients with acquired valvular heart diseases. A brief discussion on other hemodynamics will be presented only if relevant, however, specifically this paper will not discuss etiology, natural history, and treatment of these disorders. We will also assume that, for the sake of discussion, the valvular heart diseases are pure in form, i.e. the valve disease is either stenosis or regurgitation and it involves a single valve. Although, realistically, many patients have combined lesions.

In stenotic valve lesions, the relationship between flow (cardiac output), pressure gradient, and valve area is expressed by the Gorlin formula [1]. We have modified and simplified the formula [2] as follows:

$$\text{valve area (cm}^2) = \frac{\text{cardiac output (L/min)}}{\sqrt{\text{pressure gradient}}}.$$

This formula provides results comparable to the original Gorlin formula if the heart rate is in the physiological range and is applicable to patients with mitral stenosis, aortic stenosis, and pulmonic stenosis.

In regurgitant lesions, the stroke volume is described as forward (net), regurgitant, and total. The total stroke volume equals the regurgitant stroke volume plus the forward stroke volume. The total stroke volume can be measured by contrast ventriculography although other methods such as nuclear magnetic resonance, two-dimensional echocardiography, radionuclide angiography, and fast cine-computerized tomography may also be applicable. The forward stroke volume is measured by the thermodilution, dye dilution, or the Fick principle; the dye dilution is probably least reliable in the presence of regurgitation. The ratio of the regurgitant stroke volume to the total stroke volume is referred to as the regurgitant index and is a measure of severity of the regurgitation.

1. We wish to gratefully acknowledge the secretarial assistance of Joanne Vitanza.

A.-M. Salmasi and A.S. Iskandrian (eds): *Cardiac output and regional flow in health and disease*, 137–152.
© 1993 *Kluwer Academic Publishers. Printed in the Netherlands.*

Mitral stenosis

The left ventricle is either normal or even smaller in size than normal in most patients [3]. Mitral stenosis is more common in women. In our study [4], most patients with mitral stenosis were found to have small body size and low body weight; obese patients with severe mitral stenosis is indeed unusual. A possible reason for this association between body weight and severity of mitral stenosis is that the cardiac output increases with increasing body surface area for any given cardiac index. In mitral stenosis, the higher the cardiac output the higher the pressure gradient and the pulmonary artery wedge pressure. In addition, in many patients, the cardiac index may be slightly reduced or in the low normal range [5]. These are compensatory mechanisms to reduce the pulmonary artery wedge pressure towards normal. There is a unique group of patients with mitral stenosis who have a severely reduced cardiac output at rest and normal or near normal pulmonary artery wedge pressure even in the presence of severe stenosis. These patients, generally elderly, present with the main complaint of easy fatigability rather than dyspnea on exertion. Because of the low flow, the diastolic apical rumble may be soft and missed entirely, the so called "silent" mitral stenosis.

Most patients with mitral stenosis are in atrial fibrillation due to increases in left atrial size and pressure. It is also possible that atrial fibrillation, *per se*, results in further increase in left atrial size. Atrial fibrillation results in loss of atrial contribution to left ventricular filling and a decrease in cardiac output which may be appreciated by some but not all patients [6]. In some patients its possible that the left atrial contraction is ineffective because of fibrosis and, hence, the contribution to left ventricular filling is less important.

During pregnancy the increase in blood volume and cardiac output may account for worsening of symptoms and development of pulmonary edema. A rapid deterioration in clinical condition may also occur with the onset of atrial fibrillation with a rapid ventricular response because of a decrease in diastolic filling period per beat and, hence, increase in pressure gradient and pulmonary artery wedge pressure.

Cardiac output during exercise in mitral stenosis

As discussed elsewhere, the increase in cardiac output during upright exercise in normal subjects is due to increases in both heart rate and stroke volume. The increase in stroke volume is due to an increase in end-diastolic volume (Frank Starling mechanism) and a decrease in end-systolic volume (increased contractility). These changes are observed with a slight increase in pulmonary capillary wedge pressure and pulmonary artery pressure, a decrease in systemic vascular resistance and an increase in aortic pressure. The increase in oxygen consumption is due to increases in both cardiac output and oxygen extraction resulting in a decrease in oxygen saturation in the mixed venous blood. At exhaustive exercise, the mixed venous oxygen saturation may be as low as 25 to 30%.

In mitral stenosis the increase in cardiac output during exercise is associated with an increase in pulmonary capillary wedge pressure which results in dyspnea on exertion, a limiting symptom during exercise in most patients. Based on the pressure flow relationship, for any given degree of mitral stenosis, doubling of the cardiac output results in a four-fold increase in the pressure gradient. The increase in cardiac output during exercise depends on the severity of mitral stenosis and the degree of irreversible changes in the pulmonary vascular resistance and right ventricular function. The increase in cardiac output in mitral stenosis is mostly due to increase in the heart rate. Most patients, therefore, gradually adapt a more sedentary life style and avoid strenuous physical activities and many, in retrospect, after successful mitral valve repair or replacement, appreciate the degree of their physical disability before surgery.

Measurement of the cardiac output, pulmonary capillary wedge pressure, and mixed venous oxygen saturation during exercise may be useful in patients with atypical symptoms or in patients with discordant catheterization and historic data.

Left ventricular and right ventricular functions in mitral stenosis

The left ventricular ejection fraction is normal in most patients with mitral stenosis. The long standing reduction in preload, rheumatic myocarditis and associated diseases are reasons for left ventricular dysfunction in some patients. The right ventricular function depends on right ventricular afterload which is dependent on the pulmonary artery flow and pulmonary artery vascular resistance and also secondarily on volume overload due to secondary pulmonic valve insufficiency or tricuspid valve insufficiency. The right ventricular function is often depressed at rest and shows worsening of function during exercise, improvement in right ventricular function occurs after mitral valve repair or replacement. Right ventricular dilatation during exercise may affect the left ventricular function via the interaction through the septum and the confines of the pericardium. A summary of the hemodynamics at rest and exercise in mitral stenosis in Table 13.1.

In some patients the severity of mitral stenosis is better assessed during supine exercise with simultaneous measurement of the hemodynamics. In one study [7], dobutamine, was substituted for exercise in 40 patients with mitral stenosis. Dobutamine resulted in an increase in heart rate from 84 to 123 beats per minute, an increase in cardiac index from 2.4 to 3.4 L/min/m^2. Pulmonary artery pressure increased from 27 to 30 mm Hg, but the pulmonary artery wedge pressure and the mitral valve area remained unchanged. The left ventricular end-diastolic pressure, decreased from 11 to 2 mm Hg. Johnston and Kostuk [8] studied 20 patients with mitral stenosis using radi-

Table 13.1. The hemodynamic changes at rest and during exercise in mitral stenosis.

	Rest	Exercise
Heart rate	N	↑ I
Stroke volume	N, ↓ D	↔
Cardiac output	N, ↓ D	↑ I
Left ventricular		
end-diasolic volume	N, ↓ D	↔
end-systolic volume	N, ↓ D	↔, ↓ D
ejection fraction	N, ↓ D	↑ I↔ ↓ D
Right ventricular		
end-diastolic volume	N, ↑ I	↑ I
end-systolic volume	N, ↑ I	↑ I↔ ↓ D
ejection fraction	N, ↓ D	↑ I↔ ↓ D
Pul. cap. wedge	↑ I	↑ ↑ I
Pulmonary artery	↑ I	↑ ↑ I
Pul. vas. res.	N, ↑	N, ↑ I

N = normal; ↑ I = increased; ↓ D = decreased; ↔ = no change.

onuclide angiography, at rest and during exercise in the supine position. The left ventricular ejection fraction increased from 64 at rest to 74 during exercise. This increase in ejection fraction was primarily caused by a decrease in end-systolic volume. In these patients the end-diastolic volume also decreased during exercise. Therefore, the stroke volume did not change. The right ventricular ejection fraction did not rise with exercise and was worse in those with severe mitral stenosis. Klein and associates [9] studied the effect of atenolol 100 mg a day in 13 patients with mitral stenosis. Exercise performance was assessed using multistage Bruce treadmill testing after two weeks of placebo or two weeks of active therapy. Atenolol resulted in a significant decrease in heart rate at rest and during exercise and an increase in exercise time. Thus, beta blockade with atenolol appears to improve exercise capacity in patients with mitral stenosis who are in sinus rhythm conceivably by slowing the heart rate and, therefore, decreasing the cardiac output during exercise and hence the pressure gradient and, the pulmonary artery wedge pressure.

Mitral regurgitation

Doppler studies have suggested that a mild degree of valve regurgitation is present in normal subjects [10] and that the incidence, severity and the number of valves involved increase with advancing age [11]. These lesions, however, do not produce symptoms and are not associated with hemodynamic abnormalities. Mitral regurgitation may be acute or chronic. Acute mitral regurgitation is often an urgent situation associated with sudden clinical and hemodynamic deterioration often in the setting of acute myocardial infarction or rupture chordae tendineae in patients with mitral valve prolapse syndrome. The onset is often sudden with marked shortness of breath, hypotension, or shock due to low cardiac output accompanied by marked elevation in pulmonary artery wedge pressure, prominent "V" waves in the pulmonary artery pressure tracing and pulmonary edema. These patients are often in normal sinus rhythm with normal sized left ventricular cavity and normal or even supernormal ejection fraction. The left atrium is often normal sized. These patients constitute medical emergencies and often require urgent surgical intervention.

The rest of the discussion will deal with the more common entity of chronic regurgitation. The compensatory mechanisms in chronic mitral regurgitation are maintained by an increase in the force of contraction secondary to a decrease in the afterload, especially in the early stages of the disease [12]. Left ventricular dilatation occurs in the latter stages of the disease. The pressure-volume relationship of the left ventricle is shifted to the right and, hence, the filling pressure remains normal despite considerable left ventricular dilatation. It is also probably true that mitral regurgitation begets mitral regurgitation; the left ventricular dilatation causes stretching of the mitral value annulus and increasing the degree of mitral regurgitation. Eventually longstanding volume overload will result in a decrease in left ventricular function and an increase in the filling pressure and symptoms of congestive heart failure. In the initial stages of the disease the low afterload artificially increases the ejection fraction. It is probably for this reason that for the same degree of left ventricular dilatation and the same degree of regurgitation, patients with mitral regurgitation have worse contractile function of the left ventricle than patients with aortic regurgitation even though the ejection fraction might be similar [13]. Left ventricular dilatation results in increase in wall stress which is the stimulus for eccentric hypertrophy.

Cardiac output in mitral regurgitation

The resting cardiac output is normal. In the early stages, the patients are in normal sinus rhythm and the stroke volume is maintained by decreasing the end-systolic volume. In the later stages, the rhythm is atrial fibrillation and the stroke volume is maintained by left ventricular dilatation, an increase in end-systolic volume and a decrease in ejection fraction. In advanced stages of the disease the cardiac output may decrease at rest due to continued worsening of left ventricular function. In patients with mitral regurgitation and congestive heart failure, the mitral regurgitation may be dynamic such that vasodilator therapy by decreasing the systemic vascular resistance and aortic pressure may favor forward flow and decrease regurgitant flow and, thus, improve the cardiac output with minimal or no change in the ejection fraction or total flow [14].

The cardiac output during exercise depends on the degree of mitral regurgitation, and left ventricular function. Assessment of left ventricular function, cardiac output, and degree of mitral regurgitation during exercise is feasible using thermodilution, radionuclide, and two-dimensional echocardiographic and Doppler techniques or a combination of these techniques. Most studies on left ventricular function have been obtained with radionuclide angiography which can also measure the total stroke volume, the forward stroke volume, and the regurgitant stroke volume and, hence, assess changes in the regurgitant fraction and degree of mitral regurgitation. The Doppler technique is especially suited for examination of the degree of mitral regurgitation during exercise.

In the early stage, the left ventricular function may be normal during exercise. The response to exercise is manifested by an increase in end-diastolic volume and ejection fraction and a decrease in end-systolic volume resulting in an increase in stroke volume. In mitral regurgitation, although the regurgitation starts in the isovolumic contraction phase and systole is not appreciably, shortened during exercise, the degree of regurgitation may decrease. The decrease in the systemic vascular resistance may improve the forward stroke volume in favor of the regurgitant stroke volume and, therefore, decrease the regurgitant fraction and degree of mitral regurgitation and improve forward cardiac output. As progressive left ventricular dysfunction occurs, the ejection fraction decreases with exercise accompanied by an increase in end-systolic volume limiting the increase in cardiac output to only that achieved by an increase in the heart rate and redistribution of the stroke volume.

Assessment of the pulmonary capillary wedge pressure during exercise and the mixed venous (pulmonary artery) oxygen saturation is important in patients with atypical symptoms. If exercise is terminated without excessive increase in pulmonary capillary wedge pressure and if the mixed venous blood sample is not fully desaturated, a non-cardiac etiology is more likely to be responsible for the patient's symptoms. The hemodynamic responses in patients with mitral regurgitation are summarized in Table 13.2.

The right ventricular function in patients with mitral regurgitation depends on the presence and degree of pulmonary hypertension. There are several possible factors that influence right ventricular performance in patients with mitral valve disease. These include an increase in afterload, an increase in preload (because of tricuspid regurgitation or pulmonic valve regurgitation), an interaction between the left and right ventricles through the common septum, and a decrease in contractility. In some patients, rheumatic myocarditis may be a cause of depressed right ventricular function.

Iskandrian *et al.* measured intracardiac pressures and forward cardiac output during cardiac catheterization in 43 patients with mitral valve disease and measured the ejection fraction in these patients by first-pass radionuclide angiography with a multicrystal camera [15]. As previously described by Weiner and co-workers [16], a linear correlation between the pulmonary artery pressure and the right atrial pressure was found. The right ventricular

Table 13.2. The hemodynamic changes at rest and during exercise in mitral regurgitation.

	Rest	Exercise
Left ventricular		
end-diastolic volume	N, ↑ I	↔, ↑ I
end-systolic volume	N, ↓ D, ↑ I	↓ D↔ ↑ I
ejection fraction	N, ↑ I, ↓ D	↓ D↔ ↑ I
Total stroke volume	↑ I	↔ ↑ ↑ I
Forward stroke volume	N, ↓ D	↑ I↔
Regurgitant stroke volume	↑ I	↓ D
Regurgitant fraction	↑ I	↓ D
Heart rate	N	↑ I
Forward cardiac output	N	↑ I
Pul. cap. wedge	N, ↑ I	↑ I
Pulmonary artery	N, ↑ I	↑ I

N = normal; ↑ I = increased; ↓ D = decreased; ↔ = no change.

ejection fraction was abnormal in 88 percent of the patients with mitral valve disease. There was an inverse and statistically significant correlation between the right ventricular ejection fraction and the right ventricular end-diastolic volume, which may be an important compensatory mechanism to maintain cardiac output. In 22 of the 43 patients, the right ventricular circumferential wall stress was measured using the equation *Stress = pressure × radius/thickness* where the pressure is the right ventricular systolic pressure and the radius and thickness were measured by M-mode echocardiography. The circumferential wall stress of the right ventricle was abnormal in 15 patients with mitral valve disease compared to that obtained in normal subjects, and in 14 of these 15 patients the right ventricular ejection fraction was also abnormal (<40%). Therefore, an increase in afterload may be an important determinant of abnormal right ventricular performance. Several studies have examined the relationship between intracardiac pressures and the right ventricular ejection fraction in patients with valvular heart disease. Winzelberg *et al.* [17] found no significant correlation between right ventricular ejection fraction and right ventricular systolic pressure or between the right ventricular ejection fraction and right atrial pressure. Others have observed [18–20] a significant inverse relationship between mean pulmonary arterial pressure and the right ventricular ejection fraction. However, Morrison and co-workers (18) concluded that changes in resting right ventricular ejection fraction could be explained only to a minor extent by changes in the mean pulmonary artery pressure. The presence of a normal right ventricular ejection fraction (>45%) did not exclude the presence of pulmonary hypertension in patients with valvular heart disease [18].

Abnormal right ventricular reserve function during exercise in patients with mitral valve disease has also been observed. Henze and associates [21] found a significant decrease in right ventricular ejection fraction from a mean of 49% at rest to 37% during exercise. The right ventricular ejection fraction response to exercise, however, was normal in patients with aortic valve disease, increasing from 49% at rest to 64% during exercise.

The effects of mitral valve replacement on right ventricular function in patients with mitral valve disease has also been studied. In 16 patients who had radionuclide ejection fraction studies before and after mitral valve replacement, the right ventricular ejection fraction improved significantly following surgery. Such improvement substantiates the effect of alleviating abnormal wall stress on right ventricular performance. However, complete normalization of right ventricular ejection fraction was uncommon after mitral valve replacement, perhaps related to irreversible depression of right ventricular inotropy. It is tempting to postulate that persistence of symptoms in some patients after successful mitral valve replacement for mitral stenosis or mitral regurgitation may be primarily a right ventricular fault, which limits increase in cardiac output and conceivably affects the exercise tolerance in these patients.

Right ventricular ejection fraction also appears to predict cardiac morbidity and mortality in chronic mitral regurgitation. In 53 patients with chronic mitral regurgitation, treadmill exercise time correlated with right ventricular ejection fraction during exercise ($r = 0.48$, $p < 0.005$). In 23 of these patients, in whom hemodynamic data were also available, an inverse correlation between right ventricular ejection fraction and pulmonary artery wedge and pulmonary artery systolic pressures was also found [22]. Asymptomatic patients with chronic mitral regurgitation had a higher right ventricular ejection fraction both at rest and during exercise than did symptomatic patients. Of note, 5 of 35 medically treated patients died and all had a right ventricular ejection fraction below 30%.

Aortic stenosis

Concentric hypertrophy in response to increased intraventricular pressure occurs in most patients with aortic stenosis to normalize the wall stress and maintain left ventricular performance. Inappropriate hypertrophy is one reason for reduced performance. Myocardial ischemia, especially subendocardial ischemia, is common in patients with aortic stenosis due to decrease in capillary to muscle density ratio; increased distance between the vasculature and the muscle fibers; increased demand; inappropriate and reduced coronary reserve because of medial hypertrophy of the small arterioles; increased ejection time and reduced diastolic filling period during which coronary flow occurs; incomplete relaxation; myocardial bridging of the intramyocardial vessels and in patients with associated aortic regurgitation due to decrease in diastolic perfusion pressure. These two factors, hypertrophy and ischemia, are important mechanisms that determine left ventricular perfusion and function during exercise. It is, therefore, not unusual to find a decrease in ejection fraction and an increase in end-systolic volume during exercise even in patients with compensated pure aortic stenosis. The increase in muscle mass may also explain the increase in chamber stiffness with an increase in left ventricular filling pressure and pulmonary artery wedge pressure. These changes explain the symptoms of dyspnea on exertion and the importance of the atrial contribution to left ventricular filling [23]; loss of atrial kick results in underfilling of the ventricle and a decrease in cardiac output. Loss of atrial contribution may occur with both atrial and ventricular arrhythmias.

The cardiac output at rest is normal in compensated patients with aortic stenosis. The stroke volume is maintained by the atrial contribution to ventricular filling and by prolongation of the ejection time. The atrial contribution may become especially important during exercise when there is further shortening of diastolic filling period. The cardiac output during exercise increases primarily due to an increase in the heart rate with variable contribution of changes in the stroke volume. At one time it was thought that the limited cardiac output during exercise in combination with a decrease in systemic vascular resistance was the most important cause for syncope. More recent studies, however, suggest that activation of stretch receptors within the left ventricular wall is a more important mechanism. This reflex causes bradycardia or vasodilation (or both) and a decrease in systemic pressure resulting in syncope. This reflex is activated in patients with small hyperdynamic left ventricles, as those encountered in patients with aortic stenosis. Most physicians consider severe aortic stenosis as contraindication for exercise testing because of the danger of syncope or ventricular arrhythmias. However, when these patients are carefully supervised, exercise testing can be performed safely [24]. In the later stages of the disease with left ventricular dilation and dysfunction, secondary mitral regurgitation may also occur further decreasing the forward cardiac output and worsening of symptoms. In patients with severe long standing aortic stenosis and left ventricular dysfunction, the cardiac output is severely reduced at rest which also decreases the pressure gradient across the stenosis. The low flow results in a decrease in intensity of the systolic murmur and underestimation of the severity of stenosis on clinical evaluation.

Aortic regurgitation

Patients with severe aortic regurgitation often remain asymptomatic for a long period of time, however, with the onset of congestive heart failure the course is progressive and the prognosis poor without valve replacement. Surgery is often advised with the onset of deterioration in left ventricular function or when the patient becomes symptomatic. Unlike mitral regurgitation, changes in the heart rate have profound effects on the degree of

Table 13.3. Effects of atrial pacing and bicycle exercise in comparison to resting hemodynamics in patients with aortic regurgitation.

	Atrial pacing	Bicycle exercise[a]	
		Supine	Upright
Heart rate	↑ I	↑ I	↑ I
Systolic blood pressure	N.C.	↑ I	↑ I
LV ejection fraction	N.C.	N.C.	↑ I
End-diastolic volume	↓ D	N.C. or ↓ D	↓ D
End-systolic volume	↓ D	N.C.	↓ D
Total left ventricular output	N.C.	↑ ↑ I	↑ ↑ I
Forward cardiac index	↑ I[b]	↑ I	↑ ↑ I
Regurgitant fraction	N.C.	↓ D	↓ D
Regurgitant volume/stroke	↓ D	↓ D	↓ D
Regurgitant volume/minute	N.C.	N.C.	
Total stroke volume	↓ D	N.C. or ↓ D	N.C.
Forward stroke volume	↓ D	↑ I	↑ I

[a] Asymptomatic or minimally symptomatic patients.
[b] Up to a heart rate of 100 beats/min.
N.C. = no change; ↑ I = increased; ↓ D = decreased; LV = left ventricular.
(From Iskandrian [27] reproduced with permission.)

aortic regurgitation. The effects of heart rate in aortic regurgitation were first described by Corrigan in 1832 [25]: "The nature of the disease (aortic regurgitation) is in proportion to the quantity of blood that regurgitates, and the quantity that regurgitates will be large in proportion to the degree of inadequacy of the values and to the length of the pause between the contractions of the ventricle, during which the blood can be pouring back. If the action of the heart be rendered very slow, the pause after each contraction will be long and consequently the regurgitation of the blood must be considerable. Frequent action of the heart on the contrary makes the pause after each contraction short and in proportion as the pauses are shortened, the regurgitation must be lessened." Judge and colleagues [26] used atrial pacing in 8 patients with aortic regurgitation and measured left ventricular end-diastolic volume by contrast angiography. They confirmed that rapid atrial pacing caused a decrease in end-diastolic volume. The hemodynamic consequences of rapid atrial pacing in patients with severe aortic regurgitation are summarized in Table 13.3. Forward cardiac output increases with increasing heart rate but the end-diastolic volume and total and forward stroke volume typically decrease during pacing-induced tachycardia [28]. There is also a decrease in the time available per cardiac cycle for regurgitation flow [28]. Although the regurgitant volume per stoke decreases, the regurgitant volume per minute does not. Thus, the decrease in end-diastolic volume produced by rapid atrial pacing is accompanied by a decrease in regurgitant flow per stoke but not in regurgitant fraction [28].

Left ventricular function with exercise in aortic regurgitation

Exercise provides a potentially useful condition for detecting early evidence of left ventricular dysfunction as well as of early symptoms in patients with aortic regurgitation. Multiple hemodynamic mechanisms are involved because dynamic exercise produces important changes in myocardial contrac-

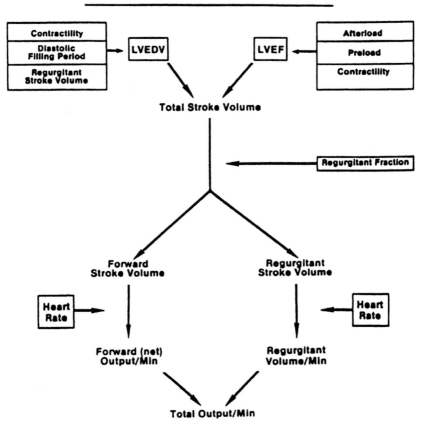

Figure 13.1. The regulation of the cardiac output during upright exercise in patients with aortic regurgitation. LVEDV = left ventricular end-diastolic volume; LVEF = left ventricular ejection fraction. (From Iskandrian *et al.* [29] with permission.)

Table 13.4. Hemodynamic data at rest and during exercise in 15 asymptomatic or minimally symptomatic patients with aortic regurgitation and in 10 normal subjects.

	Normal (n = 10)			Aortic regurgitation (n = 15)			NL vs. AR	
	R	Ex	p	R	Ex	p	R	Ex
HR	78 ± 12	153 ± 22	0.0001	74 ± 15	133 ± 20	0.0001	NS	0.03
SBP	127 ± 21	192 ± 26	0.0001	146 ± 26	191 ± 23	0.0001	NS	NS
DBP	86 ± 10	89 ± 18	NS	73 ± 24	83 ± 16	0.0001	NS	NS
EF	63 ± 7	73 ± 8	0.0001	47 ± 10	53 ± 12	0.003	0.0002	0.0001
EDVI	79 ± 27	82 ± 23	NS	153 ± 61	132 ± 39	0.02	0.003	0.002
ESVI	31 ± 16	23 ± 15	0.0001	85 ± 47	65 ± 35	0.003	0.003	0.002
TCI	3.8 ± 1.2	8.9 ± 1.9	0.0001	4.9 ± 1.1	8.9 ± 2.3	0.0001	0.03	NS
FCI	3.6 ± 1.0	8.1 ± 2.1	0.0001	2.2 ± 0.7	4.9 ± 1.1	0.0001	0.002	0.0001
RF	9 ± 7	9 ± 6	NS	53 ± 15	45 ± 15	0.03	0.0001	0.0001
FSVI	44 ± 9	53 ± 10	0.002	31 ± 10	36 ± 11	0.06	0.003	0.0007
TSVI	48 ± 13	59 ± 10	0.007	68 ± 19	66 ± 14	NS	0.009	NS
Ex dur	–	10.8 ± 4.0	–	–	7.5 ± 3.0	–	–	0.03

AR = aortic regurgitation; DBP = diastolic blood pressure, mm Hg; EDVI = end-diastolic volume index, ml/m^2; EF = ejection fraction, %; ESVI = end-systolic volume index, ml/m^2; Ex = exercise; Ex dur = exercise duration, min; FCI = forward cardiac index, Lmin^{-1}m^{-2}; FSVI = forward stroke volume index, ml/m^2; HR = heart rate; NL = normal; p = probability; R = rest; RF = regurgitant fraction, %; SBP = systolic blood pressure, mm Hg; TCI = total cardiac index, Lmin^{-1}m^{-2}; TSVI = total stroke volume index, ml/m^2.
(From Iskandrian et al. [30] reproduced by permission of the American Heart Journal.)

tility, loading conditions and heart rate. These changes are summarized in Figure 13.1 and Table 13.4.

In patients with aortic regurgitation, the response of left ventricular volumes to exercise has been related to patient selection, changes in systemic vascular resistance [31], the use of supine versus upright exercise, and the presence or absence of cardiac symptoms. For example, Dehmer et al. [32] found that left ventricular diastolic volume index increased by 6 ml/m^2 body surface area (p < 0.05) and left ventricular systolic volume index increased by 33 ml/m^2 (p < 0.05) with supine bicycle exercise in patients with aortic regurgitation and definite cardiac symptoms.

In patients with minimal or no symptoms, no change in left ventricular volume was observed in response to exercise. A decrease in left ventricular diastolic volume [33–35], is more likely to be observed with upright exercise [33], in younger patients [34, 35], in patients with normal exercise tolerance [35], and in patients with large end-diastolic volumes at rest. It is possible that a decrease in end-diastolic volume with exercise may limit the increase in end-diastolic pressure in these patients and therefore preserve the exercise capacity. The directional changes in end-diastolic volume in response to exercise are not necessarily similar to the directional changes in ejection fraction Figure 13.2.

The cardiac output in aortic regurgitation is determined by changes in the heart rate, total stroke volume, and regurgitant fraction. The stroke volume

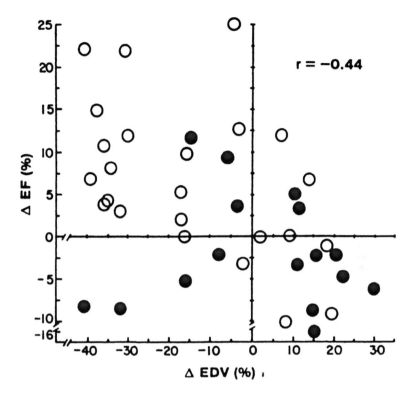

Figure 13.2. Comparison between the change in left ventricular ejection fraction (ΔEF) and the change in end-diastolic volume (ΔEDV) from rest to exercise in patients with aortic regurgitation. ●, Patients with normal exercise tolerance; ○, patients with exercise intolerance. (From Iskandrian *et al.* [35] reproduced by permission of the American College of Cardiology.)

measured by radionuclide angiography (end-diastolic volume times ejection fraction) represents the total left ventricular stroke volume; therefore, to measure the net forward stroke volume, the regurgitant fraction must also be determined.

In contrast to findings during atrial pacing, forward stroke volume may increase during exercise in patients with aortic regurgitation and normal left ventricular function. This may be related to the inotropic effects associated with exercise. Also, in contrast to findings during atrial pacing, numerous studies have demonstrated that the regurgitant fraction decreases with dynamic exercise [29, 36, 37]. Although total stroke volume is unchanged (or may even fall due to decreasing left ventricular end-diastolic volume), forward stroke volume may increase in the face of a decreasing regurgitant fraction. These findings may further explain the preservation of exercise capacity in many patients with aortic regurgitation.

In summary, left ventricular function at rest is normal in patients with aortic regurgitation. Abnormal response to exercise may be seen even in the asymptomatic patient but, *per se*, is not an indication for valve replacement. Recent studies [38, 39] have suggested that long term vasodilator therapy may decrease the regurgitation, improve left ventricular function, and decrease the left ventricular size. These findings may have important indications on patient management and timing of surgical intervention. Cardiac output at rest is maintained by left ventricular dilatation and increase in total stroke volume. With exercise, the total cardiac output may not change but the forward cardiac output increases because of the decrease in systemic vascular resistance resulting in a decrease in the regurgitant fraction and regurgitant volume per beat. In patients with far advanced degree of aortic regurgitation, left ventricular dysfunction becomes severe with equalizations of diastolic pressures in the aorta and left ventricle, reduced flow or cardiac output even at rest. Parenthetically, tachycardia is a compensatory mechanism in patients with acute aortic regurgitation to decrease the degree of regurgitation. This coupled with premature closure of the mitral value tend to decrease the pulmonary artery wedge pressures.

References

1. Gorlin R, Gorlin SG. Hydraulic formula for calculation of the area of stenotic mitral valve, other cardiac valves and central circulatory shunts. Am Heart J 1951;41:1.
2. Hakki A-H, Kimbiris D, Iskandrian AS et al. Angina pectoris and coronary artery disease in patients with severe aortic valvular disease. Am Heart J 1980;100:441.
3. Kennedy JW. The use of quantitative angiocardiography in mitral valve disease. In: Duran C, Angell WW, Johnson AD et al. (eds.), Recent progress in mitral valve disease. London: Butterworths, 1984:149.
4. Nestico PF, Iskandrian AS, Hakki A-H et al. Relation of body habitus to the severity of mitral stenosis in women. Am J Cardiol 1984;55:857.
5. Gash AK, Carabello BA, Cepin D et al. Left ventricular ejection performance and systolic muscle function in patients with mitral stenosis. Circulation 1983;67:148.
6. Stott DK, Marpole DGF, Bristow JD et al. The role of left atrial transport in aortic and mitral stenosis. Circulation 1970;41:1031.
7. Hwang MH, Pacold I, Piao ZE et al. The usefulness of dobutamine in the assessment of the severity of mitral stenosis. Am Heart J 1986;111:312.
8. Johnston DL, Kostuk WJ. Left and right ventricular function during symptom-limited exercise in patients with isolated mitral stenosis. Chest 1986;89:186.
9. Klein HO, Sareli P, Schamroth CL et al. Effects of atenolol on exercise capacity in patients with mitral stenosis with sinus rhythm. Am J Cardiol 1985;56:598.
10. Yoshida K, Yoshikawa J, Shakudo M et al. Color Doppler evaluation of valvular regurgitation in normal subjects. J Electrocardiol 1988;21:31.
11. Akasaka T, Yoshikawa J, Yoshida K et al. Age-related valvular regurgitation: a study by pulsed Doppler echocardiography. Circulation 1987;76:262.
12. Braunwald E: Mitral regurgitation: physiological, clinical and surgical considerations. N Engl J Med 1969;281:425.
13. Wisenbaugh T, Spann JF, Carabello BA. Differences in myocardial performance and load

between patients with similar amounts of chronic aortic versus chronic mitral regurgitation. J Am Coll Cardiol 1984;3:916.

14. Keren G, Bier A, Strom JA *et al.* Dynamics of mitral regurgitation during nitroglycerin therapy: a Doppler echocardiographic study. Am Heart J 1986;112:517.

15. Iskandrian AS, Hakki AH, Ren JF *et al.* Correlation among right ventricular preload, afterload and ejection fraction in mitral valve disease: radionuclide, electrocardiographic and hemodynamic evaluation. J Am Coll Cardiol 1984;3:1403.

16. Weiner BH, Alpert JS, Dalen JE *et al.* Response of the right ventricle to exercise in patients with chronic heart disease. Am Heart J 1983;105:386.

17. Winzelberg GG, Boucher CA, Pohost GM *et al.* Right ventricular function at rest and during exercise in aortic and mitral valve disease. J Am Coll Cardiol 1985;5:21.

18. Morrison DA, Lancaster L, Henry R *et al.* Right ventricular function at rest and during exercise in aortic and mitral valve disease. J Am Coll Cardiol 1985;5:21.

19. Grose, R, Strain J, Yipintosoi T. Right ventricular function in valvular heart disease: relation to pulmonary artery pressure. J Am Coll Cardiol 1983;2:225.

20. Korr KS, Gandsman EJ, Winkler ML *et al.* Hemodynamic correlates of right ventricular ejection fraction measured with gated radionuclide angiography. Am J Cardiol 1982;49:71.

21. Henze E, Schelbert Hr, Wisenberg G *et al.* Assessment of regurgitant fraction and right and left ventricular function at rest and during exercise: a new technique for determination of right ventricular stroke counts from gated blood pool studies. Am Heart J 1982;104:953.

22. Hochreiter C, Niles N, Devereux RB *et al.* Mitral regurgitation: relationship of noninvasive descriptors of right and left ventricular performance to clinical and hemodynamic findings and to prognosis in medically and surgically treated patients. Circulation 1986;73:900.

23. Murakami T, Hess OM, Gage JE *et al.* Diastolic filling dynamics in patients with aortic stenosis. Circulation 1986;73:1162.

24. Anderson FL, Tsagaris TJ, Tikoff G *et al.* Hemodynamic effects of exercise in patients with aortic stenosis. Am J Med 1969;46:872.

25. Corrigen DJ: On permanent patency of the mouth of the aorta or inadequacy of the aortic valves. Edinburgh Med Surg J 1832;37:225.

26. Judge TP, Kennedy JW, Bennett LJ *et al.* Quantitative hemodynamic effects of heart rate in aortic regurgitation. Circulation 1971;44:355.

27. Iskandrian AS. Valvular heart disease. In: Gerson MC (ed.), Cardiac nuclear medicine. New York: McGraw-Hill, Inc, 1987.

28. Firth BG, Dehmer GJ, Nicod P *et al.* Effect of increasing heart rate in patients with aortic regurgitation: effect of incremental atrial pacing on scintigraphic, hemodynamic and thermodilution measurements. Am J Cardiol 1982;49:1860.

29. Iskandrian AS, Hakki AH, Amenta A *et al.* Regulation of cardiac output during upright exercise in patients with aortic regurgitation. Cathet Cardiovasc Diag 1984;10:573.

30. Iskandrian AS, Hakki AH, Kane SA *et al.* Left ventricular pressure-volume relationship in aortic regurgitation. Am Heart J 1985;110:1026.

31. Kwanishi DT, McKay CR, Chandraratna AN, *et al.* Cardiovascular response to dynamic exercise in patients with chronic symptomatic mild-to-moderate and severe aortic regurgitation. Circulation 1986;73:62.

32. Dehmer GJ, Firth BG, Hillis LD *et al.* Alterations in left ventricular volumes and ejection at rest and during exercise in patients with aortic regurgitation. Am J Cardiol 1981;48:17.

33. Johnson LL, Powers EF, Tzall WR *et al.* Left ventricular volume and ejection fraction response to exercise in aortic regurgitation. Am J Cardiol 1983;51:1379.

34. Peter CA, Jones RH: Cardiac response to exercise in patients with chronic aortic regurgitation. Am Heart J 1982;104:85.

35. Iskandrian AS, Hakki AH, Manno B *et al.* Left ventricular function in chronic aortic regurgitation. J Am Coll Cardiol 1983;1:1374.

36. Steingart RM, Yee C, Weinstein L *et al.* Radionuclide ventriculographic study of adaptations to exercise in aortic regurgitation. Am J Cardiol 1983;51:483.

37. Gerson MC, Engel PJ, Mantil JC *et al.* Effects of dynamic and isometric exercise on the

radionuclide-determined regurgitant fraction in aortic insufficiency. J Am Coll Cardiol 1984;3:98.

38. Greenberg B, Massie B, Bristow JD *et al*. Long term vasodilator therapy of chronic aortic insufficiency. A randomized double-blinded, placebo-controlled clinical trial. Circulation 1988;78:92.

39. Scognamiglio R, Fasoli G, Ponchia A *et al*. Long-term nifedipine unloading therapy in asymptomatic patients with chronic severe aortic regurgitation. J Am Coll Cardiol 1990;16:424.

14. Cardiac output in heart failure

MARIELL JESSUP

Chronic heart failure (CHF) is the pathophysiologic state in which the heart is unable to pump blood commensurate with the metabolic needs of the body, provided there is adequate venous return to the heart. It is a constellation of signs and symptoms that result when a host of compensatory mechanisms fail to maintain cardiac output. Over the past decade, the increasing incidence of the syndrome, coupled with an often alarmingly high mortality rate, has ushered in an intensity of research productive of newer pathophysiologic insights and near miraculous therapies [1]. This chapter will briefly review the determinants of myocardial function and how they are altered by heart failure. The peripheral, as opposed to cardiac, adaptations to a decreased effective blood volume will also be outlined. However, the focus of this chapter will be to explore more recently developed concepts in our understanding of heart failure. These concepts include an examination of the structural abnormalities of the myocardium in heart failure, clinical and hemodynamic correlates of myocardial dysfunction, central mechanisms responsible for the impaired exercise response characteristic of the clinical syndrome, and the myocardial response to newer inotropic and vasodilator therapies.

Determinants of myocardial performance

The four major determinants of myocardial function are preload, afterload, contractility, and heart rate [2]. Preload is the passive force that imparts a given stretch to the ventricular muscle, which thereby determines myocardial end-diastolic fiber length. Ventricular preload is directly related to end-diastolic pressure, which in turn is a reflection of end-diastolic volume. The concept of end-diastolic wall stress calculates the effect of pressure and volume on a given thickness of myocardial wall. Under most physiologic circumstances, an increase in preload, or wall stress, results in sarcomeres stretched to greater lengths, allowing more actin-myosin interactions to take place, thus increasing the force of contraction.

The Frank–Starling relationship states that an intact ventricle has the capacity to vary the force of contraction as preload or ventricular filling increases, an obvious adaptive mechanism. One of the hallmarks of the

A.-M. Salmasi and A.S. Iskandrian (eds): Cardiac output and regional flow in health and disease, 153–168.
© 1993 *Kluwer Academic Publishers. Printed in the Netherlands.*

failing ventricle is the inability to deliver an adequate stroke volume despite what in the normal heart would be an adequate preload. Accordingly, in heart failure, compensatory mechanisms are activated to increase preload, including sodium and water retention and venoconstriction mediated via the sympathetic nervous system. Thus, the Frank–Starling curve is altered so that any increase in stroke volume is accomplished by a concomitant increase in end-diastolic volume and pressure. Ultimately, ventricular and atrial filling pressures exceed those in the pulmonary and systemic venous circuits, and extravasation of fluid into the extracellular space occurs, resulting in dyspnea, pulmonary or peripheral edema.

Afterload is the sum of forces opposing ejection or myocardial shortening. It describes the tension that must be developed by the myocardium to eject the cardiac output volume. Afterload changes throughout the cardiac cycle and is determined not only by myocardial wall thickness, ventricular pressure and volume, but also the impendence imposed by the elastic and recoil properties of the aorta, as well as the viscosity of the ejected blood. In the normal and failing heart, stroke volume is decreased as afterload is increased. However, the failing ventricle is exquisitely sensitive to minute changes in afterload, whereas stroke volume can be maintained by a normal myocardium despite marked augmentation in afterload forces.

Contractility describes the extent of myocardial fiber shortening at a given afterload and preload, but is a determinant of function independent of load. Contractility is the intrinsic property of the myocardium, dependent on myocardial cell structure and the chemical perfusate which supplies the cells. For example, hypoxemia or norepinephrine will effect a decrease or increase in myocardial contractility, respectively. Ultimately, the amount of force developed depends upon the number of actin-myosin cross bridges that interact, an energy-dependent process requiring ATP and adequate intra-cellular calcium. In the failing heart, there are multiple cellular abnormalities which have been described [3]. Moreover, biochemically there is a shift in myosin isoenzymes, cellular hypertrophy, impaired calcium use, and abnormal function of the sarcoplasmic reticulum. A number of newer observations relating to myocardial dysfunction will be discussed later in the chapter. The end effect of these alterations is decreased contractility, and, hence, a decreased cardiac output.

Cardiac output is critically affected by heart rate. For a given stroke volume, cardiac output increases with higher heart rates, until diastolic filling time is so shortened that preload is compromised. Rapid heart rates also require augmented myocardial energy requirements that often exceed oxygen delivery. Conversely, extremely low heart rates, or bradycardia, may likewise have a negative effect on cardiac output because of the limited number of ventricular contractions per minute.

Compensatory mechanisms

In the presence of myocardial dysfunction, the resultant fall in cardiac output or effective arterial blood volume serves to stimulate a number of compensatory mechanisms, the primary goal of which is to maintain adequate flow to the cerebral, coronary and renal circulations. These mechanisms include utilization of the Frank-Starling relationship, activation of the sympathetic nervous system and of the renin-angiotensin-aldosterone axis, secretion of arginine vasopressin, and the development of myocardial hypertrophy. Although these mechanisms help to preserve cardiac output and sustain systemic blood pressure, in chronic myocardial failure, the persistence of these pathophysiologic alterations have long-term deleterious effects on cardiac performance. The understanding of these neurohormonal mechanisms has greatly enhanced our ability to develop more specific pharmacotherapies for the patient with symptomatic heart failure. Nevertheless, it is obvious that if our therapy is directed at the alteration of the compensatory mechanisms, the natural course of the disease will not be substantially altered. This, in fact, describes the state of the art in the treatment of chronic heart failure. Our best drugs postpone mortality, and enhance myocardial performance, but do little to improve myocardial dysfunction. Newer efforts to understand the relationship between myocardial structure and function, cardiac function and peripheral vascular vasomotor regulation, and the effect of exercise on these relationships are reviewed below.

Structural alterations

The initiating stimulus for the cascade of compensatory mechanisms in heart failure is a decreased cardiac output. In this section, a number of different structural abnormalities are described which impact on the development of myocardial dysfunction.

Idiopathic dilated cardiomyopathy is the second most common etiology of congestive symptoms in patients with abnormal systolic ventricular function. For years, circumstantial evidence has implicated immune mechanisms in the pathogenesis of dilated cardiomyopathy. More recently, a growing body of experimental work suggests that abnormalities in cellular and humoral immunity may be implicated in the initiation or progression of the disease. A number of autoantigens have been described, that is, specific cardiac proteins that are targets of circulating autoantibodies in dilated cardiomyopathy. These targets have included the mitochondrial adenine nucleotide translocator, thus inhibiting calcium entry into the cardiac myocyte [4], the cardiac beta-adrenergic receptor [5], and adenylate cyclase [6]. For example, Caforio and coworkers (1990) performed indirect immunofluorescence on human heart and skeletal muscle to test sera from 200 normal subjects, 65 patients with dilated cardiomyopathy, 41 with chronic heart failure due to myocardial infarction, and 208 with other cardiac disease [4]. Organ-specific cardiac autoantibodies (IgG) were more frequent in patients with dilated cardiomyopathy (in 26%) than in those with other cardiac disease (1%), or heart failure from myocardial infarction (0%) or in normal subjects (3.5%). Circulating autoantibodies could theoretically modulate the function of critical components in the cardiac myocyte and account for waxing and waning of cardiac performance, virulent forms of the disease, particularly in young adults and peripartum women, and the not uncommonly observed total reversal of cardiac function in a patient with previously documented poor systolic contraction. Diagnostic tools that will allow detection of these immunogenetic mechanisms at an early stage of the disease will profoundly alter our therapy of these patients in the future.

A second area of active research has focused on the role of myocyte hypertrophy in the pathogenesis of heart failure, reviewed superbly by Dr. Arnold Katz [7]. Different disease states place increased work on active myocardial cells, whether due to abnormal hemodynamic stress, as in aortic coarctation, or to the loss of functional myocardium, as occurs after myocardial infarction. The subsequent development of hypertrophy unloads the cells by adding new sarcomeres, decreasing the rate of mechanical-energy expenditure by the individual sarcomere. However, the long-term cost of hypertrophy to the overall balance between energy demand and energy production is disadvantageous because of architectural changes in the hypertrophied heart. These changes include an increase in the distance between capillaries, resulting in relative hypoperfusion of individual cells, most pronounced in the subendocardial region of the left ventricle. Moreover, hypertrophy increases the cell volume occupied by myofibrils, which increases the need for ATP supplied by the mitochondrion, again exacerbating the energy deficit. Synthesis of new proteins is not confined to overall stimulation of muscle growth, but for the creation of isoforms of several myofibrillar proteins, lactate dehydrogenase, creatine kinase and the sarcolemmal sodium pump. In short, an acute compensatory mechanism ie. myocyte hypertrophy, serves to distribute load more equally on all the cells, but overall myocardial performance deteriorates because of chronic energy imbalance and the creation of a myocardial cell with impaired contractility.

Another focus of research emerging as critical to our understanding of cardiac performance is the role of the extracellular matrix, or cardiac interstitium. Dr. Karl Weber has summarized the several functions of the interstitium as: (1) support for the myocytes and vasculature; (2) lateral connections between cells and muscle bundles to coordinate the delivery of force to the ventricular chamber; and (3) an important determinant of diastolic and systolic myocardial stiffness which serves to resist myocardial deformation [8]. Volume or pressure overload of the heart has been shown to increase collagen concentration and effect a structural and biochemical remodeling of the collagenous matrix of the left ventricle [9]. For example, in patients with aortic valve stenosis and symptomatic heart failure myocardial collagen concentration is increased three-to-sixfold. The diverse functional consequences of interstitial remodeling on both diastolic and systolic function are now being examined. Hoeven and Factor compared the microscopic and histochemical findings of hearts obtained at autopsy of 67 patients with hypertension, diabetes mellitus or both [10]. Significant differences in heart weight, interstitial fibrosis, replacement fibrosis, and perivascular fibrosis were found among the groups. Total fibrosis correlated with heart weight and was significantly greater among patients with congestive heart failure. The amount of microscopic fibrosis increased between the groups, the lowest in hypertensive hearts, midrange in diabetic hearts, and highest in hypertensive-diabetic hearts. The authors speculated that the myocardial fibrosis contributed to the diastolic dysfunction typically seen in a diabetic, hypertensive patient with associated cardiomyopathy. In a related study, Bortone and colleagues measured passive diastolic properties of the left ventricle in 10 control subjects and 12 patients with dilated cardiomyopathy, and correlated these calculations with morphometry from right ventricular endomyocardial biopsies [11]. As expected, left ventricular end-diastolic pressure and muscle mass index were significantly higher in the cardiomyopathy patients, while left ventricular ejection fraction was lower, as compared to the control subjects. The constant of chamber stiffness was only slightly abnormal between patients and subjects. However, the constant of myocardial stiffness distinguished a division between the cardiomyopathy patients: 7 patients with a normal constant of myocardial stiffness and 5 with a significantly increased constant. Interstitial fibrosis was 19% in the first group and markedly increased to 43% in the second group. There was an exponential relation between the diastolic constant of myocardial stiffness and interstitial fibrosis. Thus structural abnormalities of the myocardium are translated into subtle, dysfunctional hemodynamic parameters which probably impact on symptoms, and undoubtedly influence prognosis.

A more obvious clinical example of the importance of distinguishing pathologic differences in patients with dilated, congestive cardiomyopathy was reviewed by Dr. Iskandrian and his co-worker [12]. They performed resting thallium-201 imaging in three groups of patients, all of whom had severe left ventricular dysfunction as evidenced by a left ventricular ejection fraction of less than 35%: 15 patients with primary cardiomyopathy and normal coronary arteries (Group I), 20 with documented coronary artery disease (group II), and 25 with an acute Q wave myocardial infarction (group III). The thallium distribution pattern was different among the three groups. Extensive perfusion defects were present in only one patient in group I but were seen in 95% of patients in group II and 100% of group III. Redistribution of thallium was not seen in group I, but in 3 patients of both group II and III. A number of population studies have now suggested that prognosis is substantially different in patients with coronary disease and poor left ventricular function compared to patients with normal coronaries. Simple hemodynamic indices, such as cardiac output determinations, may not have differentiated these three groups of patients, but other easily performed tests are now allowing us to detect important structural alterations which influence function and survival.

Clinical and hemodynamic correlates of myocardial dysfunction

Over the past two decades, the ease of obtaining bedside hemodynamic monitoring in critically ill patients has substantially enhanced our understanding of the relationship between central hemodynamics and regional blood flow in patients with heart failure. A number of important observations have been made. Leithe and his associates described the redistribution of regional blood flow in 64 patients with congestive heart failure [13]. The patients were divided into subgroups of those with mild, moderate, and severe disease on the basis of respective reduction in cardiac indexes of greater than 2.5, 2.5 to 2.0, and <2.0 liters/min/m². Mean hepatic and renal blood flow were significantly reduced compared to normal subjects for each of the three subgroups. They found a good linear correlation between individual cardiac index and both renal and hepatic flow measurements. Mean limb blood flow was substantially reduced below normal values, and for each subgroup was significantly reduced below that in each preceding subgroup of patients with less severe disease. Thus, a decrease in regional blood flow is proportional and linearly related to the severity of disease as reflected by the reduction in cardiac output. Moreover, they found little or no correlation between systemic blood pressure and hepatic, renal, or limb blood flow.

The reduction in cardiac output attendant with increasing severity of disease has other functional and hemodynamic correlates. Investigators from Belgium studied left ventricular filling characteristics in 34 patients with dilated cardiomyopathy, 16 of whom were in New York Heart Association functional class I or II (group 1) and 18 patients in functional class III or IV (group /2) [14]. No differences were observed between groups with regard to heart rate, blood pressure and M-mode echocardiographic-derived indexes of systolic function. However, peak early filling velocity was higher and atrial filling fraction was lower in group 2 than in group 1. In addition, the duration of the isovolumetric relaxation period and the time to peak filling rate were significantly shorter in group 2. All these differences occurred at a time when mean pulmonary capillary wedge pressure was higher, stroke index was lower and the grade of mitral regurgitation was larger in group 2 patients. Thus, the authors concluded that in patients with dilated cardiomyopathy, diastolic transmitral filling is determined by left atrial pressure and the severity of mitral regurgitation, and correlates better with functional class than more traditional indexes of left ventricular systolic function. Other hemodynamic descriptors of severely symptomatic heart failure have been elucidated by Hirota and colleagues [15]. They studied 32 patients with dilated cardiomyopathy, 12 of whom had only mild symptoms while 20 were markedly decompensated. There were significant differences between the two groups in left ventricular end- diastolic pressure and cavity size, ejection fraction, end-diastolic stress and end-systolic stress. No significant differences were observed in left ventricular wall thickness or muscle mass between the two groups. A significant inverse correlation was seen between ejection fraction and end-systolic stress. However, in the mildly symptomatic patients, ejection fraction was reduced but afterload was normal, indicating depressed contractility as the primary abnormality. The further reduction in ejection fraction in the decompensated patients was associated with an elevation of afterload and the absence of adequate hypertrophy, so-called afterload mismatch. Thus, a progression of symptoms in patients with dilated cardiomyopathy involves first a depression of contractility, and then an inappropriate elevation of systolic stress. This sequence of events helps to explain the striking reduction of symptoms and mortality seen with vasodilator therapy in patients with at least moderately severe heart failure [16, 17].

In addition to the classic symptoms of fatigue and dyspnea which usually prompts a patient with dilated cardiomyopathy to seek medical attention, approximately 50% of patients will experience anginal-type chest pain, often in the absence of significant coronary artery obstruction. Cannon and co-workers studied 26 patients with dilated cardiomyopathy and angiographically normal coronary arteries, half of whom gave a history of anginal chest pain [18]. During treadmill exercise testing, patients with an anginal history showed worse effort tolerance and a lower peak systolic blood pressure-heart rate product than those patients with angina. During rapid atrial pacing after ergonovine, 11 of the 12 patients with a history of angina experienced their typical chest pain, in contrast to only 1 of 12 patients in the other group. The angina group had significantly lower great cardiac vein flow and higher coronary resistance, significant widening of the cardiac arterial-venous oxygen difference and a significant fall in cardiac index during pacing. The investigators concluded that patients with dilated cardiomyopathy and chest pain exhibited impaired vasodilator responses to both metabolic and pharmacologic stimuli and an increased sensitivity to the vasoconstriction effects of ergonovine. Thus, functional abnormalities superimposed on structural cardiac dysfunction can evoke differing clinical symptoms.

The systolic and diastolic hemodynamic abnormalities discussed above are those observed at rest. More recently, functional and structural changes at both the cardiac and peripheral level have been described during exercise in heart failure.

Exercise intolerance in heart failure

Physical activity requires an augmentation of cardiac output so that adequate oxygen is delivered to the exercising muscles. In patients with heart disease, cardiac output may not rise appropriately during exercise. In a classic paper,

Dr. Weber and his associates assessed the hemodynamic response to exercise in 62 patients with heart failure, correlating the noninvasive determinations of aerobic capacity with measurements of cardiac output, oxygen extraction and lactate production [19]. The degree of circulatory dysfunction was graded according to the maximum oxygen uptake ($\dot{V}O2max$) achieved during exercise. Four classes were defined: class A ($\dot{V}O2max > 20\,ml/kg/min$), class B ($16-20\,ml/kg/min$), class C ($10-15\,ml/kg/min$) and class D ($< 10\,ml/kg/min$). Interestingly, there was no difference in cardiac index at rest for class B, C or D patients. However, exercise cardiac output was significantly different between the classes. Moreover, although resting systemic oxygen extraction was greater in the sickest patients (class D) compared to class B or C patients, maximal values for oxygen extraction were greater than 70% in each class. Since $\dot{V}O2max$ is determined by maximal cardiac output and by maximal oxygen extraction, this landmark paper provided investigators with an objective, reproducible, non-invasive means of approximating peak cardiac output in patients with heart failure. In the absence of significant pulmonary disease or anemia, and, assuming that oxygen extraction is maximal at the end of symptom-limited exercise, $\dot{V}O2max$ measured during exercise with rapidly responding O2 and CO2 analyzers is equivalent to maximal cardiac output. The authors also suggested that improvements in $\dot{V}O2max$ following an intervention, such as drug therapy or a regurgitant valve repair, could be used to document non-invasively an overall salutary hemodynamic effect of the intervention.

With the recognition that severity of CHF could be correlated with maximal cardiac output, which in turn could be assessed by the measurement of $\dot{V}O2max$, a number of important observations were made with regard to the mechanisms of exercise intolerance in CHF. Colucci *et al.* investigated the pathophysiology responsible for the attenuated heart rate response during exercise in patients with CHF [20]. They found that peak exercise heart rate and the increment in heart rate from rest to peak exercise was decreased in CHF, and both correlated strongly with peak $\dot{V}O2$. Peak exercise norepinephrine level and the increment in norepinephrine from rest to peak exercise were not attenuated in these same patients, however, although resting norepinephrine was elevated and correlated inversely with peak $\dot{V}O2$. The authors interpreted these data to suggest that the attenuated heart rate response to exercise in CHF patients is due to post-synaptic desensitization of the beta-adrenergic receptor pathway. As will be discussed later, modulation of the beta-adrenergic sympathetic nervous system is an important marker for the severity of chronic heart failure.

Sullivan and his associates studied the central hemodynamic, leg blood flow, and metabolic responses to maximal upright bicycle exercise in 30 patients with CHF and in 12 normal subjects [21]. At peak exercise, patients demonstrated reduced oxygen consumption, ($\dot{V}O2max$ 15.1 versus 32.1 ml/kg/min), cardiac output and mean systemic arterial blood pressure compared with normal subjects. Leg blood flow was decreased in patients at rest; peak exercise leg blood flow was related to peak exercise cardiac output in CHF patients. Mean systemic arterial blood pressure was no different in the two groups at rest or at matched submaximal work rates, whereas leg vascular resistance was higher in patients compared with normal subjects. Thus, in patients with CHF, skeletal muscle perfusion is decreased at rest and during exercise, and local vascular resistance is increased. The authors suggested a role for reflex-mediated peripheral vasoconstriction in linking the cardiac output and skeletal muscle blood flow response to exercise in patients with heart failure.

There is a large body of evidence to suggest that exercise intolerance in CHF is due not only to limitations of cardiac output but by peripheral maladaptive mechanisms as well, reviewed in another chapter of this book. Intense research has focused on the central cardiopulmonary response to exertion in patients with left ventricular dysfunction, however. For example, Roubin and colleagues examined hemodynamic and metabolic changes at rest and during exercise in 23 patients with chronic heart failure and in 6 control subjects [22]. At rest, heart rate, right atrial and pulmonary wedge pressure were higher in patients compared to controls; cardiac output, stroke volume, work indexes and ejection fraction were lower; mean arterial and systemic resistance were similar. During all phases of exercise, patients exhibited higher pulmonary wedge pressure, systemic vascular resistance and pulmonary vascular resistance. Cardiac output was consistently lower during exercise in the CHF patients. Femoral venous lactate and pH values were higher than values in control subjects but when normalized for respective levels of maximal exercise were similar between patients and subjects. Ventilation in relation to oxygen consumption was higher in patients with failure than in control subjects. Keren *et al.* studied left ventricular performance in 17 patients with severe CHF during isometric exercise [23]. Isometric exercise at 30% of maximum resulted in a decrease in stroke volume index with a significant increase in heart rate and in systemic vascular resistance. A significant rise in pulmonary capillary wedge pressure was associated with a marked increase in mitral regurgitant volume. The increase in mitral regurgitant volume induced by isometric exercise was correlated with the fall in forward stroke volume. Thus, they observed that the rise in systemic arterial pressure which accompanied isometric exercise is associated with a decrease in cardiac performance attributable to redistribution of total left ventricular output with an increase in mitral regurgitation and a decrease in forward cardiac output. Other investigators have, likewise, examined the effect of various forms of exercise on central hemodynamics. Gibbs and colleagues utilized long-term continuous pulmonary artery pressure monitoring during normal daiiy activities in 9 patients with chronic heart failure [24]. They found that the mean maximal pulmonary diastolic pressure was 27.8 mm Hg on treadmill exercise, 25.5 mm Hg on bicycle exercise, 24.9 mm Hg walking up and down stairs and 20.4 mm Hg walking on a flat surface. The increase in pulmonary artery pressure did not correlate with the severity of the limiting symptoms except during walking on a flat surface. Moreover, they noted that neither symptoms nor pulmonary artery pressure during maximal exercise is the same as during daily activities. In summary, it is clear that an examination of only cardiac output changes during exercise in patients with heart failure would be misleading with respect to the host of other central and peripheral adaptations which are occurring.

The sympathetic nervous system in heart failure

Congestive heart failure is associated with marked dysfunction of the sympathetic nervous system which contributes importantly to the clinical expression of the syndrome. As reviewed by Daly and Sole [25], the content of cardiac norepinephrine stores becomes depressed as heart failure progresses. However, the depletion of catecholamines is non-uniform throughout the myocardium. The noradrenergic loss is so sustained in some areas of the failing heart that there is even destruction of the cardiac sympathetic nerve terminals, whereas other areas of the myocardium are richly innervated. The pathogenesis of the destruction of cardiac sympathetic nerve terminals in CHF is unknown. Adrenergic receptors are also affected by myocardial dysfunction. The number of beta-1-receptors are reduced in patients with CHF, whereas beta-2 and alpha-1-receptors do not appear to be subject to this same down regulation process. Receptor down regulation may result from the chronic exposure of beta-1-receptors to high circulating norepinephrine levels or norepinephrine from adjacent nerve terminals. The functional importance of the decreased receptor number is demonstrated by the attenuated contractile response observed when isoproterenol is applied *in vitro* to myocardium taken from patients with heart failure [26].

Cardiac sympathetic tone is regulated by a stream of afferent neural signals that are integrated in the cardiovascular centers of the central nervous system [25]. The increase in sympathetic activity seen in heart failure partially reflects a breakdown in this control system. Moreover, although circulating levels of norepinephrine appear to correlate with survival [27] they do not accurately relate to the etiology of heart failure or to the extent of hemodynamic abnormalities observed. Excessive sympathetic stimulation may be responsible in part for both the systolic and diastolic dysfunction seen in CHF. Cardiac diastolic function may be adversely affected by catecholamine-induced sinus tachycardia which shortens the diastolic filling period [28]. In animal models, catecholamines stimulate myocardial hypertrophy and predispose to atrial and ventricular arrhythmia [29]. The heterogeneous sympathetic innervation of the failing heart might be expected to produce minute areas of asynchronous myocardial contraction. In short, the failing heart exhibits both anatomic and functional defects in its sympathetic innervation and adrenergic receptor function. Understanding these pathogenetic mechanisms has ushered in an exciting new approach to the management of patients with symptomatic heart failure.

The use of long-term beta-blockade in some forms of dilated cardiomyopathy was first introduced by Dr. Waagstein in 1975 [30]. A number of subsequent studies published have confirmed the original observations. Most recently, Dr. Waagstein and his colleagues have published a detailed study of 33 patients with dilated cardiomyopathy and severe heart failure to evaluate the short and long-term effect of beta-adrenergic blockade with metoprolol [31]. Twenty-six of 33 patients survived more than 6 months. Mean functional class improved from 3.3 to 1.8, while left ventricular ejection fraction increased from 24% to 42%. Likewise, there was a significant decrease in left-ventricular end-diastolic dimension, mitral regurgitation, pulmonary wedge pressure, left ventricular end-diastolic pressure and systemic vascular resistance. These salutary results were accompanied by a significant increase in systolic blood pressure, cardiac index and left ventricular stroke work index. Withdrawal of metoprolol resulted in a decrease in ejection fraction, followed by an improvement with readministration of metoprolol. Patients had a low number of ventricular beta-adrenergic receptors compared with healthy control subjects, but long-term treatment with metoprolol caused a moderate up regulation. The authors concluded that metoprolol had a beneficial clinical and hemodynamic long-term effect in these severely ill patients.

Bucindolol, a nonselective beta-antagonist with mild vasodilatory properties, was equally effective in 15 patients with various degrees of heart failure after 3 months of therapy [32]. Left ventricular ejection fraction increased from 23% to 29%, and end-systolic elastance, a relatively load-independent determinant of contractility, significantly increased from 0.60 to 1.11 mm Hg/ml. Moreover, the time constant of left ventricular isovolumic relaxation was significantly reduced by bucindolol therapy. Eichhorn and associates concluded that beta-blockade significantly improves myocardial contractility and minute work, but not at the expense of myocardial oxygen consumption. In addition, bucindolol appeared to improve myocardial relaxation. These data promise to expand our ability to alter the neurohormonal consequences of a depression in cardiac output so that the symptoms of CHF are delayed or even prevented. Ongoing, multicenter trials will elucidate further the number of patients who may benefit from this form of therapy.

Cardiac response to drug therapy

The goals of therapy in the management of patients with symptomatic left ventricular dysfunction are to identify and reverse exacerbating or precipitating factors; improve central hemodynamics; alleviate orthopnea and edema; enhance exercise performance; and prolong survival. The determinants of a response to a given therapy are multiple, complex, and not completely understood, and are the focus of intense investigation. For the purpose of this chapter, the central hemodynamic characteristics of given pharmacologic interventions will be discussed.

As mentioned earlier, one of the hemodynamic hallmarks of the failing heart is a maintenance of a normal cardiac output by the augmentation of end-diastolic volume or preload. This dependence on an expanded intravascular volume results in the clinical symptoms of dyspnea and edema. The premise upon which vasodilator therapy is based is that alteration in load will allow a decrease in filling pressures without a concomitant drop in forward cardiac output. This was explored in a study by Warner–Stevenson and Tillisch [33]. They followed the hemodynamic response to vasodilator and diuretic therapy in 25 patients with severe CHF symptoms and poor left ventricular function to determine the lowest ventricular filling pressure which could be achieved while maintaining cardiac output. In 20 of 25 patients, normal pulmonary capillary wedge pressures were achieved, while stroke volume increased from 39 ml at baseline to 60 ml at the peak hemodynamic response. For each patient, stroke volume and stroke work index were maintained and were often maximal at the lowest wedge pressure obtained. This study demonstrates the marked responsiveness of the failing ventricle to manipulations of the loading conditions imposed upon it.

However, there are factors which have been shown to interfere with a beneficial or significant response to therapy. Feldman and associates studied the effects of different classes of inotropic drugs on human myocardium *in vitro*, taken from patients with end-stage heart failure, and compared the responses to muscle from nonfailing, control hearts [34]. They found that the peak isometric force developed with added extracellular calcium reached control levels in the myocardium from patients with CHF, but the time course of contraction and rate of relaxation was greatly prolonged. The inotropic effectiveness of the beta-adrenergic agonist isoproterenol and the phosphodiesterase inhibitors milrinone and caffeine were markedly reduced in the failing muscles. In contrast, the effectiveness of inotropic stimulation with acetylstrophanthidin and the adenylate cyclase activator forskolin was preserved. Acetylstrophanthidin acts by mechanisms independent of cyclic AMP, while forskolin increased intracellular cyclic AMP levels through direct activation of adenylate cyclase. On the other hand, drugs which act via sarcolemmal receptors to increase intracellular cyclic AMP show diminished effectiveness, as seen with extracellular calcium, isoproterenol and milrinone. The authors concluded that an abnormality in cyclic AMP production may be a fundamental defect present in patients with severe heart failure which impacts greatly on the response to a given inotropic agent.

In addition to a down-regulation or reduction of beta-adrenoceptors, discussed earlier, which occurs in the failing heart, there is accumulating evidence that other alterations take place as well. The G-proteins play a pivotal role in the regulation of a number of physiologic processes, such as inhibition or stimulation of adenylate cyclase activity or gating of ionic channels [35]. The G-proteins can be divided into the inhibitory quanine-nucleotide-binding protein α-subunits (Giα) and stimulatory α-subunits (Gsα). Bohm and his colleagues designed a study to investigate whether there were alterations of Giα that depend on the underlying pathogenesis of heart failure [36]. They found an increase of Giα from hearts with idiopathic dilated cardiomyopathy but not from hearts with ischemic cardiomyopathy, despite the reduction in number of beta-adrenoceptors being similarly reduced in both groups. In both types of heart failure there was a marked reduction of the positive inotropic responses to isoproterenol and milrinone, but there was a further reduction in the dilated cardiomyopathic hearts compared to the ischemic ones. It was concluded that the increase of Gi is accompanied by a reduction of basal and guanine-nucleotide-stimulated adenylate cyclase activity, and is more functionally relevant in dilated cardiomyopathy than in ischemic cardiomyopathy. These findings may account for the differing effects of inotropic agents often observed in the two disease states.

Other functional alterations in cardiac performance determine response to therapy besides those described at the sub-cellular level. Keren and co-workers examined the effect of mitral regurgitation during treatment with dobutamine or intravenous nitroglycerine in 12 patients with severe CHF [37]. They found that both dobutamine, a positive inotrope, and nitroglycerine, a pure vasodilator, significantly decreased mitral regurgitant volume from 18 to 11 ml at rest, while forward stoke volume significantly increased from 46 to 55 ml. Moreover, in patients with at least moderately severe mitral regurgitation, both drugs decreased mitral regurgitant volume during exercise, counteracting the normal deleterious effect of exercise on the degree of mitral regurgitation in patients with severe failure. Thus, the presence and severity of functional mitral regurgitation seems to be a determinant of the hemodynamic response to acute inotropic and vasodilator therapy.

A potential disadvantage of the use of inotropic agents to improve contractility in the failing heart is that myocardial oxygen consumption may be adversely elevated and cause myocardial anaerobiosis. Sundram *et al.* examined myocardial energetics and efficiency in patients with idiopathic dilated cardiomyopathy during incremental dosing with dobutamine alone and with dobutamine in combination with amrinone [38]. They found that despite a marked augmentation of cardiac index and minute work, myocardial oxygen consumption remained constant. Myocardial lactate extraction rose significantly but no patient had net lactate efflux into the coronary sinus, and myocardial efficiency continuously improved. The investigators summarized their work by noting that dobutamine and the combination of amrinone and dobutamine had additive beneficial effects on ventricular performance without adversely effecting myocardial oxygen consumption or lactate production and with a resultant improvement in efficiency.

The above studies and numerous other investigations have documented that, even in patients with severe left ventricular dysfunction, a substantial amount of myocardial reserve can be stimulated by appropriate inotropic or vasodilator therapy so that cardiac hemodynamics are significantly improved.

However, these hemodynamic changes must translate into an enhanced delivery of oxygen to the metabolizing tissues in order to reverse the clinical symptomatology of patients with heart failure. Increasing evidence suggests that not all forms of therapy result in short or long-term relief of dyspnea, fatigue or exercise intolerance for patients. For example, Mancini *et al.* examined the effect of dobutamine on skeletal muscle metabolism at rest and during exercise using phosphorus-31 magnetic resonance spectroscopy and femoral vein blood flow in 7 patients with CHF [39]. During exercise, dobutamine increased femoral venous blood flow and femoral venous oxygen saturation, indicative of improved total leg blood flow. However, dobutamine did not change the relation between systemic oxygen uptake and the leg inorganic phosphate to phosphocreatine relation, and did not change muscle pH, suggesting no improvement in blood flow to active skeletal muscle. It appears, therefore, that our next important challenge will be more than the augmentation of cardiac output at rest with various forms of therapy. Our goal will be to insure that oxygen delivery to the exercising skeletal muscles is improved simultaneous to the increased cardiac output following pharmacologic intervention.

References

1. Braunwald E, Colucci WS. Evaluating the efficacy of new inotropic agents. J Am Coll Cardiol 1984;3:1570–4.
2. Coralli RJ, Gravanis MB. Heart failure. In: Gravanis (ed), Cardiovascular pathophysiology. New York: McGraw-Hill Book Company; 1987: 379–418.
3. Parmley WW. Pathophysiology and current therapy of congestive heart failure. J Am Coll Cardiol 1989;13:771–85.
4. Caforio ALP, Bonifacio E, Stewart JT *et al*. Novel organ-specific circulating cardiac autoantibodies in dilated cardiomyopathy. J Am Coll Cardiol 1990;15:1527–34.
5. Limas CJ, Goldenberg IF, Limas C. Effect of cardiac transplantation on anti-beta-receptor antibodies in idiopathic dilated cardiomyopathy. Am J Cardiol 1989;63:1134–7.
6. Goff S, Andersen D, Hansson V. Beta adrenoceptor density and adenylate cyclase response in right atrial and left ventricular myocardium of patients with mitral valve disease. Cardiovasc Res 1986;20:331–6.
7. Katz AM. Cardiomyopathy of overload. A major determinant of prognosis in congestive heart failure. N Engl J Med 1990; 322: 100–0.
8. Weber KT. Cardiac interstitium in health and disease. The fibrillar collagen network. J Am Coll Cardiol 1989;13:1637–52.
9. Weber KT, Clark WA, Janicki JS *et al*. Physiologic versus pathologic hypertrophy and the pressure-overloaded myocardium. J Cardiovasc Pharmacol 1987;10(Suppl 6):537–49.
10. Hoeven KH van, Factor SM. A comparison of the pathologic spectrum of hypertensive, diabetic, and hypertensive-diabetic heart disease. Circulation 1990;82:848–55.
11. Bortone AS, Hess OM, Chiddo A *et al*. Functional and structural abnormalities in patients with dilated cardiomyopathy. J Am Coll Cardiol 1989;14:613–23.
12. Iskandrian AS, Hakki AH, Kane S. Resting Thallium-201 myocardial perfusion patterns in patients with severe left ventricular dysfunction: Differences between patients with primary cardiomyopathy, chronic coronary artery disease, or acute myocardial infarction. Am Heart J 1986;111:760–7.

13. Leithe ME, Margorien RD, Hermiller JB *et al.* Relationship between central hemodynamics and regional blood flow in normal subjects and in patients with congestive heart failure. Circulation 1984;69:57–64.
14. Vanoverschelde JJ, Raphael DA, Robert AR *et al.* Left ventricular filling in dilated cardiomyopathy: relation to functional class and hemodynamics. J Am Coll Cardiol 1990;15:1288–95.
15. Hirota Y, Shimizu G, Kaku K *et al.* Mechanisms of compensation and decompensation in dilated cardiomyopathy. Am J Cardiol 1984;54:1033–8.
16. Cohn JN, Archibald DG, Ziesche S *et al.* Effect of vasodilator therapy in mortality in chronic congestive heart failure: results of a veterans administration cooperative-study (V-HeFt). N Engl J Med 1986;314:1547–52.
17. The CONSENSUS Triai Study Group. Effects of enalapril on mortality in severe congestive heart failure. N Engl J Med 1987;316:1429–35.
18. Cannon RO, Cunnion RE, Parrillo JE *et al.* Dynamic limitation of coronary vasodilator reserve in patients with dilated cardiomyopathy and chest pain. J Am Coll Cardiol 1987;10:1190–200.
19. Weber KT, Kinasewitz GT, Janicki JS *et al.* Oxygen utilization and ventilation during exercise in patients with chronic cardiac failure. Circulation 1982;65:1213–23.
20. Colucci WS, Ribeiro JP, Rocco MB *et al.* Impaired chronotropic response to exercise in patients with congestive heart failure. Role of postsynaptic B-adrenergic desensitization. Circulation 1989;80:314–23.
21. Sullivan MJ, Knight JD, Higginbotham MB *et al.* Relation between central and peripheral hemodynamics during exercise in patients with chronic heart failure. Muscle blood flow is reduced with maintenance of arterial perfusion pressure. Circulation 1989;80:769–81.
22. Roubin GS, Anderson SD, Shen WF *et al.* Hemodynamic and metabolic basis of impaired exercise tolerance in patients with severe left ventricular dysfunction. J Am Coll Cardiol 1990;15:986–94.
23. Keren G, Katz S, Gage J *et al.* Effect of isometric exercise on cardiac performance and mitral regurgitation in patients with severe congestive heart failure. Am Heart J 1989;118:973–9.
24. Gibbs JSR, Keegan J, Wright C *et al.* Pulmonary artery pressure changes during exercise and daily activities in chronic heart failure. J Am Coll Cardiol 1990;15:52–61.
25. Daly PA, Sole MJ. Myocardial catecholamines and the pathophysiology of heart failure. Circulation 1990;82(Suppl I):I35–43.
26. Colucci WS. *In vivo* studies of myocardial beta-adrenergic receptor pharmacology in patients with congestive heart failure. Circulation 1990;82(Suppl I):I44–51.
27. Cohn JN, Levine TB, Olivari MT *et al.* Plasma norepinephrine as a guide to prognosis in patients with congestive heart failure. N Engl J Med 1984;311:819–23.
28. Walsh RA. Sympathetic control of diastolic function in congestive heart failure. Circulation 1990;82(Suppl I):I52–8.
29. Podrid PJ, Fuchs T, Candinas R. Role of the sympathetic nervous system in the genesis of ventricular arrhythmia. Circulation 1990;82(Suppl I):I103–13.
30. Waagstein F, Hjalmarson A, Varnauskas E *et al.* Effect of chronic beta-adrenergic receptor blockade in congestive cardiomyopathy. Br Heart J 1975;37:1022–36.
31. Waagstein F, Caidahl K, Wallentin I *et al.* Long-term Beta-blockade in dilated cardiomyopathy. Effects of short and long-term metoprolol treatment followed by withdrawal and readministration of metoprolol. Circulation 1989;80:551–63.
32. Eichhorn EJ, Bedotto JB, Malloy CR *et al.* Effect of beta-adrenergic blockade on myocardial function and energetics in congestive heart failure. Improvements in hemodynamic, contractile, and diastolic performance with bucindolol. Circulation 1990;82:473–83.
33. Warner-Stevenson L, Tillisch JH. Maintenance of cardiac output with normal filling pressures in patients with dilated heart failure. Circulation 1986;74:1303–8.
34. Feldman MD, Copelas L, Gwathmey JK *et al.* Deficient production of cyclic AMP pharmacologic evidence of an important cause of contractile dysfunction in patients with end-stage heart failure. Circulation 1987;75:331–9.

35. Gilman AG. G proteins and dual control of adenylate cyclase. Cell 1984;36:577–9.
36. Bohm M, Gierschik P, Jakobs K *et al*. Increase of Gi in human hearts with dilated but not ischemic cardiomyopathy. Circulation 1990;82:1249–65.
37. Keren G, Katz S, Strom J. *et al*. Dynamic mitral regurgitation. An important determinant of the hemodynamic response to load alterations and inotropic therapy in severe heart failure. Circulation 1989;80:306–13.
38. Sundram P, Reddy HK, McElroy PA *et al*. Myocardial energetics and efficiency in patients with idiopathic cardiomyopathy: response to dobutamine and amrinone. Am Heart J 1990;119:891–8.
39. Mancini DM, Schwartz M, Ferraro N *et al*. Effect of dobutamine on skeletal muscle metabolism in patients with congestive heart failure. Am J Cardiol 1990;65:1121–6.

15. Cardiac output in systemic hypertension

ABDUL-MAJEED SALMASI

Systemic hypertension is a complicated syndrome resulting from a complicated and widely distributed pathophysiological mechanism involving the cardiovascular system. A wide variety of changes do take place in various parts or systems namely the blood volume, intravascular volume, peripheral resistance and cardiac output. Other systems may also be involved such as those associated with renin and aldosterone secretion.

The arterial blood pressure is a hemodynamic variable and its elevation as a pathophysiological entity takes place as a result of failure of one or more of such variables which under normal physiological circumstances interplay in such a way in order to keep the arterial blood pressure under a control level of normal range. Hence an elevated arterial blood pressure is only a clinical sign of a rather widely distributed "syndrome" that could involve, and may well result from changes in different systems of the body. Whatever the cause for the elevated blood pressure (except in the case of coarctation of the aorta), the basic mechanism will be a failure to control the vascular resistance. This, in turn, will result in damaging the arteries, hence vascular diseases do result; the latter is responsible for the morbidity as a consequence of involvement of these organs such as the heart, kidneys, brain and the retina.

Hemodynamic changes are not only noted in the arterial system; however, veins and capillaries are involved too. Proximal capillary pressure and venular tone are determined by the degree of arteriolar constriction. Veins below heart level act as capacitance vessels and help in determining central blood volume which correlates well with cardiac output.

Mechanisms which play an important role in determining the hemodynamic changes associating systemic hypertension are sympathetic activity and renal mechanism in addition, in certain circumstances, to certain diseases with which hypertension is associated. The sympathetic activity is the major factor that determines many of the hemodynamic variables observed in hypertension as it influences myocardial contractility and heart rate and hence the cardiac output. It also influences arteriolar tone, outflow resistance, venous capacity and central blood volume. The renal mechanisms, on the other hand, regulate the extracellular fluid volume while angiotensin II is produced by the juxtaglomurular apparatus which in turn increases arteriolar tone, influences sympathetic nervous function and affects aldosterone production.

A.-M. Salmasi and A.S. Iskandrian (eds): Cardiac output and regional flow in health and disease, 169–173.
© 1993 *Kluwer Academic Publishers. Printed in the Netherlands.*

The latter *per se* provides an obvious influence on the fluid and electrolyte balance and bears an independent effect on the renal excretion of salt and water. These mechanisms are closely interrelated as can be seen from that the activity of the nervous system influences renin release. The renal pressor system in turn plays a role in determining the degree of sympathetic nervous activity both centrally and peripherally [1].

The main determinants of the mean arterial blood pressure (MABP) are cardiac output (CO) and peripheral resistance (PR) as can be seen from the formula

$$MABP = CO \times PR.$$

Therefore one can assume that under normal physiological circumstances, in the presence of an increased cardiac output, the blood pressure can be kept under control only if there is a fall in the peripheral resistance. Cardiac output can rise due to an increase in myocardial contractility (which is the case in borderline and mild hypertension) and an elevated pulmonary volume in relation to the total blood volume. Peripheral resistance, on the other hand, is controlled by local humoral and neural factors. All arteries are profusely supplied by adrenergic nerves which provide for vasoconstriction and an increased neural tone has been noted in mild, but not in severe, hypertension [1].

In this chapter, only changes in cardiac output and related factors will be discussed in various types of hypertension.

Essential hypertension

Borderline or mild hypertension

Although it is not a constant hemodynamic change, cardiac output rises but only slightly in a substantial number of patients. This takes place against a normal peripheral resistance [1]. An increase in both the stroke volume and the heart rate contributes to the elevated cardiac output noted in this class of hypertensives [2, 3]. It has been reported that cardiopulmonary blood volume/total blood volume ratio (CPBV/TBV) increases in this class of hypertensives. This is mainly due to redistribution of intravascular volume from peripheral veins to cardiopulmonary capacitance bed [3].

Moderate and severe hypertension

The hemodynamic changes in these two types of hypertension depend very much upon the presence or absence of cardiac enlargement and the degree of vasoconstriction [4]. In moderate hypertension without cardiac enlargement cardiac output is kept within normal limits while there is an increase in the peripheral resistance. A progressive decrease in the cardiac output and increase in the peripheral resistance are noted when hypertension becomes more severe and becomes associated with cardiac enlargement.

Following regression of left ventricular hypertrophy in patients with essential hypertension as a result of treatment with antihypertensive medications, Panayiotou and associates (1991) reported no change in left ventricular function [5]. The authors reported regression of left ventricular mass in 9 out of 13 hypertensive patients within 6 months of therapy with methyldopa and enalpril; this was associated with a significant reduction in blood pressure. However no significant change was reported in the ejection fraction or cardiac output both at rest and at maximal exercise as measured by radionuclide ventriculography.

The status of left ventricular function in normotensives with a positive family history of hypertension has not been studied until the report of Graettinger and associates in 1990 [6]. The authors studied 16 adolescents with positive family history of hypertension compared to 21 subjects without such a history. Although body weight was higher in the group with a positive family history of hypertension than in the group without a family history of hypertension, no significant difference was noted between the two groups in left ventricular wall thickness or left ventricular mass. However a lower stroke volume and a higher peripheral resistance were noted in the subjects with a positive family history of hypertension.

When hypertension becomes severe one of the regional circulations which will suffer most is the renal circulation when renal flow becomes reduced. This in turn will lead to a further enhancement of the renin production hence further vasoconstriction will result.

In moderate and severe hypertension there is a reduction in plasma volume [7] while the extracellular fluid volume remains unchanged. Therefore a diminished plasma volume/interstitial fluid volume ratio results [1]. This reflects an overall decrease in vascular capacity.

In patients with severe hypertension the plasma renin activity is elevated [8]. However in some patients with established hypertension plasma renin activity is low although there is no clear knowledge of its significance [1].

Renovascular hypertension

The incidence of this type of hypertension is variable and depends upon the population studied. The severity of the elevation of the blood pressure is also variable and can range from a borderline to a severe or even accelerated type.

In renovascular hypertension there is a slight increase in cardiac output even in severe cases of this type of hypertension. This is associated with a slight elevation in the peripheral resistance [9]. The hypertension is not due to the increase in cardiac output because it was noted that following renal revascularisation the decrease in the peripheral resistance is not associated with a change in the cardiac output [1]. There is a slight increase in heart rate and stroke volume. Plasma volume is decreased [10].

Hypertension associated with renal parenchymal disease

In acute glomerulonephritis the hypertension results from fluid retention [1] and a hyperdynamic circulation therefore results in elevated cardiac output. The peripheral resistance is a factor of much variation and vary according to different studies; it is either normal or slightly increased or slightly decreased. In acute glomerulonephritis failure of the peripheral circulation to respond to the increased cardiac output is another hemodynamic mechanism [11, 12]. This is because the plasma volume which is expected to be elevated as a result of the edema is normal. In renal parenchymal disease with normal renal function, a normal cardiac output and elevated peripheral resistance were reported [13].

In uremic patients with renin-dependant hypertension there is a decrease in cardiac output with rather raised peripheral resistance [14]. However in uremic patients with salt and water dependant hypertension, cardiac output is increased and the peripheral resistance is slightly elevated.

Hypertension associated with primary aldosteronism

As expected due to the excess aldosterone this type of hypertension is salt and water dependant. Cardiac output is elevated but negatively correlated with the level of the blood pressure [1]. The increase in plasma volume and total blood volume is positively correlated with cardiac output but negatively correlated with arterial blood pressure and peripheral resistance. In patients with mild to moderate hypertension due to primary aldosteronism an elevated cardiac output and raised plasma volume are thus expected. The elevated cardiac output is mainly due to increased heart rate and a normal stroke volume. A normal plasma catecholamine could suggest that the increased heart rate represents an increased sympathetic drive to the heart. In severe hypertension, on the other hand, a normal cardiac output and elevated peripheral resistance will be noted.

Pheochromocytoma

Orthostatic hypotension is a common finding in this type of hypertension. This is because the neural control of the blood pressure and the circulation is taken over by the increased circulating catecholamines. Cardiac output is either normal or elevated. The plasma renin activity is elevated [15]. The generalized vasoconstrictor effect of the catecholamines results in a reduced plasma volume.

References

1. Dustan HP. Pathophysiology of hypertension. In: Hurst JW (ed), The heart. 6th ed. New York: McGraw Hill Book Company, 1986:1038–48.
2. Julius S, Esler MD, Randall OS. Role of the autonomic nervous system in mild human hypertension. Clin Sci Mol Med 1975;48:234s.
3. Safar M, Weiss YA, London GM *et al*. Cardiopulmonary blood volume in borderline hypertension. Clin Sci Mol Med 1974;47:153.
4. Frolich ED, Kozul VJ, Tarazi RC *et al*. Physiological comparison of labile and essential hypertension. Circ Res 1970;26(Suppl 1):55.
5. Panayiotou H, Benjamin F, Kroenberg MW. Regression of hypertrophy causes no change in ventricular function in patients with essential hypertension. J Am Coll Cardiol 1991;17(Suppl A):177A.
6. Graettinger WF, Cheung DG, Neutel JM *et al*. Cardiovascular characteristics of normotensive adolescents with a family history of hypertension. J Am Coll Cardiol 1990;15:184A.
7. The 1984 report of the Joint National Committee on detection evaluation and treatment of high blood pressure. Arch Intern Med 1984;Vol 144.
8. Laragh JH. Vasoconstriction-Volume analysis for understanding and treating hypertension: the use of renin and aldosterone profiles. Am J Med 1973;55:261.
9. Dustan HP, Tarazi RC, Bravo EL. Physiologic characteristics of hypertension. Am J Med 1972;52:610.
10. Dustan HP, Tarazi RC, Frolich ED. Functional correlates of plasma renin activity in hypertensive patients. Circulation 1970;41:555.
11. DeFazio V, Cristensen RC, Regal TJ *et al*. Circulatory changes in acute glomerulonephritis. Circulation 1959;20:190.
12. Fleisher DS, Voci G, Garfunkel J *et al*. Hemodynamic findings in acute glomerulonephritis. J Pediatr 1966;69:1054.
13. Frolich ED, Tarazi RC, Dustan HP. Hemodynamic and functional mechanisms in two renal hypertensions: arterial and pyelonephritis. Am J Med Sci 1971;261:189.
14. Onesti G, Kim KE, Greco JS *et al*. Blood pressure regulation in end-state renal disease and anephric man. Circ Res 1975;36/37(Suppl 1):145.
15. Maebashi M, Miura Y, Yoshinaga K *et al*. Plasma renin activity in pheochromocytoma. Jpn Cir J 1968;32:1427.

PART FOUR

Cardiac output in the critically ill patient

16. Cardiac output in the critically ill surgical patient

FAWZI P. HABBOUSHE

It is important to recognise that oxygen delivery at a cellular level is a paramount function of the cardiovascular system. To the extent that it is a function of the cardiac output and can be estimated or measured it makes for a valuable trackable sign in the relevant situation. This chapter assumes an understanding of monitoring methods and techniques, cardiovascular physiology and pathology well illustrated in other chapters. To a great extent, it avoids lengthy discussions of cardiogenic, septic, pulmonary embolic and neurogenic mechanisms of shock and dysfunction better detailed elsewhere. Suffice it to say that a thorough and longitudinal continuous consideration of the state of all the systems, relevant medications and fluid balance antecedent, during and subsequent to the surgical event and a posture of intelligent anticipation are essential to proper resolution and recovery.

Hard data as to the incidence and strict indications of various monitoring, withholding and discontinuing of the same, across the board, in a group of heterogenous set of patients is not available. Because of the increasing sophistication of medical care and the escalating medicolegal considerations on the one hand and the determined pressures by third parties and others to constrict the financial purse on the other, have all resulted in organized screening of medical care evidenced by supervisory organizations and functions such as utilization reviews and the National Practitioners' Data Bank in the United States. All these considerations not withstanding, there has been medically legitimate reason for classifications of patients according to severity from different perspectives. These classifications have the effect, taken singly or collectively, of providing the basis for the decisions relating to the indications for monitoring. The ultimate in management is the most indispensable physician attribute which is that of clinical judgement.

The reader is encouraged to be familiar with these various classifications of severity of illness. Some of the prevailing classifications are The Therapeutic Intervention Scoring System (TISS) [1, 2]. The Injury Severity Scale (ISS), a primarily anatomical classification modified to include physiologic parameters called (TRISS) [3] and the APACHE (Acute Physiology and Chronic Health Evaluation) scores, directed to the intensive care setting has correlated well with the TISS system [4] and has been updated to the APACHE III [5]. The French have used (SAPS), Simplified Acute Physiologic Score, which has

A.-M. Salmasi and A.S. Iskandrian (eds): Cardiac output and regional flow in health and disease, 177–194.
© 1993 *Kluwer Academic Publishers. Printed in the Netherlands.*

helped in prognostication and therefore implicitly suggesting the use of monitoring [6].

Relevant to the understanding for the need to monitor, it has become a standard during surgery among other things to monitor oxygen saturation by pulse oximetry [7]. This is a non invasive method and obtains important information regarding oxygen content of the blood. Together with the amount of hemoglobin, oxygen saturation are the prime determinants of oxygen content as pO2 otherwise figures very little in this regard. This is so because further increases in pO2 essentially only increases the dissolved oygen, which is negligable.

In many instances, therefore, because of adequate preload and good cardiac function, the cardiac output is assumed to be normal. In these instances clinical assessment and monitoring of vital signs and the above measurements may be adequate. In other instances when information as to preload, cardiac function, and afterload, singly or in combination, are in doubt, or likely to become otherwise unassessable, then further information is needed to determine the adequacy of oxygen delivery to the tissues.

Oxygen delivery, oxygen consumption and oxygen demand

Oxygen delivery, DO2, is the oxygen content (approximated by $13 \times$ Gm Hb $\times$ % Oxygen saturation) multiplied by the cardiac output thus providing the amount of oxygen delivered to the tissues per minute. To obtain this information it is necessary to measure cardiac output with a pulmonary artery (Swan-Ganz) catheter. In addition this device provides for measurements of wedge pressure and to help assess preload as well as provide for mixed venous samples needed in measuring oxygen uptake, which is the amount of oxygen actually utilized by the tissues. This Oxygen uptake (VO2, otherwise also called oxygen consumption to be distinguished from oxygen demand) as measured is very useful in the critically ill. Thus oxygen uptake:

1. Varies as a result of metabolic rate and temperature, 13% for each degree centigrade. Fever increases it and hypothermia decreases it such as might occur with infusion of unwarmed fluids and when the body is exposed or cavities are open for prolonged periods of time as is frequently seen in the operating theater.
2. Decreases with compensatory mechanisms in the hypovolemic and critically ill incident to vasoconstriction and hypoperfusion of vasoactive beds. In this instance oxygen debt is incurred despite increase in the venous oxygen extraction, which is the immediate response of hypoxic tissues. This debt has to be repaid as resuscitation proceeds and the previously constricted vascular beds become better perfused when VO2 increases ultimatlly to levels higher than normal (Figure 16.1).

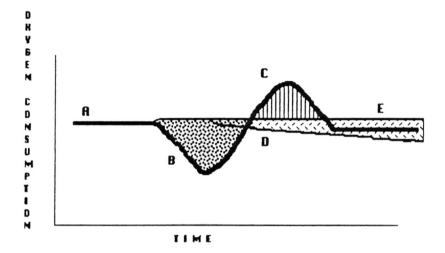

Figure 16.1. Oxygen consumption normal in (A) is reduced as a result of the hypovolemic insult thereby incurring oxygen debt in (B). This deficit is repaid following adequate fluid resuscitation in (C). Exposure and unwarmed fluid replacement causes hypothermia with resulting decrease in oxygen requirement in (D). This shift in oxygen demand incident upon hypothermia biases in favour for a more rapid oxygen repayment. The stippled area (A) should be approximately matched by the vertically hatched area in (B). The cross hatched area between (D) and (E) represents repayment equivalent. Adapted from Siegel JH, Linbeg SE, Wiles III CE. Therapy of low-flow-shock states (Chapter 9). In: Siegel JH (ed), Trauma: emergency surgery and critical care. Churchill Livingstone (publisher, 1987).

3. It is also increased in the well controlled septic patient and in the normal stress response to trauma or surgery (by 15–35%).
4. In the unstable septic patient, the severe critically ill patient and in the severe burn, venous extraction becomes fixed leading to increasing debt that can only be limited by increasing cardiac output. This is very common and is referred to as the flow dependent state of oxygen uptake seen in serious illness (Figure 16.2).
5. Oxygen debt has been shown to be a good predictor of survival at least in the dog hemorrhagic model [8].
6. Unsatisfied oxygen demand is reflected, over time, in oxygen debt and accumulating acid metabolites of anerobic metabolism (Lactate/pyruvate ratio or lactate). Plasma lactate levels underestimates what is in the tissues that are deprived of active perfusion.

Clinical evidence for adequate cardiac output

1. Appropriate mental status.
2. Good skin perfusion as judged by color, capillary refill and absence of perspiration.
3. Good urinary output.

THE RELATIONSHIP OF OXYGEN UPTAKE AND DELIVERY

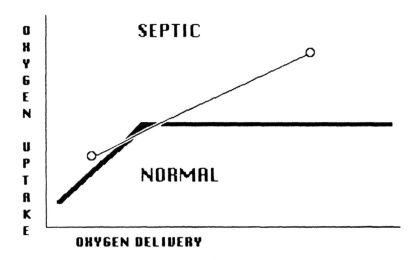

Figure 16.2. In the normal individual oxygen uptake plateaus beyond a certain level of oxygen delivery (bold line). Thus unless significant delivery is curtailed oxygen requirements are met over a large range of delivery values. In the septic patient however oxygen uptake appears to continue to be required despite abundance of oxygen delivery as in (plain line). This probably reflects regional hypoperfusion and areas of yet unmet oxygen debt. Adapted from Danek SJ, Lynch JP, Weg JG *et al.* The dependance of oxygen uptake on oxygen delivery in the adult espiratory distress syndrome. Am Rev Respir Dis 1980; 122:387.

4. Stable cardiovascular function as judged by vital signs.
5. Reliable records of fluid intake and output with consideration for insenssible losses and sequestrations of fluid.

Estimation of blood loss

To simplify estimation of blood volume losses and their effect on hemodynamics, it is convenient to assume an adult blood volume of about five liters and therefore the equivalent of ten units of whole blood. Thus every pint of blood loss represents approximately ten percent of the blood volume, and would ultimately result in a drop of the hematocrit, after fluid repletion, of about three points. The prevalent changes in the vital signs and the state of the subject with graded losses are listed in Table 16.1, simplified from the classes according to the American College of Surgeons classification.

Table 16.1. Classes in acute hemmorhage. Adapted from the classification by the American College of Surgeons.

	N	I	II	III	IV
			Classes		
% Loss	0	15	20	30	40
H.R.	70	>80	>100	>120	>140
B.P.	120/80	118/82	110/80	80/50	>50
Pulse pr.	40	35	30	25	20
Urine O.P. ml/hr.	50	30	25	10	5
Mental		Anxiety		Anxious Confused Lethargic	
Fluids		Crystalloids		Crystalloid and blood	

HR = heart rate (beats per minute); BP = blood pressure in mm Hg; O.P. = output; N = normal; % Loss = percentage of blood volume loss (Pulse pr. = Pulse pressure).

Based on initial presentation of the hypovolemic patient, one unit blood loss (10%) is tolerated well in the normal adult as is frequently observed in the blood donor [9]. Venous capacitance contributes as an autotransfusion and is exhausted by the first 10% of volume loss resulting in small but definite drop in cardiac output. As the loss is increased to 15%, however changes in the vital signs and urinary output begin to reflect compensatory cardiovascular changes with minimal changes in the heart rate and pulse pressure (class I). Loss of 20% (class II) then causes significant drop of urinary output to about half normal (from 50 to 25 cc per hour) assuming no use of diuretics, the heart rate increases by 20 bpm (to >100 bpm) and the pulse pressure further decreases slightly. The patient becomes fairly anxious.

It may be of practical importance to separate classes I & II above from classes III & IV to be described below, in that the former set usually has normal blood pressure in the recumbent position, fair to good urinary output, no mental confusion and require only crystalloid replacement, while the last two have low recumbent blood pressure, poor urinary output, mental confusion and usually require both crystalloid as well as blood.

A severe loss of 30% (class III) causes increase of heart rate by another 20 bpm (to >120 bpm) and the pulse pressure drops by 15 mm Hg but the blood pressure, despite this increment in heart rate of 40–50 bpm, reaches the ranges of the breaking point of an average of 70–90 mm Hg, which is close to the threshold for autoregulation of the brain and the kidneys (about 60 mm Hg). This therefore is responsible for mental confusion and a drop of the urinary output to about 20% of normal (10 cc/hr). Finally an exsanguinating loss of 40% or more of the blood volume (class IV, 4 or more units) results in the shut down blood pressure of 50 or less despite increment in the heart rate of another 20 bpm or more (to 140 or more). Urinary output becomes near nil and the patient becomes lethargic as well as confused.

It is apparent from this table that incremental loss of blood volume and decrease of venous return and stroke volume is compensated for by a fairly linear increase in the heart rate and increases in the systemic vascular resistance (S.V.R.), thereby maintaining a fairly normal blood pressure, in the recumbant position, in classes I and II. Net cardiac output drops from the outset [10]. Despite further contribution of heart rate and S.V.R. and the decrease in pulse pressure in classes III and IV however, would not be sufficient to maintain blood pressure, which begins to fail thereby, infringing on the autoregulatory capacities of the brain and the kidneys. Diastolic pressure fails less quickly due to severe increases in the S.V.R. as reflected in the decrease in pulse pressure. This in the normal heart maintains an edge for cardiac perfusion as coronary perfusion is significantly dependent on diastolic pressure.

Relative to patient assessment in this regard, it is important to note the following:

1. The earliest changes in hypovolemic shock is coolness of the skin and tachycardia. The latter may be blunted in certain individuals, the elderly or due to certain medications such as beta blockers where cardiovascular compensation is limited.
2. These events described are true when hemorrhage occurs in a fairly rapid manner. Thus specific deviations of signs and symptoms, therefore, become blunted or delayed as blood loss occurs more slowly, due to fluid redistribution into the intravascular space or if volume replacement is in progress.
3. Average blood volume is probably closer to five and one half liters rather than five. The simplification is meant to help in rapid assessment rather than for exactness and when blood volumes are to be estimated, one should take into account sex, body habitus, height and weight.
4. The magnitude and distribution of compensatory mechanisms are somewhat variable from subject to subject, particularly when considering all ages. Some might overly vasoconstrict maintaining a relatively normal blood pressure on the expense of oxygen debt and *vice versa* [11].
5. The above classification of blood losses holds best for acute events in the otherwise healthy patient who is not on medications and best typified by the trauma patient entering the emergency department. In this setting the response calls for rapid assessment and management with large bore peripheral lines and fluid administration in addition to and after instituting other vital resuscitative measures such as airway and ventilation frequently referred to as the ABCs of resuscitation.
6. Palpable pulses of the radial, femoral and carotid disappear sequentially

with diminishing blood pressure such that the radial disappears below 80 mm Hg, femoral below 70 mm Hg, and carotid below 60 mm Hg thus allowing for quick assesment of blood pressure.
7. In the trauma patient, in addition to the need to immobilize fractures, their presence signifies possible serious volume losses [12].

(a) Extremities: As the extremity swells with blood it assumes a less cylindrical and a more spherical shape the geometry of which allows for greater hidden looses. A fractured tibia (or humerus) or femur can thus be associated with more than a unit and two units of blood respectively. Assuming even the normal cylindrical shape of an average thigh an increase of 1 cm and 2 cm in radius computes to 2L and 4.5L net volume gain respectively. (b) Thorax: More concealed losses can occur in the chest where up to exsanguinating volumes can be lost. Each hemithorax may contain 2–3 liters of blood. There should be no hesitation therefore to the placement of bilateral chest tubes if necessary to detect losses and replace them, expand the lungs and decide on surgical intervention. (c) Abdomen: Abdominal girth changes can be effected by fluid or gas and reliance on these assessments can be misleading. Suffice it to say that a gain of 1 cm and 2 cm in radius can compute to 3L and 6L gain respectively. Therefore a patient can exsanguinate before measurements can be of any help. (d) Pelvis: Because of the concealed retroperitoneal nature of pelvic bleeding 3 to 4L of blood can be lost without any external manifestations. (e) The cranium cannot be the site of significant loss as minimal losses produce significant central nervous system changes that become the source for attention.

Emergency surgery

In as much as central venous pressure is a reflection of venous return and the performance of the right heart only, great discrepancy may be realized between such measurement and that of blood volume and cardiac output. None the less its measurement and trends can be helpful in the critical setting providing its limitations are recognized. A low reading or minimal change, or decline with fluid administration signifies low blood volume and ongoing losses, respectively. A rapid increase in the C.V.P. or an initial high reading signifies volume repletion or cardiac dysfunction, cardiac tamponade or tension pneumothorax or a combination of all these factors.

Noteworthy is that an initial high reading may be due to rapid volume repletion in the face of peripheral vasoconstriction (reflex from hypovolemia and endogenous or exogenous sources of vasoconstrictors). It is therefore, important to recognize the dynamic changes active at the time and not to ascribe to this measurement impulsive and unwarranted implications as to volume or cardiac function.

Decision making in the patient with acute blood loss, who is otherwise healthy such as in trauma, can be made with central venous pressure measurement and amounts of fluid repletion sufficient to bring about a restitution of volume as judged by vital signs, color, mental status and urinary output:

1. A prompt and sustained response is realized with blood loss of less than 20% of blood volume. In this case crystalloids are sufficient and if stability is maintained no further monitoring to establish cardiac output or other hemodynamic parameters will be necessary barring other compelling factors.
2. A transient response, on the other hand, signifies losses of 20–40%, the patient showing clinical signs of deterioration. In this case further crystalloids and probably blood transfusion is needed with a further evaluation as to the need for operative intervention based on evidence of continued blood loss. Pulmonary artery catheter may be indicated.
3. If minimal response to initial fluid therapy results then a normal or high central venous pressure may imply cardiac or pulmonary causes of shock, such as tamponade, tension pneumothorax, cardiac or valvular failure or pulmonary obstructive condition. Immediate diagnosis and resolution of the cause is imperative. If on the other hand the central venous pressure is low then volume loss and exsanguination is assumed necessitating blood transfusion and immediate surgery. Pulmonary artery catheter may be decided upon after control of the bleeding is accomplished.

The urge to obtain more interpretable hemodynamic readings such as wedge pressure and cardiac output, as indicated above, may have to be temporarily tempered by the frequent activity around the patient, particularly as it relates to the determining of the need for initial stabalization and the execution of operative intervention. When the bleeding source is being actively controlled and observable losses repleted, the surgeon or more usually the anesthesiologist may access with a pulmonary artery catheter thereby wedge pressures, cardiac output and oxygen delivery can be obtained. These are more necessary in the case of significant gastrointestinal bleeds but more particularly in the patient with ruptured aortic aneurysm, where coronary artery disease is a frequent accompaniment.

Not without complications of possible pneumothorax, vascular injury, embolization, thrombosis and infection, the central line can frequently be rapidly inserted, under sterile conditions, and can be later converted, with minimal additional morbidity if certain precautions are observed, to a pulmonary artery catheter, a more nearly useful and faithful tool for hemodynamic monitoring in the critically ill.

The elective surgical patient

Most of the surgery performed every day are of such nature and the effort taken preoperatively is thorough enough that extensive monitoring, particularly invasive types, are deleted. The patient's fluid balance, preoperative and intraoperative such as evaporative and urinary losses as well as blood losses are fairly tightly controlled and replaced appropriately. Fluid and blood losses postoperatively are also fairly well estimated and replaced. In this regard adequate venous access, intake and output records and oximetry along with hemoglobin determination can provide the necessary requisits. Oximetry is the standard of care in the surgical patient who undergoes sedation or anesthesia [7].

More extensive monitoring of wedge pressures, cardiac output and other parameters might be indicated in the following categories:

1. Major intrathoracic, central vascular, or extensive intrabdominal procedures or extensive surgery on an extremity.
2. Cases in which calculations of fluid deficits are subject to errors such as the patient with long prior undeterminable or ongoing fluid losses, long procedures in which evaporative losses and blood loss estimations become doubtful or patients in which interstitial fluid accumulation becomes very significant.
3. Significant cardiac dysfunction, or renal dysfunction present or anticipated, such as coronary artery, valvular disease or cardiac failure or renal failure in the patient undergoing major surgery.
4. The aged undergoing extensive surgery.
5. The malnourished and debilitated, particularly with cancer.
6. The patient with sepsis.
7. Reoperation with major anticipated surgery and protracted recovery.
8. Surgery for extensive burns.

Fluids

Fluid replacement is generally thought of as consisting of two major types:

1. Maintenance fluids.
2. Replacement fluids.

Fluids for *maintainance* generally dextrose 5% or dextrose 5% in 1/2% normal saline, are used to replenish losses from insensible loss due to evaporation incident to respiration, perspiration and urinary output. Intraoperative evaporative loss from an open cavity as well may be included in this category.

Fluids of *replacement* are balanced salt solutions (BSS) with composition near that of the extracellular fluid at least with regard to sodium. Thus so called normal sodium chloride solution or Ringer's lactate solution with or without 5% dextrose are fairly standard. The addition of glucose however, while supplying some calories increases the osmotic load considerably. These fluids are used to replace gastrointestinal losses, third space sequestrational losses and when blood loss is being replaced with crystalloids. When this is done to replace blood loss, three times the volume lost is used because crystalloids diffuse throughout the extracellular space, and also, due to dilution, because of the reduction of intravascular oncotic pressure incident upon this non colloid type of fluid replacement.

Fluid sequestration

In addition to the normal intracellular and extracellular spaces of fluid, operative and trauma sites can contain another space of tissue fluid accumulation. Depending on the magnitude of the inciting cause, as much as 15% of the body weight in fluid could be lost in this manner. This space has to be reckoned with in the calculation for replacement or possible serious volume deficits result. This sequestration begins from the time of the surgery or trauma and continues on for 48 to 72 hrs. Thereafter resolution or persistence of this fluid would depend in large part on whether or not visceral leak or infection ensues that may cause persistence or further accumulation. In the favorable situation this fluid space resolves by absorbtion into the vascular space and excreted in the urine by the third to fifth day postoperatively. Lack of this expected resolution, as judged by an intelligent longitudinal review of the fluid balance, should alert the surgeon of possible complications of leak or infection, or could be used with other available evidence for such possible complications. Similarly the magnitude of its replacement in any case will depend on the magnitude of the surgery and of the deviations in the monitoring parameters chosen for the case along with review of the patient's fluid balance. It is also important to realize that resolution of this fluid space involves temporary expansion of the intravascular volume with its possible risks of overload.

Crystalloid versus colloid

The choice of the type of fluid best suited to the circumstance has been argued intensively and continues to be a heated discussion. In particular this relates to the choice between balanced salt solution versus colloid, as is the main controversy seen in the United States scene. In Europe the controversy more intensively surrounds the type of colloid best suited [13].

In hemorrhagic shock

To be able to understand the rationale of the use of BSS, it is necessary to note that in hemorrhagic volume loss the intravascular volume deficit reflects itself into the extracellular space. This deficit is automatically replaced by the use of BSS, which diffuses fairly freely throughout the extracellular compartments. Contrariwise, transfusion of colloid will fill essentially only the intravascular space. When hypovolemia is accompanied by significant hypotension, cellular dysfunction ensues. This dysfunction consists at least in part of a disorder in the ATPase dependant sodium pump of the cell membrane, thereby causing escape of some of the extracellular sodium with its attendant water into the cell. In this state BSS given in amounts that correct the hemodynamic parameters is about three times the volume of blood lost and corrects this membrane pump dysfunction unless given late in the derangement when a variable degree of irreversible membrane damage will have become prevalent.

It is important to remember that current evidence from the literature would show that if blood loss is replaced by equal volumes of either colloid or crystalloids, that the colloid group would result in higher cardiac index, cardiac work, A–a O2 gradient and mean arterial pressure than the crystalloid resuscitated group. On the other hand if the cryastalloid replacement is made to be three times the volume, these negative changes observed are prevented and the hemodynamic parameters are normalized. The emphasis in resuscitation with crystalloids is to obtain normal or preincident parameters. With this criterion no difference in the mortality and postoperative pulmonary dysfunction result in either the hemodynamically stable [14] or patients in shock postoperatively [15], when comparing colloid to crystallold resuscitation.

Transfusion of albumin is capable of causing a very transient increase of plasma volume with subsequent decrease of intravascular volume. The extravascular volume however, is not repleted with apparent consequences in organ function. There is marked antidiuresis and lower urinary output. Total fluid requirements become greater [16] and renal recovery is delayed. Adequate volumes of crystalloid resuscitation to normalize hemodynamics, on the other hand results in early diuresis and normalizes renal tubular function [17]. A post resuscitation systolic and diastolic hypertension with renal, pulmonary and central nervous system deficits result in the severely injured patient with shock, and found to be more sustained in the albumin group [16] can be best prevented by the earlier diuretic phase seen with crystalloid therapy.

In severe shock

In the more severe shock models however, particularly in ischemic shock, 3% albumin could exceed preshock blood volumes by 20%, a feature that seemed to correlate with better survival. Ringer's lactate on the other hand, despite a 4.4 fold infusion was only able to obtain 80% of the preshock blood volumes [18]. Albumin has been perceived to have unique features that make it preferable over balanced salt solution. It is thought to be a scavenger for free radicals, binds toxic products in disease states and regulates plasma concentration of drugs and substances. It is also thought that it reduces microvascular permeability to protein and has an inhibitory effect on pathological platelet aggregation [19]. On the other hand albumin binds free calcium with possible resulting myocardial depression. It is also thought that it has the theoretical disadvantage of binding immune globulins with possible immune suppression. Finally, as cost has become an increasingly important topic in the practice of medicine today, issues of its possible true competence well considered, 500 cc of 5% albumin costs 137 times a liter of crystalloid.

In septic states

In septic states as systemic vascular resistance decreases, cardiac index increases. This is particularly true if preload is corrected. A low cardiac index in the septic patient spells concomitant fluid deficits and significant fluid requirements. This phenomenon of high, or potentially high cardiac putput, is seen early in sepsis and seems to continue until either recovery ensues or drops preterminally, except in a small subset of patients in whom cardiac index declines slowly till death. The predominant terminating defect in most subjects is either intractible hypotension or, if the process proceeds for more than a week without signs of recovery, frank multiple organ failure occurs [20]. In the lung the normally somewhat leaky capillaries to protein tend to be even more so with resulting increase in lung water. While the dynamics involves the difference in pulmonary capillary pressure (approximated by PCWP + 0.4[Pa − PCWP]) (PCWP = Pulmonary capillary wedge pressure; Pa = Pulmonary artery pressure) and the colloid osmotic pressure, infusion of albumin in an attempt to reduce fluid exudation in ARDS has not proven to be of benefit [21].

Management

In the *hypovolemic* patient the essential defect is that of preload, low cardiac output and peripheral vascular resistance is elevated. Correction with appropriate fluids is predicated by the estimation of deficits and needs for maintainance indicated above. This is monitored in the emergent situation by following clinical signs of hypovolemia and repletion and possibly with the use of a central venous line. This however, as indicated, is subject to limitations. As time allows and only if deemed necessary, preload can best be assessed with the use of a pulmonary arterial catheter measuring pulmonary capillary pressure. A reading of 12−18 mm Hg is targetted with due attention to the all important clinical signs of shock. Cardiac output can also be obtained directly by the thermodilution method providing therefore in addition calculations of oxygen delivery:

$DO2 = Oxygen\ content \times C.O.;$

Oxygen content being approximated by ($13 \times Hb \times oxygen\ saturation$).

Oxygen saturation is easily obtained continuously by oximetry.

In the *septic* patient several defects prevail. (1) Preload deficits is frequently present or subsequently occurs, requiring well monitored fluid replacement. (2) Cardiac defects of dilatation of both ventricles with diminished ejection fractions. (3) Derangement of the Frank-Starling curves. (4) Oxygen uptake continues to increase despite a supernormal oxygen delivery. These can best be primarily corrected, in part, by eliminating the source for sepsis and treating it with antiibiotics.

Again preload is always addressed first in the treatment of sepsis. Preload to the left ventricle is most nearly approximated, in the clinical setting, by the pulmonary capillary wedge pressure. In an investigational setting, or under special clinical circumstances, a more accurate set of measurements is the end diastolic left ventricular volume, usually obtained with use of nuclear studies [22]. In addition ventricular ejection fraction is the more accurate reflection of ventricular function than PCWP, particularly in the patient with coronary artery disease [23].

Weisel and coworkers [24] reported their findings resulting from preload of fluid administration in septic states, where PCWP was plotted against left ventricular stroke work index (LVSWI), which is a reflection of left ventricular function. Ognibene *et al.* [25] plotted LVEDVI (left ventricular end diastolic volume index), considered a better measure of left ventricular preload, against LVSWI in three groups of patients. Controls, sepsis without shock and sepsis with shock cases were given incremental volume loads. Their findings showed that increasing preload increased ventricular performance as measured by the LVSWI in all the groups. The curve was steeper in the controls and started from a higher level of performance with lower LVEDVI than the patients with septic shock, with the septic patients without shock manifesting an intermediate position (Figure 16.3). Similar results were obtained from the work of Rackow *et al.* [26]. These studies taken together have also shown that some patients, upon fluid administration, responded with dilatation of the ventricle with limited increase in ventricular contractility, thus an abnormal Frank-Starling curve, while others had limited ventricular compliance and therefore did not dilate their ventricles despite full preloading.

It becomes necessary therefore, to caution against preloading to beyond 15 cm mm Hg PCWP, since the septic patient is prone to the adult respiratory distress syndrome, as any greater increases in PCWP may not translate into increasing left ventricular preload in some patients (diminished ventricular compliance), or in others where ventricular compliance is near normal, further fluid loading may not increase ventricular performance. These observations underscore the importance of detailed and informed monitoring in the critically ill septic patient.

The patient with coronary artery disease, valvular disease and the patient in failure require special management. In the first place it is important to know that most patients with known heart disease are on various medications

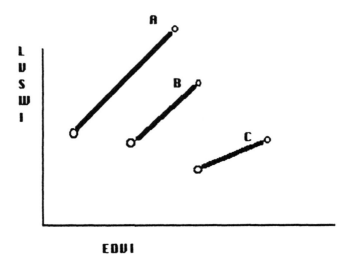

Figure 16.3. LVSWI = left ventricular stroke work index; EDVI = left ventricular end-diastolic index, before and after fluid loading in controls (A), septic patients without shock (B) and in septic patients with shock (C). Simultaneous pulmonary arterial pressures measurements and radionuclide cineangiography were done to calculate left ventricular parameters. Adapted from Ognibene FP, Parker MM, Natanson C *et al*. Depressed left ventricular performance: response to volume infusion in patients with sepsis and septic shock. Chest 1988;93:908.

and possibly specific diets. Their medications, in the usual instance, should be continued to the day of surgery and restarted soon thereafter whenever possible, unless contraindicated. This is particularly true for the patient on beta blockers as rebound on withdrawal of this type of agent might occur [27]. Hemodynamic responses in the prevailance of B blockade may continue to be appropriate [28]. Prophylactic antibiotics should be used specially in valvular disease, to prevent endocarditis. Anticoagulants have to be stopped or replaced by heparin which is stopped 6 hours prior to the procedure and restarted 12–14 hours after it. Resumption of oral anticoagulation can then be done when oral intake allows. Prophylactic heparinization and other measures against thromboembolism is undertaken. Digitalis prophylaxis may be indicated in the elderly undergoing major pulmonary resection. Digoxin a rather weak inotropic drug, except for atrial fibrillation is frought with serious side effects, especially that of ventricular irritability, particularly because of its very long half life. Digoxin immune Fab is now available as an antidote for potentially life threatening digitalis intoxication [29]. Overdiuresis and hypokalemia should be avoided or corrected prior to the procedure. Symptomatic heart block has to be managed with a pacemaker. The need for steroids in the patient on such medications and cognizance of the patient's thyroid status are attended to.

Table 16.2. Cardiac risk in the surgical patient classified based on a cumulative point system. See text for percentage risk for each of the four classes. Adapted from Goldman L, Caldera DL, Nussbaum SR *et al.* Multifactorial analysis of cardiac risk in non cardiac surgical procedurs N Engl. J Med 1977;297:845.

Goldman cardiac risk index	
S3 Gallup, jugular distention, CHF	11 points
MI < 6 months	10 points
Non-sinus rhythm, >5 PUCs/min. – each	7 points
>70 years of age	5 points
Emergency surgery	4 points
Intrathoracic, intrabdominal,	
Aortic surgery – each	3 points
Aortic stenosis	3 points
Bedridden, BUN > 50, CR. > 3 – each	3 points
PO2 < 60, PCO2 > 50, K < 3 – each	3 points
Class I (0–5 pts); Class II (6–12 pts)	
Class III (13–25 pts); Class IV (>25pts)	

The cardiac patient who is undergoing a non cardiac surgical procedure does not have the benefit of the correction in cardiac function incident with open heart surgery. Therefore stricter vigil should be taken in their monitoring and if the general proedure is elective in a patient with significant coronary artery or valvular disease, then serious consideration should be given to correcting the cardiac problem first.

Surgical risk

Cardiac dyfunction and disease presents a host of various considerations for the surgical team for analysis and deliberation. Cardiac risk evaluations in view of anesthesia and surgery has been attempted quantitatively. A point system by Goldman *et al.* in 1977 [30], taking multiple factors with different point weighting classifies cases into four classes. Class I was 99% major cardiac risk free, while class II had 5% and 2% major cardiac risk and cardiac death respectively. The same figures for class III were 11% and 2%. The figures for class IV, however, were 22% and 56% (Table 16.2). It is interesting to note that from the cardiac risk assessment standpoint, factors frequently assessed in favour of risk do not have an independent risk in this study. These include hypertension, hyperlipidemia, smoking diabetes, peripheral vascular disease, stable angina and MI more than six months. The patient with recent myocardial ischemia has a very high morbidity and mortality. Recurrent myocardial infarction or cardiac death is 30% and 15% if

Table 16.3. Frequency of mortality and respiratory complications in the five classes according to the American Society of Anesthesiologists' physical status classification. Mortality in 48 hours;' adapted from Vacanti CJ, Van Houten RJ, Hill RC. A statistical analysis of the relationship of physcial status to postoperative mortality in 68,388 cases. Anesth Analg 1970;49:564. Respiratory postoperative complications adapted from Seymour DG, Pringle R. Postoperative complications in the elderly surgical patient. Gerontology 1983;29:262.

	Classes				
	I	II	III	IV	V
Mortality 48 hrs (percent)	0.08	0.27	1.8	7.8	9.4
Respiratory complications (percent)	18	33	49	48	100

major surgery is done within 3 and 6 months postinfarct respectively. The rate plateaus at 5% after 6 months [31, 32]. It is therefore prudent to delay the procedure (unless emergency surgery is necessary) up to six months when the complication rate drops considerably. The rate of reinfarction is probably lower now with improved perioperative care but the relative importance of timing of the surgery postinfarction, remains.

The American Society of Anesthesiologists (ASA) according to the physical status of the patient has a five class risk scale based on a large collective study by Vacanti et al. (1970) [33]. Mortality rates at 48 hrs reported by these authors and respiratory complications in a series of elderly patients in 1983 [34] based on the same classification are listed in Table 16.3.

A more recent study by Del Guercio and associates (1980) [35] in 148 elderly patients were classified into four groups based on physiologic parameters of ventricular, pulmonary and oxygen transport. With a view for perioperative monitoring for correction of significant derangements classes II and III when corrected physiologically resulted in mortality of 8.5%. Those that were in class IV and uncorrectable resulted in 100% mortality unless other modalities of anesthesia or nonoperative intervention were chosen.

In those cases deemed to be in a high surgical risk it is imperative that consideration for vigorous monitoring is understaken with a view to correcting preload, reducing afterload, maximizing cardiac output and increasing coronary flow. This would have the effect of shifting the risk class to a lower one especially if this "fine tuning" is proceeded with preoperatively, with anticipated better outcome. The use of nitroglycerine drip and other vasoactive agents such as dobutamine and dopamine in this regard, to maintain hemodynamics and improve coronary flow thereby dealing with cardiovascular dysfunction is fairly well founded [36, 37].

References

1. Cullen DJ, Civetta JM, Briggs BA *et al*. Therapeutic intervention scoring system: a method for quantitative comparison of patient care. Crit Care Med 1974;2:57.
2. Keene AR, Cullen DJ. Therapeutic intervention scoring system: update. Crit Care Med 1983;11:1.
3. Guirguis EM, Hong C, Liu D *et al*. Trauma outcome analysis of two Canadian centers using the TRISS method. J Trauma 1990;30:426–9.
4. Knaus WA, Zimmerman JE, Wagner DP *et al*. APACHE: acute physiology and chronic health evaluation: a physiologically based classification system. Crit Care Med 1981;9:591.
5. APACHE III study design: analytic plan for evaluation of severity and outcome. Zimmerman JE (ed), Crit Care Med Dec 1989; Vol 17, No 12, part 2, suppl.
6. French Multicenter Group of ICU: Loiral P, Lechevallier H, Guilmet D *et al*. Factors related to outcome in intensive care: French multicenter study. Crit Care Med 1989;17:305–8.
7. Tremper KK, Barker SJ. Pulse oximetry. Anesthesiology 1989;70:98–108.
8. Crowell JW, Smith EE. Oxygen deficit and irreversible hemorrhagic shock. Am J Physiol 1964;206:313.
9. Wong DH, O'Connor D, Tremper KK *et al*. Changes in cardiac output after acute blood loss and position change in man. Crit Care Med 1989;17:979–83.
10. Shoemaker WC, Czer LS. Evaluation of the biologic importance of various hemodynamic and oxygen transport variables: Which variables should be monitored in postoperative shock? Crit Care Med 1979;7:424.
11. Siegel JH. Pattern and process in the evolution of and recovery from shock. In: Siegel JH, Chodoff PD (eds), The aged and high risk surgical patient. New York: Grune & Stratton, 1976:381.
12. Trunkey DD, Sheldon GF, Collins JA. The treatment of shock. In: Zuidema GD, Rutherford RB, Ballinger II WB (eds), The treatment of trauma. Philadelphia: WB Saunders; 1979.
13. Dawidson I. Fluid resuscitation of shock. Current controversies. Crit Care med 1989;17:1078–9.
14. Lowe RJ, Moss GS, Jilek J *et al*. Crystalloid vs. colloid in the etiology of pulmonary failure after trauma: A randomized trial in man. Surgery 1977;81:676.
15. Moss GS, Lowe RJ, Jilek J *et al*. Colloid or crystalloid in the resuscitation of hemorrhagic shock: a controlled clinical trial. Surgery 1981;89:434.
16. Ledgerwood AM, Lucas CE. Postresuscitation hypertension, etiology morbidity and treatment. Arch Surg 1974;108:531.
17. Moss GS, Proctor HJ, Herman CM *et al*. Hemorrhagic shock in the baboon I. Circulatory and metabolic effects of dilutional therapy: preliminary report. J Trauma 1968;8:837.
18. Dawidson I, Ottosson J, Reisch J. Infusion volumes of Ringer's lactate and 3% albumin soution as they relate to survival after resuscitation of a lethal intestinal ischemic shock. Circ Shock 1986;18:277.
19. Emerson ThE Jr. Unique features of albumin: a brief review. Crit Care Med 1989;17:690–4.
20. Parker MM, Shelhamer JH, Natanson C *et al*. Serial cardiovascular variables in survivors and nonsurvivors of human septic shock: heart rate as an early predictor of prognosis. Crit Care Med 1987;15:923.
21. Jing DL, Kohler JP, Rice CL *et al*. Albumin therapy in permeability pulmonary edema. J Surg Res 1982;33:482–8.
22. Joel K, Kahn JK, Sills MN *et al*. What is the current role of nuclear cardiology in clinical medicine? Chest 1990;97:442–6.
23. Harris PJ, Harrel FE, Lee KL *et al*. Survival in medically treated coronary artery disease. Circulation 1979;60:1259.

24. Weisel RD, Vito L, Dennis RC *et al.* Myocardial depression during sepsis. Am J Surg 1977;133:512.
25. Ognibene FP, Parker MM, Natanson C *et al.* Depressed left ventricular performance: response to volume infusion in patients with sepsis and septic shock. Chest 1988;93:903.
26. Rackow EC, Kaufman BS, Falk JL *et al.* Hemodynamic response to fluid repletion in patients with septic shock: evidence for early depression of cardiac performance. Circ Shock 1987;22:11.
27. Goldman L. Noncardiac surgery in patients on propranolol: case reports and recommended approach. Arch Intern Med 1981;141:193–6.
28. Kopriva CJ, Brown ACD, Pappas G. Hemodynamics during general anesthesia in patients receiving propranolol. Anesthesiology 1978;48:28–33.
29. Wenger TL. Clinical experience with digoxin immune Fab(ovine). Prim Cardiol 1988;1 (spec ed):19–23.
30. Goldman L, Caldera DL, Nussbaum SR *et al.* Multifactorial index of cardiac risk in noncardiac surgical procedures. N Eng J Med 1977;297:845–50.
31. Goldman L. Cardiac risks and complications of noncardiac surgery. Ann Int Med 1983;98:504–13.
32. von Knorring J. Postoperative myocardial infarction: a prospective study in a risk group of surgical patients. Surgery 1981;90:55–60.
33. Vacanti CJ, Van Houten RJ, Hill RC. A statistical analysis of the relationship of the physical status to postoperative mortality in 68,388 cases. Anesth Analg 1970;49:564.
34. Seymour DG, Pringle R. Postoperative complications in the elderly surgical patient. Gerontology 1983;29:262.
35. Del Guercio LRM. Cohn JD. Monitoring operative risk in the elderly. J Am Med Ass 1980;243:1350.
36. Ayers SM. The prevention and treatment of shock in acute myocardial infarction. Chest 1988;93(Suppl 1):7S–21S.
37. Roberts R. Inotropic therapy for cardiac failure associated with acute myocardial infarction. Chest 1988;93(Suppl 1): 22S–24S.

17. Cardiac performance and systemic oxygen transport after cardiopulmonary bypass surgery

PAUL L. MARINO and JAMES D. SINK

The success of cardiopulmonary bypass (CPB) surgery is limited primarily by the risk for mutiorgan damage, which can occur either during the procedure or in the early postoperative period. Intraoperative sources of organ injury include the extracorporeal circuit [1–3], the period of systemic hypothermia [4], and the cardioplegic arrest [5, 6]. The early postoperative period can lead to multiorgan damage if oxygen deficits sustained during the procedure are not corrected [7], or when ischemic areas release toxic metabolites that produce widespread reperfusion injury in the major organ systems [8]. Finally, the postoperative period can be a source of organ damage when the rate of oxygen delivery in arterial blood is inadequate to serve the needs of aerobic metabolism [9].

The performance of the heart in the early period after cardiopulmonary bypass surgery is a marker of organ injury (both cardiac and systemic) sustained during the procedure. In addition, the cardiac output is a marker of the risk for further organ injury during the postoperative recovery period. This chapter will focus on the changes in cardiac performance expected after cardiopulmonary bypass and will emphasize the relationship between cardiac output, organ failure, and clinical outcome in the postoperative period.

Clinical outcome

The relationship between cardiac output, organ failure, and mortality after cardiopulmonary bypass surgery is shown in Figure 17.1. The data in this figure is taken from a large cohort consisting of 4,179 bypass procedures performed over a 10 year period from 1977 to 1986 [10]. Low cardiac output syndrome (LOS), defined as a cardiac output less than 2.2 L/min/m2 (indexed to body surface area) requiring inotropic or mechanical support, was identified in 884 patients (21%) in the early postoperative period. The mortality in patients without LOS was 0.9%, whereas the patients who developed low cardiac output after bypass surgery had a mortality of 5.2%. Of the 884 patients with LOS, 553 (62%) also developed failure in one of the major organ systems, and the appearance of organ failure boosted mortality considerably. As shown in Figure 17.1, low cardiac output associated with failure of the lungs, kidneys or central nervous system carried a seven-fold or higher

A.-M. Salmasi and A.S. Iskandrian (eds): Cardiac output and regional flow in health and disease, 195–211.

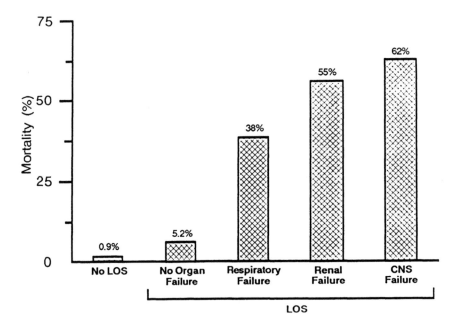

Figure 17.1. Mortality recorded in 4,179 cardiopulmonary bypass procedures in relation to postoperative cardiac output and organ failure. LOS = low output syndrome, defined as a cardiac index <2.2 L/min/m2 requiring pharmacologic or mechanical assistance. Redrawn from reference 10.

risk for mortality than did a low cardiac output without faliure in these organ systems. This indicates that mortality is determined more by the presence of organ failure than by a low cardiac output in the early postoperative period, emphasizing the distinction between "low" cardiac output and "insufficient" cardiac output (i.e., insufficient to support function in the vital organ systems) as the principal determinant of survival after cardiopulmonary bypass surgery. This distinction will be presented in more detail later in the chapter.

Cardiac performance

The influence of cardiopulmonary bypass on cardiac function involves several issues, and will be presented using the determinants of cardiac output; i.e., ventricular preload, intrinsic cardiac function, and ventricular afterload.

Hypothermia and rewarming

Systemic hypothermia is routine during cardiopulmonary bypass surgery, and is aimed reducing the risk for widespread organ damage. The blood is cooled to 25 °C as it circulates through the extracorporeal circuit using a heat exchanger in the oxygenator apparatus.

The cooling process is rapid, and is usually complete in 10 or 15 minutes [11]. The rewarming process, on the other hand, can take hours to complete [12]. The longer time for rewarming is the result of cold-induced peripheral vasoconstriction, which retards temperature equilibratation between the circulating blood and tissue compartments. Any process that creates a low cardiac output, such as hypovolemia, will aggravate the vasoconstrictionand produce a prolonged rewarming period.

Cardiac output

The relationship between temperature and cardiac output following uncomplicated cardiopulmonary bypass surgery is shown in Figure 17.2. The mean body temperature for all patients on admission to the ICU was 90 °F, and rewarming was complete at 8 hours after ICU admission. The pattern of change in cardiac output is similar to the pattern of change in body temperature, suggesting that the two are causally linked (i.e., the temperature changes are responsible for the cardiac output changes). However, the increase in cardiac output during rewarming is exaggerated; i.e., the final level exceeds the baseline preoperative levels. This suggests that rewarming involves more than the removal of cold-induced cardiac depression. This notion is supported by the behavior of the stoke volume and ventricular filling pressures (PCWP and RAP) during rewarming; i.e., the stroke volume does not return to baseline after rewarming while the PCWP and RAP are either unchanged or elevated. This indicates tha there is some degree of ventricular dysfunction that developed during the hypothermia or rewarming period.

The exaggerated rise in cardiac output during rewarming is partly due to cold-induced activation of the sympathetic nervous system [13]. The sympathetic activation represents a response to injury, so that the hyperdynamic state after bypass surgery can be used as a marker of ischemic organ damage sustained during the procedure. This is referred to as an "oxygen debt", a concept that will be developed later in the chapter.

Preload

The relationship between body temperature and ventricular filling pressures during bypass surgery is illustrated in Figure 16.2, using the right atrial pressure (RAP) and the pulmonary capillary wedge pressure (PCWP) as the filling pressures of the right and left ventricles, respectively. Note that the RAP increases during the rewarming period while the PCWP is unchanged.

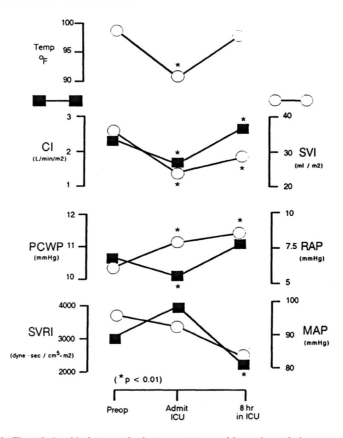

Figure 17.2. The relationship between body temperature and hemodynamicsin coronary artery bypass surgery. Graphs indicate mean values for each parameter in 17 patients with uncomplicated bypass surgery, and asterisks denote a difference in relation to preoperativevalues. Abbreviations: CI = cardiac index; SVI = stroke volume index; PCWP = pulmonary capillary wedge pressure; RAP = right atrial pressure; SVRI = systemic vascular resistance index; MAP = mean arterial pressure. Redrawn from data in reference 12.

This discrepancy is explained by the limitations of end-diastolic pressure (EDP) as a measure of ventricular filling; i.e., preload is defined as the degree of stretch on resting muscle, so that the end-diastolic volume (EDV) is the measure of preload in the intact heart. However, EDV is not easily obtained in the clinical setting, and EDP is the clinical measure of ventricular preload.

The problem with the end-diastolic pressure as a measure of ventricular filling is illustrated in Figure 17.3. The graphs in this figure show the changes in left atrial pressure (LAP) and left ventricular end-diastolic volume index (EDVI) during the rewarming period following uncomplicated coronary artery bypass surgery [14]. The end-diastolic volume was obtained in these

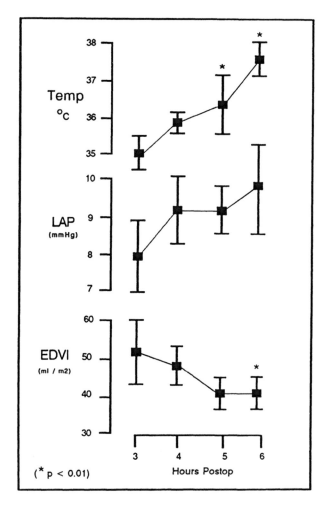

Figure 17.3. Changes in end-diastolicvolume (EDVI) and left atrial pressure (LAP) during rewarming period after bypass surgery. Squares and crossbars indicate means and standard deviation for 8 patients who underwent uncomplicated coronary artery bypass surgery. Asterisks indicate a difference in relation to the initial measurementat 3 hours after surgery. Redrawn from data in reference 14.

patients by measuring the stroke volume using thermodilution, and the ejection fraction (EF) measured by nuclear ventriculography. The relationship between the variables is given by the formula: $EDV = SV/EF \times 100$. Note that the end-diastolic pressure in Figure 17.3 (LAP) does not change significantly as the temperature rises (as was the case with the PCWP in Figure 17.2), but the EDVI (which is the EDV corrected for body surface area) falls during rewarming. In other words, ventricular filling (EDVI) falls during rewarming, but this is not indicated by the changes in the end-diastolic pressure (EDP). The discrepancy between the pressure and volume changes during rewarming is explained by the compliance (distensibility) of the ventricles. That is, the ventricular compliance, defined as the ratio of change in EDV to change in EDP, is reduced during the rewarming period. This indicates that the ventricle is less distensible after rewarming, and further, that the EDP is unreliable as a measure of ventricular filling after bypass surgery [15].

Hypovolemia

The drop in ventricuiar filling volume after bypass surgery is partly the result of hypovolemia, since bypass surgery is usually associated with a 10–20% decrease in blood volume [16, 17]. Several factors can contribute to this hypovolemia, including blood loss during the procedure, osmotic diuresis from colloid hemodilution, diuretic administration, and enhanced sodium excretion from the release of atrial natriuretic factor after bypass surgery [18]. Whatever the mechanism, the combination of hypovolemia and a less compliant ventricle (see Figure 16.3) emphasizes the value of maintaining the intravascular volume after cardiopulmonary bypass surgery.

Rewarming is associated with peripheral vasodilatation, and this could reduce venous return and contribute to the decrease in ventricular filling volume seen during the rewarming period. The administration of nitroglycerin, which serves as a venodilator at low doses, can aggravate this problem and lead to increased requirements for volume in the rewarming period [19]. The popularity of nitroglycerin for preventing coronary artery spasm after bypass surgery should be tempered by the ability of this drug to aggravate the decrease in ventricular filling that occurs during the rewarming period.

Diastolic performance

The decline in ventricular distensibility that occurs during rewarming can be explained by two mechanisms. The first is impaired ventricular relaxation, which could be the result of ischemic cell damage with calcium influx into the cells producing an exaggerated muscle tone [15]. The second explanation for the drop in ventricular distensibility after bypass surgery is the accumulation of edema fluid in the walls of the ventricles [20, 21]. Laks and colleagues [20] shown that the wet-to-dry weight of the heart can increase by 30% when crystalloid fluid is used for hemodilution. Reperfusion injury to the endothelium might play a role in promoting edema after bypass surgery [8], and the possible role of oxygen metabolites in this process creates a variety of possible therapeutic maneuvers to help alleviate this problem.

Systolic performance

Surprisingly few studies are available on the systolic function of the heart after bypass surgery, and the studies that have been performed are limited by the use of ejection fraction (EF) as a measure of systolic function. Gray and colleagues [22] studied 23 patients with uncomplicated coronary artery bypass surgery and found that the EF fell from 58% to 41% during bypass surgery but increased to preoperative levels by the end of the second postoperative day. Ivavnov and associates [14] reported similar findings in 6 adults with uncomplicated bypass surgery. The load-dependence of the EF limits the interpretation of these results, but the prevailing notion is that systolic function is preserved after uncomplicated bypass surgery.

Afterload

The clinical measure of ventricular afterload is the systemic vascular resistance, and the changes in vascular resistance that occur in association with bypass surgery are shown in Figure 17.2. The increase in vascular resistance during hypothermia represents cold-induced vasoconstriction. This is reversed during rewarming, but the vascular resistance at the end of rewarming is lower than the preoperative levels. This indicates active vasodilatation, which is a common finding after periods of reduced flow (e.g., reactive hyperemia). There are several mediators released during bypass that could exlain the vasodilatation, including the prostaglandin vasodilator, prostacyclin [23]. We have recorded elevated endotoxin levels in blood in 6 randomly selected adults after uncomplicated coronary artery bypass surgery (unpublished observation) and inflammatory mediators like the endotoxins or the interleukins may also play a role in the vasodilatation seen after bypass surgery.

Low output syndrome

Low output syndrome is defined as a cardiac output below 2.0–2.2 L/min/m2 requiring inotropic or mechanical support [10]. This condition is reported after 20 to 30% of cardiopulmonary bypass procedures [1, 5, 10]. The culprit here is inadequate protection of the myocardium during bypass [5], while infarction and tamponade are less common offenders. The major risk factors for impaired cardiac function after bypass surgery are a prolonged time on bypass [1] and a prolonged aortic cross-clamp time [5, 23]. Abnormal cardiac function prior to surgery is not a documented risk factor for postoperative cardiac dysfunction [1, 3, 5]. As stated earlier in the chapter and illustrated in Figure 17.1, patients with impaired cardiac function after bypass surgery carry a much higher risk for not surviving the experience.

Myocardial infarction

An NIH Consensus Conference in 1981 stated that acute myocardial infarction (MI) can be expected after coronary bypass surgery in 5% to 10% of patients [24]. However, the incidence of perioperative MI is not certain because of the limitations associated with the usual diagnostic tests for MI after open heart surgery. For example, the electrocardiogram is neither sensitive nor specific after bypass surgery, as shown by an autopsy report indicating that 23% of patients with transmural infarction on postmortem exam did not have Q waves on the ECG, while 20% of patients with new Q waves did not have a transmural infarction on postmortem examination [25]. Diagnosis of MI by cardiac isoenzymes can also be misleading after cardiac surgery, since the surgical procedure itself can produce elevated levels of cardiac enzymes. Regional wall motion abnormalities can be helpful if combined with ECG changes, but isolated changes in the echocardiogram are nonspecific and can be misleading [26]. The limitation of the diagnostic tests for MI after bypass surgery has led to the recommendation that the diagnosis be based on a series of complimentary tests rather than a single test used in isolation.

Risk factors for MI after bypass surgery include prolonged bypass time, occlusion of the left main coronary artery, and prior evidence for abnormal cardiac function [27]. The hemodynamic consequences are variable, however one study reported that 74% of patients with perioperative MI developed multiorgan failure [5]. Management is primarily aimed at the hemodynamic consequences of the infarction, and is similar to the management of low cardiac output states that result from nonischemic damage to the myocardium. Tachycardia is the exception, since aggressive measures are recommended to reduce tachycardia of any magnitude in the presence of acute infarction.

Pericardial tamponade

Pericardial tamponade is reported in fewer than 5% of bypass procedures [3], but the incidence may be higher [5]. The diagnosis of tamponade in the immediate postoperative period can be perplexing because of the atypical behavior of the cardiac compression. Postoperative tamponade is caused by mediastinal blood clots and the compression can be localized rather than diffuse. The traditional criteria for diagnosis, such as equalization of pressures in the thorax and pulsus paradoxus, are neither sensitive nor specific for tamponade in the early postoperative period [28]. Conventional echocardiography with precordial transducers can be problematic after open heart surgery because air in the mediastinum interferes with penetration of ultrasound waves. The transesophageal approach is promising, and provides better visualization of clots surrounding the right atrium. A recent clinical study of LOS after bypass surgery found tamponade in 9 of 88 patients (10.2%)

using transesophageal probes, while precordial probes revealed tamponade in only 2 patients (2.2%). Despite the promising results with the transeso-phageal method, the diagnosis of tamponade in the early postoperative pe-riod often must be based on clinical judgement without echocardiography results. The diagnosis is entertained in any patient with refractory cardiogenic shock after bypass surgery in the absence of evidence for acute infarction, and the definitive procedure for both diagnosis and therapy is to reopen the median sternotomy.

Hypertension
Hypertension, defined as a mean arterial pressure above 104mm Hg, is pre-sent in at least one-third of patients in the first 24 hours after bypass surgery [29]. This is primarily due to an increase in circulating catecholamines [30], which is magnified in patients with a prior history of hypertension. Systolic hypertension usually predominates, and since this is due to reflected waves that move back toward the heart, this form of hypertension should not promote small vessel disruption or microvascular bleeding. Instead, it serves to increase left ventricular afterload and can compromise stroke output. Therefore, monitoring stroke volume will aid in determining if acute therapy is necessary. If therapy is warranted, there are several parenteral agents available. Therapy with nitroprusside, once popular in this setting, is now being questioned because of recent reports of cyanide accumulation in the blood during nitroprusside infusion in roiutine doses after bypass surgery [31]. The pharmacologic approach to acute hypertension is beyond the scope of this chapter, but there are several excellent reviews on the subject [32].

Systemic oxygen transport

The purpose of oxygen transport monitoring is to identify an oxygen debt in the early postoperative period, and to determine if the cardiac output is adequate for the aerobic needs of the individual patient. The goal here is to maintain tissue oxygenation and thereby help limit the risk for peripheral ischemia and multiorgan failure [7, 9].

Oxygen transport variables

The transport of oxygen from the lungs to metabolically active tissues IS described with four parameters: (1) the oxygen content of arterial blood; (2) the oxygen delivery in arterial blood; (3) the oxygen uptake from the microcirculation; and (4) the fractional extraction of oxygen from arterial to venous blood.

   The oxygen content of arterial blood (CaO_2) is derived with the serum hemoglobin concentration (Hb) and the oxyhemoglobin saturation (SaO_2) using the following equation: CaO_2 (ml/100 ml) = 1.39 × Hb × SaO_2. The

Table 17.1. Influence of $\dot{V}O_2$ on clinical outcome after cardiopulmonary bypass surgery

Study variables	$\dot{V}O_2$ ml/min m^2	
	> 100	< 100
# Subjects	8	8
Age < 65/≥ 65	3/5	2/6
Cardiac index	2.38 20.28)	2.41 (0.29)
Organs failed	0.4 (0.4)	2.4 (0.8)*
Alive @ 4 wks	8	6*

(*p < 0.01).

oxygen content of "mixed venous" blood (CvO2) is derived in the same fashion, using the oxyhemoglobin saturation in a blood sample obtained from the pulmonary artery (SvO2). The oxygen delivery rate in arterial blood (D02) is calculated as the product of cardiac output (Q) and the oxygen content of arterial blood: i.e., D02 (ml/min) = Q × CaO2. The oxygen uptake (VO2), also called the oxygen consumption, is determined with the Fick equation using cardiac output and the areriovenous oxygen content difference; VO2 (ml/min) = Q × (CaO2 − CvO2). Finally, the oxygen extraction ratio (02ER) is used to determine the fractional uptake of oxygen across the microcirculation using the ratio: O2ER = VO2/DO2. These variables are readily obtained at the bedside using pulmonary artery catheters, and any one of several microcomputer programs will generate these calculations to simplify the task [33].

Predictive value of VO2

The value of monitoring the VO2 in the postoperative period following bypass surgery is shown in Table 17.1 This table contains two groups of patients, both with cardiac output above 2 L/min/M2, adequate urine output and no other evidence for organ hypoperfusion in the first 24 hours after surgery. The only difference is that one group has a VO2 below 100 ml/min/m2 and the other has a VO2 above this level. Note that patients with low VO2 had a higher mortality and a higher organ failure score than the patients with normal VO2. This suggests that a low VO2 can identify patients with ongoing ischemia and therapy directed to correcting the ischemia may help to prevent the appearance of organ failure later in the postoperative course.

The DO2–VO2 relationship

Figure 17.4 shows the relationship between O2 delivery and O2 uptake in healthy subjects with an adjustable oxygen extraction, and in critically ill

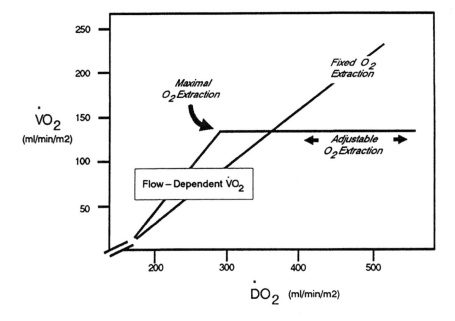

Figure 17.4. Relationship between oxygen delivery (DO2) and oxygen uptake (VO2) in normal subjects (with adjustable O2 extraction) and in critically ill patients with fixed O2 extraction. See text for further explanation.

patients with a fixed oxygen extraction. As DO2 decreases from the normal level of 500 ml/min/m2 in normal subjects, there is an increase in O2 extraction from the capillaries, and this enhanced O2 extraction maintains VO2 constant in states of reduced blood flow. However, O2 extraction eventually reaches a maximum (usually at 50%) and further decreases in DO2 will result in a similar decrease in VO2, leading to a state of inadequate tissue oxygenation (i.e., shock). The point at which VO2 starts to decrease is called the "critical level of oxygen delivery", indicated in Figure 17.4 as the point of maximal oxygen extraction. As shown in the figure, this level has been recorded at 300 ml/min/m2 following open heart surgery [35]. The straight line in Figure shows that a fixed oxygen extraction results in a linear relationship between DO2 and VO2. The inability to adjust oxygen extraction and maintain tissue oxygenation in low cardiac output states creates a "flow-dependent" VO2, and this lack of protection from tissue ischemia in low flow states carries a reduced survival value. This condition is common in patients who have sustained ischemic organ damage during surgery [35], and the appearance of a flow-dependent VO2 should prompt agressive measures to maintain cardiac output.

Hypothermia

The major benefit from hypothermia is considered to be a decrease in metabolic rate, which would protect against anoxic injury [34]. The problem here is that the effects of hypothermia are measured as a decrease in VO2, and a decrease in VO2 may be a reflection of defective oxygen extraction from capillaries (which can lead to tissue ischemia) instead of a drop in the metabolic rate. Some studies have documented that hypothermia produces a defect in oxygen extraction by noting that VO2 declines more than DO2 [4, 36–38]. This is shown in Figure 17.5, which is taken from a study of 8 adults who were cooled to a body temperature of 26 degrees centigrade during bypass surgery. There is a 41% decrease in DO2, but the VO2 decreases by 61%, so that the O2 extraction from the microcirculation drops by 21%. The drop in O2 extraction creates tissue ischemia, as evidenced by the rise in tissue lactate shown in Figure 17.3. Note also that the lactate continues to accumulate after the bypass procedure is completed and the DO2 and VO2 have returned to normal levels, suggesting that tissue ischemia is persisting into the postoperative period.

Oxygen debt

Hypothermia-induced tissue ischemia during bypass surgery can create an "oxygen debt", which must be "repayed" in the early postoeative period to reduce the risk of multiorgan failure [7]. Figure 17.6 illustrates the concept of oxygen debt and its relation to multiorgan damage after major surgery. The total oxygen debt is the area bounded by the VO2 curve and the lower limit of the normal range for VO2 (shaded area in the Figure 17.6). This accumulated deficit or debt can be counterbalanced or "repayed" by achieving a supranormal VO2, as indicated by the upper curve in Figure. Failure to achieve the overshoot carries a risk for postoperative multiorgan failure 17.6, as shown by the lower curve in Figure 17.6. Shoemaker and associates [7] have shown that failure to correct or repay oxygen deficits within 24–36 hours after major surgery can lead to mutiorgan failure.

Management strategies

The approach to the patient fresh from bypass surgery can be separated into two steps. The first step centers on the cardiac output and the systemic vascular resistance (i.e., blood flow and blood pressure). If the cardiac output is reduced but the blood pressure is adequate, volume is given if the pulmonary capillary wedge pressure (PCWP) is below 15 mm Hg. The colloid osmotic pressure of plasma has been reported at 15 m Hg after bypass surgery [39], and this level is chosen as the upper limit for the PCWP to prevent hydrostatic pulmonary edema. Furthermore, the response to volume loading

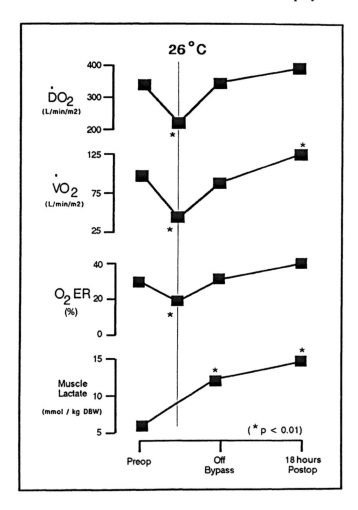

Figure 17.5. Influence of hypothermia on oxygen delivery (DO2), oxygen uptake (VO2), and oxygen extraction ratio (O2ER). Solid squares indicate mean values for 8 patients who had aortic valve replacement surgery, and asterisks mark a difference in relation to the preoperative values. Muscle lactate is expressed in millimoles per kilogram dry body weight (mmol/kg DBW). Data taken from reference 4.

after bypass surgery is greatest when the ventricular filling pressures are increased from low to normal levels [40], which would correspond to a PCWP of 12–15 mm Hg. The choice of fluid is a matter of personal preference. Crystalloid fluids are less expensive, but colloids are more effective for promoting blood volume [41].

Low cardiac output with adequate or excessive filling pressures can be

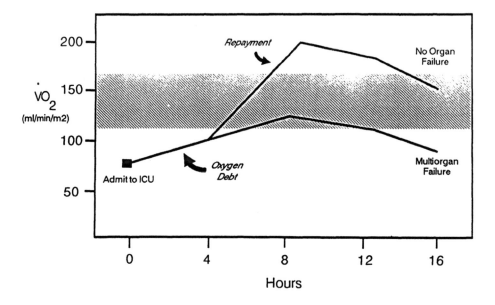

Figure 17.6. Schematic illustration of the oxygen debt concept and the patterns of oxygen uptake (VO2) in the early postoperative period in patients with and without postoperative multiorgan failure. The shaded area denotes the normal range for VO2. See text for further explanation.

managed according to the blood pressure. Hypotension is treated with dopamine and, if neccessary, intraaortic balloon counterpulsation. Dobutamine is reserved for low output syndromes with normal blood pressure, since this agent often causes a proportional decrease in systemic vascular resistance and does not increase blood pressure [42, 43]. Vasodilator therapy for normotensive heart failure is generally not favored early after bypass surgery because of the propensity for vasodilatation during rewarming. Amrinone, introduced as a combined inotropic agent and vasodilator, has variable inotropic effects in individual patients [44], and should be used with caution because of the risk of hypotension. Amrinone can be valuable in combination with dobutamine for patients who are refractory to dobutamine [45].

When cardiac output and blood pressure are satisfactory, the VO2 is used to dictate decisions in the second stage of the approach. A low VO2 after the patient has rewarmed is an ominous sign, and should be corrected as soon as possible. Since patients with an oxygen debt have a flow dependent VO2 (see Figure 17.4), the VO2 is increased by increasing cardiac output with volume or inotropic agents [7, 9, 46]. Volume is preferred whenever possible because many hemodynamic drugs stimulate both O2 delivery and metabolic rate, and this combination may cancel any beneficial effect from improving O2 delivery. Finally, a VO2 in the normal range (100–

160 ml/min/m2) does not ensure adequate tissue oxygenation in the early postoperative period because of the hypermetabolism that characterizes this setting [13]. Therefore, when the VO2 is in the normal range, a serum lactate should be measured to assess the balance between oxygen delivery and the aerobic metabolism. A serum lactate above 4 mEq/L is used as evidence for organ ischemia, and therapy in this situation involves increasing cardiac output with volume and dobutamine [7, 9], even if cardiac output is in the normal range. In fact, Shoemaker *et al.* [47] have shown that attaining supranormal levels of cardiac output and oxygen delivery to match the hypermetabolism of the postoperative state is associated with improved survival and fewer postoperative complications. This raises several questions about the exact requirements for nutrients, drug doses, or any other intervention in critically ill patients, and this area must be explored further.

References

1. Kirklin JK, Westaby S, Blackstone EH *et al.* Complement and the damaging effects of cardiopulmonary bypass. J Thorac Cardiovasc Surg 1983;86:845–57.
2. Westaby S. Organ dysfunction after cardiopulmonary bypass. A systemic inflammatory reaction initiated by the extracorporeal circuit. Intensive Care Med 1987;13:89–95.
3. Kuan P, Bernstein SB, Ellestad MH. Coronary artery bypass surgery morbidity. Am Coll Cardiol 1984;3:1391–7.
4. Fiaccadori E, Vezzani A, Coffrini E *et al.* Cell metabolism in patients undergoing major valvular heart surgery: relationship with intra and postoperative hemodynamics, oxygen transport, and oxygen utilization patterns. Crit Care Med 1989;17:1286–92.
5. Beppu S, Sakakibara H, Tanaka N *et al.* Prediction and diagnosis of low cardiac output syndrome after open heart surery: an echocardiographic study. In: Manabe H, Zweifach BW, Messmer K (eds), Microcirculation in circulatory disorders. New York: Springer-Verlag, 1988:95–102.
6. Buckberg GD, Olinger GN, Mulder DG *et al.* Depressed postoperative cardiac performance. Prevention by adequate myocardiac protection during cardiopulmonary bypass. J Thorac Cardiovasc Surg 1975;70:974–88.
7. Shoemaker WC, Appel PL, Kram HB. Tissue oxygen debt as a determinant of lethal and nonlethal postoperative organ failure. Crit Care Med 1988;16:1117–20.
8. Forman MB, Puett DW, Virmani R. Endothelial and myocardial injury during ischemia and reperfusion: pathogenesis and therapeutic implications. J Am;Coll Cardiol 1989;13:450–9.
9. Vincent JL, DeBacker D. Initial management of circulatory shock as prevention of MOF. Crit Care Clin 1989;5:369–78.
10. Kumon K, Tanaka K, Hirata T *et al.* Multiple organ failure in low cardiac output syndrome after cardiac surgery. In: Manabe H, Zweifach BW, Messmer K (eds), Microcirculation in circulatory disorders. New York:Springer-Verlag, 1988:79–85.
11. Blanche C, Matloff J, MacKay DA. Technical aspects of cardiopulmonary bypass. In: Gray RJ, Matloff JM (eds.), Medical management of the cardiac surgical patient. Baltimore: Williams & Wilkins, 1990:55–68.
12. Czer L, Hamer A, Murphy F *et al.* Transient hemodynamic dysfunction after myocardial revascularization. J Thorac Cardiovasc Surg 1983;86:226–34.
13. Chiara O, Giomarelli PP, Bagioli B *et al.* Hypermetabolic response after hypothermic cardiopulmonary bypass. Crit Care Med 1987;15:995–1000.

14. Ivanov J, Weisel RD, Mickelborough LL *et al.* Rewarming hypovolemia after aortocoronary bypass surgery. Crit Care Med 1984;13:1049–54.
15. Gilbert JC, Glantz SA. Determinants of left ventricular filling and of the diastolic pressure-volume relation. Circ Res 1989;64:827–52.
16. Karanko M. Severely depressed blood volume after coronary bypass [letter]. Crit Care Med 1987;15:182.
17. Beattie HW, Evans G, Garnett ES *et al.* Sustained hypovolemia and extracellular fluid volume expansion foilowing cardiopulmonarybypass. Surgery 1972;71:891–96.
18. Schaff H, Mashburn JP, McCarthy PM *et al.* Natriuresisduring and after cardiopulmonary bypass: relationship to atrial natriuretic factor, aldosterone, and antidiuretic hormone. J Thorac Cardiovasc Surg 1989;98:979–86.
19. Calvin JE, Driedger AA, Sibbald WJ. The hemodynamiceffect of rapid fluid infusion in critically ill patients. Surgery 1981;90:61–76.
20. Laks H, Standeven J, Blair O *et al.* The effects of cardiopulmonary bypass with crystalloid and colloid hemodilution on myocardial extravascularwater. J Thorac Cardiovasc Surg 73:129–38.
21. Erdmann AJ, Geffin GA, Barrett LV *et al.* Increased myocardial water content with acute Ringer's lactate (RL) hemodilution in dogs. Circulation 1974;50(Suppl II):18.
22. Gray R, Maddahi J, Berman D *et al.* Scintigraphic and hemodynamic demonstration of transient left ventricular dysfunction immediately after uncomplicated coronary artery bypass grafting. J Thorac Cardiovasc Surg 1979;77:504–10.
23. Reves JG, Croughwell N, Jacobs JR *et al.* Anesthesia during cardiopulmonary bypass: does it matter? In: Tinker JH (ed), Cardiopulmonary bypass: current concepts and controversies. Philadelphia: W.B. Saunders, 1989:69–98.
23. Schraut WH, Kampman K, Lamberti JL *et al.* Myocardial protection from permanent injury during aortic cross-clamping: effectiveness of pharmacologic cardiac arrest combined with topical cardiac hypothermia. Ann Thorac Surg 1981;31:224–39.
24. National Institutes of Health Consensus-Development Conference Statement. New Engl J Med 1981;304:681–4.
25. Bukley BH, Hutchins GM. Myocardial consequences of coronary artery bypass graft surgery. Circulation 1977;56:906–13.
26. Force T, Bloomfield P, O'Boyle J *et al.* Quantitative two-dimensional echocardiographic analysis of regional wall motion in patients with perioperative myocardial infarction. Circulation 1984;70:233–41.
27. Bauer HR, Peterson TA, Arnar O *et al.* Predictors of perioperative myocardial infarction in coronary artery operation. Ann Thorac Surg 1981;31:36–44.
28. D'Cruz IA, Callaghan WE. Atypical tamponade: clinical and echocardiographic features. Internal Med Special 1988;9:68–78.
29. Hoar PF, Hickey RF, Ulyot DJ. Systemic hypertension following myocardial revascularization. J Thorac Cardiovasc Surg 1976;71:859–64.
30. Reed HL, Chernow B, Lake GR *et al.* Alterations in sympathetic nervous system activity with intraoperative hypothermia during coronary artery bypass surgery. Chest 1989;95:616–22.
31. Patel CB, Laboy V, Venus B *et al.* Use of sodium nitroprusside in post-coronary bypass surgery. A plea for conservatism. Chest 1986;5:663–7.
32. Rubenstein EB, Escalante C. Hypertensive crisis. Crit Care Clin 1989;5:477–98.
33. Marino PL, Krasner J. An interpretive computer program for analysing hemodynamicproblems in the ICU. Crit Care Med 1984;12:601–3.
34. Morray JP, Pavlin EG. Oxygen delivery and consumption during hypothermia and rewarming in the dog. Anesthesiol 1990;72:510–6.
35. Komatsu T, Shibutani K, Okamoto K *et al.* Critical level of oxygen delivery after cardiopulmonary bypass. Crit Care Med 1987;15:194–8.
36. Willford DC, Hill EP, Moores WY. Theoretical analysis of oxygen transport during hypothermia. J Clin Monit 1986;2:30–43.

37. Willford DC, Hill EP, White FC *et al*. Decreased critical mixed venous oxygen tension and critical oxygen transport during induced hypothermia in pigs. J Clin Monit 1986;2:155–68.
38. Schumaker PT, Rowland J, Saltz *et al*. Effects of hyperthermia and hypothermia on oxygen extraction by tissues during hypovolemia. J Appl Physiol 1987;63:1246–52.
39. Klancke KA, Assey ME, Kratz JM *et al*. Postoperative pulmonary edema in postcoronary artery bypass graft patients. Relationship of total serum protein and colloid oncotic pressures. Chest 1983;84:529–34.
40. Weisel RD, Burns RJ *et al*. Optimal postoperative volume loading. J Thorac Cardiovasc Surg 1983;85:552–63.
41. Karanko MS, Klossner JA, Laaksonen VO. Restoration of volume by crystalloid versus colloid after coronary artery bypass: hemodynamics, lung water, oxygenation, and outcome. Crit Care Med 1987;15:559–66.
42. Saloman NW, Plachetka JR, Copeland JG. Comparison of dopamine and dobutamine following coronary artery bypass grafting. Ann Thorac Surg 1982;33:48–53.
43. Cohn LH. Dobutamine in the postcardiac surgery patient. In: Chatterjee K (ed), Dobutamine: a ten year review. Indianapolis: Eli Lilly & Co, 1989:123–38.
44. Franciosa JA. Amrinone:advance or wrong step? Ann Int Med 1985;102:399–400 (editorial).
45. Guimond JG, Matuschak GM, Meyers *et al*. Augmentation of cardiac function in end-stage heart failure by combined use of dobutamine and amrinone. Chest 1986;90:302–4.
46. Vincent JL, Roman A, De Backer D *et al*. Oxygen/supply dependency. Effects of short-term dobutamine infusion. Am Rev Respir Dis 1990;142:2–7.
47. Shoemaker WC, Appel PL, Kram HB *et al*. Prospective trial of supranormal values of survivors as therapeutic goals in high-risk surgical patients. Chest 1988;94:1176–86.

18. Cardiac output and hemodynamics of septic shock

GARY J. VIGILANTE

Septic shock is a complex syndrome caused by the interaction of an infectious agent with host defense mechanisms. The sepsis syndrome is defined as the systemic response to infection including tachycardia, fever or hypothermia, tachypnea and evidence of circulatory abnormalities [1] Septic shock occurs when the sepsis syndrome is accompanied by hypotension and end-organ dysfunction due to impaired tissue perfusion or oxygen utilization unresponsive to fluid therapy [1, 2]. This hemodynamic abnormality often results in significant morbidity and mortality [3].

Epidemiology

Patients with septic shock are commonly found in a wide variety of settings. This syndrome is one of the most commonly encountered problems and causes of death in intensive care units in the United States and Europe [4, 5]. The incidence of sepsis and septic shock is rising secondary to an increase in the population subgroups at risk. These subgroups include the elderly, diabetics, immunosuppressed and cancer patients, intravenous drug abusers, patients with invasive medical devices, patients using broad spectrum antibiotics and those undergoing high risk surgery [6]. Shock occurs in about 40% of patients with the sepsis syndrome. There is estimated to be a 50% to 90% death rate in those patients who actually develop shock [7, 8]. This high mortality rate has continued despite great improvements in antibiotic therapy, invasive monitoring and aggressive fluid therapy [9]. There is a death rate of approximately 10% in patients with sepsis who do not develop shock [7]. There are several factors which predispose a patient with the sepsis syndrome to develop shock. These include increasing age, hypothermia, delayed treatment, immunosuppression, congestive heart failure, renal failure, hepatic insufficiency, hematologic malignancies and infection due to enterococci or gram-negative bacilli [2, 10].

Septic shock is most commonly noted in patients with gram-negative infections. Frequently cultured organisms include *Escherichia coli*, *Klebsiella pneumoniae*, *Pseudomomas aeruginosa*, *Serratia marcescens* and *Proteus* species [11]. Endotoxin, a lipopolysaccharide liberated from the membrane of these gram-negative bacteria, was once thought to be a major cause of the

A.-M. Salmasi and A.S. Iskandrian (eds): Cardiac output and regional flow in health and disease, 213–221.
© 1993 Kluwer Academic Publishers. Printed in the Netherlands.

septic shock syndrome. However, other microbes without endotoxin have been frequently noted to elicit shock [4]. Such organisms include gram-positive cocci (especially *Staphylococcus aureus* and Group D *Streptococci*), anaerobes, fungi, rickettsiae, and viral infections [6, 11, 12]. Therefore, a complex number of initiating mediators appear to be important in the development of septic shock. Substances proposed to modify the cardiovascular response to septic shock include bradykinin (through activation of the kinin system), histamine, complement proteins, prostaglandins, endorphins and cytokines released from leukocytes.

Cardiovascular pattern

Septic shock is considered to be the classic example of a distributive form of shock. Other examples of distributive shock include anaphylaxis, neurogenic shock, the toxic shock syndrome and endocrinologic shock [4]. These types of shock are often manifested by volume sequestration, a severe decrease in systemic vascular resistance, and redistribution of a normal or elevated cardiac output to different organ systems [2, 6]. These hemodynamic abnormalities contrast with the cardiogenic, extracardiac obstructive and hypovolemic forms of shock which produce significant hypotension because of reduced cardiac output.

For a number of reasons, the hemodynamics of septic shock in humans are difficult to study. One of the major factors is that many patients with sepsis have underlying chronic cardiac and other systemic diseases with baseline hemodynamic abnormalities. These findings may significantly alter one's cardiovascular response to sepsis [6]. In addition, many hemodynamic studies of septic shock are flawed by incomplete data bases due to the lack of invasive monitoring with such devices as pulmonary artery catheters, arterial lines and thermodilution cardiac output thermistors. Also, it has been unusual to closely document the serial hemodynamic changes in patients with septic shock. Finally, an acceptable animal model which mimics cardiovascular changes seen in human sepsis has been difficult to produce [6]. In spite of these problems, the hemodynamic patterns in septic shock have become well defined in recent years.

Early clinical studies divided septic shock into two phases. The early or warm form consisted of a high cardiac output with peripheral vasodilation. The late or cold form of shock demonstrated significant vasoconstriction and a low cardiac output [13, 14]. The late form was associated with a very poor prognosis. It is now clear that the "phases" of septic shock are actually part of a continuum [9]. In fact, it is uncommon to encounter low cardiac outputs in patients with sepsis without hypovolemia in the absence of underlying chronic cardiac abnormalities. Ninety percent of patients with septic shock will demonstrate normal or elevated cardiac outputs when aggressively volume loaded [15]. It is unusual to measure low cardiac outputs even in the

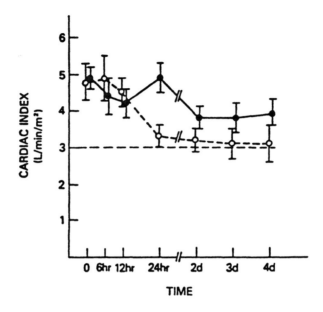

Figure 18.1. Serial mean cardiac index plotted against time for survivors and nonsurvivors of septic shock. The dashed line correlates with normal mean resting cardiac index. The open circles represent survivors while the closed circles represent nonsurvivors. (Reproduced, with permission, from reference 15.)

late stages of septic shock [4] (Figure 18.1). In fact, a recent study of hemodynamic variables in septic shock demonstrated that the major difference between the survivors and non-survivors was that the cardiac output quickly decreased into the normal range in survivors. However, most non-survivors continued to have high cardiac outputs within 24 hours of death. Thus, the mechanism of demise was either a low systemic vascular resistance unresponsive to aggressive fluid and vasopressor therapy or complications of multiple organ system dysfunction in the majority of non-survivors [41].

Shock occurs in sepsis when the decreased systemic vascular resistance is not completely compensated by the increase in cardiac output. This blood flow is inadequate to appropriately perfuse and meet the increased metabolic demands of the essential organs. Therefore, relative heart failure occurs [13]. This is manifested by lactic acidemia with hepatic and renal failure, adult respiratory distress syndrome, mental status changes and peripheral vascular insufficiency. There is a narrowed arteriovenous oxygen difference reflecting the inadequate peripheral use of oxygen (reduced tissue oxygen consumption).

The causes of the decrease in systemic vascular resistance with poor tissue perfusion are probably multifactorial. The release of vasoactive mediators such as bradykinin, histamine, prostaglandins, cytokines and endorphins may lead to inadequate flow to some tissues [2]. Perfusion of organs may also be adversely affected by leukocyte aggregation within capillaries caused by compliment activation. This may result in arteriovenous shunting. Another important mechanism may be capillary leaking with interstitial fluid accumulation resulting from a vascular endothial injury [6]. Most likely, all of these mechanisms are active to some degree in contributing to the hemodynamic response in septic shock.

Venous tone is also an important contributor to cardiac output in septic shock. In some situations, sepsis may involve active venoconstriction and an increase in venous resistance. This may result in a decreased cardiac output. More often, active venodilation is encountered early during sepsis with an increase in venous compliance. Again, a low cardiac output syndrome will occur unless fluid therapy is initiated [16]. The changes in venous tone appear to be mediated by the same factors which alter systemic vascular resistance. In most cases, aggressive intravenous volume loading will increase the cardiac output to normal or above normal levels [15, 16]. The addition of a vasoconstrictor such as norepinephrine may occasionally be required to increase preload. In the uncommon situation when active venoconstriction occurs, the addition of venodilators such as nitrates, calcium blockers or beta-2 sympathetic agonists may further augment cardiac output [16].

Although cardiac output is normal or increased in the majority of patients with septic shock, there is general agreement that myocardial dysfunction occurs in a high percentage of cases [4, 17]. Cardiac output is usually maintained because of the significant reduction in systemic vascular resistance with a lowering of the mean arterial pressure. This reduction in vascular resistance may be part of an adaptive and compensatory response to metabolic abnormalities in the presence of cardiac dysfunction [18]. Myocardial depression has not been shown to be an important feature of the sepsis syndrome without shock [13].

Ejection fractions and ventricular volume measurements derived from radionuclide gated blood pool scans have been used to evaluate relative load independent measures of cardiac function in septic shock. In the initial stages of human septic shock, the left ventricular ejection fraction is usually significantly reduced with an increase in both end-diastolic and end-systolic volumes [19] (Figure 18.2). These abnormalities of left ventricular function are usually global, but may occasionally be segmental [20]. It appears that the increase in left ventricular volume may occur without a significant rise in left ventricular pressure reflecting an increase in ventricular compliance. The left ventricular dilation may be a compensatory response to sepsis and help to maintain stroke volume and cardiac output via the Frank-Starling mechanism [4]. Therefore, septic shock appears to produce both systolic and diastolic cardiovascular dysfunction. This myocardial depression is reversible in most survivors of the disease, with the ejection fraction returning towards normal 7 to 10 days after the episode of septic shock. Interestingly, in

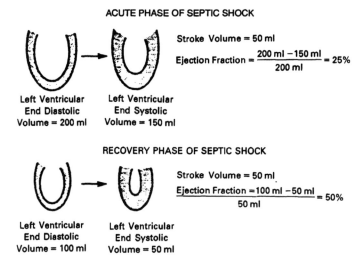

Figure 18.2. Schematic representation of cardiac performance changes during the acute and recovery phases of septic shock. (Reproduced, with permission, from reference 19.)

many non-survivors of septic shock, the left ventricle does not appear to significantly dilate which may lead to the inability to maintain stroke volume and cardiac output [21]. This inability to increase left ventricular diastolic size may be related to myocardial edema [17]. However, most patients who succumb to septic shock still appear to die as a result of persistent peripheral vascular vasodilatation rather than myocardial failure [22].

Right ventricular function is also adversely affected in patients with septic shock. Right ventricular dilation and decreased ejection fraction occur in most of these patients. Parker *et al.* [23] demonstrated significant reductions in both right and left ventricular ejection fractions which returned toward normal at recovery. In addition, both dilated ventricles became smaller after shock resolved.Their conclusion was that cardiac dysfunction is a biventricular occurrence in septic shock.

In contrast to the systemic circulation, pulmonary vascular resistance is abnormally elevated with prolonged septic shock. This pulmonary hypertension may occur by a number of mechanisms. Postulated mediators of increased pulmonary vascular resistance include acidemia, hypoxemia, histamine, prostaglandins and angiotensin [2]. The findings of Kimchi and associates [24] suggested that right sided cardiac abnormalities are caused by elevated right ventricular afterload in some patients and reduced myocardial contractility in others. However, it appears likely that both the increased afterload produced by elevated pulmonary vascular resistance and depressed myocardial contractility combine to cause right ventricular dysfunction [25]. These findings are important in planning the treatment strategies in patients with septic shock. Therapies which augment preload, reduce pulmonary vascular resistance and enhance right ventricular contractility would be expected to significantly improve right ventricular dysfunction. Currently, the only major practical therapy available to reduce pulmonary vascular resistance without adversely affecting the systemic circulation is the use of supplemental oxygen to reduce potential hypoxic vasoconstriction [26].

Two major theories have been proposed to explain the cardiac dysfunction found in septic shock. One theory is based upon the hypothesis of altered coronary hemodynamics causing myocardial ischemia. However, Cunnion and colleagues [27] demonstrated excellent myocardial blood flows in patients with septic shock and myocardial depression. Abnormal autoregulation of coronary flow was noted. Since reduction in the ejection fraction was not associated with a reduction in coronary blood flow nor elevated myocardial lactate production, myocardial ischemia was not implicated as a cause of cardiac dysfunction in this study. However, this conclusion is not completely shared by all investigators [28].

The second theory to explain the cardiac dysfunction of septic shock involves the presence of direct circulating mediators of myocardial depression. Fascinating studies have demonstrated the presence of a circulating myocardial depressant substance or substances in most patients with septic shock manifesting significant cardiac dysfunction [4, 29]. The chemical nature of this depressant activity remains unknown. Endotoxin has not been found to cause this myocardial depression *in vitro*. However, tumor necrosis factor, a cytokine released by leukocytes, does cause significant myocardial depression *in vitro* and may play a role in cardiac dysfunction.

Effects on other organ systems

In addition to the severe effects on the cardiovascular system, septic shock often causes significant dysfunction of other organ systems. The major pulmonary complication is development of the adult respiratory distress syndrome (ARDS). This syndrome describes the pulmonary edema induced by increased capillary permeability which may contribute to further hemodynamic deterioration. ARDS results in refractory hypoxemia and diffuse infiltrates in patients with normal left ventricular filling pressures. Approximately 50% of patients in septic shock develop this syndrome [9]. Other major organ and metabolic derangements which may modify the complex cardiovascular patterns found in septic shock include disseminated intravascular coagulation, renal failure, liver failure, gastrointestinal hemorrhage and cerebrovascular dysfunction.

Management

The mainstay in treatment of septic shock is control of the infectious process. Improvement and survival are dependent on the irradication of the septic focus with appropriate therapies. Initially, broad spectrum antimicrobial agents may be utilized until the specific infectious agent or agents are identified.

Restoration of an adequate intravascular volume remains one of the first major therapies to be instituted in patients with septic shock [4, 9]. Close hemodynamic monitoring is needed during fluid resuscitation. Due to the poor correlation of central venous pressure measurements with actual left ventricular filling pressures, the early use of a pulmonary artery catheter should be strongly considered [30]. Patients with septic shock are rapidly given intravenous fluids until either the hemodynamics significantly improve or the pulmonary capillary wedge pressure exceeds 10 to 15 mm Hg. Unfortunately, these patients often show markedly reduced myocardial responses to volume expansion with the inability to dilate or increase contractility of the ventricle [31]. In addition, the ability to administer volume may be tempered by development of the adult respiratory distress syndrome. The need for mechanical ventilation and positive end-expiratory pressure (PEEP) often occurs [9].

There remains controversy as to whether crystalloid or colloid fluids should be used in resuscitating septic shock patients. Colloid solutions have the advantage of achieving desired filling pressures rapidly. However, these fluids are expensive, difficult to titrate and may be associated with a substantial increase in the adult respiratory distress syndrome [10]. In addition, a recent study suggested that volume expansion with crystalloid fluids did not promote development of pulmonary edema [32]. Due to these considerations, the use of crystalloid fluids must be favored over colloid solutions.

If a patient with septic shock remains hypotensive after appropriate administration of fluids, vasoactive drug therapy is then instituted. Dopamine is usually considered the preferred vasopressor agent due to it's ability to raise blood pressure by increasing the systemic vascular resistance and myocardial contractility while improving renal and mesenteric blood flow at moderate doses. Dobutamine is sometimes added to further improve cardiac function. The use of norepinephrine is indicated when a markedly decreased systemic vascular resistance and hypotension remain refractory to dopamine. This potent vasoconstrictor has been demonstrated to reverse refractory septic shock resulting in a reasonable survival rate [33] Norepinephrine has been shown to improve arterial pressure, cardiac output and urine output in those patients who remain hypotensive despite volume and dopamine infusions [34].

Several other therapies have been used or are in various stages of investigation for the treatment of septic shock. Corticosteroid use had been advocated in this disorder. However, recent evidence has demonstrated no improvement in survival compared to placebo when high dose steroids were instituted [35, 36]. Super-infections were also a problem in these steroid treated patients. Therefore, routine corticosteroid use can no longer be recommended in patients with septic shock.

Theoretically, naloxone may be useful in the therapy of septic shock by inhibiting endorphin receptors. Although it has not been shown to improve survival, use of naloxone has been associated with a significant improvement in blood pressure in patients with sepsis [37]. Unfortunately, antihistamines have not been proven efficacious in the treatment of septic shock. Other experimental therapies such as prostaglandins and prostaglandin inhibitors, endotoxin antisera and anticomplement antibodies await clinical trials.

Summary

Septic shock remains a major problem encountered in today's medical practice associated with high morbidity and mortality rates. Decreased systemic vascular resistance and significant myocardial depression are the major cardiovascular abnormalities noted in this syndrome. The use of antibiotics, fluid resuscitation and vasopressor medications are the mainstays of therapy. Future investigations may lead to improvement in treatment and survival in patients with septic shock.

References

1. Bone RC, Fisher CJ, Clemmer TP *et al*. Sepsis syndrome: a valid clinical entity. Crit Care Med 1989;17:389–93.
2. Ellrodt AG. Sepsis and septic shock. Emer Med Clin North AM 1986;4 809–40.
3. Abboud FM. Pathophysiology of hypotension and shock. In: Hurst JW, Logue RG, Rackley CE *et al*. The heart. 6th ed. New York: McGraw Hill, 1985:370–82.
4. Parrillo JE, Parker MM, Nathanson C *et al*. Septic shock in humans-advances in the understanding of pathogenesis, cardiovascular dysfunction, and therapy. Ann Intern Med 1990;113:227–42.
5. Kazda A. Sepsis-metabolic changes and their development. Czech Med 1988;11:10–9.
6. Parker MM, Parillo JE. Septic shock-hemodynamics and pathogenesis. J Am Med Assoc 1983;250:3324–7.
7. Kreger BE, Craven DE, McCabe WR. Gram-negative bacteremia-re-evaluation of clinical features and treatment in 612 patients. Am J Med 1980;68:344–55.
8. Parrillo JE. Cardiovascular dysfunction in septic shock: new insights into a deadly disease. Inter J Card 1985;7:314–21.
9. Luce JM. Pathogenesis and management of septic shock. Chest 1987;91:883–8.
10. Karakusis PH. Considerations in the therapy of septic shock. Med Clin North Am 1986;70:933–44.
11. Abraham E, Bland RD, Cobo JC *et al*. Sequential cardiorespiratory patterns associated with outcome in septic shock. Chest 1984;85:75–80.
12. Okrent DG, Abraham E, Winston D. Cardiorespiratory patterns in viral septicemia. Am J Med 1987;83:681–6.

13. Schremmer B, Dhanaut JF. Heart failure in septic shock: effects of inotropic support. Crit Care Med 1990;18:s49–55.
14. Weil MH, Nishijima H. Cardiac output in bacterial shock. Am J Med 1978;64:920–2.
15. Parker MM, Shelhamer JH, Nathanson C et al. Serial cardiovascular variables in survivors and nonsurvivors of human septic shock: heart rate as an early predictor of prognosis. Crit Care Med 1987;15:923–9.
16. Bressack MA, Raffin TA. Importance of venous return, venous resistance and mean circulatory pressure in the physiology and management of shock. Chest 1987;92:906–12.
17. Ledingham IM, Messmer K, Thijs L. Report on the European conference on septic shock of the European society of intensive care medicine and the European shock society. Intens Care Med 1988;14:181–4.
18. Chiarla C, Giovannini I, Boldrini G et al. Pathophysiological correlates of cardiac overperformance in sepsis and septic shock. Prog Clin Biol Res 1989;308:259–63.
19. Parker MM, Shelhamer JH, Bacharach SL et al. Profound but reversible myocardial depression in patients with septic shock. Ann Intern Med 1984;100:483–90.
20. Ellrodt AG, Riedinger MS, Kimchi A et al. Left ventricular performance in septic shock:reversible segmental and global abnormalities. Am Heart J 1985;110:402–9.
21. Parker MM, Suffredini AF, Nathanson C et al. Responses of left ventricular function in survivors and nonsurvivors of septic shock. J Crit Care 1989;4:19–25.
22. Groeneveld AB, Bronsveld W, Thijs LS. Hemodynamic determinants of mortality in human septic shock. Surgery 1986;99:140–53.
23. Parker MM, McCarthy KE, Ognibene FP et al. Right ventricular dysfunction and dilatation, similar to left ventricular changes, characterize the cardiac depression of septic shock in humans. Chest 1990;97:126–31.
24. Kimchi A, Ellrodt AG, Berman DS et al. Right ventricular performance in septic shock:a combined radionuclide and hemodynamic study. J Am Coll Cardiol 1984;4:945–51.
25. Dhainaut JF, Lanore JJ, DeGournay JM et al. Right ventricular dysfunction in human septic shock. Prog Clin Biol Res 1988;264:343–8.
26. Schneider AJ. Right ventricular performance in sepsis and septic shock. Neth J Med 1988;33:187–204.
27. Cunnion RE, Schaer GL, Parker MM et al. The coronary circulation in human septic shock. Circulation 1986;73:637–44.
28. Archer LT. Myocardial dysfunction in endotoxin and *E.coli* induced shock: pathophysiological mechanisms. Circulation Shock 1985;15:261–80.
29. Reilly JM, Cunnion RE, Whitman CBC et al. A circulating myocardial depressant substance is associated with cardiac dysfunction and peripheral hypoperfusion (lactic acidemia) in patients with septic shock. Chest 1989;95:1072–80.
30. Redl G, Zadrobilek E, Schindler I et al. Judgement of central hemodynamics with and without Swan-Ganz catheter in septic shock states. Prog Clin Biol Res 1987;236B:123–8.
31. Ognibene FP, Parker MM, Nathanson C et al. Depressed left ventricular performance-response to volume infusion in patients with sepsis and septic shock. Chest 1988;93:903–10.
32. Zadrobilek E, Hackl W, Sporn P et al. Effect of large volume replacement with crystalloids on extravascular lung water in human septic shock syndrome. Prog Clin Biol Res 1989;308:809–13.
33. Meadows D, Edwards JD, Wilkins RG et al. Reversal of intractible septic shock with norepinephrine therapy. Crit Care Med 1988;16:663–6.
34. Desjars P, Pinaud M, Potel G et al. A reappraisal of norepinephrine therapy in human septic shock. Crit Care Med 1987;15:134–7.
35. Bone RC, Fisher CJ, Clemmer TP et al. A controlled clinical trial of high dose methylprednisolone in the treatment of severe sepsis and septic shock. N Engl J Med 1987;317:653–8.
36. Hinshaw L, Peduzzi P, Young E et al. Effect of high dose glucocorticoid therapy on mortality in patients with clinical signs of systemic sepsis. N Engl J Med 1987;317:659–65.
37. Hackshaw KV, Parker GA, Roberts JW. Naloxone in septic shock. Crit Care Med 1989;18:47–51.

PART FIVE

Cardiac output: effect of intervention

19. Effect of medications on cardiac output

JOHN G. F. CLELAND and DAVID P. MOORE

The purpose of the cardiovascular system is to provide a flexible, variable mechanism for the provision of oxygen to and removal of waste products from metabolising tissue. Previous chapters have outlined the enormous capacity of the heart to modify output according to physiological requirements such as exercise and have dealt with the changes in cardiac function which result from cardiovascular disease states. Precisely because of its role in homeostasis, the cardiovascular system is susceptible to a wide range of pharmacological interventions, which may result in an increase or reduction in cardiac output as a result of direct pharmacological effects on heart muscle, effects on vasomotor tone, or through the neural and hormonal mediators which influence cardiovascular function. Moreover, the haemodynamic effects of any intervention will depend on the patients disease (e.g. A patient with heart failure may respond to a pressor agent with a fall in cardiac output and little change in arterial pressure, whereas a subject with normal ventricular function will maintain cardiac output and arterial pressure will rise) and pre-existing haemodynamic state (e.g. reducing pre-load in a patient with heart failure and markedly elevated filling pressures will not affect cardiac output, but in a patient in whom the filling pressure is low due to diuretic-induced dehydration cardiac output and arterial pressure may fall).

The purpose of this chapter is to discuss the mechanisms and effects of the principal categories of agents which havepossible clinically useful or significant action on cardiovascular function. However, a word of caution is appropriate at this juncture. The isolated correction of a haemodynamic abnormality, whether hypertension or chronic heart failure, may be of little clinical benefit. Diuretics reduce the risk of stroke in hypertension and this is probably due to a reduction in blood pressure, but it is doubtful if they normalise haemodynamics. Beta-blockers also reduce the incidence of stroke in hypertension and reduce the risk of re-infarction and sudden death in patients after myocardial infarction, but this may be related directly to their effects on adrenergic receptors rather than to haemodynamic effects.

Angiotensin converting enzyme inhibitors have proved useful in the management of chronic heart failure, but this may be due to correction of metabolic and neuro-endocrine disturbances and not related to haemodynamic effects. Other vasodilators have generally failed to show benefit in heart failure except in the context of acute pulmonary oedema, where nitrates

A.-M. Salmasi and A.S. Iskandrian (eds): *Cardiac output and regional flow in health and disease*, 225–250.

have a clearly defined role. Conclusive proof that inotropic agents should be given to patients with chronic heart failure does not exist, even for digoxin. Newer inotropic agents may reduce survival despite significant haemodynamic benefit. It is important to appreciate that the haemodynamic effects of pharmacological agents in chronic heart failure are only a surrogate endpoint for other more important measures such as a reduction in symptoms and improvement in survival.

Clearly, a different approach is justified in the management of chronic heart failure compared with acute pulmonary oedema, where haemodynamic end points are of more practical importance, if only because of the controlled environment in which such measurements are made.

Agents with a positive inotropic action (Figure 19.1)

Many physiological and pharmacological agents have positive inotropic actions. Thus, a variety of endogenous catecholamines, histamine and angiotensin II all increase the contractility of isolated muscle preparations. Because the effects of such inotropic agents are not confined to changes in cardiac contractility, the net effect of such agents depends on the capacity of the cardiac muscle to respond to stimulation:substances such as angiotensin II and noradrenaline elevate vascular resistance, so that cardiac output is maintained and blood pressure rises if ventricular function is normal, but in patients with poor ventricular function cardiac output may decline with little change in arterial pressure. Obviously, many patients will exhibit effects intermediate between these two extremes; however it is important to bear in mind that the response to a pharmacological agent is the result of a complex interaction between patient and drug factors.

Inotropic agents have largely been developed for use in heart failure and shock. However, major difficulties arise in determining whether drugs that have shown to be effective inotropic agents *in vitro* retain their effect in the intact, though diseased, cardiovascular system. The net response to both inotropic agents and arterial vasodilators is an increase in stroke volume. Correction for stroke work does not reliably differentiate an inotropic agent from a vasodilator because this equation does not take into account those components of myocardial loading unrelated to the blood pressure; for instance the end-diastolic volume. In the case of agents with combined dilator and inotropic actions (e.g. phosphodiesterase inhibitors) the relative importance of each component in the clinical setting is largely undetermined.

Digitalis

The cardiac glycosides were introduced to medical practice in 1785 by Sir William Withering [1]. Digoxin continues to be the most widely used positive

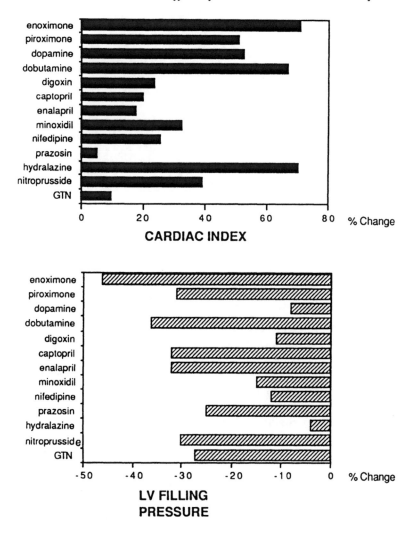

Figure 19.1. Effect on cardiac index and left ventricular filling pressure 'of short term administration of vasodilator and inotropic agents.

inotropic agent, and possibly the only orally active inotropic agent effective in the long term.

The cellular mechanism of inotropy is based upon inhibition of Na/K ATPase, the so-called sodium pump, causing enhanced transient increases in intracellular sodium in the region of the sarcolemma. The presence of increased sodium in turn activates the sodium-calcium exchange mechanism, and the consequent increase in cytosolic calcium concentration, results in increased myocardial contractility (Figure 19.2). Digoxin increases parasym-

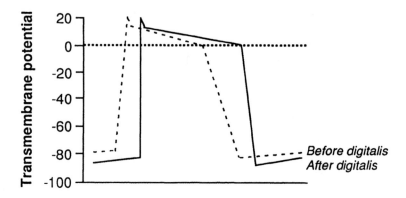

Figure 19.2. Effect of digitalis on actual potential in cardiac Purkinje cells. Adapted from Bresnehan *et al.* Mayo Clin Proc 1979;54:675–84.

pathetic activity, reducing the discharge rate of the sinus node and slowing atrio-ventricular conduction, while it enhances arterial baroreceptor reflexes and in high doses may increase central sympathetic drive [2] (Figure 19.3).

Digoxin is of undoubted clinical benefit in patients with atrial fibrillation and heart failure, providing rate control without depressing cardiac function. Controversy persists over the role of digoxin in patients with heart failure who remain in sinus rhythm, when beneficial haemodynamic effects cannot be attributed to control of ventricular rate [3–5].

When ventricular function is normal the acute administration of digoxin enhances cardiac contractility, but concomitant direct (mediated through increased smooth muscle cell sodium and calcium) and reflex systemic vaso-constriction results in little change or a decline in cardiac output [6].

McMichael and Sharpey-Schafer [7], in an early series of studies showed that acute adminsitration of digoxin increased cardiac output and reduced the venous pressure in patients with heart failure. The rise in cardiac output in this situation facilitates a reflex decline in sympathetic tone and a secondary reduction in vascular resistance and venous tone.

More recent longer-term studies have confirmed that digoxin leads to sustained increases in resting left ventricular ejection fraction [8] echocardio-graphic indices of ventricular function and cardiac output [10]. However, there is less information on the long term effects on symptoms, some reports indicating benefit [9, 10], but others failing to show a significant difference from placebo [8, 11].

Intravenous digoxin and captopril have similar acute effects on resting left ventricular filling pressures and systemic vascular resistance [12], although digoxin increases ejection fraction, while captopril has a neutral effect [8].

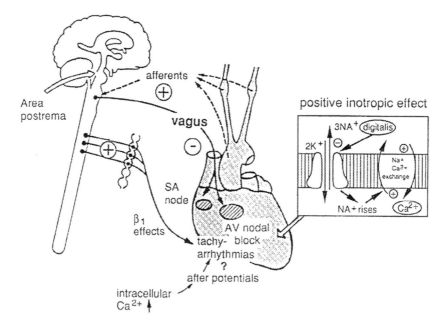

Figure 19.3. The inotropic effect of digitalis is best explained 'by inhibition of the sodium pump. Slowing of the heart rate and inhibition of the atrioventricular node is explained by vagal stimulation (a direct effect of nodal tissue may also play a role). Toxic arrhythmias are less well understood, but may be caused 'by a combination of sympathomimetic stimulation (β_1 = beta, adrenoceptor stimulation) and the development of calcium-dependent afterpotentials.

Sympathomimetic amines

The group of drugs which exert their positive inotropic effects on the myocardium through activation of the myocardial adrenergic receptors are classified as sympathomimetic amines. Most of these agents also exert effects on the peripheral circulation, and in some cases the direct myocardial effects may be negligible (Figure 19.4). The concept of a receptor system mediating inotropic and vasoactive functions within the cardiovascular system was introduced by Ahlquist [13]. Distinct α and β receptors are recognised, mediating predominantly arterial vasoconstriction and arterial and venodilation accompanied by an inotropic effect respectively. Manipulation of the chemical structure of these archetypal sympathetic agonists has led to the development of a range of synthetic agents (see Table 19.1) and to the recognition of discrete receptor subgroups, as well as the extension of the classification to include the so called dopaminergic receptors, δ_1 and δ_2.

Adrenergic receptors in heart failure

The sympathetic nervous system is intimately concerned with the responses to myocardial insufficiency, and the adrenergic receptor status of the myocar-

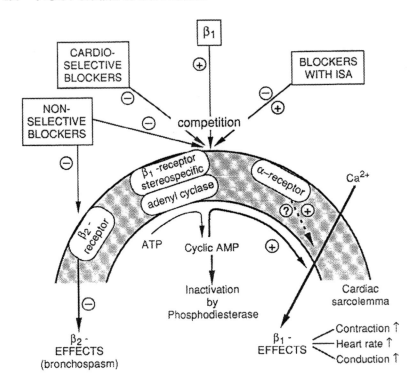

Figure 19.4. Cardiac adrenergic receptors. β_1-agonists acxt on the β_1-selective recep;tor in the heart cell membrane. Nonselective blockade by propranolol gives β_1 plus β_2-blockade. Cardioselective blockers at low doses are relatively β_1-specific. Agents with ISA (intrinsic sympathomimetic activity, Figure 19.6) simultaneously block and stimulate the receptor with the blockade dominating during states of enhanced sympathetic tone.

dium differs from normal in patients with pump failure. In healthy human myocardium, adrenergic agents are capable of increasing the maximum force of contraction to the same extent as exposure to Ca^{++}. In the failing myocardium, however, cAMP dependent agents are less effective than Ca^{++}. The *in vitro* observation that the myocardium of experimental animal models of

Table 19.1. Sympathomimetic amines in current clinical use.

Drug	Receptor
Dopamine	$\beta 1$, $\delta 1$, $\alpha 1$, ? $\alpha 2$, $\delta 2$
Dobutamine	$\beta 1$, $\beta 2$, $\alpha 1$
Isoprenaline	$\beta 1$
Ibopamine	$\delta 1$, $\delta 2$, $\beta 1$
Adrenaline	$\beta 1$, $\beta 2$
Noradrenaline	α
Dopexamine	$\delta 1$, $\beta 2 \gg \beta 1$

heart failure, and of patients with end stage cardiomyopathy exhibited less than predicted response to beta-adrenergic agonists coupled with the discovery that beta receptors are sharply reduced in number in proportion to the severity of dysfunction [14] suggests that chronic exposure to elevated plasma catecholamines can down regulate the receptors [15]. In support of this apparent tachyphylaxis to β adrenergic agonists is a study by Unverferth in which it was demonstrated that less than 60% of the initial hemodynamic effect of a given dose of dobutamine remains after 4 days intravenous infusion [16]. The β_1 partial agonist xamoterol, which is discussed below, has favourable haemodynamic effects during short term usage,and has been demonstrated to confer sustained benefit in mild to moderate heart failure [17], while *in vitro* studies have shown no evidence of beta receptor down regulation [18]. Myocardial β_2 and α_1–receptors are less prone to down-regulation in heart failure and may therefore become relatively more important in mediating the inotropic action of some sympathomimetic amines in this condition.

Dopamine

Dopamine is the natural precursor in the synthesis of noradrenaline. Its principal effects are mediated through increased noradrenaline synthesis and release, and stimulation of peripheral δ_1 and δ_2 receptors. The haemodynamic effects of dopamine administration are dose dependent, with activation of dopaminergic receptors at rates of 1–5 µg/kg/min, leading to reduced peripheral vascular resistance and increased cardiac output [19, 20]. A specific reduction in renal vascular resistance and therefore increase in renal blood flow occurs at these low doses. Alpha receptor stimulation occurs with increasing dose, and this is manifest not only by increasing peripheral vascular resistance, but also by enhanced venous return due to venoconstriction. The increase in resistance leads to increases in both systolic and diastolic arterial pressures, and reduction in renal blood flow. The absence of chronotropic response at low doses may represent an inhibitory δ_2 effect on the conduction system [21] the increment in cardiac output being entirely due to augmented contractility and attenuated PVR. At higher doses of dopamine, a chronotropic response is usual however. Due to its prominent effects on myocardial contractility, dopamine increases myocardial oxygen consumption and coronary blood flow in a dose-dependent fashion. At low doses in congestive cardiac failure, however, the principal cause of haemodynamic improvement is reduction of peripheral vascular resistance with concomitant effects in reducing myocardial wall tension, and hence there is little or no increase in myocardial oxygen consumption despite significant increases in cardiac output [22]. At higher doses, peripheral vascular resistance rises and there is a substantial rise in myocardial oxygen consumption, with the potential for development of myocardial ischemia and increased infarct size in experimental models [23].

Levo-dopa

The search for orally active sympathomimetic agents has led to interest in the use of levo-dopa, the biochemical precursor of dopamine: there is evidence that levo-dopa at a dose of 1–1.5 g has equal potency with dopamine at 2–4 μg/kg/min [24]. Whether the improved haemodynamics primarily reflect increased myocardial contractility or peripheral vasodilation remains to be established. Widespread use of levo-dopa has been limited by the high incidence of gastrointestinal side effects.

Bromocriptine

This drug facilitates the release of noradrenaline from sympathetic nerve terminals via δ_1 and δ_2 receptors and has vasodilator actions without direct inotropic effect [25].

Ibopamine

Ibopamine is a combined δ_1, δ_2 and β_2 agonist. Preliminary clinical studies in heart failure have shown that it increases resting cardiac output while reducing preload and afterload [26].

Dopexamine

Dopexamine is a newly developed synthetic catecholamine which combines dopaminergic δ_1 and adrenergic β_2 actions, with only weak β_1 effects. This combination of actions provides preferential renal vasodilation and reduced overall PVR, with consequent increases in cardiac output. Short term administration of dopexamine has been associated with reduction in both systemic and pulmonary vascular resistance and increased cardiac output. High doses produce a marked chronotropic response, which result in increased myocardial oxygen consumption: the long term effects of dopexamine therapy are unknown though tachphylaxis has been reported [27].

Beta₁ agonists

Dobutamine

Pharmacological modifications of isoprenaline in an attempt to isolate the inotropic functions of the synthetic amines led to the development of dobutamine, a predominantly β_1 agonist agent which also has weak effects on β_2 and α_1 receptors. The diverse effects of this agent are attributable to the presence of a racemic mixture of *l* and *d* isomers possessing differing pharmacological effects. The *l*-isomer has α_1 agonist properties, whereas the β effects

Table 19.2. Comparison of dopamine and dobutamine effects on hemodynamics in patients with congestive heart failure.

	Dopamine	Dobutamine
Cardiac output		
Low dose	↑	↑ ↑
High dose	↑	
Arterial blood pressure		
Low dose	→	→
High dose	↑	↑
Heart rate		
Low dose	→	→
High dose	↑	Δ ↑
LV filling pressure		
Low dose	→	→ ↓
High dose	↑	↓
Peripheral vascular resistance		
Low dose	→ ↓	→ ↓
High dose	↑	↓

are characteristic of the *d*-isomer [28]. At low doses in cardiac failure, dobutamine increases cardiac output with a small decline in SVR and little effect on mean arterial pressure or left ventricular filling pressure, effects which are best explained by β_1 mediated increase in myocardial contractility, possibly with a contribution from α_1 mediated effects [29]. With increasing doses, both preload and afterload do however decline, as a consequence of β_2 stimulation. Combination with an alpha-1 antagonist may result in hypotension indicating that vascular resistance is held in equilibrium by opposing beta-2 (vasodilator) and alpha-1 (constrictor) influences. Dopamine causes more vasoconstriction at higher doses which may desirable in some cases of hypotension.

Chronotropic responses are minimal below 15 μg/kg/min, but may be prominent above this dose. Dobutamine does not directly influence renal blood flow in low output conditions, but increased renal sodium and water losses may be consequent upon the improvement in hemodynamics [30]. Table 19.2 demonstrate a comparison between dopamine and dobutamine.

The largest increases in cardiac output are seen in patients with the most severely depressed cardiac output [29]. The duration of inotropic effect of dobutamine is controversial: in one study inotropic effect appeared to be sustained during continuous IV therapy up to 72 hrs in duration [30], while in another a 40% reduction in inotropic effect occurred within 4 days [16]. Dopamine and dobutamine are only effective as intravenous infusions; their capacity to augment cardiac output in the short term is undoubted, but their long term effects are uncertain. Adrenergic receptor down regulation might be expected on theoretical grounds to lead to attenuation of the improved hemodynamics achieved with their short term administration, but initial enthusiasm for long term intermittent administration has now been tempered with caution due to possible adverse effects on prognosis, and attention has been focussed on newer oral adrenergic receptor agonists and inotropic agents with alternative mechanisms.

Xamoterol

Whether an adrenergic agent possesses full adrenergic efficacy or has only partial agonist properties may influence its long term haemodynamic potential. The β_1 partial agonist xamoterol has 43% of the sympathomimetic activity of isoprenaline [18]. In mild heart failure when prevailing sympathetic activity is low xamoterol acts as an adrenergic agonist. In severe heart failure at rest, or milder degrees of heart failure during strenuous exercise the prevailing endogenous sympathetic activity is high and xamoterol acts as a beta-adrenergic receptor antagonist.

In mild heart failure acute administration is accompanied by a rise in cardiac index and reduction in pulmonary wedge pressure; several studies have shown significant improvements in short term exercise tolerance. The haemodynamic benefits are maintained during long term oral administration for up to 12 months [17]. However, an excess mortality associated with an deterioration in the underlying condition has been noted in patients with more severe heart failure [31].

Beta antagonists

Beta blockers cause a reduction in rest and exercise cardiac output in normal subjects and in patients with heart failure [32], and their use in congestive heart failure remains controversial: nevertheless, there is evidence of haemodynamic benefit associated with their use in some categories of heart failure [33]. The down regulation of beta receptors attributable to feedback inhibition from chronic overstimulation by catecholamines may be reversible, resulting in an increased response to intravenous β stimulants, and increased resting ejection fraction [34]. Recent studies suggest that hemodynamic benefits are maintained during long term treatment. Long term metoprolol therapy was associated in one study with an increase in resting cardiac index from $2.17 - 2.58 \, l/min/m^2$ and an increase in stroke work index from 31 to $65 \, g \, m/m^2$ and drug withdrawal was associated with a haemodynamic deterioration. These changes were accompanied by evidence for modest β receptor up-regulation [35].

Adrenaline

Adrenaline (US Epinephrine) is a mixed β stimulant which also has some α mediated effects. Although positive inotropic effects are prominent, resulting in increased cardiac output due to both increased myocardial contractility and peripheral vasodilation, as with isoprenaline, tachyarrhythmia limits its clinical application as a therapeutic agent for this purpose.

Isoprenaline

Isoprenaline (US Isoproterenol) has both β_1 and β_2 activity and like adrenaline has prominent chrontropic and potentially arryhthmogenic actions which limit its application as an inotropic agent.

Selective β_2 agonists

Salbutamol causes peripheral vasodilatation and hence an increase in cardiac output, especially in the failing ventricle. At doses of 0.5 µg/kg/min this agent has been shown to improve indices of contractility in patients heart failure already optimally treated with digitalis and diuretics [36], though in the intact circulation it is difficult to be certain whether this represents changes in ventricular loading or a true inotropic effect.

Alpha agonists

Noradrenaline, Metaraminol, Methoxamine

Vascular alpha-1 adrenoceptors are concentrated in the region of postsynaptic sympathetic nerve terminals.Their stimulation causes increased smooth muscle contraction, membrane permeability changes leading to reduced depolarisation threshold probably being the responsible mechanism. Myocardial α receptors may facilitate Ca^{++} entry or have a role in calcium release from the sarcoplasmic reticulum, leading to increased contractile force [37].

Peripheral vasoconstriction tends to predominate with alpha agonists with the effect of limiting any potential increase in cardiac output attributable to the improved cardiac contractility. Hypertension may also cause reflex bradycardia with further reductions in cardiac output. In patients witl heart failure the increased afterload results in a fall in stroke volume as well so that alpha agonists have a net negative effect on cardiac output. These agents have an established therapeutic role in the maintenance of blood pressure in patients with non-cardiogenic shock or post operative hypotension.

Alpha antagonists

The alpha-1 antagonists reduce peripheral arterial and venous constriction mediated by the sympathetic nervous system. Prazosin and terazosin increase resting and exercise cardiac index, accompanied by improvements in LV preload, afterload and coronary blood flow [38]. Tachyphylaxis due to enhanced sympathetic activity, a result of α-2 inhibition, may occur with long-term use [39]. The effects of these agents may be enhanced during submaximal exercise as sympathetically mediated vasoconstriction may be important in preventing exercise induced falls in vascular resistance at this time.

Phosphodiesterase inhibitors

The shortcomings of cardiac glycosides and sympathomimetic amines, and the increasing recognition of the fundamental role of cAMP in the mediation of extracardiac influences on myocardial contractility have stimulated the search for alternative positive inotropic agents (Figure 19.5). This quest has led to the development of a group of agents, which although structurally dissimilar, share the capacity to inhibit phosphodiesterase-III, which is a cAMP specific cardiac phosphodiesterase. A number of these agents have

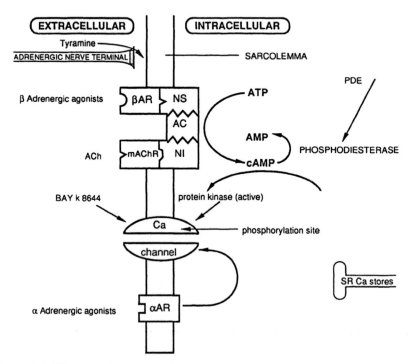

Figure 19.5. Diagrammatic representation of some of the sites of action of positive inotropic agents. βAR: beta adrenoceptor; αAR: alpha adrenoceptor; ACh: acetyl choline; mAChR: muscarinic ACh receptor; Ni: guanine inhibitory subunit; Ns: guanine stimulatory subunit; SR: sarcoplasmic reticulum.

now undergone extensive clinical trials, and have been licensed for use in heart failure, principally for short term intravenous hemodynamic support: studies of their long term effects are in progress.

The effects of increased myocyte cAMP are similar with each of the phosphodiesterase inhibitors: peak developed tension and rate of maximum tension development are increased; the duration of systolic contraction is reduced, and simultaneously the maximal rate of myocardial relaxation is enhanced.

PDE inhibitors increase the rate of inward calcium flux into the myocyte [40], and this appears to be their major mode of action, for extracellular Ca $^{++}$ or blockade of the Ca^{++} channels markedly attenuates their inotropic effect [41]. However, even when extracellular calcium concentrations are raised high enough to obviate the role of the slow Ca^{++} channels, phosphodiesterase inhibitors retain some additional effect, implying the existence of at least one additional inotropic mechanism [42].

Amrinone and milrinone

Amrinone was the first PDE inhibitor to undergo extensive clinical trials. The oral or intravenous administration of amrinone in heart failure is marked by increased cardiac output and reduced left ventricular preload and systemic vascular resistance, although despite its clear vasodilator effect there is little change in heart rate or blood pressure except at high doses [43]. Some investigators have suggested that it posesses little or no inotropic activity in patients with severe heart failure and that haemodynamic effects are due solely to vasodilatation[44, 45]. The occurrence of hypotension is potentiated by its use in the setting of low ventricular filling pressure, most likely because of the prominent venodilator effect possessed by this agent.

Initial experience with the phosphodiesterase inhibitors has indicated that although effective in the short term, long term administration may lead to attenuation of the beneficial hemodynamic effect. In a study of the effects of long term oral amrinone therapy, it was found that although stroke volume and stroke work indices improved markedly at 48 hrs after initiation of oral therapy, subsequent reinvestigation at 2–10 weeks demonstrated a return to pretreatment values despite maintenance therapy. Furthermore, withdrawal of the agent led to a deterioration in these variables to below baseline values [46]. The basis of the deterioration in left ventricular function in these patients is unclear. Although perhaps attributable to natural progression of the underlying disease, these patients demonstrated progressive activation of plasma renin and a decline in plasma Na^{++} which may have caused vascular resistance to increase.

Milrinone is approximately 15 times as potent as amrinone [47], and though gastro-intestinal upset is common with higher doses the side effect profile is generally superior to amrinone [48]. In a study comparing milrinone with dobutamine in the treatment of severe heart failure, milrinone caused relatively more reduction in SVR than the β_1 agonist for a similar increase in dP/dT [49].

Studies in man in which milrinone was administered as an intracoronary infusion indicate that it has a direct effect on myocardial contractility: when intravenous milrinone was subsequently administered to the same patients, a further improvement in stroke volume and pre and afterload was observed [50]. The overall effect of milrinone in heart failure is to increase cardiac output without changes in myocardial oxygen consumption. The sparing of myocardial oxygen requirement reflects the vasodilator effect which reduces O2 demand thereby balancing the effects of increased contractility. Publication of the "promise" study that demonstrated an excess mortality with little clinical benefit with the active agent has terminated the development of milrinone for long-term clinical use [104].

Enoximone and piroximone

Enoximone belongs to a structurally distinct category of PDE inhibitors, the imidazolones: the pharmacologic action again appears to be inhibition of phosphodiesterase-III, and the drug has a similar hemodynamic profile to the bipyridine agents, with reductions in peripheral vascular resistance and improvements in cardiac output and peak dP/dt. Preliminary studies with enoximone [51] and a related drug, Piroximone, MDL 19,205 [52] have indicated sustained improvements in aerobic capacity during oral therapy of more than 4 months duration as well as acute improvements in cardiac output and left ventricular preload in some but not all studies. Piroximone has been shown also to have persistent hemodynamic benefit after two months oral treatment [53]. The effect of PDE inhibitors depend on the rate of cAMP production, which in turn depends on the level of sympathetic activity. PDE inhibition sufficient to cause hemodynamic effects at rest in patients with chronic heart failure may be excessive during exercise. Reports of increased mortality during chronic therapy with phosphodiesterase inhibitors [54] may be attributable in part to inappropriate selection of dose. Studies are now being conducted with lower doses of enoximone and piroximone which may be more appropriate for chronic use.

Diuretics

The most widely prescribed therapeutic agents for congestive cardiac failure are diuretics, although their precise hemodynamic effects are poorly understood. Intravenous frusemide administration is associated with a prompt decline in right atrial pressure before the onset of diuresis, an effect mediated by the prostglandin/bradykinin system [55, 56]. Reports vary as to the acute effects on cardiac output. Neuro-endocrine activation may result in vaso-constriction and a fall in cardiac output with elevated left ventricular filling pressure immediately after intravenous administration [57]. However, relief

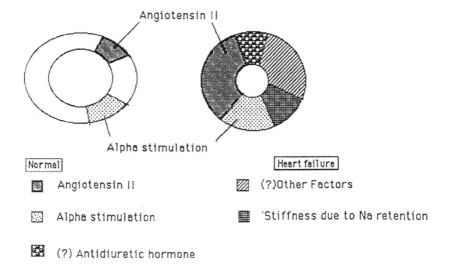

Figure 19.6. Fiagrammatic representation of a normal arteriole (L) and one in cardiac failure (R) indicating vasoconstrictor influences.

of pulmonary oedema and distress tend to result in a fall in sympathetic activity and vascular resistance with a consequent increase in cardiac index [58]. In patients with massive oedema, vascular wall sodium loading and increased tissue pressure may contribute to vascular resistance (Figure 19.6). Reduction of oedema causes a substantial increase in maximal vasodilator capacity in patients with congestive heart failure [59] this effect will potentiate the vasodilator effects of other drugs.

Vasodilators (Figure 19.7)

The effect of a vasodilator depends critically on the underlying cardiovascular state. In patients with normal ventricular function the predominant effect of arterial vasodilator agents is to reduce arterial pressure, as the stroke volume is dependent on venous return. Venodilator agents are likely to cause a fall in cardiac output if cardiac function is normal because the ventricle is working at or below the optimal filling pressure at rest (Figure 19.7).

The failing ventricle responds to a fall in vascular resistance with a rise in cardiac output, because the stroke volume is much more dependent on afterload. If filling pressure is high venodilation may be reduced with little effect on cardiac output.

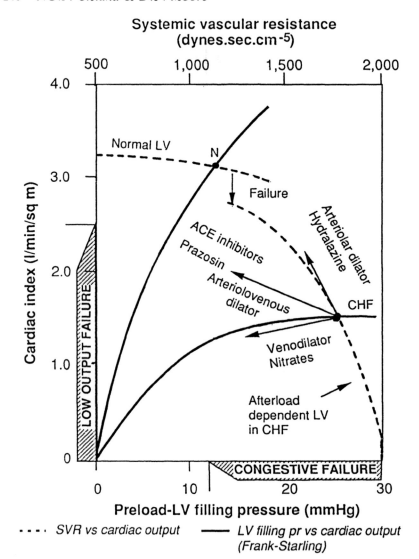

Figure 19.7. A high left ventricular (LV) end-diastolic pressure causes congestive symptoms, i.e., dyspnea. A low cardiac output causes symptoms of forward failure, i.e. fatigue. Two basic therapies are vasodilators reducing the LV end-diastolic pressure; and agents increasing contractile activity of the heart such as digitalis. In normal heart (point N), cardiac output (CO) is principally regulated by changes in impedance ("afterload-dependent"); alterations in preload are of minor importance. In CHF, the pure arteriodilator, hydralizine, raises lowered CO markedly with mild decline of elevated left ventricular end-diastolic pressure (LVEDP); the angiotensin-converting enzyme inhibitors and prazosin act on both venous and arterial systems to raise the lowered CO and to decrease elevated LVEDP; and pure venodilator, sublingual nitroglycerin, decreases elevated LVEDP markedly with little or no improvement of lowered CO.

Nitroprusside

The nitrates, both organic and inorganic are thought to mediate their effects through a mechanism analogous to that of endothelium derived relaxing factor (EDRF).

Sodium nitroprusside is a powerful, short acting vasodilator agent with direct actions on vascular smooth muscle. It has equivalent vasodilator effects on the venous and arterial circulations. Nitroprusside is extensively used in the management of low-output states especially after cardiac surgery. The increase in cardiac output in the presence of severe mitral regurgitation may be especially impressive as the fall in aortic impedance will lead to a reduction in regurgitant fraction. Nitroprusside is also a valuable anti-hypertensive agent in the peri-operative period and after aortic dissection. Its rapid onset and offset of action are used to advantage in this context. The increase in cardiac output observed with nitroprusside is exclusively the result of reduced systemic vascular resistance and is achieved through an increase in stroke volume. As noted above, if filling pressures are already low venodilatation will result in a fall in cardiac output.

Organic nitrates

Organic nitrates act principally on venous capacitance vessels, though they also have arterial dilating effects. In acute pulmonary oedema, sublingual nitroglycerine 0.8–2.4 mg can achieve a significant improvement in cardiac output, reduce right and left atrial pressure and lead to the rapid resolution of edema [60]. Similar hemodynamic effects are reported with intravenous and oral preparations of nitrates in acute studies [61]. Long term administration of nitrates leads to the development of tolerance [62].

Hydralazine

This direct-acting arterial vasodilator has been widely used in the treatment of hypertension and heart failure. In patients with hypertension with or without heart failure there is a decrease in SVR, and an increase in stroke volume and cardiac output: little effect is observed on pulmonary wedge pressure or right atrial pressure. There is evidence that patients with severely dilated ventricles (>60 mm) benefit more than others from haemodynamic improvements, but this awaits confirmation [63]. Tolerance to hydralazine occurs in 30% of patients with favourable initial haemodynamic responses, and explains the lack of significant long-term benefit in a number of patients [64].

Minoxidil

Minoxidil is a potent arterial vasodilator, principally utilised for the control of severe hypertension. Like other arterial vasodilators its effects on arterial resistance lead to an increased cardiac output in congestive heart failure [65]. During exercise, minoxidil has been shown to significantly increase maximal cardiac output in patients with severe chronic heart failure during short term administration, although left ventricular filling pressures were not affected [66]. Usage of this drug in heart failure is restricted by its tendency to cause massive fluid retention [67].

Flosequinan

This agent is a direct acting vasodilator presently undergoing clinical trials in the management of congestive heart failure. Short term haemodynamic improvements without hypotension or arrhythmogenic side effects have been reported [68]. Flosequinan has been shown, in a further study to both increase resting cardiac output while reducing left ventricular preload, and to improve exercise capacity during a 4 week placebo controlled trial [69]. Comparative data between flosequinan and other vasodilators are not available.

Calcium antagonists

Calcium antagonists cause arterial vasodilatation and have negative inotropic effects mediated through reduced availability of calcium for excitation contraction coupling. Effects on the venous circulation are more controversial and possibly indirect.

Verapamil has the greatest negative chronotropic and inotropic effects, nifedipine and diltiazem less so. Nicardipine, felodipine, amlodipine and isradipine have even less.

The myocardial depressant effect leads to little or no change in cardiac output in normal individuals despite peripheral vasodilation [70].

Verapamil, diltiazem and nifedipine have all been studied in heart failure because of the possibly beneficial effects observed with other vasodilator agents. Isolated reports have suggested minor benefit with nifedipine but the arterial vasodilation seen with nifedipine is offset by the negative inotropic effect of this drug [71]. Felodipine, which has negligible negative inotropic effect, has been shown to significantly increase both rest and exercise cardiac output in heart failure, although there was no change in exercise tolerance after 3 weeks treatment [72]. Nifedipine has been compared with captopril in heart failure; exercise time improved, with reduced pulmonary wedge pressure and increased cardiac output on captopril but not with nifedipine: ventricular dimensions enlarged on nifedipine but declined with captopril despite similar effects on peripheral resistance. With the possible exception of amlodipine [74] the results of controlled trials in heart failure have shown minimal benefit or deterioration with the use of calcium antagonists [75], and the use of this class of drug in the management of heart failure, should be restricted to those patients with relatively well-preserved left ventricular function and concomitant angina.

ACE inhibitors

Although angiotensin II has positive inotropic actions this effect is more than offset by arterial constriction and sympathetic nerve activation. Angiotensin converting enzyme inhibitors (ACEI) act on the renin-angiotensin-aldosterone system by preventing the formation of angiotensin II, either systemically or locally in vascular tissue. The fall in angiotensin II leads to a secondary decline in sympathetic activity, aldosterone, atrial natriuretic peptide and anti-diuretic hormone. Heart rate falls, a result of the decline in sympathetic activity and a rise in parasympathetic tone. The net consequence of these effects is one of mixed arterial and venous vasodilation. Venodilatation is believed to be due to a reduction in sympathetically mediated venoconstriction. Although a potentiating effect of ACE inhibitors on Bradykinin is also possible.

Haemodynamic effects of acute administration are a fall in systemic and pulmonary vascular resistance and pressures, and an increase in cardiac output. The perfusion of vital organs is maintained despite the reduction in arterial pressure [76]. In the long-term ACE inhibitors have sustained vasodilator effects. This combined with their ability to limit salt and water retention in response to vasodilatation is probably the reason for their clinical efficacy (Table 19.3).

Acute and chronic administration of captopril in heart failure is accompanied by modest increases in cardiac index (in the range of 0.0.4 L/min) accompanied by quite marked reduction in arterial blood pressure [77, 78]. The increase in output is exclusively due to increase in stroke volume: heart rate declines due to a fall in sympathetic activity and the vagotonic effects of angiotensin II withdrawal. An increase in renal blood flow is the predominant effect on the peripheral circulation [79, 80]. No changes in limb blood flow occur with acute administration, although the effects with chronic captopril therapy are controversial. Occasionally severe first dose hypotension occurs with ACE inhibitors; this is probably due to venodilation resulting in a fall in cardiac output compounded by the reduction in systemic vascular resistance due to reduced angiotensin II [77, 82].

Table 19.3. Currently available angiotensin-enzyme inhibitors.

Captopril	Perindopril	Fosinopril
Enalapril	Ramipril	Cilazapril
Lisinopril	Quinapril	

Captopril produces no significant effect on pulmonary vascular resistance [78, 83]. Enalapril, lisinopril, ramipril, quinapril and perindopril all share many of the characteristics of captopril, with similar improvements in cardiac output following acute administration and sustained benefit with long term oral use. Enalapril and captopril have been shown to reduce mortality during long term follow-up [84].

The results of large scale clinical trials have now shown that ACE inhibitors improve the prognosis of patients with systolic left ventricular dysfunction regardless of whether heart failure is present or not. ACE inhibitors delay the onset of heart failure either by retarding progressive impairment of ventricular function or by resetting the haemodynamic baseline from which the patient will deteriorate [105–107]. ACE inhibitors also reduce the risk of recurrent myocardial infarction [105–107].

Potential therapeutic interventions

A large number of vasoactive compounds is currently being evaluated for therapeutic potential. The most exciting of these are the endogenously occurring vasoactive peptides, which may have a future role in modifying cardiac output and peripheral resistance either through direct administration, or through inhibition of synthesis or breakdown. Their study has provided many of the answers in the long running debate over the mechanism of homeostasis of systemic vascular resistance and cardiac output.

A number of endogenously occurring peptides have been shown to be active on the cardiovascular system (Table 19.4); the effects of angiotensin, and bradykinin are more fully understood than those of the remaining peptides, whose physiologic role is not yet fully understood.

Bradykinin, Substance-P and the related neurokinins are amongst the most potent vasodilator agents known, primarily acting directly on the endothelium to facilitate EDRF production as well as that of prostanoids and especially prostacyclin.

Table 19.4. Vasoactive peptides and their physiological effect(s).

Peptide	Effect on vascular smooth muscle
Angiotensin	contraction
Vasopressin	contraction
Endothelin	contraction
Bradykinin	relaxation/contract
Calcitonin-gene related peptide	relaxation
Substance-P	relaxation
Neurokinin-A	relaxation/contraction
Opioids	inhibition of NAD release
Somatostatin	inhibition of NAD release
Bombesin	relaxation
Neurotensin	relaxation
Atial natriuretic peptide	relaxation

Calcitonin-gene related pepide (C-GRP)

C-GRP is a peptide possessing both smooth muscle relaxing and positive inotropic properties [85, 86]. Significantly, it also has positive chronotropic effects, and it appears that both the inotropic and chronotropic actions are mediated through modulation of intracellular calcium in a way which mimics the effects of beta adrenergic agonists [87].

Angiotensin II Angiotensin acts both directly and indirectly to increase SVR, acting via AII receptors on vascular smooth muscle and through enhanced synthesis and release of noradrenaline as well as through a possible effect on vascular wall sodium content [88].

There is evidence that vasoconstrictor peptides, such as *neuropeptide Y* are elevated in congestive heart failure compared with normal controls [89]. Inhibition of ACE may cause vasodilatation partly through increased levels of vasodilator peptides such as bradykinin+VIP [90].

Arginine vasopressin is also a potent vasopressor agent which is increased in congestive cardiac failure [91]. Its relationship to increased SVR is unknown, as plasma levels are not high enough to exert a substantial vasoconstrictor effect. Blockade of the vascular effect of AVP appears to have little effect on cardiac output even in congestive heart failure [92]. In experimental models, however, the vascular and antidiuretic effects of AVP have been discriminated, and it appears that if the vasoconstrictor effects are blocked, that peripheral resistance falls and cardiac output rises [93].

Endothelins are a family of powerful vasoconstrictor peptides, for which an increasing number of physiological roles is emerging. In addition to their important effects on SVR, at least one endothelin, ET-1 has been shown to exert a positive inotropic effect [94].

Atrial natriuretic peptide (ANP) causes vascular smooth muscle relaxation through an endothelium independent mechanism [95]. *In vivo* studies in man have shown that it is an arterioselective vasodilator which produces dose dependent increases in skin and muscle blood flow at doses producing plasma levels equivalent to those found in patients with heart failure [96]. Short term intravenous infusion of ANP in congestive heart failure has been reported to increase cardiac output and reduce left ventricular preload [97, 98]. However, reduced right atrial pressure due to venodilation or fluid shifts has also been reported to reduce cardiac output during prolonged ANP infusion [99, 100].

Atriopeptidase inhibitors. Experiments in animal models with inhibitors of neutral endopeptidase have failed to show any effect of the increased increased levels of ANP on left atrial pressure or cardiac output, though preliminary studies in human heart failure appear promising.

Prostaglandins. PGE-1 has been shown to increase cardiac output in patients with left ventricular dysfunction following myocardial infarction due largely to a reduction in SVR, but accompanied by reductions in left ventricular filling pressure and pulmonary vascular resistance [102].

Anti arrhythmic agents. Class 1 All anti-arrhythmic agents in Vaughan

Williams Class 1 have negative inotropic effects. These may be profound in the case of flecainide and disopyramide. Lignocaine, quinidine and procainamide have less marked negative inotropic effects, which may be further offset by vasodilatation in the case of procainamide.

Class 2. The haemodynamic effects of β blockage are dealt with above.

Class 3. Amiodarone is generally well tolerated haemodynamically. In patients with heart failure only slight cardiac depression is generally observed [103]. A reduction in heart rate may result in an artefactual increase in left ventricular ejection fraction which probably accounts for its apparent beneficial effect on ventricular function in heart failure.

Bretylium tosylate has powerful vasodilator actions due to ganglionic blockade and hence may cause increased cardiac output despite a negative inotropic tendency.

References

1. Withering W. An account of the foxglove and some of its medicinal uses: with practical remarks on dropsy and other diseases. London: GGJ Robinson.
2. Somberg J, Smith T. Localisation of the neurally mediated arrhythmogenic properties of digitalis. Science 1979;204:323–3.
3. Johnston G, McDevitt D. Is maintenance digoxin neccessary in patients with sinus rhythm? Lancet 1979;(1):564–70.
4. Sommers D, Reitz C, Koch Z. Digoxin withdrawal in patients with sinus rhythm. S Afr Med J 1981;60,:239–40.
5. Pugh S, White N, Aronson J et al. Clinical, haemodynamic and pharmacological effects of withdrawal and reintroduction of digoxin in patients with heart failure in sinus rhythm after long term treatment. Br Heart J 1989;61:529.
6. Braunwald E, Bloodwell R, Goldberg L et al. Studies on digitalis. IV. Observations in man on the effects of digitalis preparations on the contractility of the non-failing heart and on total vascular resistance. J Clin Invest 1961;40:529.
7. McMichael M, Sharpey-Schafer E. The action of intravenous digoxin in man. Q J Med 1944; 13: 123–35.
8. The Captopril-Digoxin Multicenter Research Group. Comparative effects of therapy with captopril and digoxin in patients with mild to moderate heart failure. J Am Med Assoc JAMA 1988;259:539–44.
9. Griffiths B, Penny W, MJL, Henderson A. Maintenance of the inotropic effect of digoxin on long term treatment. Br Med J 1982;284:1819–22.
10. Murray R, Tweddel A, Martin W et al. Evaluation of digitalis in cardiac failure. Br Med J 1982;284:1526–8.
11. The German and Austrian Xamoterol Study Group. Double blind placebo controlled comparison of digoxin and xamoterol in chronic heart failure. Lancet 1988;i:489–93.
12. Gheorghiade M, Hall V, Lakier JSG. Comparative haemodynamic and neurohumoral effects of intravenous captopril and digoxin and their combinations in patients with severe heart failure. J Am Coll Cardiol 1989;13:134–42.
13. Ahlquist R. A study of the adrenotropic receptors. Am J Physiol 1948;153:586–600.
14. Erdmann E, Bohm M. positive inotropic stimulation in the normal and insufficient human myocardium. Basic Res Cardiol 1989;84(Suppl 1):125–33.
15. Bristow M, Ginsburg R, Minobe W et al. Decreased catecholamine sensitivity and beta adrenergic receptor density in failing human hearts. N Engl J Med 1982;307:205–11.

16. Unverferth D, Blanford M, Kates R *et al*. Tolerance to dobutamine after a 72 hr continuous infusion. Am J Med 1980;69:262–6.
17. Kayanakis J, Coutaul L, Fauvel J *et al*. Changes in exercise tolerance and resting haemodynamics during long term treatment of heart failure with xamoterol. Eur Heart J 1990;11(Suppl A):52–53.
18. Nuttall A, Snow H. The cardiovascular effects of ICI118587: a betal adrenoceptor partial agonist. Br J Pharmacol 1982;77:381–8.
19. Beregovich J, Bianchi C, D'Angelo R *et al*. Haemodynamic effect of a new inotropic agent (dopamine) in chronic cardiac failure. Br Heart J 1975;37:629–33.
20. Beregovich J, Bianchi C, Rubler S *et al*. Dose related renal and hemodynamic effects of dopamine in congestive heart failure. Am Heart J 1974;87:550–7.
21. Clarke B. Dopamine receptor stimulants in hypertension. Acta Med Scand 1977;606(Suppl):95–9.
22. Crexells C, Bourassa M, Biron P. Effects of dopamine on myocardial metabolism in patients with ischaemic heart disease. Cardiovasc Res 1973;7:438–45.
23. Maroko P, Kjekshus J, Sobel B *et al*. Factors influencing infarct size following experimental coronary artery occlusion. Circulation 1971;72:67–82.
24. Goldberg L, Rajfer S. Dopamine receptors: applications in clinical cardiology. Circulation 1985;43:245–8.
25. Opie L. Drugs for the heart. 2nd ed. Orlando: Grune and Stratton,1987:102.
26. Taylor S. Pharmacotherapeutic profile of ibopamine in heart failure. J Cardiovasc Pharmacol 1989; 14(Suppl 8): S1118–S23.
27. Einertz T, Drexler H. Dopexamine in congestive heart failure: how do the pharmacological activities translate into the clinical situation? Basic Res Cardiol 1989;84(Suppl 1): 177–86.
28. Ruffolo R, Spradlin G, Pollock G *et al*. Alpha and beta effects of the stereoisomers of dobutamine. J Pharmacol Exp Ther 1981;219:447–52.
29. Sonnenblick E, Fishman W, LeJemtel T. Dobutamine: a new synthetic cardioactive sympathetic amine. New Engl J Med 1979;300:17–22.
30. Leier C, Webel J. The cardiovascular effects of the continuous infusion of dobutamine in patients with severe cardiac failure. Circulation 1977;56:468–72.
31. The Xamoterol in Severe Heart Failure Study Group. Xamoterol in severe heart failure. Lancet 1990;336:1–6.
32. Taylor S, Silke B. Haemodynamic effects of beta-blockade in ischaemic heart failure. Lancet 1981;2:835–7.
33. Englemeier R, O'Connell J, Walsh R *et al*. Improvement in symptoms and exercise tolerance by metoprolol in patients with dilated cardiomyopathy: a double blind, randomised, placebo controlled trial. Circulation 1985;72:536–46.
34. Heilbrunn S, Shah P, Bristow M *et al*. Increased beta receptor density and improved hemodynamic response to catecholamine stimulation during long term metoprolol therapy in heart failure from dilated cardiomyopathy. Circulation 1989;79:483–90.
35. Waagstein F, Caidahl K, Wallentin I *et al*. Long term Beta blockade in dilated cardiomyopathy: effects of short and long term metoprolol therapy followed by withdrawal and readministration of metoprolol. Circulation 1989;80:551–63.
36. Sharma B, Goodwin J. Beneficial effects of salbutamol on cardiac function in severe congestive cardiomyopathy. Effect on systolic and diastolic function of the left ventricle. Circulation 1978;58:449–60.
37. Exton J. Mechanisms involved in alpha adrenergic effects of catecholamines. New York: John Wiley & Sons, 1981: 117–29.
38. Agorien R, Sinnathamby S, Leier C *et al*. Rest and exercise effects of terazosin in congestive heart failure. Am J Cardiol 1990;65:638–43.
39. Colucci W, Williams G, Braunwald E. Clinical, haemodynamic and neuroendocrine effects of chronic prazosin therapy for congestive heart failure. Am Heart J 1981;102:615–21.
40. Adams H, Rhody J, Sutko J. Amrinone activates depolarised atrial and ventricular myocardium of guinea pigs. Circ Res 1982;51:662–5.

41. Kondo N, Shibata S, Kodama I et al. Electrical and mechanical effects of amrinone on isolated guinea pig ventricular muscle. J Cardiovasc Pharmacol 1983;5:903–12.
42. Rendig S, Amsterdam F. Positive inotropic effect of amrinone: effect of elevated external Ca^{++} Cardiovasc Pharmacol 1984;6:293–9.
43. Wynne J, Malacoff R, Benotti J et al. Oral amrinone in refractory congestive cardiac failure. Am J Cardiol 1980;45:1245–9.
44. Wilmshurst P. Hemodynamic effects of intravenous amrinone in patients with impaired left ventricular function. Br Heart J 1983;49:77–82.
45. Franciosa J. Intravenous amrinone: an advance or a wrong step? Ann Intern Med 1985;102:399–400.
46. Packer M, Medina N, Yushak M. Haemodynamic and clinical limitations of long term inotropic therapy with amrinone in patients with severe chronic heart failure. Circulation 1984;70:1038–47.
47. Alousi A, Carter J, Cicero F et al. Pharmacology milrinone. In: Braunwald E, Sonnenblick E, Chakrin L et al. (eds), Milrinone: investigation of new inotropic therapy for congestive heart failure. New York: Raven Press, 1984:21–48.
48. LeJemtel T, Maskin C, Chadwick B et al. Clinical response to long term milrinone therapy in patients with severe congestive heart failure. In: Braunwald E, Sonnenblick E, Chakrin L et al. (eds), Milrinone: investigation of new inotropic therapy for congestive heart failure. New York: Raven Press, 1984:177–90.
49. Colucci W, Wright R, Jash B et al. Milrinone and dobutamine in heart failure: differing hemodynamic effects and individual patient responses. Circulation 1986;73(3 Pt 2 Suppl):175–183.
50. Manrad E, McKay R, Baim D et al. Improvement in indexes of diastolic performance in patients with congestive heart failure. Circulation 1984;70:1030–37.
51. Crawford M, Richards K, Sodums M et al. Positive inotropic and vasodilator effects of MDL 17403 in patients with reduced left ventricular performance. Am J Cardiol 1984;53:1051–3.
52. Petein M, Levine B, Cohn J. Persistent haemodynamic effects without long term clinical benefits in response to oral piroximone (9MDL 19,205) in patients with congestive heart failure. Circulation 1986;173(Suppl III):III–230–6.
53. Weber K, Janicki J, Maskin C. Effects of new inotropic agents on exercise performance. Circulation 1986;73(Suppl III):III–196.
54. Uretsky B, Jessup M, Konstam M et al. Multicenter trial of oral enoximone in patients with moderate to moderately severe congestive heart failure. Circulation 1990;82:774–80.
55. Yeung Laiwah A, Mactier R. Antagonistic effect of non-steroidal anti-inflammatory drugs on frusemide-induced diuresis in cardiac failure. Br Med J 1981;283:714.
56. Atallah A. Interaction of prostaglandins with diuretics. Prostaglandins 1979;18:369–72.
57. Francis G, Siegel R, Goldsmith S et al. Acute vasoconstrictor response to intravenous furosemide in patients with chronic congestive heart failure. Ann Intern Med 1985;103:1–6.
58. Nikolic V, Omcikus M, Mihatov S et al. Daily administration of furosemide in dilated cardiomyopathy – yes or no? Acta Med Austriaca 1990;15:17–22.
59. Sinoway L, Minotti J, Musch T et al. Enhanced metabolic vasodilation secondary to diuretic therapy in decompensated congestive heart failure secondary to coronary artery disease. Am J Cardiol 1987;60:107.
60. Bussmann W-D, Schupp D. Effect of sublingual nitroglycerine in emergency treatment of severe pulmonary edema. 1978;41:931–6.
61. Nelson G, Silke B, Ahuja R et al. Haemodynamic advantages of isosorbide dinitrate over frusemide following myocardial infarction. Lancet 1983:730–3.
62. Packer M, Medina N, Yushak M et al. Haemodynamic factors limiting the response to transdermal nitroglycerine in chronic congestive heart failure. Am J Cardiol 1986;57:260–7.

63. Chatterjee K, Parmley W, Massie W *et al.* Oral hydrallazine therapy for chronic refractory heart failure. Circulation 1976;54:879–83.
64. Packer M. Vasodilator and inotropic therapy for severe chronic heart failure: passion and scepticism. J Am Coll Cardiol 1983;2:841–52.
65. McKay C, Chatterjee K, Ports T *et al.* Minoxidil therapy in chronic congestive heart failure: acute plus long term haemodynamic and clinical study. Am Heart J 1982;104:575–80.
66. Nathan M, Rubin S, Siemienczuk D *et al.* Effects of acute and chronic minoxidil administration on rest and exercise hemodynamics and clinical status in patients with severe chronic heart failure. Am J Cardiol 1982;50:960–6.
67. Markham R, Gilmore A, Pettinger W *et al.* Central and regional hemodynamic effects and neurohumoral consequences of minoxidil in severe congestive heart failure and comparison to hydralazine and nitroprusside. Am J Cardiol 1983;52:774–81.
68. Schneeweiss A, Wynne R, Marmor A. The effect of flosequinan in patients with acute-onset heart failure complicating acute myocardial infarction. Jpn Heart J 1989;30:627–34.
69. Cowley A, Wynne R, Stainer K *et al.* Flosequinan in heart failure: acute haemodynamic and longer term symptomatic effects. Br Med J 1988;297:169–73.
70. Chew C, Hecht H, Collett J *et al.* Influence of severity of ventricular dysfunction on haemodynamic responses to intravenously administered verapamil in ischaemic heart disease. 1981;47:917–22.
71. Matsumoto S, Ito T, Sada T. Haemodynamic effects of nifedipine in congestive heart failure. Am J cardiol 1980;46:476–80.
72. Tan L, Murray R, Littler W. Felodipine in patients with chronic heart failure: discrepant haemodynamic and clinical effects. Br Heart J 1987;58:122–8.
73. Agostoni P, De Cesare N, Doria E *et al.* Afterload reduction: a comparison of captopril and nifedipine in dilated cardiomyopathy. Br Heart J 1986;55:391–9.
74. Packer M, Nicod P, Khanderia B. Randomised multi-center placebo controlled evaluation of amlodipine in patients with mild to moderate heart failure. J Am Coll Cardiol 1991;17(Suppl 1):274A.
75. (Editorial) Calcium antagonist caution, Lancet 1991;33:885–6.
76. Ader R, Chatterjee K, Ports T *et al.* Immediate and sustained hemodynamic improvement in chronic heart failure by an oral angiotensin converting enzyme inhibitor. Circulation 1980;61:931–7.
77. Cleland J, Semple P, Hodsman P *et al.* Angiotensin II levels, haemodynamics and sympathoadrenal function after low dose captopril in heart failure. A J Med 1984;77:880–6.
78. Packer M, Meller J, Medina M *et al.* Quantitative differences in the haemodynamic effects of captopril and nitroprusside in severe chronic heart failure. Am J Cardiol 1983;51:183–8.
79. Cleland J, Dargie H, Hodsman G *et al.* Captopril in heart failure: a double blind controlled trial. Br Heart J 1984;52:530–5.
80. Cleland J, Dargie H, Ball S *et al.* Effects of enalapril in heart failure. Br Heart J 1985;54:305–12.
81. Faxon D, Halperin J, Creager M *et al.* Angiotensin inhibition in severe heart failure: Acute central and limb hemodynamic effects of captopril with observations on sustained oral therapy. Am Heart J 1981;51:183–8.
82. Cleland J, Dargie H, McAlpine H *et al.* Severe hypotension after first dose of enalapril in heart failure. Br Med J 1985;291:1309–12.
83. Packer M, Medina N, Yusak M *et al.* Hemodynamic patterns of response during long-term captopril therapy for severe chronic heart failure. Circulation 1983;68:803–12.
84. The CONSENSUS Trial Study Group. Effects of enalapril on mortality in severe congestive heart failure. N Engl J Med 1988;316:1429–35.
85. Kawasaki H, Takasaki K, Saito A *et al.* Calcitonin-gene related peptide acts as a novel vasodilator neurotransmitter in mesenteric resistance vessels of the rat. Nature 1988;335:164–7.

86. Miyauchi T, Ishikawa T, Sugishitsa Y *et al.* Effects of capsaicin on nonadrenergic noncholinergic nerves in the guinea pig atrium: role of calcitonin gene related peptide as cardiac neurotransmitter. J Cardiovasc Pharmacol 1987;10:675–82.

87. Ono K, Delay M, Nakajima T *et al.* Calcitonin gene-related peptide regulates calcium current in heart muscle. Nature 1989;340:721–4.

88. Opie L. The Heart. Physiology, Metabolism, Pharmacology and Therapy. Orlando and London: Grune and Stratton 1984.

89. Maisel A, Scott N, Motulsky H *et al.* Elevation of plasma neuropeptide Y levels in congestive heart failure. Am J Med 1989;86:43–6.

90. Woie L, Dickstein K, Kaada B. Increase in vasoactive polypeptides (VIP) by the angiotensin converting enzyme (ACE) inhibitor lisinopril in congestive heart failure. Relation to haemodynamic and hormonal changes. Gen Pharmacol 1987;18:577–87.

91. Goldsmith S, Francis G, Cowley A *et al.* Increased plasma arginine vasopressin levels in patients with congestive cardiac failure. J Am Coll Cardiol 1983;1:1385–90.

92. Nicod P, Waeber B, Bussien J-P *et al.* Acute haemodynamic effects of a vascular antagonist of vasopressin in patients with congestive cardiac failure. Am J Cardiol 1985;5:1043–7.

93. Liard J-F. Cardiovascular effects of vasopressin: some recent aspects. J Cardiovasc Pharmacol 1986;8(Suppl 7):S61–S65.

94. Ishikawa T, Yanagisawa M, Kimura S *et al.* The positive inotropic action of a novel vasoconstrictor peptide endothelin. Am J Physiol 1988;255:H970–73.

95. Murad F. Cyclic guanosine monophosphate as a mediator of vasodilatation. J Clin Invest 1986;78:1–5.

96. Webb D, Benjamin N, Allen M *et al.* Vascular responses to local atrial natriuretic peptide infusion in man. Br J Clin Pharmacol 1988;26:245–51.

97. Cody R, Atlas S, Laragh J *et al.* Atrial natriuretic factor in normal subjectsand heart failure patients; plasma levels and renal, hormonal and hemodynamic responses to peptide infusion. J Clin Invest 1986;78:1362–74.

98. Molina C, Fowler M, McCrory S *et al.* Hemodynamic, renal and endocrine effects of atrial natriuretic peptide infusion in severe heart failure. J Am Coll Cardiol 1988;12:175–176.

99. Marks E, Zukowska-Grojec Z, Ropchak T *et al.* Alterations in systemic haemodynamics induced by atriopeptin III. J Hypertension 1987;5:39–46.

100. Almeida F, Suzuki M, Maack T. Atrial natriuretic factor increases haematocrit and decreases plasma volume in nephrectomised rats. Life Sci 1986;39:1193–9.

101. Cavero P, Margulies K, Winaver J *et al.* Cardiorenal actions of neutral endopeptidase inhibition in experimental congestive heart failure. Circulation 1990;82:196–201.

102. Popat K, Pitt B. Hemodynamic effects of prostaglandin E1 infusion in patients with acute myocardial infarction and left ventricular failure. Am Heart J 1982;103:485–9.

103. Cleland J, Dargie H, Findlay I *et al.* Clinical, haemodynamic and antiarrhythmic effects of long term treatment with amiodarone of patients in heart failure. Br Heart J 1987;57:436–45.

104. Packer M, Carver JR, Rodeheffer RJ *et al.* Effect of oral milrinone on mortality in severe chronic heart failure. N Engl J Med 1991;325(21):1468–75.

105. Swedberg K, Held P, Kjekshus J *et al.* Effects of the early administration of enalapril on mortality in patients with acute myocardial infarction. Results of the Coperative New Scandinavian Enalapril Survival Study II (CONSENSUS II). N Engl J Med 1992;327:678–84.

106. The SOLVD Investigators. Effect of enalapril on mortality and the development of heart failure in asymptomatic patients with reduced left ventricular ejection fractions. N Engl J Med 1992;327:685–91.

107. Pfeffer M, Braunwald E, Moye LA *et al.* Effect of captopril on mortality and morbidity in patients with left ventricular dysfunction after myocardial infarction. N Engl J Med 1992;327:669–77.

20. Changes in cardiac output during rapid atrial pacing

ABDULMASSIH S. ISKANDRIAN

The changes in cardiac output in patients with permanent pacemakers will be discussed in a separate chapter (Chapter 24). This chapter will deal with pacing as a stress test and will discuss the results in normal subjects, patients with coronary artery disease, patients with aortic regurgitation, and finally patients with congestive heart failure.

Abnormality in the site of impulse generation and sequence of activation may affect ventricular filling and stroke volume. The ideal situation is exemplified in subjects with normal sinus rhythm; the activation of the ventricles is in an organized fashion and atrial contraction contributes to ventricular filling. Loss of atrial contraction or inappropriate coupling (too short or too long P-R intervals) may affect left ventricular filling especially in the presence of a stiff left ventricle such as in patients with ischemia or hypertrophy. Loss of normal synchrony of activation may also impede left ventricular contraction and emptying. The worse scenario is probably seen in patients with ventricular pacing whereby the sequence of activation is abnormal and there is no atrial contribution; there may even be mitral regurgitation because of the abnormal sequence of contraction [1].

Atrial pacing approaches normal physiology by maintaining both atrial contraction and the synchrony of activation. However, with fast pacing rate, the P-R interval gradually prolongs, and the P-wave may coincide with the T-wave, therefore decreasing the effectiveness of atrial contribution to ventricular filling.

Atrial contraction may contribute 10–15% to left ventricular filling in normal subjects but as much as 50% in patients with stiff left ventricles. The pacing tachycardia may by itself have a positive inotropic effect, the so called "treppe effect" [1–3].

In normal subjects as well as in patients with coronary heart disease, atrial pacing may result in Wenchebach type first degree A-V block which may even occur at a low pacing rate. Atropine is often used to accelerate conduction through the A-V node which by its vagolytic effect may also enhance ventricular function. Finally, the anxiety associated with the procedure may increase sympathetic activity and contribute to enhancement of ventricular filling and emptying as well.

A.-M. Salmasi and A.S. Iskandrian (eds): Cardiac output and regional flow in health and disease, 251–259.

Methods

A pacing catheter is positioned in the high right atrium or into the coronary sinus (via the femoral vein or the antecubital vein). For measurement of the cardiac output, a Swan-Ganz thermodilution catheter is advanced into the pulmonary artery. The blood pressure is measured by the cuff method or via an arterial line. The usual parameters measured during a pacing study include changes in the electrocardiogram (ST-segment shifts); hemodynamic measurements (pulmonary artery wedge pressure, pulmonary artery pressure, right ventricular and right atrial pressures and the cardiac output); left ventricular function studies including pressure/volume relationship using either contrast ventriculography or more often radionuclide angiography; assessment of the perfusion pattern using thallium-201; measurement of the coronary blood flow (most often by the thermodilution technique) and metabolic measurements such as measurement of the coronary sinus lactate. One electrocardiographic lead or more is continuously monitored during pacing, the blood pressure is obtained at every minute or is monitored constantly if an arterial line is used. Pacing is started at a rate of 10 beats/minute above the baseline heart rate, and is increased by 10 beats every 2–3 minutes until a maximum pacing rate is reached (usually 150 beats/minute) or when angina pectoris of at least moderate severity, ST-segment depression, hypotension or marked abnormalities in hemodynamics are observed.

When radionuclide angiography is combined with pacing, a portable gamma camera may be used in the cardiac catheterization laboratory or alternatively after the catheters are placed in position, the patient is transferred to the nuclear cardiology laboratory where the final measurements are performed. More recently transesophageal pacing has been used in combination with thallium-201 or two-dimensional echocardiography in patients undergoing transoesophageal echocardiographic studies.

The most common method for measuring the cardiac output during pacing is the thermodilution technique. The combination of the thermodilution-derived stroke volume and the radionuclide-derived ejection fraction permits precise assessment of left ventricular end-diastolic and end-systolic volumes because both the stroke volume and ejection fraction are derived by methods independent on geometric assumptions and have been proven to be accurate and reproducible [1–4]. The equations used are as follows:

$$\text{Stroke volume} = \frac{\text{Cardiac out (thermodilution)}}{\text{Heart rate}}$$

$$\text{EF} = \frac{\text{SV}}{\text{EDV}} \times 100,$$

where EF is ejection fraction, SV is stroke volume and EDV is end-diastolic volume. Assuming that the right and left ventricular stroke volumes are equal, the right ventricular end-diastolic and end-systolic volumes can be similarly calculated. The rest of the discussion therefore will be based on this combination of techniques unless otherwise stated.

Normal subjects

The cardiac output with rapid atrial pacing in normal subjects either does not change or increases slightly. The effect of tachycardia is neutralized by a proportionate decrease in stroke volume because of the reduction in the diastolic filling period. The slight increase in cardiac output observed in some normal subjects may be secondary to inotropic effect secondary to pacing tachycardia, excitement or effect of medications.

There is also a decrease in end-diastolic volume and end-systolic volume of both the left and right ventricles because of the decrease in the diastolic filling period. The ejection fraction often remains unchanged despite a decrease in the preload. Maintenance of the ejection fraction is most likely related to the decrease in the systolic blood pressure (decrease in afterload), and enhanced contractility because of the "treppe effect" discussed earlier. In fact, the systolic blood pressure/end-systolic volume ratio increases with pacing suggesting enhanced contractility.

Although the systolic blood pressure decreases, the mean aortic pressure does not change, and there is a decrease in the pulse pressure reflecting the reduction in the stoke volume. The left ventricular end-diastolic pressure decreases because of the decrease in end-diastolic volume, although the wedge pressure remains unchanged [1–3] (Table 20.1).

Pacing results in no wall motion abnormalities in normal subjects, and the myocardial metabolism remains aerobic as reflected by lactate extraction, with a slight increase in coronary flood flow.

Patients with coronary artery disease

Atrial pacing may be used in combination with radionuclide angiography or thallium-201 to detect coronary artery disease in patients who are not ideal candidates for exercise testing such as those with peripheral vascular disease neuro-musculo-skeletal disease, chronic obstructive pulmonary disease or other contraindications for exercise testing. More recently however, the availability of potent coronary vasodilators such as dipyridamole and adenosine which are used in conjunction with thallium-201 or the newer technetium labelled perfusion agents have decreased the need for pacing studies as a screening test for coronary artery disease. However, pacing may remain an appropriate approach in patients with bronchospasm in whom adenosine and dipyridamole studies are contraindicated.

In the catheterization laboratory pacing studies have been extremely important to the understanding of the pathophysiology of ischemia heart disease, and in the study of the pharmacologic effect of various drugs [2, 3, 5–8].

Table 20.1. Hemodynamic data at rest and during pacing in normal subjects and patients with coronary artery disease.

	Normal (n = 8)		CAD (n = 10)		
	Baseline	Pacing	Baseline	Submaximal	Maximal
HR	72 ± 8	123 ± 11[a]	67 ± 9	99 ± 4[a]	130 ± 10[a]
PA	16 ± 5	16 ± 6	19 ± 4	18 ± 5	23 ± 5[b]
AO	96 ± 7	101 ± 5	106 ± 8	114 ± 13	118 ± 12[b]
CI	3.2 ± 0.6	3.3 ± 0.6	2.9 ± 0.4	3.2 ± 0.6	3.0 ± 0.6
EDVI	79 ± 13	47 ± 8[a]	102 ± 26	76 ± 26[a]	65 ± 26[a]
ESVI	35 ± 6	21 ± 5[a]	58 ± 20	44 ± 21[a]	42 ± 24[a]
EF	54 ± 3	56 ± 5	45 ± 7	45 ± 8	40 ± 12
ESP/ESV	1.5 ± 0.4	2.6 ± 0.8[a]	1.2 ± 0.6	1.7 ± 0.8[a]	2.0 ± 1.4[b]

AO = mean aortic pressure (mm Hg); CAD = coronary artery disease; CI = cardiac index (liters/min/m²); EDVI = end-diastolic volume index (ml/m²); EF = left ventricular ejection fraction; (%); ESP/ESV = end-systolic pressure/end-systolic volume, ESVI = end-systolic volume index (ml/m²); PA = mean pulmonary artery pressure (mm Hg); EDVI and ESVI were derived from the thermodilution and radionuclide angiographic measurements.
[a] $p < 0.001$.
[b] $p < 0.01$ (baseline vs pacing).
Note: there is no significant change in cardiac output with pacing. The decrease in EDV is progressive. The patients with CAD are different from patients reported in Table II. (Source: Iskandrian *et al.* Am J Cardiol 1983;51:1057.)

It should be noted that the stress of atrial pacing is less than that that of exercise testing because unlike exercise, there is a decrease in systolic blood pressure, a decrease in end-diastolic volume, and hence lower myocardial oxygen demand. Nevertheless, atrial pacing may cause hemodynamic abnormalities even in the absence of symptoms. In fact, the presence or absence of chest discomfort during pacing is not a reliable predictor of the presence and extent of ischemic abnormality.

The cardiac output during pacing in patients with coronary artery disease either does not change or increases slightly (similar to the observations in normal subjects) as long as ischemia is not induced (such as submaximal pacing). At peak pacing and with the development of myocardial ischemia, the cardiac output may decrease due to deterioration in left ventricular function and a decrease in ejection fraction resulting in a further decrease in stroke volume. The development of myocardial ischemia can also be manifested as ST-segment depression; increase in pulmonary capillary wedge pressure; decrease in cardiac output; new or worsening wall motion abnormality; decrease in ejection fraction, decrease in contractility (such as a decrease in systolic pressure/end-systolic volume ratio) and lactate production. In severe cases of ischemia, pulsus alternans may develop. Pacing-induced ischemia may result not only in systolic left ventricular dysfunction, but also in diastolic dysfunction with an increase in left ventricular stiffness which contributes to the elevation of the left ventricular filling pressure resulting from a shift in the left ventricular diastolic pressure-volume relation-

Table 20.2. Hemodynamic data at baseline and during rapid pacing in 12 patients with coronary artery disease.

Variable	Baseline	Pacing	p
HR (bpm)	72 ± 11	139 ± 12	<0.0001
CO (L/min)	5.4 ± 0.9	6.0 ± 1.7	NS
BP (mm Hg)			
Systolic	148 ± 19	149 ± 25	NS
Diastolic	78 ± 12	95 ± 20	<0.01
Mean	104 ± 12	116 ± 19	NS
PAW (mm Hg)	9 ± 4	16 ± 8	<0.004
PA (mm Hg)	17 ± 3	23 ± 7	<0.009
RV systolic (mm Hg)	26 ± 6	29 ± 7	<0.004
RA (mm Hg)	7 ± 4	9 ± 4	<0.04
LVEF (%)	45 ± 10	41 ± 14	<0.04
LVEDV (ml)	179 ± 58	118 ± 48	<0.0006
LVESV (ml)	107 ± 56	78 ± 44	NS
RVEF (%)	35 ± 7	31 ± 7	<0.05
RVEDV (ml)	229 ± 75	145 ± 45	<0.001
RVESV (ml)	153 ± 68	102 ± 35	<0.04

BP = blood pressure; CO = cardiac output; EDV = end-diastolic; EF = ejection fraction; ESV = end-systolic volume; HR = heart rate; LV = left ventricular; NS = not significant; PA = mean pulmonary artery pressure; RA = mean right atrial pressure, RV = right ventricle.

Table 20.3. Comparison of hemodynamics during pacing in a coronary artery disease in patients with ischemia (#1) or without ischemia (#2).

	Pt #1			Pt #2		
	Rest	Submaximal pacing	Peak pacing	Rest	Submaximal pacing	Peak pacing
HR (bpm)	78	104	151	66	102	153
AO (mm Hg)	180/90 (110)	184/97(135)	135/107(121)	140/70(98)	140/80(104)	150/100(120)
CO(L/min)	3.8	4.8	2.8	5.0	5.6	4.9
PA(mm Hg)	30/8(18)	32/7(18)	35/22(30)	24/9(16)	16/8	20/20(16)

HR: heart rate; AO: aortic pressure; CO: cardiac output; PA: pulmonary artery pressure.

ship upwards and to the left. Obviously, the denominator for all these abnormalities is the failure to increase the coronary blood flow proportionate to the increase in myocardial oxygen demand. Furthermore, with the development of myocardial ischemia, papillary muscle dysfunction may occur resulting in mitral regurgitation and a decrease in forward cardiac output (Tables 20.1–20.3).

Importantly, these hemodynamic derangements promptly return to baseline upon discontinuation of the pacing. Ischemia is a function of a disparity in the myocardial oxygen supply and demand, the demand being determined by the pacing tachycardia. It's also possible that there is an actual reduction in coronary blood flow with rapid pacing due to vasospastic changes at the site of coronary stenosis. In some, but not all patients, similar abnormalities may be seen in the right ventricular function.

Patients with aortic regurgitation

Pacing studies in patients with aortic regurgitation are fascinating because of the complex nature of the hemodynamic abnormalities that involve changes in pressures, volumes, forward output, regurgitant volume, and total cardiac output.

To begin with, the regurgitant fraction equals to the regurgitant stroke volume divided by the total stroke volume. Let us assume that the total left ventricular stroke volume is 150 cc/beat, of which 80 cc/beat reflects the forward (or net) volume/beat, and 70 cc is the regurgitant volume/beat. The regurgitant fraction equals 47% (70/150 × 100) Let us also assume that the resting heart rate was 75 beats/min. The total cardiac output = 75 × 150 = 11.25 liters/min; the regurgitant flow = 75 × 70 = 5.25 liters/min, and the net (or forward) cardiac output = to 75 × 80 = 6 liters/min.

The regurgitant volume depends on the gradient between aortic pressure and the left ventricular pressure during diastole, size of the aortic valve, diastolic filling period and the total cardiac output which depends on the left ventricular end-diastolic volume and ejection fraction [1, 4].

Pacing will cause a decrease in left ventricular end-diastolic volume, a decrease in total stroke volume, a decrease in forward stroke volume, and a decrease in regurgitant stroke volume, but no change in the total cardiac output, net cardiac output, and net regurgitant flow, because the pacing tachycardia compensates for the reduction in the stroke volume. The regurgitant fraction does not change but as mentioned above, the regurgitant volume/beat decreases. In the above example let's assume that pacing was performed to a rate of 150 beats/min. which resulted in a decrease in the total stroke volume to 75 cc, regurgitant stroke volume to 35 cc, and the forward stroke volume to 40 cc. Hence, the total cardiac output remains 11.25, the regurgitant volume 5.25, the forward cardiac output 6 liters/min, and the regurgitant fraction 47%. The reduction in the total stroke volume reflects the reduction in the end-diastolic volume due to a decrease in diastolic filling period. The above assumptions are valid if pacing does not result in additional changes in left ventricular performance, i.e. if the ejection fraction remains unchanged. However, in many patients the marked decrease in the preload will result in a decrease in ejection fraction which will result in a further reduction in the total and the net cardiac outputs.

A clinically important observation from the above hemodynamic changes can be applied to patients with hemodynamic compromise due to acute aortic regurgitation. Pacing tachycardia, by reducing the left ventricular end-diastolic volume, will result in a decrease in end-diastolic pressure and pulmonary artery wedge pressure and clearance of the pulmonary edema. This

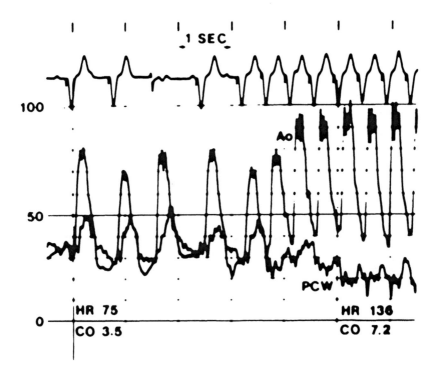

Figure 20.1. Simultaneous tracings of the aortic pressure and pulmonary artery wedge pressure in a patient with severe acute aortic regurgitation due to endocarditis. This patient developed high degree A-V block because of the spread of infarction to the conduction system. Rapid pacing resulted in a decrease in wedge pressure (PCW), increase in aortic pressure (AO) and increase in cardiac output (measured by thermodilution) (courtesy of Gary Mintz, M.D.).

may be a lifesaving measuring before urgent surgery can be undertaken (Figure 20.1).

Patients with congestive heart failure

A compensentary mechanism in patients with congestive heart failure and severe left ventricular dysfunction is left ventricular dilatation. The dilation maintains normal or near normal the resting stroke volume and cardiac output. The dilation however, may result in an increase in wall stress, and secondary hypertrophy in order to normalize the wall stress and maintain the left ventricular performance. We have observed that in patients with one-vessel coronary artery disease and localized scar due to old infarction, that the wall motion abnormality extends to areas remote from infarcted myocardium, even though such areas are nourished by normal coronary arteries. This is indeed unexpected since such areas should be supernormal or at least normal to maintain reasonable left ventricular performance. In patients with acute myocardial infarction, the remodelling process similarly results in dilatation and hypofunction of remote areas.

I have suggested that this dilatation may be detrimental because of the slippage in the actin-myosin junctions, resulting in a decrease in the developed tension, i.e. the fiber stretch exceeds the L-max length-tension relationship [9]. Since pacing uniformly causes a decrease in left ventricular dimension by decreasing the diastolic filling period, it may decrease the slippage and optimize fiber length and improve left ventricular function, stroke volume and cardiac output. Because the remodelling may be a slow process, the beneficial effects may not be detected immediately.

Thus, pacing in patients with congestive heart failure may be looked upon as a therapeutic rather than a diagnostic approach. I have suggested also that the ideal candidates for this kind of treatment are patients who have bradycardia at rest (either spontaneously or induced by medications) and patients without extensive coronary artery disease who may tolerate pacing rates in the range of 100–110 beats/min without development of myocardial ischemia. Additional advantages of pacing include a decrease in wall stress, and a decrease in mitral or tricuspid regurgitation and optimization of atrial contribution to ventricular filling.

A recent report by Hochteitner et al. [10] showed improvement in symptoms in small and selected group of patients with severe congestive heart failure. Obviously, further studies are needed to define the role of pacemaker therapy in such patients.

References

1. Iskandrian AS. Atrial pacing. In:.Iskandrian AS (ed.), Nuclear cardiac imaging: principles and applications. Philadelphia: F.A. Davis, 1987:344–50.
2. Iskandrian AS, Hakki AH, Bemis CE et al. Left ventricular end-systolic pressure-volume relation: combined radionuclide and hemodynamic study. Am J Cardiol 1983;51:1057.
3. Iskandrian AS, Bemis CE, Hakki AH et al. Ventricular systolic and diastolic impairment during pacing-induced myocardial ischemia in coronary artery disease: simultaneous hemodynamic, electrocardiographic and radionuclide angiographic evaluation. Am Heart J 1986;112:382–91.
4. Iskandrian AS, Hakki AH, Kane SA et al. Quantitative radionuclide angiography in assessment of hemodynamic changes during upright exercise: observations in normal subjects, patients with coronary artery disease and patients with aortic regurgitation. Am J Cardiol 1981;48:239–46.
5. Bourdillon PD, Lorell BH, Mirsky I et al. Increased regional myocardial stiffness of the left ventricle during pacing-induced angina in man. Circulation 1983;67:316.
6. Parker J.O, Chlong MA, West RO et al. Sequential alternations in myocardial lactate metabolism, ST segments, left ventricular function during angina induced by atrial pacing. Circulation 1969;40:113–31.
7. McLaurin LP, Rolette EL, Grossman W. Impaired left ventricular relaxation during pacing-induced ischemia. Am J Cardiol 1973;32:751.

8. Mann JT, Brodie RR, Grossman W *et al*. Effect of angina on left ventricular diastolic pressure-volume relationships. Circulation 1977;55:761.

9. Iskandrian AS. Pacemaker therapy in congestive heart failure. Am J Cardiol 1990;66:223–4.

10. Hochleitner M, Hortnagl H, Ng CK *et al*. Usefulness of physiologic dual-chamber pacing in drug-resistant idiopathic dilated cardiomyopathy. Am J Cardiol 1990;66:198–202.

21. The hemodynamics of cardiac pacing

WALTER R. HEPP and LEONARD N. HOROWITZ

One of the greatest advances in medical technology in the twentieth century was the advent of the permanent implantable pacemaker. Until that time, patients suffering from conduction abnormalities, symptomatic brady-arrhythmias, and some tachyarrhythmias, had no reliable form of medical treatment. These patients were often symptomatic presenting with fatigue, weakness, shortness of breath, mental status changes, near syncope, and syncope.

In 1958, the first permanent pacemaker was implanted. The pacemaker functioned with fixed-rate asynchronous ventricular pacing. The constant rate provided by the pacemaker greatly improved the cardiac performance and sense of well-being in patients suffering with symptomatic bradyarrhythmias. Although these pacemakers marked a great advance in medical technology, they were far from the ideal "physiologic pacemaker."

Over the past 32 years, pacemakers have evolved from single chamber asynchronous devices to current multiprogrammable dual chamber pacemakers capable, with sensor technology, of adjusting the pacing rate based upon changes in certain measured physiologic parameters.

In this chapter we will review the determinants of cardiac performance and how pacemaker therapy has evolved to improve the hemodynamics of cardiac pacing.

The circulation and cardiac dynamics

The purpose of the circulatory system is to continuously deliver oxygen-rich blood to the body while at the same time to remove waste and transport blood to the lungs for gas exchange. The circulatory system requires an integrated response between the heart, systemic arteries and veins, lungs, and pulmonary artery and veins. The heart itself is central to the flow of blood in this system, continuously pumping blood throughout the circulation.

Normally, the driving force behind the heart is the sinoatrial (SA) node. The SA node discharges rhythmically under autoregulatory control. The cardiac impulse traverses the atria resulting in atrial depolarization and subsequent atrial contraction. The impulse continues through the atrioventricular

A.-M. Salmasi and A.S. Iskandrian (eds): Cardiac output and regional flow in health and disease, 261–271.
© 1993 Kluwer Academic Publishers. Printed in the Netherlands.

node and the bundle of His to the Purkinje system by which ventricular depolarization and ventricular contraction are initiated.

Atrial contraction in late diastole serves normally as a "booster pump" following passive ventricular filling and further elevates ventricular end diastolic volume. As the ventricular pressure rises above the atrial pressure, the atrioventricular valves close and the aortic and pulmonic valves open. Blood is ejected during ventricular systole until the aortic pressure exceeds the left ventricular pressure. This results in aortic and pulmonic valve closure.

During diastole, the ventricular pressures fall below the atrial pressures and the atrioventricular valves open allowing passive filling of the ventricle. Atrial contraction from the next sinoatrial node depolarization again causes active filling of the ventricle in late diastole and the cardiac cycle begins again.

Determinants of cardiac performance at rest

There are three major determinants of cardiac performance – preload, afterload, and contractility. Cardiac performance is commonly measured in terms of the amount of blood pumped through the heart over a period of time. When measured in liters per minute, this performance measurement is termed the cardiac output. The cardiac output is the multiple of the heart rate and stroke volume (amount of blood expelled from the heart with each systole). Preload, afterload, and myocardial contractility are the physiologic factors that determine the cardiac output.

Preload

Preload is the load or force which stretches the myofibers in diastole and determines the end diastolic filling pressure. Increases in preload have been shown to augment stroke volume as well as the extent and velocity of myocardial shortening. Additionally, a linear relationship exists between ventricular end diastolic pressures and volumes. Simply stated, as end diastolic pressure rises, the end diastolic volume rises in a linear fashion and preload is increased.

There are several factors that contribute to preload. One of the most obvious factors is volume status. A fall in venous return due to dehydration or blood loss will be associated with a lowering of the ventricular end diastolic pressure and hence preload. Decreased fiber stretch will be associated with a lower stroke volume which will result in a lower cardiac output.

Venous return is the second determinant of preload. Preload can be significantly reduced under conditions of low peripheral vascular resistance such as fever, sepsis, and anemia. Other conditions associated with decreased venous return include elevations in intrathoracic pressure and position changes from supine to upright posture. Catecholamine and muscular activity tend to augment venous return to the heart.

When properly timed, atrial contraction is the third factor that augments ventricular filling and preload. Atrial systole during late diastole results in increased ventricular end diastolic pressure and volume. This also results in lower mean atrial pressures than those observed during atrial fibrillation or poorly timed atrial contractions.

Patients with severe left ventricular dysfunction appear to benefit least in cardiac performance from atrial systole. It appears that these patients with dilated ventricles and high end diastolic pressures gain very little in stroke volume from the atrial systole due to already high end diastolic pressures. On the other hand, those patients with diastolic dysfunction, as seen with ventricular hypertrophy and decreased diastolic compliance, appear to be very dependent on the atrial contribution to ventricular filling. Atrial systole has been shown to contribute as much as 30% to the cardiac output. Clinical deterioration is often seen when patients with decreased ventricular compliance develop atrial fibrillation.

Afterload

Afterload is the second factor that contributes to cardiac performance. Afterload is defined as that force or load which acts on the myofibers after the onset of shortening. Hence afterload represents those forces that resist ventricular emptying.

Elevations in afterload have been shown to reduce myofiber shortening and stroke volume. Afterload therefore is a major determinant of the amount of blood ejected by the ventricle.

The most important determinant of afterload is the aortic impedance. Aortic impedance is influenced by the peripheral arterial resistance, the condition of the arterial vasculature system, and the volume of blood.

Contractility

Cardiac contractility is the third factor that influences cardiac performance. Contractility represents the inherent ability of the cardiac contractile elements to generate force when stimulated independent of changes resulting from afterload or preload. Improved contractility results in significantly greater cardiac performance. Factors that augment cardiac contractility include sympathetic nerve stimulation, circulating catecholamines, and heart rate.

Cardiac performance during exercise

With the onset of exertion, several physiologic changes occur. An increase in metabolic rate increases tissue needs and utilization of oxygen. Local products of increased metabolism are generated and there is an increase in CO_2 production. These influences affect the circulatory system by increasing the cardiac output.

Elevation of the cardiac output is accomplished primarily by an increase in heart rate. The increase in heart rate may be threefold over resting heart rates. To a lesser extent, the stroke volume also increases up to 150%. As can be seen by the elevations in heart rate and stroke volume, the cardiac output may increase by 4.5 times over resting levels.

Heart rate is increased by heightened sinus node automaticity secondary to neurohumoral stimulation.

Stroke volume is augmented by several factors. Increased heart rate increases myocardial contractility independent of circulating catecholamines. Peripheral vasodilatation reduces afterload, which improves systolic function and increases stroke volume. Muscular activity augments venous return which elevates end diastolic volume and preload. This results in augmented stroke volume. Therefore with the onset of exertion, physiologic demands are met by augmented rate response primarily with a smaller contribution from augmented stroke volume.

Pacing and cardiac performance

When a pacemaker is determined to be clinically indicated, there are a host of decisions to be made regarding pacemaker selection. The type of arrhythmia or conduction abnormality often dictates which pacemaker modality will be most advantageous in restoring the normal physiologic functioning of the heart. Ideally, physiologic function of the heart is preserved when AV synchrony and rate responsiveness are maintained with pacemaker therapy.

There are many combinations of pacemaker modalities. Because of the complexity of these modalities, a better code has been devised. This letter code in the past has consisted of three positions, each referring to a specific functioning modality. Recently, two positions have been added due to the expanding capabilities of today's pacemakers.

The first letter code position refers to the cardiac chamber(s) which be paced. An A, V, or D in this position indicates that the atrium, ventricle, or both the atrium and ventricle are paced.

The second letter code position refers to the cardiac chamber(s) which the pacemaker senses spontaneous electrical activity. An A, V, or D in this position again refer to atrial, ventricular, or both atrial and ventricular chambers have sensed electrical activity. The letter 0 in this position indicates that sensing spontaneous electrical activity is not present.

The third letter code position refers to the way the pacemaker will respond to sensed electrical activity. The letter 0 in this position indicates that activity is not sensed and therefore the pacemaker will pace at a fired rate irrespective of spontaneous cardiac activity. An I or T in this position indicates that sensed spontaneous activity will inhibit pacemaker activity or trigger the pacemaker to deliver a stimulus respectfully. The letter D in this position indicates that a sensed electrical event will either inhibit or trigger a pacemaker stimulus.

The fourth letter code position refers to the noninvasive programmability of the pacemaker. The fifth letter code position refers to the tachyarrhythmia functions of antitachycardia pacemakers. The fourth and fifth letter code positions will not be used in this chapter.

Rate responsive pacemakers have sensors which monitor specific physiologic parameters. During exercise and changes in these physiologic parameters, the pacemaker sensor controls pacemaker rate changes. This programmable function will be designated by a hyphenated R after the standard three letter position code.

Asynchronous pacemakers (AOO, VOO)

Pacemakers in the late 1950s and early 1960s functioned in the asynchronous pacing mode. These pacemakers currently have no clinical indication and may be considered "obsolete" due to the availability of alternative and more adaptive pacing modalities. Asynchronous pacing modes pace at a fixed rate irrespective of the underlying cardiac activity. These pacemakers were single chamber devices and capable of pacing in the atrium or ventricle. Many single chamber demand pacemakers revert to the asynchronous mode whenever a magnet is placed over the pacemaker generator.

The advent of the asynchronous permanent pacemaker greatly improved the resting hemodynamics in patients suffering from bradyarrhythmias. The increased cardiac performance was a direct result of the increased heart rate provided by the fixed rate pacing over the resting bradyarrhythmia. Increased cardiac demands and subsequent increased heart rate response was not possible with asynchronous pacing. These conditions resulted in limited exertional effort due to lack of heart rate response. Cardiac output increases with fixed rate pacing was limited and due to increased stroke volume.

Demand pacemakers

Demand atrial and ventricular pacemakers were the second generation system developed with the application of sensor technology. Analogous to the asynchronous pacemakers, the demand pacemakers are a single chamber device capable of pacing the atrium or ventricle. Sensor technology, however, now allowed the pacemaker to stimulate the heart on demand when no appropriately timed spontaneous electrical activity was detected. This advancement eliminates competitive pacing found with asynchronous pacing devices.

Demand pacemakers function in the triggered (T) or inhibited (I) mode. Both modes are designed to deliver a pacing stimulus at a specific pacing interval if no appropriately timed spontaneous cardiac impulse is detected. The triggered mode additionally will deliver a pacing stimulus immediately after each sensed spontaneous impulse and reset its pacing timing cycle. The triggered mode was not as frequently used as the inhibited mode.

In the inhibited mode, the pacemaker will withhold a stimulus in response to any appropriately timed sensed impulse. Following a sensed event, the pacemaker resets its pacing cycle. If a spontaneous event is not sensed at the end of the programmed pacing cycle, the pacemaker will deliver a stimulus.

Atrial demand pacemakers are indicated in some forms of sick sinus syndrome associated with normal AV conduction. This pacing mode preserves AV synchrony with fixed atrial rate pacing and ensured an adequate cardiac output at rest.

The importance of AV synchrony at rest can be demonstrated by comparing identical rate pacing in the AAI and VVI mode. For a given patient with symptomatic sinus bradycardia and normal AV conduction, AAI pacing can increase the resting cardiac output by as much as 30% over VVI pacing at identical rates. Of note, the maximal increases in cardiac output during both AAI and WI pacing generally occurs with pacing rates between 60 and 100 beats per minute.

The augmented cardiac output with AAI pacing is due to the increased stroke volume which is the result of the atrial contribution to ventricular filling. Increased end diastolic ventricular volume or preload results in increased myocardial contractility which augments stroke volume. However, under conditions of left ventricular dysfunction and already elevated end diastolic pressures, the atrial contribution to ventricular filling is less effective in augmenting cardiac output.

Ventricular demand pacing is generally indicated in patients with symptomatic bradyarrhythmias with underlying atrial fibrillation, atrial flutter, or some form of sick sinus syndrome with AV block. Under these circumstances, atrial pacing with preservation of AV synchrony is not possible or feasible. Ventricular demand pacing under these circumstances provides a basal heart rate allowing for an adequate cardiac output at rest.

Some patients, however, suffer hemodynamic deterioration with WI pacing. There are several potential reasons for this. In patients with atrial fibrillation, the loss of the atrial contribution to ventricular filling results in a decrease in stroke volume and cardiac output. Adaptive measures, such as elevations in the mean atrial pressure during atrial fibrillation, usually ensures adequate ventricular filling pressures to maintain the cardiac performance, but this is not always observed.

Dissociated atrial contractions also occur in some patients with ventricular demand pacemakers. When this occurs, the atrial contribution to ventricular filling is again lost, as often times P waves occur during or after the paced ventricular complex. When the P waves are physiologically timed 100 to 250 msec before the paced complex, a marked rise in systolic pressure and force of contraction is noted.

Retrograde VA conduction is another important cause for hemodynamic deterioration with ventricular demand pacemakers. The presence of VA conduction is found in over half of the patients studied with sick sinus syndrome. Ventricular demand pacing in patients with fixed VA conduction results in adverse hemodynamic consequences. A clinical clue to the presence of VA conduction in patients with ventricular demand pacemakers and sinus node dysfunction is the presence of cannon A waves during ventricular pacing. This physical finding represents forceful atrial contraction simultaneously with ventricular contraction. Atrial pressure generated with atrial contraction is not nearly high enough to open the atrioventricular valves closed by the forces of ventricular contraction. This results in forcing blood retrogradely back into the pulmonary veins as well as the superior and inferior vena cava. Hemodynamically this results in a lowering of the ventricular end diastolic volume since blood will take time to reenter the atria. As a result, stroke volume, myocardial contractility, cardiac output, and systemic pressures are all reduced. Higher pulmonary vascular pressures result in a higher incidence of congestive heart failure patients with VVI pacing and retrograde VA conduction.

Additionally, atrial stretch receptors are stimulated by the large waveform created as the atria contract against closed mitral and tricuspid valves. These receptors when stimulated result in peripheral vasodilatation and an acute fall in systemic vascular resistance. This results in decreased venous return and preload which lowers stroke volume and cardiac output.

An associated finding in patients who have sinus node dysfunction and the recent insertion of a VVI pacemaker is the increased incidence of developing atrial fibrillation. Statistics have shown a 10 to 20% increased risk of developing atrial fibrillation after VVI pacing is initiated.

Hemodynamic deterioration with VVI pacing may result in numerous symptoms. These include weakness, fatigue, diaphoresis, mental status changes, shortness of breath, and near syncope. These symptoms, when associated with the hemodynamic and electrophysiologic findings described above, is called the "pacemaker syndrome."

Rate responsive demand pacemakers (AAI-R, VVI-R)

The major limitation with both atrial and ventricular demand pacing is the lack of rate responsiveness. Demand pacemakers provide adequate basal heart rates which satisfy the cardiac output needs at rest but not during exertion. An appropriate chronotropic response is necessary for an adequate cardiac output during exercise. For patients with symptomatic bradyarrhythmias, chronotropic incompetence, and an active lifestyle, an alternative method of increasing the heart rate became necessary.

With the onset of exercise, certain physiologic parameters are altered. By developing sensor technology to monitor these parameters and adjust pacing rates based upon changes in these parameters, adaptive rate responsive pacemakers were developed. These sensors monitor one of many parameters such as blood pH, temperature, QT interval and activity.

Hemodynamic studies have demonstrated that heart rate response is the primary determinant of cardiac performance during exercise. When atrial synchronous ventricular pacing was compared to demand ventricular pacing at identical heart rate, blood pressure, and exercise workloads, no significant difference was observed in cardiac performance. Ventricular volume measurements demonstrated identical stroke volumes during exercise; however, ventricular pacing was associated with lower end diastolic and end systolic volume. The stroke volume during exercise with ventricular pacing was maintained at atrial synchronous pacing levels due to enhanced myocardial contractility as evident by an increased ejection fraction. Additionally, patients were found to have improved exercise tolerance with rate responsive ventricular pacing when compared to fixed rate ventricular pacing.

Dual chamber pacemakers

Dual chamber (atrial and ventricular) pacemakers provide a nearly ideal "physiologic" pacing by preserving AV synchrony and rate responsive capabilities. There are several modes of pacing, each with specific advantages and disadvantages.

Atrial synchronous ventricular pacemakers (VAT, VDD) were designed for those patients with normal SA node function and impaired AV conduction. The VAT mode of pacing senses atrial activity with the atrial lead and paces the ventricle via the ventricular lead after a preset physiologic delay interval. In this mode, the atrium cannot be paced and the ventricular spontaneous electrical activity cannot be sensed. In the VDD or DDD mode, atrial activity is sensed.

Advantages with atrial synchronous pacing include preserved AV synchrony and rate responsiveness with ventricular pacing, sensing acceleration of the sinus rate by the atrial lead. With exercise, cardiac performance is the result of increased heart rate and stroke volume with increases in preload and myocardial contractility. Afterload either remains unchanged or may decrease during exercise.

Disadvantages with this mode of pacing is the potential initiation of "pacemaker mediated tachycardia (PMT)." Pacemaker mediated tachycardia is a potential problem in dual chamber pacemakers when VA conduction is present. The tachycardia is initiated when a ventricular impulse has associated VA conduction to the atrium where the atrial electrogram is sensed by the atrial lead. Following the preset physiologic AV delay interval, the pacemaker paces the ventricle. This ventricular impulse is again conducted retrogradely with intact VA conduction to the atrium where the atrial impulse is detected by the pacemaker and following the AV delay the ventricle is again paced. This initiated an endless loop tachycardia termed pacemaker mediated tachycardia. These tachycardias may be associated with hemodynamic deterioration, especially in patients with ischemic heart disease, left ventricular dysfunction, and decreased diastolic compliance.

In order to avoid the possibility of initiating PMT, patients should be evaluated for the presence of VA conduction. If VA conduction is present, the atrial refractory period (portion of pacing cycle when atrial activity will not result in ventricular pacing) must be programmed to a longer time interval then the VA conduction time to ensure that retrograde atrial activity is not sensed by the pacemaker.

The second disadvantage to atrial synchronous ventricular pacing is a problem common to all dual chamber devices. In order to have rate responsiveness with exertion, normal SA node function must be present. If the SA node demonstrates chronotropic incompetence, all dual chamber pacemakers will function in the fixed rate mode.

AV sequential pacemakers

In the AV sequential pacing mode (DVI), AV synchrony is preserved but spontaneous atrial activity is not sensed, resulting in lack of rate responsiveness with exercise. This mode of pacing was designed to be used in patients with sinus node dysfunction with associated abnormal AV conduction. During DVI pacing, only ventricular activity is sensed but both the atrium and ventricle are capable of being paced. Following a sensed spontaneous ventricular electrogram, the pacemaker escape pacing interval is reset. If no subsequent ventricular impulse is sensed during the escape pacing interval, the pacemaker will pace the atrium. Following a preset AV delay interval if no ventricular impulse has been sensed, the ventricle will also be paced.

By not sensing atrial activity and with the presence of sinus node dysfunction and chronotropic incompetence, this mode of pacing is incapable of altering its pacing rate when increases in cardiac performance are needed during exercise.

Hemodynamically, patients with constant rate AV sequential pacing increase cardiac output during exercise through increases in stroke volume. The stroke volume is augmented through increases in venous return (preload) and myocardial contractility. Afterload generally remains the same or may be slightly decreased.

The lack of rate responsiveness is the major disadvantage of this pacing mode. Utilization of compensatory mechanisms such as increases in preload and contractility to augment stroke volume and cardiac output with exercise has been demonstrated to increase myocardial oxygen consumption and increase wall stress. Chronic DVI pacing has been associated with cardiac dilatation due to chronically elevated end diastolic volumes necessary to augment cardiac output.

Universal (DDD) pacemakers

The DDD mode of dual chamber pacing is referred to as the "universal" mode because of the ability to reprogram the pacemaker to any other mode. Available modes include ventricular inhibited pacing, atrial pacing, atrial synchronous pacing, and AV sequential pacing. The DDD mode is able to provide AV synchrony and rate responsiveness in patients with normal SA node function in either DDD, VAT, VDD, or AAI modes.

During exercise, DDD pacing results in improved cardiac performance primarily by rate responsiveness but also through enhanced stroke volume due to increased preload and force of contractility from AV synchrony.

The ability of the DDD pacemaker to be reprogrammed to another mode is a distinct advantage since one-third of the patients with DDD pacemakers have required an alternative mode after four years following implantation. Disadvantages with the universal DDD mode is again appreciated in patients with sinus node dysfunction and chronotropic incompetence. Under these circumstances, rate responsiveness is not possible and the pacemaker will function with fixed rate pacing.

Rate responsive universal pacemakers (DDD-R)

The rate responsive universal pacemaker (DDD-R) provided appropriate chronotropy in patients with sinus node dysfunction, bradyarrhythmias, and AV block. The rate responsive sensor technology is the same as that previously described with rate responsive demand single chamber pacemakers. During exertion utilizing DDD-R pacing modes, cardiac performance is enhanced through increasing heart rate response as well as increased stroke volume by increases in preload and contractility.

References

1. Ausubel K, Furman 5. The pacemaker syndrome. Ann Int Med 1985;103:420–9.
2. Braunwald E. Heart disease - a textbook of cardiovascular medicine. Philadelphia: WB Saunders Co, 1988.
3. Coskey R, Feit T, Plaia R *et al*. AV pacing and LV performance. PACE 1983;6:631–40.
4. Fananapazir L, Bennett D, Monks P. Atrial synchronized ventricular pacing: contribution of the chronotropic response to improved exercise performance. PACE 1983;6:601–8.
5. Fananapazir L, Venkateswaren S, Bennett D. Comparison of resting hemodynamic indices

and exercise performance during atrial synchronized and asynchronous ventricular pacing. PACE 1983;6:202–9.

6. Fearnot N, Smith H, Geddes L. A review of pacemakers that physiologically increase rate:DDD and rate-responsive pacemakers. Prog Cardiovasc Dis 1986;26:145–64.
7. Furman S, Gross J. Dual-chamber pacing and pacemakers. Current problems in cardiology 1990;15:119–79.
8. Hauser R. Techniques for improving cardiac performance with implantable devices. 1984;7:1234–9.
9. Humen D, Kostuk W, Klein G. Activity-sensing, rate-responsive pacing: improvement in myocardial performance with exercise. PACE 1985;8:52–9.
10. Janusik D *et al*. The hemodynamic benefit of differential atrioventricular delay intervals for sensed and paced events during physiologic pacing. J Am Coll Cardiol 1989;14:499–507.
11. Karlsson D, Kristensson B. The importance of different atrioventricular intervals for exercise capacity. PACE 1988;11:1051–62.
12. Klementowicz P *et al*. An analysis of DDD pacing mode survival: the first 5 years. PACE 1987;10:699(A 279).
13. Leman R, Kratz J. Radionuclide evaluation of dual chamber pacing: comparison between variable AV intervals and ventricular pacing. PACE 1985;8:408–14.
14. McMeekin J *et al*. Importance of heart rate response during exercise in patients using atrioventricular synchronous and ventricular pacemakers. PACE 1990;13:59–68.
15. Nitsch J, Seiderer M, Bull U *et al*. Evaluation of left ventricular performance by radionuclide ventriculography in patients with atrioventricular versus ventricular demand pacemakers. Am Heart J 1984;107:908–11.
16. Norlander R, Pehrsson S, Astrom H Myocardial demands of atrial-triggered versus fixed-rate ventricular pacing in patients with complete heart block. PACE 1987;10:1154–9.
17. Reiter M, Hindman M. Hemodynamic effects of acute atrioventricular sequential pacing in patients with left ventricular dysfunction. Am J Cardiol 1982;49:687–92.
18. Rossi P *et al*. Respiration-dependent ventricular pacing compared with fixed ventricular and atrial-ventricular synchronous pacing: aerobic and hemodynamic variables. J Am Coll Cardiol 1985;6:646–52.
19. Videen J *et al*. Hemodynamic comparison of ventricular pacing, atrioventricular sequential pacing, and atrial synchronous ventricular pacing using radionuclide ventriculography. Am J Cardiol 1986;57:1305–8.
20. Wirtzfeld A, Schmidt G, Himmler F *et al*. Physiological pacing: present and future developments. PACE 1987;10:41–57.

22. Cardiac output and coronary blood flow during pharmacologic stress testing

THACH N. NGUYEN, J. DAVID OGILBY and
ABDULMASSIH S. ISKANDRIAN

The coronary circulation is regulated by several control mechanisms. The dominant factors are metabolic demand, autoregulation and extravascular compressive forces. Of lesser importance are humoral and neural control mechanisms. There is a tight coupling between myocardial oxygen consumption and coronary blood flow in normal hearts. A change in oxygen demand elicits almost instantaneous proportional changes in coronary blood flow and coronary vascular resistance. Furthermore, the coronary circulation is autoregulated over a wide range of perfusion pressures (40 to 170 mm Hg). Autoregulation is defined as the ability to maintain constant coronary blood flow despite changes in perfusion pressure as long as myocardial oxygen demand is unaltered. When coronary perfusion falls as a result of proximal coronary stenosis the distal small arterioles vasodilate in an attempt to maintain constant flow. Autoregulatory reserve varies across the different layers of the myocardium, more exhausted in the subendocardium than the epicardium; the subendocardial microvasculature is subject to higher intracavitary compressive forces and, therefore, is more vasodilated at base line and has less vasodilatory reserve. The normal subendocardial-to-subepicardial flow ratio is approximately 1.2:1.0. This ratio may decrease to 1:2 with severe ischemia or increase to as high as 3:1 during adenosine infusion [1].

Humoral control is another important factor in the regulation of myocardial perfusion. The coronary endothelium can modulate the vascular effects of a number of humoral substances. The normal coronary arteries with intact endothelium vasorelax in response to an increase in coronary blood flow and to the local administration of acetylcholine. The normal vasodilating mechanism is lost when the endothelium is damaged, leaving the underlying smooth muscle cells exposed to vasoconstrictive stimuli. The endothelium modulates the coronary vascular tone by releasing the endothelium-derived relaxing factor (EDRF) which is thought to be nitric oxide. Many factors elicit the release of EDRF such as ADP, serotonin, vasopressin, norepinephrine, increased shear stress and others. It appears that the endothelial cells can sense and respond to the mechanical forces generated by increased blood flow. On the other hand, atherosclerosis, and hyperlipidemia have been demonstrated to impair the functional capacity of the endothelium [2, 3].

A.-M. Salmasi and A.S. Iskandrian (eds): Cardiac output and regional flow in health and disease, 273–285.
© 1993 *Kluwer Academic Publishers. Printed in the Netherlands.*

Dipyridamole and adenosine

Dipyridamole is a complex pyrimidine derivative that inhibits cellular reuptake and capillary endothelial transport of endogenously produced adenosine, and blocks its inactivation by adenosine deaminase in red cells, lungs and myocardial tissues. Dipyridamole has indirect vasodilatory effects on the small coronary arterioles or resistance vessels. The mechanism of coronary hyperemia appears to be related to elevated plasma adenosine levels [4, 5]. Adenosine is a direct and potent mediator of vaso-relaxation in most vascular beds except in the renal afferent arterioles and hepatic venous system where it causes vasoconstriction. Adenosine appears to exert its vasodilating effects through activation of membrane receptors (adenosine A_1, and A_2). The exact mechanism of trans-membrane signal transduction has not been fully elucidated. There is evidence to support both the activation of adenylate cyclase through A_2–receptors in smooth muscle cells, and the inhibition of intracellular calcium influx, possibly through the inositol phosphate pathway [6]. Adenosine may also decrease vascular tone by modulating sympathetic neurotransmission. Recent studies [7, 8] suggested that adenosine also stimulated guanylate cyclase in vascular smooth muscle cells to increase cyclic GMP production that ultimately mediates vasodilation by complex intracellular mechanisms. The interaction between the vascular endothelium, EDRF and adenosine in the regulation of coronary blood flow is not fully understood. Vasodilation may occur even in the absence of the endothelium. However, a recent study [8] demonstrated that mechanical removal of the endothelium attenuated adenosine-induced dilation of rat aorta. In addition, hemoglobin and methylene blue which inhibited the effect of EDRF, partly reversed adenosine-induced vasodilation.

Dipyridamole and adenosine act more selectively on the small arterioles than the large epicardial arteries. They do not dilate the epicardial vessels as much as nitroglycerin. However, there appears to be a flow-mediated dilation of the large coronary vessels probably due to EDRF released by the signal of increased blood flow and shear stress. Hintze et al. [9] demonstrated that intravenous dipyridamole produced vasodilation of both the resistance vessels (or small arterioles) and the large epicardial arteries. Cox and associates [10] studied the effect of adenosine delivered into the middle segment of the left anterior descending artery (LAD) on the coronary blood flow and the dimension of the proximal segment in patients with angiographically normal looking LAD arteries and those with luminal irregularities, using quantitative angiography and Doppler flow catheter. Flow-mediated dilation was observed in angiographically normal LAD segments but was markedly impaired in arteries with luminal irregularities despite a greater increase in coronary blood flow in the latter group. However, both groups responded with equal vasodilation to intracoronary nitroglycerin. The evidence suggested the diminution of flow-mediated dilation of mildly atherosclerotic arteries may reflect impaired endothelial vasodilator function.

Pharmacokinetics

Following intravenous infusion of dipyridamole, plasma levels rapidly decline in a triexponential pattern with an initial alpha half-life of 3–12 minutes, beta half-life of 33–62 minutes, and a terminal disposition half-life of 6–15 hours [11].

Approximately 95% of dipyridamole is bound to plasma α_1–glycoprotein and albumin. Dipyridamole is metabolized in the liver to glucuronic acid conjugate and excreted in the bile.

Following intravenous administration, adenosine is rapidly taken up from plasma by erythrocytes and vascular endothelium via a specific transmembrane nucleoside carrier. Intracellular adenosine is rapidly metabolized either via phosphorylation to adenosine monophosphate by adenosine kinase or via deamination to inosine by adenosine deamination in the cytoplasm. Adenosine kinase has a lower Km and Vmax than adenosine deaminase, and hence the predominant pathway is the phosphorylating pathway at physiologic adenosine concentration. However, when the intracellular adenosine is increased deamination plays a more significant role. Clearance of adenosine from plasma is extremely rapid with half-life of about 10 seconds [6].

The effect of dipyridamole and adenosine is antagonized by aminophylline, caffeine, or other xanthine-containing products through a direct competitive inhibition. Aminophylline competes directly with adenosine at the receptor site. Therefore, plasma adenosine level tends to rise after aminophylline infusion as adenosine is displaced from the receptor [12].

Hemodynamics

Dipyridamole and adenosine are potent coronary vasodilators, producing three to five times increase in coronary blood flow in normal arteries compared to 1.7 to 2.5 times increase with maximal exercise. Intravenous administration elicits a modest increase in heart rate, cardiac output, and a mild decrease in blood pressure [13, 14]. However, no significant systemic changes are observed with intracoronary injection. Marchant and associates [15] notes a 73% increase in coronary sinus flow (thermodilution) with intracoronary dipyridamole (0.5 µg/kg). When this injection was followed by a same dose given intravenously, there was an additional 88% increase in coronary sinus flow. It appears that the mechanism for the coronary blood flow augmentation with intravenous route is related to both the primary coronary vasodilations and the modest increase in rate-pressure product. Dipyridamole decreased coronary vascular resistance more than systemic resistance, suggesting a more selective effect on the coronary circulation. The optimal dosage of dipyridamole for effective vasodilation is 0.142 mg/kg/min infused intravenously over 4 minutes. Peak coronary flow response occurs approximately 7 minutes (3 to 9 minutes) from the start of the 4–minute infusion.

Coronary flow returns to baseline level by about 30 minutes after infusion. A small percentage of patients (10 to 25%) fail to achieve maximal coronary dilation with this conventional dose. Flow augmentation may occur with an additional 0.284 mg/kg dose.

Brown and colleague [16] suggested that handgrip exercise increased the coronary dilator response to dipyridamole. Coronary sinus flow was 68% greater with combined stresses than with intravenous dipyridamole alone. However, subsequent study [17] using more accurate coronary Doppler flow measurement did not document further increase in coronary blood flow with the addition of handgrip. It is likely that the difference in techniques used to measure coronary flow or patient selection may account for the different results.

The effects of adenosine on coronary hemodynamics have been evaluated by Wilson and associates [18]. Adenosine produces a dose-dependent vasodilation. Maximal coronary vasodilation, i.e. greater than four-fold increase above baseline was achieved in 84% of normal arteries at an intravenous dose of 140 mcg/kg/min. In the group with submaximal hyperemia, increasing the infusion rate to 180–200 mcg/kg/min failed to elicit any greater vasodilation. At a lower dose (70–100 mcg/kg/min) coronary flow velocity fluctuated significantly. The average interval from onset of infusion to peak effect was 84 ± 46 seconds (range, 23–125 sec). The time from termination of infusion until coronary flow returned to baseline was 145 + 67 seconds (range, 54–310 seconds). Intracoronary bolus of 15 mcg adenosine in the left coronary artery or 12 mcg in the right coronary artery or continuous intracoronary infusion of 80 mcg/kg/min also caused maximal hyperemia. Rossen and associates [19] compared the dilating effects of IV adenosine (140 mcg/kg/min), IV dipyridamole (140 mcg/kg/min over 4 minutes) and maximally dilating dose of intracoronary papaverine in a small group of patients without significant CAD. Coronary flow responses were assessed by measuring the change in Doppler flow velocity and calculating the coronary resistance index. Both adenosine and dipyridamole produced comparable increases in coronary blood flow, more than three times resting flow, but a little less than papaverine. Adenosine caused a greater reduction in coronary resistance and had a more rapid onset of action than dipyridamole (55 ± 34 vs. 287 ± 101 sec).

At standard doses of 140 mcg per kg per minute intravenous dipyridamole and adenosine produce similar hemodynamic changes e.g. 5 to 15% decrease in systolic and diastolic blood pressures, 20 to 40% increase in heart rate, and 30 to 50% increase in cardiac output (as a result of greater increase in heart rate than stroke volume). Systemic vascular resistance decreased by 25 to 35% [20–24]. The mean rate-pressure product increased by 10 to 28%, but not to the same level as that achieved by dynamic or isometric exercise. The effect on heart rate is probably due to adenosine-induced activation of reflex autonomic mechanisms. Occasionally, adenosine (<5%) and rarely, dipyridamole (0.3%) are associated with sinus bradycardia and atrioventricular block because adenosine depresses the pacemaker activity of sino-atrial node and atrioventricular conduction [25]. The difference in the incidence of atrioventricular block of these two agents is probably related to the direct effect and rapid onset of action of adenosine. The SA and AV nodes are exposed to a high dose of exogenously administered, direct acting adenosine for a brief duration whereas endogenous adenosine level rises more slowly after dipyridamole infusion.

Sinus bradycardia and AV block tend to occur early, within 2 minutes after the start of adenosine infusion, last about 2 minutes, and frequently disappear during the infusion in the majority of patients [25]. Occasionally, intravenous adenosine produces high grade AV block with hypotension, requiring premature termination of adenosine and reversal with aminophylline. AV block appears unrelated to the presence or absence of ischemia but may be potentiated by concomitant dromotropic medications (beta and calcium blockers) and dipyridamole.

Dipyridamole/adenosine lowers coronary vascular resistance via its primary action on the small arterioles. Total coronary vascular resistance is made up of three different components: the resistance of the large epicardial vessels (R_1), the small arterioles (R_2) and the intramyocardial capillaries (R_3). The small arterioles (R_2) usually play a predominant role in the control of total coronary vascular resistance in the normal hearts $(R_2 > > R_1)$. However, in the presence of a hemodynamically significant coronary stenosis, the increased large vessel resistance (R_1) is partially offset by a proportional decrease in arteriolar resistance (R_2) up to a certain limit. Once the vasodilating reserve capacity of the small arterioles is exhausted, the resistance of the large vessel stenosis becomes flow-limiting $(R_2 > > R_1)$ [26] (Figure 22.1). Coronary flow reserve is, therefore, a useful functional measure of stenosis severity. It is the ratio of maximal or peak hyperemia to resting flow. The ratio is about 4:1 or 5:1 under normal conditions. Coronary flow reserve is a measure of the ability of coronary vasculature to augment blood flow in response to vasodilatory stimuli independent of changes in myocardial oxygen consumption. Although resting coronary flow is not affected by less than 85% diameter stenosis, the maximal coronary flow begins to decline with stenosis of 50 to 60% diameter [27]. It is important to recognize that coronary flow reserve may be influenced by multiple factors other than coronary stenosis, such as loading conditions, heart rate, left ventricular hypertrophy, anemia, etc. Since the coronary flow reserve is a ratio of maximal (or hyperemic) to resting flow, conditions that change the resting flow may affect the flow reserve. Increases in heart rate increase resting flow but do not significantly affect hyperemic flow. Thus, coronary flow reserve decreases [1].

Dipyridamole/adenosine creates disparities in regional myocardial perfusion in the setting of a significant coronary stenosis. The heterogeneity of perfusion is due to the relative abilities of the small vessels to dilate and augment flow to a greater extent in myocardial regions supplied by a normal

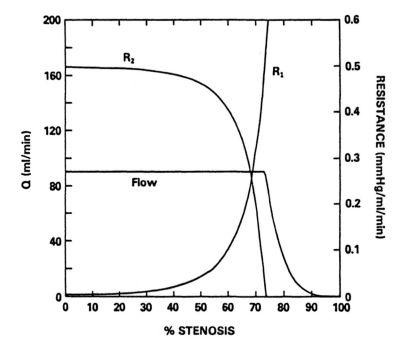

Figure 22.1. Influence of degree of stenosis on coronary flow and resistance. As the epicardial coronary artery resistance (R_1) increases with increasing stenosis severity, the arteriolar resistance (R_2) decreases proportionally to maintain total resistance and flow at constant normal levels. Once the vasodilating reserve capacity of the small arterioles (R_2) is exhausted the resistance of the epicardial arteries (R_1) becomes flow limiting. Reprinted with permission from Am J Cardiol [26].

artery than in those regions subtended by a stenotic artery because of the limited vasodilatory reserve of the latter [28, 29].

The severity of coronary stenosis is probably best defined in terms of the relationship between the stenosis pressure gradient and coronary flow velocity regardless of the geometry and length, the percent or absolute dimension of the stenosis, the degree of streamlining, or the size of the coronary artery. For a fixed stenosis the pressure gradient increases in a curvilinear fashion as flow velocity increases in response to any stimulus, whether exercise or coronary vasodilator (Figure 22.2).

With more severe stenosis, the pressure gradient-flow velocity relationship becomes steeper and the whole curve shifts to the left. It can be appreciated from the Figure 22.2 that resistance is the slope of the tangent line relating pressure to flow, resistance is not fixed but increases linearly with increasing

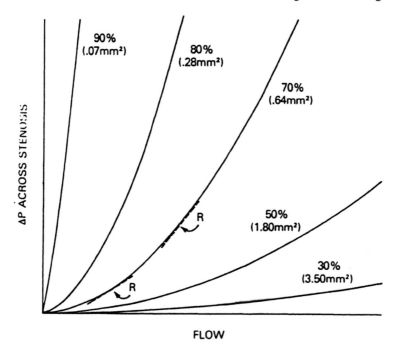

Figure 22.2. Relation between pressure drop (AP) and flow (Q) across j the stenosis. Curves are plotted for stenoses of 30%, 50%, 70%, 80%, and 90% internal diameter. Tangents to the curves (R) represent stenosis resistance. For any given flow the resistance increases with increasing per cent stenosis. The resistance also increases linearly with increasing flow despite no change in stenosis severity. (Newsletter of the Council on Clinical Cardiology of the American Heart Association, Inc 1982, Vol 7, No 3. With permission from the AHA, Inc.)

flow despite no significant alteration in the anatomic severity of the stenosis [26].

Therefore, adenosine-induced coronary hyperemia in the presence of a critical stenosis will result in an increased transtenotic pressure gradient and a decrease in distal perfusion pressure with a consequent reduction in subendocardial flow despite mild increase in subepicardial flow. This transmural redistribution of flow or "transmural steal" occurs because the resting distal perfusion to the subendocardium is significantly reduced and these subendocardial arterioles nearly exhaust their vasodilatory reserve whereas the subepicardial arterioles have more capacity to dilate and augment flow in response to dipyridamole and adenosine (Figure 22.3). Thus, subendo to subepicardial flow ratio falls significantly [30–32]. The transmural redistribution of coronary flow and decrease in systemic blood pressure may result in worsening of subendocardial ischemia.

In myocardial regions perfused by normal arteries, blood flow increases

TRANSMURAL FLOW

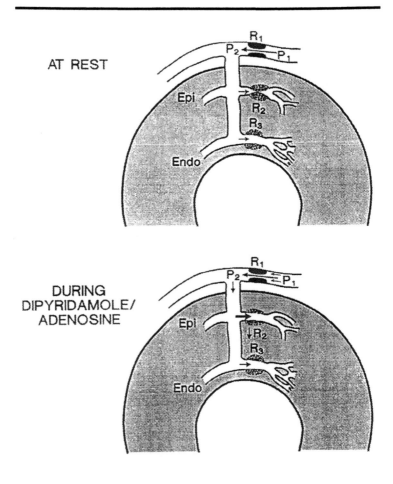

Figure 22.3. Effects of a stenosis on endo-and epicardial flow at rest and during dipyridamole/adenosine. The epicardial arterioles are less vasodilated than endocardial arterioles at resting state. Adenosine-induced flow augmentation will cause a greater pressure drop across the stenosis and a decrease in distal perfusion pressure (P_2) as long as the fall in resistance in subepicardial vessels (P_2) is greater than the fall in perfusion pressure (P_2), subepicardial flow will increase. However, because of limited subendocardial vasodilatory reserve the fall in perfusion pressure (P_2) will not be accompanied by a fall in resistance (R_2). Hence, subendocardial flow decreases. Modified with permission from Am J Cardiol [26].

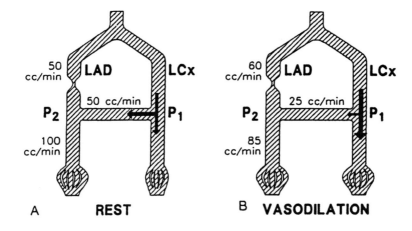

Figure 22.4. Hydraulic model illustrating possible mechanism of intercoronary (collateral) steal. In this model the LAD has a severe proximal stenosis with its distal vessel supplied by collaterals from the LCX. P_1 is the perfusion pressure at the origin of the collaterals from the circumflex branches. P_2 is the perfusion pressure of the distal LAD vascular territory. In A the recipient vascular bed vasodilates to maintain normal resting perfusion ($P_1 > P_2$). In B, during high flow state induced by pharmacologic vasodilation, there is increased pressure loss across the donor LCX, resulting in a lower distal perfusion pressure ($P_1 > P_2$). Hence, the collateral driving pressure falls. (Reprinted with permission from Prog Cardiovasc Dis 1988;30:312.)

substantially in both endocardial and epicardial layers, reflecting normal coronary reserve.

Myocardial ischemia may also occur in the presence of collateral vessels. In the resting state, myocardial beds distal to a severe stenosis receive most of their blood supply through collateral channels from a normal or less diseased vessel. The collateral flow may be sufficient to avert resting ischemia. Furthermore, there is minimal pressure gradient (<5 mm Hg) from the coronary ostium to the most distal areas of the normal donor epicardial artery. During high flow states induced by dipyridamole/adenosine there is increased pressure loss across the donor epicardial arteries due to proximal stenosis or proximal viscous friction in normal arteries. The pressure gradient across the donor epicardial artery may substantially increase, exceeding 20 mm Hg and may decrease the distal perfusion pressure at the origin of the collateral vessels, effectively reducing collateral flow (Figure 22.4). The phenomenon has been termed "collateral steal" [33–35]. Actually, there is no backward flow or true steal through collateral channels to the donor vascular bed. The absolute collateral flow decreased below resting level during coronary arteriolar dilation, thereby producing ischemia. Changes in resistance in collateral vessels may also be an important mechanism contributing to steal. ST depression as a marker of ischemia during dipyridamole/adenosine studies appears to correlate with the presence of collateral vessels and a modest increase in rate-pressure product [36, 37].

Dipyridamole/adenosine creates disparities in regional myocardial perfusion that can be detected by blood flow tracer imaging such as thallium-201, technetium-99m complexes, rubidium-82, etc. Some of the regional perfusion defects are due to the heterogeneity of flow and tracer uptake in different myocardial regions because of differential flow reserve. This concept does not require the implication of myocardial ischemia. However, other defects may reflect true ischemia, especially in patients with severe coronary artery disease. Evidence for ischemia is suggested by ischemic ST depression and changes in both global and regional indices of left ventricular function. An improvement in left ventricular ejection performance manifested as increased cardiac output and transient hyperkinesis on echocardiography or contrast ventriculography is the usual response to dipyridamole and adenosine infusion in normal subjects and some patients with CAD, and is probably secondary to the combined effects of increased heart rate and decreased afterload [24, 38]. Whether increased myocardial blood flow enhances contractile function (Gregg's phenomenon) remains controversial. Recent studies, however, demonstrated that increased myocardial perfusion induced by intracoronary adenosine does not enhance regional systolic wall thickening or segmented shortening, left ventricular (LV) positive and negative dp/dt, or LV end diastolic pressure (LVEDP) in animals without coronary stenosis [39–41].

The hemodynamic and functional changes are more variable in patients with coronary artery disease. New or worsening of preexisting regional wall motion abnormalities may occur when the transmural ischemia threshold is reached. A wall motion abnormality that newly developed, worsened, or remained unchanged compared to baseline was observed in about 40 to 80% of patients with coronary artery disease during dipyridamole or adenosine studies. The explanation for a wide variation in the sensitivities of two-dimensional echocardiography in the detection of CAD by angiography or thallium perfusion defects is not clear, but may be related to patient selection, expertise of the observers, methods of assessment (consecutive versus digitized side-by-side comparison), doses of vasodilators (0.56 mg/kg versus 0.84 mg/kg dipyridamole), addition of handgrip exercise [24, 38, 42–47] and personal biases. Furthermore, the criteria for defining abnormality may vary in different studies, e.g., failure to become hyperkinetic versus worsening segmental wall motion. A regional wall motion may not actually worsen compared to baseline but appear hypokinetic relative to the other hypercontractile segments. In general, patients with multi-vessel disease are more likely to develop wall motion abnormality than those with single-vessel disease.

Other evidence of ischemia is supported by the finding of transient left ventricular dilation in some patients with CAD during dipyridamole or adenosine thallium imaging. We and others reported that the LV inner cavity dilated much more than its outer chamber, suggesting that wall thinning is due to subendocardial ischemia [48, 49]. The degree of cavity dilation correlated positively with the extent and severity of scintigraphic perfusion defects and lung/hear thallium ratio [48].

Significant hemodynamic alterations are also observed during pharmacologic stress testing. Picano and associates [50] correlated the central hemodynamic changes with dipyridamole-echocardiography in patients with and without CAD. Patients with abnormal or positive dipyridamole-echo tests had significantly higher LVEDP, lower + and − LVdp/dt during IV dipyridamole infusion than those with normal or negative echo test.

In our laboratory we are currently evaluating the mechanisms of the hemodynamic, scintigraphic, and angiographic changes during intravenous adenosine in patients with and without CAD. Hemodynamic data are obtained before and during intravenous adenosine infusion of 140 mcg/kg/min. There was approximately 50% increase in cardiac output in normal subjects and slightly less in patients with CAD. Some but not all patients with CAD exhibited a marked transient elevation in pulmonary arterial and wedge pressures with prominent V-waves. These findings suggest a transient ischemia-induced diastolic dysfunction or possibly secondary mitral regurgitation due to papillary muscle dysfunction in some cases. There was no significant change in coronary stenosis dimensions or passive collapse on quantitative angiography. Transmural and/or collateral steals are most likely the mechanism of myocardial ischemia [51]. The tachycardia and hyperkinesis suggest that the mechanism of increase in cardiac output involve increases in heart rate and stroke volume. Unlike exercise, however, the increase in cardiac output is modest and is not associated with regional redistribution. As discussed earlier, the increase in coronary blood flow is much more than the increase in cardiac output. This finding is of special interest to nuclear imaging procedures as it increases myocardium tracer concentration that result in high image quality.

References

1. Marcus ML, Harrison DG. Physiologic basis for myocardial perfusion imaging. In:.Cardiac imaging. Philadelphia: WB Saunders, 1991:8–23.
2. Freiman PC, Mitchell GG, Heistad DD *et al*. Atherosclerosis impairs endothelium dependent vascular relaxation to acetylcholine and thrombin in primates. Circ. Res 1986;58:783–89.
3. Henderson AH. Endothelium in control. Br Heart J 1991;65:116–23.
4 Fitzgerald GA. Dipyridamole. N Engl J Med 1987;316:1247–56.
5. Knabb RM, Gidday JM, Ely SW *et al*. Effects of dipyridamole on myocardial adenosine and active hyperemia. Am J Physiol 1984;247:804–10.
6. Belardinelli L, Linden J, Berne RM. The cardiac effects of adenosine. Prog Cardiovasc Dis 1989;32:73–97.
7. Kurtz A. Adenosine stimulates guanylate cyclase activity in vascular smooth muscle cells. J Biol Chem 1987;262:6296–302.

8. Moritoki H, Matsugi T, Takase *et al*. Evidence for the involvement of c-GMP in adenosine-induced, age-dependent vasodilation. Br J Pharmacol 1990;100(3):569–75.
9. Hintze TH, Vatner SF. Dipyridamole dilates large coronary arteries in conscious dogs. Circulation 1983;68:1321–7.
10. Cox DA, Vita JA, Treasure CB *et al*. Atherosclerosis impairs flow-mediated dilation of coronary arteries in man. Circulation 1989;80:458–65.
11. Mahony C, Wolfram KM, Cocchetto DM *et al*. Dipyridamole kinetics. Clin Pharmacol Ther 1982;31:330–3.
12. Alfonso S. Inhibition of coronary vasodilating action of dipyridamole and adenosine by aminophylline in dogs. Circ. Res 1970;26:743–52.
13. Fuller RW, Maxwell DL, Conradson TBG *et al*. Circulatory and respiratory effects of infused adenosine in conscious man. Br J Clin Pharmacol 1982; 4:309–17.
14. Bush A, Busst CM, Clarke B *et al*. Effects of infused adenosine on cardiac output and systemic resistance in normal subjects. Br J Clin Pharmacol 1989;27:265–71.
15. Marchant E, Pichard A, Rodriguez JA *et al*. Acute effect of systemic versus intracoronary dipyridamole on coronary circulation. Am J Cardiol 1986;57:140–4.
16. Brown BG, Josephson MA, Peterson RD et al. Intravenous dipyridamole combined with isometric handgrip for near maximal acute increase in coronary flow in patients with coronary artery disease. Am J Cardiol 1981;48:1077–85.
17. Rossen JD, Simanetti I, Marcus ML *et al*. Coronary dilation with standard dose dipyridamole and dipyridamole combined with handgrip. Circulation 1989;79:566–72.
18. Wilson RF, Wyche K, Christensen BSN *et al*. Effects of adenosine on human coronary arterial circulation. Circulation 1990;82:1595.1606.
19. Rossen JD, Stenberg RG, Lopez AG *et al*. Coronary dilation with intravenous adenosine and dipyridamole: a comparative study. Circulation 1990;82:2906.
20. Leppo JA. Dipyridamole-thallium imaging: the lazy man's stress test. J Nucl Med 1989;30:281–7.
21. Miller DD, Scott RA, Reismeyer JS *et al*. Acute hemodynamic changes during intravenous dipyridamole thallium imaging early after infarction. Am Heart J 1989;118:686–94.
22. Gould KL. Noninvasive assessment of coronary stenosis by myocardial perfusion imaging during pharmacologic coronary vasodilation I. Physiologic basis and experimental validation. Am J Cardiol 1978;41:267–78.
23. Verani MS, Mahmarian JJ, Hixson JB *et al*. Diagnosis of CAD by controlled coronary vasodilation with adenosine and thallium-201 scintigraphy in patients unable to exercise. Circulation 1990;82:80–7.
24. Nguyen TN, Heo J, Ogilby JD *et al*. Single-photon emission computed tomography with thallium-201 during adenosine-induced coronary hyperemia: correlation with coronary arteriography, exercise thallium imaging and two-dimensional echocardiography. J Am Coll Cardiol 1990;16:1375–83.
25. Nguyen TN, Heo J, Paugh B *et al*. Atrio-ventricular block during adenosine thallium imaging. Circulation 1990;82:2905.
26. Epstein SE, Cannon RO III, Talbott TL. Hemodynamic principles in the control of coronary blood flow. Am J Cardiol 1985;56:4E.
27. Gould KL, Lipscomb K, Hamilton GW. A physiologic basis for assessing critical coronary stenosis. Am J Cardiol 1974;33:87–94.
28. Iskandrian AS, Heo J, Askenase A *et al*. Dipyridamole cardiac imaging. Am Heart J 1988;115:432–43.
29. Gould KL. Pharmacologic intervention as an alternative to exercise stress. Seminars in Nuclear Medicine 1987;17:121–30.
30. Meerdink DJ, Okada RD, Leppo JA. The effects of dipyridamole on transmural blood flow gradients. Chest 1989;96:400–5.
31. Gallagher KP, Folts, JD, Shebuski RJ *et al*. Subepicardial vasodilator reserve in the presence of critical coronary stenosis in dogs. Am J Cardiol 1980;46:67–3.

32. Bache RJ, Schwartz JS. Effect of perfusion pressure distal to coronary stenosis on transmural myocardial blood flow. Circulation 1982;65:928–35.
33. Becker LC. Conditions of vasodilator-induced coronary steal in experimental myocardial ischemia. Circulation 1978;57:1103–10.
34. Demer L, Gould KL, Kirkeeide R. Assessing stenosis severity: coronary flow reserve, collateral function, quantitative coronary angiography, positron imaging, and digital subtraction angiography. A review and analysis. Prog Cardiovasc Dis 1988;30:307–22.
35. Patterson RE, Kirk ES. Coronary steal mechanisms in dogs with one-vessel occlusion and other arteries normal. Circulation 1983;67:1009–15.
36. Chambers CE, Brown KA. Dipyridamole-induced ST segment depression during thallium-201 imaging in patients with CAD: angiographic and hemodynamic determinants. J Am Coll Cardiol 1988;12:37–41.
37. Nishimura S, Mahmarian JJ, Verani MS. Adenosine-induced ST-segment depression during thallium-201 scintigraphy in patients with CAD: angiographic and hemodynamic determinants. J Am Coll Cardiol 1991;17(Suppl)78A.
38. Picano E, Distante A, Masini M et al. Dipyridamole-echocardiography test in effort angina pectoris. Am J Cardiol 1985;56:452–6.
39. Christensen CW, Rosen LB, Gal RA et al. Comparison of the effects of papaverine and adenosine on coronary flow, ventricular function, and myocardial metabolism. Circulation 1991;83:294–303.
40. Schulz R, Guth BD, Heusch G. No effect of coronary perfusion on regional myocardial function within autoregulatory range in pigs: evidence against Gregg phenomenon. Circulation 1991;83:1390–1403.
41. Kiesz S, Gehman JD, Copenhaver GL et al. Increased myocardial blood flow induced by intracoronary vasodilators does not enhance myocardial systolic function. J Am Coll Cardiol 1990;15(Suppl):48A.
42. Picano E, Masini M, Distante A et al. High dose dipyridamole echocardiography test in effort angina pectoris. J Am Coll Cardiol 1986;8:848–54.
43. Margonato A, Chierchia S, Cianflone D et al. Limitations of dipyridamole-echocardiography in effort angina pectoris. Am J Cardiol 1987;59:225–30.
44. Trakhtenbroit AD, Cheirif J, Kleiman N et al. Adenosine echocardiography in the diagnosis of CAD: comparison with coronary angiography [abstract]. Circulation 1990;82:763.
45. Martin T, Seaworth J, Johns J et al. Comparison of adenosine, dipyridamole and dobutamine stress echocardiography for the detection of coronary artery disease. J Am Coll Cardiol 1991;17(Suppl):277A.
46. Wilson VE, Schwaiger M, Allman KC et al. Adenosine echocardiography for the detection of CAD: correlation with SPECT-thallium scintigraphy. J Am Coll Cardiol 1991;17(Suppl):277A.
47. Baker WB, Trakhtenbroit AD, Desir R et al. Adenosine echocardiography with or without handgrip in the diagnosis of CAD comparison with exercise echocardiography. J Am Coll Cardiol 1991;17(Suppl):278A.
48. Iskandrian AS, Heo J, Nguyen T et al. ventricular dilation and pulmonary thallium uptake after SPECT using thallium-201 during adenosine-induced coronary hyperemia. Am J Cardiol 1990;66:807–11.
49. Takeishi Y, Tono-oka I, Ikeda K et al. Dilatation of left ventricular cavity on dipyridamole thallium-201 imaging: a new marker of triple-vessel disease. Am Heart J 1991;121:466–75.
50. Picano E, Simanetti I, Carpeggiani C et al. Regional and globular biventricular function during dipyridamole stress testing. Am J Cardiol 1989;63:429–32.
51. Ogilby D, Mercuro J, Nguyen T et al. Correlation between hemodynamics, coronary stenosis dimensions, and myocardial perfusion SPECT thallium images during adenosine-induced coronary hyperemia [abstract]. European Nuclear Cardiology Meeting, March 22–23, 1991.

23. Cardiac output during anesthesia

JEFFREY J. SCHWARTZ

The perioperative period is associated with large changes in hemodynamic performance. Cardiovascular function is altered perioperatively not only by the physiologic effects of surgery, but by the direct and/or indirect depressant effects of anesthetics and adjuvants as well. In addition, cardiac function may be altered by a number of factors, such as the intense sympathetic stimulation found with laryngoscopy and sternotomy, or changes in ventilation, patient position, etc. The integration of overall cardiovascular function manifested as cardiac output (CO), is highly important to those involved in the perioperative management of patients.

Effect of ventilation

The patient's ventilation is usually controlled during general anesthesia. Positive pressure ventilation decreases cardiac output by raising pleural pressure and decreasing the pressure gradient between extrathoracic and intrathoracic veins that returns venous blood to the heart [1]. During inspiration, filling of the right ventricle is reduced. The decrease in CO correlates with mean airway pressure [2]. High airway pressures reduce CO by 17–25%. Decreased inspiratory time lowers mean airway pressures. Consequently, the inspiratory:expiratory ratio can affect CO. This circulatory depression is worsened by hypovolemia [3]. Reflex venoconstriction, as a normal response to increased intrathoracic pressure, may be impaired by anesthesia or disease. A change from spontaneous to controlled ventilation in healthy volunteers during halothane anesthesia causes a decrease in CO, heart rate (HR) and mean arterial pressure (MAP) [4]. Positive pressure ventilation increases pulmonary vascular resistance as well, which may impair cardiac output in patients with right ventricular dysfunction. Positive end-expiratory pressure (PEEP) is used for the management of certain patients with respiratory failure as well as those exhibiting hypoxia intraoperatively. PEEP raises the impedance to right ventricular ejection and decreases venous return to the right atrium. A reduction occurs in CO almost linearly related to the applied pressure [5]. Volume infusion increases CO during PEEP therapy [6].

Occasionally, patients are allowed to breathe spontaneously. This, however, is usually associated with some degree of hypoventilation as all currently

A.-M. Salmasi and A.S. Iskandrian (eds): Cardiac output and regional flow in health and disease, 287–305.
© 1993 *Kluwer Academic Publishers. Printed in the Netherlands.*

used anesthetics are respiratory depressants, capable of producing apnea. Hypercarbia has several circulatory effects. Carbon dioxide (CO_2) is a direct myocardial depressant *in vitro* [7]. Similarly, hypercarbia depresses myogenic activity in the peripheral vasculature particularly in precapillary resistance vessels [8]. Finally, hypercarbia stimulates the sympathetic nervous system through peripheral and central chemoreceptors. There is an almost linear relationship between plasma catecholamines concentration and $PaCO_2$ [9], which in the awake patient causes a rise in MAP, HR and CO [10]. The increase in CO is approximately 0.2 liter/min per mm Hg increase in $PaCO_2$ [11]. Anesthetic agents may either mute or enhance the sympathetically mediated response to hypercarbia. Halothane, for example, reduces the increase in CO caused by hypercarbia to approximately one third of the awake value [12].

Hyperventilation, such as employed in the anesthetic management of a neurosurgical procedure, causes a decrease of 0.5–1.0% in CO per mm Hg reduction in $PaCO_2$ in patients receiving a variety of anesthetic agents [12, 13]. This suggests the importance of the direct effects of lowering $PaCO_2$ rather than the anesthetic agent employed.

Effect of stimulation

Associated with laryngoscopy, intubation and surgical incision are strong sympathoadrenal responses, usually producing an increase in MAP and HR and occasionally causing dysrhythmias [14, 15]. Among the most intense surgical stimulations are aortic dissection and cross-clamping. Coronary vaso-constriction and myocardial ischemia may result from these [16]. Cardiac output may increase as a result of increased heart rate and contractility. However, with inadequate myocardial reserve, cardiac output may actually decrease on the basis of increased left ventricular afterload or myocardial ischemia induced changes in left ventricular compliance. In patients with valvular insufficiency, skin incision may lead to marked deterioration in hemodynamics [17].

Effect of position

Most surgery is performed with the patient in the supine position. Other positions that are employed can have hemodynamic consequences. The sitting position is utilized during neurosurgery for posterior fossa, cervical and occipital procedures. Circulatory effects of the sitting position (60° head-up tilt) in the anesthetized paralyzed patient include a 12–20% decrease in CO and a 50–80% increase in SVR [18, 19]. Intrathoracic blood volume decreases and fluid retention may occur. These effects can be blunted by slowly changing from the supine position and by bandaging the legs. Use of the kidney rest in the lateral position can cause inferior vena cava compression and may lead to considerable decreases in CO and BP. Increased intraabdominal and intrathoracic pressures may result from the prone position and can lead to decreased venous return. Likewise, reverse Trendelenburg or back-up position can decrease venous return.

Effect of inhaled anesthetics

General anesthetics are rarely administered in the *absence* of surgery for the purpose of investigation. This fact must be recognized when examining the literature on anesthetic effects on the circulation. The hemodynamic response to anesthetics is altered by numerous other factors such as adjuvant drugs, disease and drug therapy, surgery and controlled ventilation.

Only four inhalation agents are currently employed in clinical practice; halothane, enflurane, isoflurane, and nitrous oxide. Desflurane, a new inhalation anesthetic, is currently undergoing clinical and laboratory investigation.

The anesthetic potency of an inhaled agent is measured as its MAC. This is the minimum end tidal alveolar concentration at one atmosphere that prevents movement in 50% of patients in response to a skin incision. Uptake of anesthetic gas from the alveolus by pulmonary blood flow causes the alveolar concentration to always be less than the inspired concentration. When comparing the various effects of the inhaled agents, it is important to study them at the same MAC rather than the same inspired concentration.

Halothane

When given to healthy volunteers not undergoing surgery, during controlled ventilation, halothane causes a linear dose-dependent decrease in cardiac output (Figure 23.1) [20]. The change is considerable; 1.5 MAC halothane causes a 25% decrease in cardiac output while 2.5 MAC reduces cardiac output by half. The decrease is entirely due to a diminished stroke volume as HR and SVR remain constant. Both MAP and CO decrease to same degree. An increase in right atrial pressure (RAP) with a decrease in the IJ wave amplitude of the ballistocardiogram suggests the cause to be myocardial depression.

The major mechanism by which halothane reduces contractility is by direct depression of the myocardial cell [21]. Although the process by which this occurs is not entirely known, it appears most likely to be by inhibition of excitation-contraction coupling at the level of the calcium ion. Halothane also depresses myocardial metabolism. However, the maintenance of high energy phosphate levels in the myocardial cells suggests that this is not a primary mechanism.

Other mechanisms for the decrease in cardiac output are less substantiated.

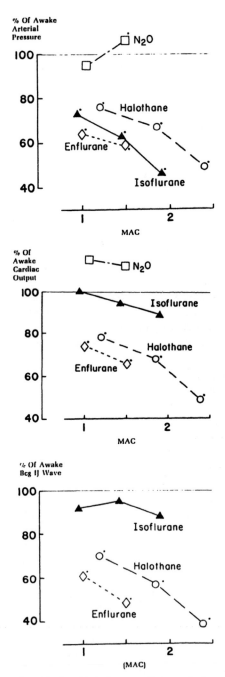

Figure 23.1. Cardiovascular effects of halothane, enflurane, isoflurane and nitrous oxide in volunteers during normocapnia. Eger EI II: Isoflurane (Forane): a compendium (Anaquest, Madison, 1985). MAC = anaesthetic potency of an inhaled agent. It is the minimum end tidal alveolar concentration at one atmosphere that prevents movement in 50% of patients in response to skin incision.

If halothane is administered solely to the CNS, both the MAP and the contractile force decrease, probably by inhibition of the medullary vasomotor center [22]. Halothane may also cause ganglionic blockade.

There is some recovery from the circulatory depressant effects of halothane after three to four hours [20], probably due to activation of cardiac adrenergic beta receptors. This effect is prevented by administration of propranolol and is not present *in vitro*.

Enflurane

Enflurane causes a linear dose-dependent decrease in MAP, CO and SV, of a magnitude somewhat greater than that caused by halothane (Figure 23.1) [23]. The decrease in MAP results from a moderate decrease in SVR and a large decrease in CO. HR does not increase enough to compensate for the decreased SV. As with halothane, CVP increases and the BcgIJ wave decreases suggesting depressed myocardial function. The mechanism for enflurane, though not as thoroughly explored as that of halothane, is probably the depression of excitation-contraction coupling.

Unlike with halothane and isoflurane, volunteers given 2.0 MAC enflurane show a progressive deterioration in cardiac output and blood pressure to unacceptable levels, reversible only by elimination of the enflurane [23]. There is some recovery of cardiovascular function with time, particularly with low concentrations, but not to the same degree as halothane.

Isoflurane

Isoflurane causes large dose-dependent decreases in MAP due almost entirely to a decrease in SVR (Figure 23.1) [24]. At 1.9 MAC SVR is reduced 50%. However, CO remains near awake levels even at 2 MAC concentrations. While all anesthetics reduce resistance to the flow of blood to the brain and skin, isoflurane also reduces resistance to flow in resting skeletal muscle. Isoflurane causes a 20% dose-independent increase in HR. Although SV decreases 20%, other measures of myocardial contractility remain unchanged. Isoflurane appears to depress the myocardium much less, if at all, than halothane and enflurane [25]. Interestingly, *in vitro*, isoflurane appears to have a depressant effect similar to that of halothane and enflurane [26]. It is unclear why this does not manifest *in vivo*. Decreased afterload may lead to improved ventricular emptying and a maintained CO. In addition, compensatory neurohumoral reflexes may be left relatively more intact. There is little change in cardiovascular function over the duration of the drug's administration.

Desflurane

Desflurane, a new volatile anesthetic, is currently undergoing laboratory and clinical study. When given in anesthetic concentrations to healthy volunteers, diastolic BP decreases 15% while the decrease in systolic BP is statistically insignificant [27]. HR remains constant and the rate-pressure product changes little. Desflurane is thought to decrease SVR while maintaining CO, despite the absence of specific measurements. In swine, desflurane causes a dose-related decrease in BP and SVR while, because of an increase in heart rate, CO remains unchanged [28].

Nitrous oxide

As a weak anesthetic, nitrous oxide is unable to provide complete anesthesia without causing hypoxia, except under hyperbaric conditions. It is used clinically in combination with potent anesthetics or narcotics which generally modify the cardiovascular effects of nitrous oxide.

Nitrous oxide appears to be a mild, direct myocardial depressant. Additionally, it increases central sympathetic outflow thereby increasing HR, SVR, MAP [29]. This can counteract its myocardial depressant effect, minimizing circulatory changes. When nitrous oxide is added to steady state halothane anesthesia, SVR and MAP increase while CO, HR and SV remain unchanged, suggesting a sympathomimetic effect [30]. No cardiovascular changes are seen, however, when nitrous oxide is added to steady state enflurane anesthesia, and its effect, when added to isoflurane, is somewhat less than that of halothane.

Clinically, nitrous oxide is most often substituted for a portion of the anesthetic requirement of the potent agent thus reducing the resultant cardiovascular depression [31].

Effect of intravenous anesthetic drugs

Thiopental

The barbiturate, thiopental, is the prototype for all intravenous induction agents. When given to healthy patients, thiopental causes a 10–15% decrease in MAP, SV and SVR [32]. Cardiac output is often unchanged, however, because of relatively intact baroreceptor reflexes and the resulting increase in heart rate. The major mechanism for these changes is venodilation leading to increased venous pooling [33]. Usual doses of thiopental cause minimal myocardial depression. More vulnerable to hypotension during thiopental induction are hypovolemic patients and those treated with central antihypertensives or beta-adrenergic antagonists.

Ketamine

Ketamine, an arylcyclohexylamine, is unique in its pharmacologic effects. Ketamine causes dose related increases in MAP, HR, SV and CO [34]. SVR does not change. There is venoconstriction and an increase in inotropy, and a considerable increase in myocardial oxygen consumption. After 2.2 mg/kg IV, CO is increased 41% [35]. The mechanism for this cardiovascular stimulation is central autonomic nervous system activation [36] and possibly a decrease in vagal tone. There may also be a cocaine-like effect whereby ketamine inhibits the reuptake of norepinephrine at adrenergic nerve terminals [37]. Ketamine has a direct myocardial depressant effect [38]. Thus, patients unable to increase sympathetic outflow because of either cervical cord transection, critical illness, high epidural anesthesia, drug effect or general anesthesia, may develop hypotension when given ketamine. The increased pulmonary vascular resistance can precipitate right heart failure in patients with decreased right ventricular reserve.

Ketamine is often used for induction of anesthesia in hypovolemic patients because of its cardiovascular stimulating effects, but must be used with caution, if at all, in patients with either coronary or myocardial disease.

Etomidate

Etomidate, a carboxylated imidazole, is associated with cardiovascular stability. When given to healthy patients, no clinically significant change is seen in SV, CO, HR, MAP, CVP, PCWP or SVR [39]. In addition, patients with cardiovascular disease or severe coronary artery disease show little change in hemodynamics on induction of anesthesia with etomidate [40, 41]. Indeed, there may be a mild nitroglycerine-like coronary vasodilatory effect [42]. Some studies do show a slight decrease in SVR and contractility with etomidate.

Etomidate has no analgesic properties and is consequently used in combination with a narcotic to achieve the anesthetic state. The combination of etomidate (0.3 mg/kg) and fentanyl (10 µg/kg) blocks the increase in HR and MAP seen with endotracheal intubation, causes bradycardia, and a decrease in both CO and the rate-pressure product [41].

Propofol

A recently introduced intravenous anesthetic, propofol is an alkyl phenol and is chemically unrelated to all previous induction agents. When administered as an induction dose of 2 mg/kg to premedicated patients, propofol causes an approximately 30% decrease in systolic BP [43–45]. Changes in heart rate are variable and not clinically significant. One study suggests the cause of hypotension to be a decrease in SVR while SV and CO are maintained [44]. In contrast, other studies show a 30% decrease in CO [43, 45].

When given to patients with good left ventricular function just prior to coronary artery bypass surgery, hypotension is found with statistically insignificant changes in CO [46]. Patients may develop coronary sinus lactate production, suggestive of myocardial ischemia.

While the data are inconsistent, propofol appears to cause more profound hypotension than other intravenous induction agents and may be detrimental to selected patients.

Effect of narcotics

Narcotics, or opioids, cause profound analgesia by selectively binding to receptors distributed unevenly throughout the central nervous system. They are utilized in anesthesia for premedication, postoperative pain relief, supplementation of general anesthetics, and as a primary anesthetic for critically ill patients. Of the large number of opioids currently in use, several enjoy the most frequent use, namely, morphine, fentanyl *and* sufentanil. A recently introduced opioid is alfentanil. Opioids differ more in terms of their pharmacokinetic profiles than their cardiovascular effects, and may thus be considered together.

Although several opioids have been reported to cause direct myocardial depression, this is generally associated with, excepting meperidine, much greater doses than would be produced clinically [47–49]. The effect of opioids on the contractility of the already impaired heart has not yet been studied. Opioids do not interfere with the effect of catecholamines on the heart.

With the exception of meperidine, opioids tend to decrease heart rate by a centrally mediated increase in vagal activity and decrease in sympathetic tone [50]. This effect may be blocked by either atropine or by vagotomy. There may also be direct effects on the sinoatrial and atrioventricular node [51].

Opioids can cause hypotension by arterial dilatation and venodilation. Several mechanisms are involved. Opioid action at the medulla decreases sympathetic activity. Histamine release, particularly when induced by morphine, can cause profound vasodilation with an accompanying increase in CO and decrease in MAP. Although weakened, this response is not prevented by blockade of H_1 and H_2 receptors [52]. Fentanyl, sufentanil and alfentanil do not cause histamine release [53]. In the presence of an opioid antagonist, morphine may still have a direct vasodilating effect on vascular smooth muscle.

The usual effects of vasodilation, negative chronotropy and normal inotropy cause minimal CO changes in healthy individuals. The administration of large doses of morphine to individuals with or without cardiac disease, does not usually cause clinically significant hemodynamic changes [54]. However, patients with increased sympathetic tone as a compensation for hypovolemia, heart failure, tamponade or chronic valvular disease, may have larger changes in hemodynamics [55].

While opioids tend to be associated with stable hemodynamics, they are not complete anesthetics as they do not cause generalized central nervous system depression. Hypertension and tachycardia, unresponsive to increasing doses, are common in response to surgical stimulation while under pure opioid anesthesia [56, 57]. Attempts to prevent this potentially adverse response by supplementing opioid anesthesia often lead to unstable hemodynamics. All hypnotic supplements to opioid anesthesia cause what may be a clinically significant decrease in blood pressure. The interaction appears to be synergistic in that small, otherwise innocuous doses of hypnotics can cause profound hypotension when added to an opioid anesthetic [58, 59]. When given to patients with coronary artery disease, diazepam and fentanyl anesthesia does not prevent the sympathetic response to stimulation, and decreases myocardial contractility, MAP, SVR, HR and CO [60, 61]. Conversely, small doses of narcotic can cause hypotension when added to an induction dose of a hypnotic. A decrease in central nervous system sympathetic activity most likely contributes largely to this effect [58]. Nitrous oxide, when added to morphine anesthesia, may cause large decreases in cardiac output and yet not sufficiently blunt cardiovascular responses to noxious stimuli [62]. The addition of low concentrations of potent inhaled agents can caused marked cardiovascular depression in patients with coronary artery disease [63, 64].

Effect of regional anesthesia

Regional anesthesia is a broad term encompassing local infiltration, nerve block, plexus block and central neuraxis anesthesia. Its circulatory effects range from minimal to profound depression and may be caused by sympathetic blockade as well as the systemic effects of absorbed local anesthetics and vasoconstrictors. Here, again, supplemental drugs such as sedatives, narcotics and general anesthetics may act synergistically with the cardiovascular effects of regional anesthesia.

Subarachnoid blockade

Subarachnoid blockade, or spinal anesthesia, is achieved by introducing a local anesthetic into the cerebrospinal fluid, generally in the lumbar region. The anesthetic spreads as a result of gravity, patient position and density of the local anesthetic solution. Blockade of motor fibers causes immobility and relaxation of skeletal muscle; blockade of sensory fibers causes analgesia; and blockade of autonomic vasoconstrictor and cardiac sympathetic fibers brings about cardiovascular changes. Spread of the anesthetic in the cerebrospinal fluid causes a segmental level of blockade. Generally, the level of sympathetic blockade exceeds that of sensory blockade by two dermatomal levels.

The extent of the cardiovascular effects is directly related to the degree of sympathetic blockade. Sympathetic outflow from the spinal cord occurs from approximately T_1 to L_2. Loss of sympathetic tone causes venodilation, arteriolar vasodilation and, if the level is higher than T_4, negative inotropic and chronotropic effects on the heart. Compensatory vasoconstriction occurs above the level of a partial sympathetic blockade [65]. When healthy volunteers are given a T_5 sensory level, MAP and CVP decrease 15–20%, while CO, HR and SV change only minimally [66]. There is a decrease in SVR of only 5%, indicating that the primary cause of these changes is venous pooling. Total sympathetic denervation causes only a moderate 15–18% decrease in SVR in normal euvolemic subjects [67]. CO is therefore mainly dependent on venous return which, in turn, is determined by the position of the patient. CO is unchanged in normovolemic subjects during high spinal anesthesia if their legs are elevated above the level of the heart. High spinal anesthesia is not tolerated as well in older or hypovolemic patients. No cardiovascular changes occur with low spinal anesthesia that avoids blockade of the upper lumbar segments. During high spinal anesthesia, coronary blood flow as well as myocardial oxygen consumption are reduced [68].

Vasoconstrictors, such as epinephrine and phenylephrine, are occasionally added to local anesthetic solutions to increase the duration of spinal anesthesia. If given intravenously, these doses would cause adverse effects. Absorption is slow from the cerebrospinal fluid and produces no systemic effects.

Epidural blockade

Epidural anesthesia is produced by introduction of a local anesthetic solution into the epidural space. Neural transmission can be blocked in either of two ways: either at the nerve roots as they traverse the epidural space or by diffusion of the local anesthetic into the subarachnoid space. As with spinal anesthesia, the degree of sympathetic blockade largely determines the resultant cardiovascular effects. Additionally, the requisite doses of local anesthetic and vasoconstrictor for epidural blockade are quite large and can themselves lead to systemic effects.

Epidural blockade below the level of T_4 preserves the function of cardiac sympathetic fibers, and also allows for compensatory vasoconstriction in unblocked segments. There is vasodilation in the pelvis, lower extremities and abdominal viscera. One liter of blood may be pooled in the venous capacitance vessels, which may lead to large decreases in venous return, RAP and CO. Sympathetic activity increases reflexively above the level of blockade causing vasoconstriction of the head, neck and upper extremities. There may be increased myocardial contractility and heart rate.

Epidural blockade above the level of T_4, generally to T_1, can be regarded as total sympathetic blockade. With this degree of epidural blockade, unmedicated patients and volunteers show a 20% decrease in MAP and SVR, and a 15% to 20% decrease in CO [69]. Some studies, however, show the CO to be either slightly increased or unchanged [70]. HR changes only slightly, implying a decrease in parasympathetic activity concomitant with the sympathetic denervation. An increase in CVP has been found without an attendant increase in SV, suggesting impairment of ventricular emptying [70]. This indicates that, during high epidural blockade, all compensatory mechanisms of the cardiovascular system may have been pushed to their limits. These patients will be more sensitive to hypovolemia, head-up positioning and vena cava obstruction. Furthermore, without the ability to increase sympathetic tone, the decreased parasympathetic tone predisposes the patient to profound vagal reflexes including transient cardiac arrest. Indeed, decreased venous return can provoke a vagal reflex that can in turn cause asystole during a high level of autonomic blockade [71, 72].

Following epidural blockade, moderate blood levels of local anesthetic (<4 μg/ml lidocaine) usually cause no measurable changes in HR, CO, MAP or SVR, even in patients with cardiovascular disease [70, 73]. There may be mild centrally-induced cardiovascular stimulation. With high blood levels of local anesthetic, as may be seen with inadvertent intravascular injection or epidural overdose, there is generalized cardiovascular depression with attendant decreases in CO, HR, MAP and SVR [70]. This is due to the negative inotropic action and the peripheral vasodilator effect of the local anesthetic. Systemic absorption of epinephrine from local anesthetic solution can lead to mild beta adrenergic stimulation. Seen with the administration of epidural epinephrine in doses of 80–130 μg without local anesthestic are a moderate increase in HR and CO, and decreased MAP [74]. When epinephrine is added to the local anesthetic solution during epidural anesthesia to T_5 level, CO increases 20% compared to plain solutions [75]. The mild vasodilatory effects of this dose may antagonize compensatory vasoconstriction above the level of blockade. Also, epinephrine appears to make more pronounced the sympathetic blockade of epidural block [76].

Epidural blockade is finding increasing popularity in combination with light general anesthesia. When thiopentone-nitrous oxide-oxygen anesthesia was followed by epidural injection of plain lidocaine some patients had no significant hemodynamic changes while others showed a 30% decrease in MAP [77]. The only decrease in CO, however, was associated with bradycardia. One study in healthy patients showed that epidural block administered before or after general anesthesia causes similar decreases in MAP [78]. Again, the greatest decreases in MAP were associated with slow heart rates and intravenous administration of atropine restored hemodynamics to awake levels.

Local blockade

Regional anesthesia of the upper extremity can be effected with a brachial plexus block, and of the lower extremity with a lumbar plexus or femoral/sciatic block. The cardiovascular effects of these blocks are minimal and related to the effects of systemically absorbed local anesthetics and epinephrine rather than sympathetic blockade of the extremity.

Effect of special techniques

Isovolemic hemodilution

Isovolemic hemodilution acutely reduces hematocrit by first removing an aliquot of blood from a patient and then replacing it with a red blood cell free substitute such as Ringers lactate or dextran. Hemodilution is most commonly used during cardiopulmonary bypass when the pump is primed without blood. It may also be used to decrease the amount of homologous blood required during an operation. With the hemorrhaging patient, isovolemic hemodilution will result when volume is replaced adequately with crystalloid or colloid rather than with blood.

Acute isovolemic hemodilution while maintaining normovolemia with a colloid causes CO and MAP to rise, and SVR to fall [79, 80]. As the colloid is removed from the vasculature over a period of several hours to several days, CO decreases, reaching a nadir at three days [81]. Increased cardiac sympathetic activity accounts for most of these circulatory changes. Left ventricular afterload is reduced as well, because of the diminished blood viscosity [82]. An acute rise in red blood cell 2,3-DPG levels facilitates unloading of oxygen to the tissues. The increased CO tends to maintain normal oxygen delivery down to a hematocrit of 25–30%. Total oxygen consumption does not become supply dependent until a hematocrit of less than 10% [83]. In its basal state the normal heart tolerates hemodilution well. In the presence of coronary artery disease or increased myocardial oxygen requirement, subendocardial ischemia may result.

Controlled hypotension

Controlled, or deliberate hypotension is induced to reduce bleeding during selected surgical procedures. For example, it is used to aid in the dissection and clipping of cerebral aneurysms. A number of drugs and techniques are used to facilitate hypotension.

In higher concentrations, halothane has been used to produce controlled hypotension. As previously discussed, dose-dependent decreases in CO and MAP attend its use. Halothane precipitated cardiac arrest in one patient during controlled hypotension [84]. Isoflurane, on the other hand, can cause hypotension while maintaining CO, which may be more desirable [85].

Trimethaphan is the only ganglionic blocker in current clinical use. A reduction in both CO and SV is the usual response to trimethaphan [86]. Myocardial contractility is reduced most likely because of reduced sympathetic tone to the heart from blocked ganglia. The agent most frequently use for controlled hypotension is sodium nitroprusside because of its rapid and evanescent action. Nitroprusside causes direct smooth muscle relaxation and vasodilatation. CO increases during nitroprusside infusion [87]. Additionally, the sympathetic nervous system and renin-angiotensin system are activated. This can cause tachycardia and resistance to nitroprusside's hypotensive effect. Interestingly, a comparison of nitroprusside and trimethaphan showed blood loss to be related to MAP rather than CO [88]. To achieve a MAP of approximately 55 mm Hg, healthy patients were given either nitroprusside or trimethaphan. Patients receiving trimethaphan had a 37% decrease in CO while patients receiving nitroprusside had a 27% increase in CO. Blood loss in both groups was similar.

Other drugs such as labetalol, esmolol, hydralazine, and adenosine have been used to induce hypotension. Although their hemodynamic effects during hypotension have not been well studied, they generally appear similar to those in the awake patient.

Occasionally, hypertension is induced perioperatively when managing cerebral vasospasm or stroke, usually with a combination of fluid loading and either dopamine or phenylephrine. This is often accompanied by large increases in cardiac output.

Intraoperative monitoring

Most patients tolerate perioperative hemodynamic changes well by virtue of compensatory mechanisms and large reserves in organ function. For most patients, blood pressure, measured either noninvasively or with an intraarterial catheter, is considered an adequate indicator of cardiovascular function and cardiac output. Certain patients, however, may benefit from more direct indicators of cardiac function, and may include those patients with heart disease and those undergoing more invasive types of surgery.

Intraoperatively, CO is most frequently measured by thermodilution utilizing a pulmonary artery (Swan-Ganz) catheter. Thermodilution is a variation of the indicator dilution technique where a bolus of 'cold' is substituted for a bolus of dye as the indicator [89]. A fixed volume of dextrose solution (D5W) is injected into the right atrium. The injectate mixes with blood and a thermistor in the pulmonary artery records the resultant decrease in temperature. A computer then integrates a time-temperature curve and, based on the physical properties of the injectate and blood, derives a CO. CO determinations may be repeated frequently, easily and reproducibly.

There is excellent correlation between thermodilution cardiac output and Fick and dye dilution methods [90, 91]. However, there are certain caveats associated with its use. Pulmonary artery temperature varies with respiration causing marked variability in measured CO [92]. Measurements are best done at a fixed point in the respiratory cycle, usually end-expiration. Regurgitant and shunt lesions, particularly tricuspid insufficiency, can cause significant recirculation of blood in the right side of the heart leading to erroneous measurements. The volume and temperature of the injectate must be measured precisely to avoid error.

Thermodilution CO, in combination with left and right sided filling pressures and mixed venous oxygen saturation, provide information to guide fluid therapy, the treatment of oliguria, the use of vasoactive drugs, the diagnosis and treatment of myocardial ischemia, and may prompt a change in anesthetic technique. Common indications for placement of a pulmonary artery catheter include a left ventricular ejection fraction of less than 40%, triple vessel coronary artery disease or its equivalent, symptomatic valvular heart disease and pulmonary hypertension. Mixed venous oxygen measurement may be used to assess the physiologic significance of a change in CO. The pulmonary artery catheter is not, however, without risk. Dysrhythmias, and cardiac and pulmonary artery rupture are among the most serious complications.

Noninvasive monitoring techniques, though not yet used commonly, are being investigated as possible additions to clinical care. Intraoperative echocardiography, usually by the transesophageal route, can image in real time all four cardiac chambers, the mitral and tricuspid valves, and regional wall function. The aortic valve and coronary arteries may also be seen. Preload, as a measure of the initial stretch on myocardial fibers, is better assessed by a volume measurement on a transesophageal echocardiogram rather than a central pressure measurement. Contractility can be assessed by a number of indices including fractional shortening [93], circumferential fractional shortening [94] and ejection fraction. CO can be calculated from measurement of end-diastolic and end-systolic volumes though the non- uniform shape of the left ventricle and the inability of the echocardiogram to visualize more than a two dimensional slice of the heart can make this determination inaccurate [95].

Pulsed doppler echocardiography can measure blood velocity in the aorta [96]. This measurement, combined with suitable assumptions or measurements of aortic cross-sectional area and systolic ejection time can determine stroke volume. A changing aortic diameter, as well as difficulties aligning the probe, can lead to inaccuracies [97].

Bioimpedance cardiography measures stroke volume on a beat-to-beat basis [98]. The change in thoracic impedance is related to changes in intrathoracic blood volume and, hence to stroke volume. The calculation makes certain assumptions about thoracic geometry that may not always be true and the measurement is sensitive to changes in hematocrit and lung water. Poor correlations between bioimpedance measured CO and thermodilution CO have been reported [99].

Summary

The most important goal of perioperative management is the maintenance of normal cellular and organ function in the face of many stresses. It is difficult, if not impossible, to measure directly organ function in clinical practice. Most attention is directed to the cardiovascular system both because of its primacy and because normal cardiovascular function sustains other vital organ function. In the early days of anesthesia, the quality of the peripheral pulse was used to assess adequacy of the circulation. Harvey Cushing introduced the concept of monitoring blood pressure and heart rate during surgical procedures. Today, in healthy patients, blood pressure is still used as a primary indicator of cardiovascular function. Blood pressure is the product of both the cardiac output and systemic vascular resistance, making it difficult to determine which variable has effected a change in blood pressure. Patients who are at risk for having severe derangements of cardiac output should have this parameter measured directly. A normal cardiac output, however, does not ensure a normal distribution of blood flow to core organs. However, a reduced cardiac output usually implies a maldistribution of blood flow or inadequate reserves.

Still, cardiac output remains one of our most useful cardiovascular parameters whether it is inferred clinically or measured directly. A thorough knowledge of the effects of anesthetic drugs, perioperative events and disease states enables the clinician to better preserve the patient's vital functions.

References

1. Werko L. The influence of positive pressure breathing on the circulation in man. Acta Med Scand 1947;193(Suppl):1.
2. Cournand A, Motley HL, Werko L et al. Physiological studies of the effects of intermittent positive pressure breathing on cardiac output in man. Am J Physiol 1948;152:162–94.
3. Morgan BC, Crawford EW, Guntheroth WG. The hemodynamic effects of changes in blood volume during intermittent positive pressure ventilation. Anesthesiology 1969;30:297–305.
4. Bahlman SH, Eger EI II, Halsey MJ et al. The cardiovascular effects of halothane in man during spontaneous ventilation. Anesthesiology 1972;36:494–502.
5. Lenfant C, Howell BJ. Cardiovascular adjustment in dogs during continuous pressure breathing. J Appl Physiol 1960;15:425–8.
6. Jardin F, Farcot JC, Boisante L et al. Influence of positive end-expiratory pressure on left ventricular performance. N Engl J Med 1981;304:387–92.
7. Pannier JL, Leusen L. Contraction characteristics of papillary muscle during changes in acid-base composition of the bathing-fluid. Arch Internat de Physiol et de Bioch 1968;76:624–34.
8. Blair DA, Glover WE, McArdle L et al. The mechanism of the peripheral vasodilatation following carbon dioxide inhalation in man. Clin Sci 1960;19:407–23.
9. Morris ME, Millar RA. Blood pH/plasma catecholamine relationships: respiratory acidosis. Br J Anaesth 1962;34:672–81.
10. Richardson DW, Wasserman AJ, Patterson JL. General and regional circulatory responses to change in blood pH and carbon dioxide tension. J Clin Invest 1961;40:31–43.

11. Cullen DJ, Eger EI II, Smith NT. The circulatory response to hypercapnia during fluroxene anesthesia in man. Anesthesiology 1971; 34:415–20.
12. Prys-Roberts C, Kelman GR, Greenbaum R et al. Hemodynamics and alveolar-arterial PO_2 differences at varying $PaCO_2$ in anaesthetized man. J Appl Physiol 1968; 25:80–7.
13. Marshall BE, Cohen PJ, Klingenmaier CH et al. Some pulmonary and cardiovascular effects of enflurane (ethrane) anaesthesia with varying $PaCO_2$ in man. Br J Anaesth 1971;43:996–1002.
14. King BD, Harris LC, Greifenstein A et al. Reflex circulatory responses to direct laryngoscopy and tracheal intubation performed during general anesthesia. Anesthesiology 1951;12:556–66.
15. Prys-Roberts C, Greene LT, Meloche R et al. Studies of anaesthesia in relation to hypertension. II: haemodynamic consequences of induction and endotracheal intubation. Br J Anaesth 1971;43:531–45.
16. Kleinman F, Henkin RE, Glisson SN et al. Qualitative evaluation of coronary flow during anesthetic induction using Thallium-201 perfusion scans. Anesthesiology 1986;64:157–64.
17. Stone JG, Faltas AN, Hoar PF. Sodium nitroprusside therapy for cardiac failure in anesthetized patients with valvular insufficiency. Anesthesiology 1978;49:414–8.
18. Coonan TJ, Hope CE. Cardiorespiratory effects of change of body position. Can Anaesth Soc J 1983;30:424–37.
19. Dalrymple DG, MacGowan SW, MacLeod GF. Cardiorespiratory effects of the sitting position in neurosurgery. Br J Anaesth 1979;51:1079–82.
20. Eger EI II, Smith NT, Stoelting RK et al. Cardiovascular effects of halothane in man. Anesthesiology 1970;32:396–409.
21. Goldberg AH, Ullrick WC. Effects of halothane on isometric contractions of isolated heart muscle. Anesthesiology 1967;28:838–45.
22. Price HL, Linde HW, Morse HT. Central nervous actions of halothane affecting the systemic circulation. Anesthesiology 1963;24:770–78.
23. Calverly RK, Smith NT, Prys-Roberts C et al. Cardiovascular effects of enflurane during controlled ventilation in man. Anesth Analg 1978;57:619–28.
24. Stevens WC, Cromwell TH, Halsey MJ et al. The cardiovascular effects of a new inhalation anesthetic, forane, in human volunteers at constant arterial carbon dioxide tension. Anesthesiology 1971;35:8–16.
25. Wade JG, Stevens WC. Isoflurane: an anesthetic for the eighties? Anesth Analg 1981;60:666–82.
26. Kemmotsu O, Hashimoto Y, Shimosato S. Inotropic effects of isoflurane on mechanics of contraction in isolated cat papillary muscles from normal and failing hearts. Anesthesiology 1973;39:470–7.
27. Jones RM, Cashman JN, Mant TGK. Clinical impressions and cardiorespiratory effects of a new fluorinated inhalation anaesthetic, desflurane (I-653), in volunteers. Br J Anaesth 1990;64:11–5.
28. Weiskopf RB, Holmes MA, Eger EI II et al. Cardiovascular effects of I-653 in swine. Anesthesiology 1988;69:303–9.
29. Eisele JH, Smith NT. Cardiovascular effects of 40 percent nitrous oxide in man. Anesth Analg 1972;51:956–63.
30. Smith NT, Eger EI II, Stoelting RK et al. The cardiovascular and sympathomimetic responses to the addition of nitrous oxide to halothane in man. Anesthesiology 1970;32:410–21.
31. Bahlman SH, Eger EI II, Smith NT et al. The cardiovascular effects of nitrous oxide-halothane anesthesia in man. Anesthesiology 1981;35:274–85.
32. Elder JD Jr, Nagano SM, Eastwood DW et al. Circulatory changes associated with thiopental anesthesia in man. Anesthesiology 1955;16:394–400.
33. Dwyer EM, Weiner L. Left ventricular function in man following thiopental. Anesth Analg 1969;48:499–505.
34. Johnstone M. The cardiovascular effects of ketamine in man. Anaesthesia 1976;31:873–82.

35. Virtue RW, Alanis JM, Mori M *et al*. An anesthetic agent: 2-orthochlorophenyl 2-methylamine cyclohexanone HCl (CI-581). Anesthesiology 1967;28:823–33.
36. Ivankovich AD, Miletich DJ, Reimann C *et al*. Cardiovascular effects of centrally administered ketamine in goats. Anesth Analg 1974;54:924–33.
37. Hill GE, Wong KC, Shaw CL *et al*. Interactions of ketamine with vasoactive amines at normothermia and hypothermia in the isolated rabbit heart. Anesthesiology 1978;48:315–9.
38. Schwartz DA, Horwitz LD. Effects of ketamine on left ventricular performance. J Pharmacol Exp Ther 1975;194:410–4.
39. Criado A, Maseda J, Navarro E *et al*. Induction of anesthesia with etomidate: hemodynamic study of 36 patients. Br J Anaesth 1980;52:803–5.
40. Gooding JM, Jen-Tsou Weng, Smith RA *et al*. Cardiovascular and pulmonary response following etomidate induction of anesthesia in patients with demonstrated cardiac disease. Anesth Analg 1979;58:40–1.
41. Tarnow J, Hess W, Kline W. Etomidate, alfathesin and thiopentone as induction agents for coronary artery surgery. Can Anesth Soc J 1980;27:338–44.
42. Kettler D, Sonntag H, Donath V *et al*. Haemodynamics, myocardial function, oxygen requirements and oxygen supply to the human heart after administration of etomidate. Anaesthesist 1974;23:116–21.
43. Coates DP, Monk CR, Prys-Roberts C *et al*. Hemodynamic effects of infusions of the emulsion formulation of propofol during nitrous oxide anesthesia in humans. Anesth Analg 1987;66:64–70.
44. Claeys MA, Gepts E, Camu F. Hemodynamic changes during anesthesia induced and maintained with propofol. Br J Anaesth 1988;60:3–9.
45. Monk CR, Coates DP, Prys-Roberts C *et al*. Haemodynamic effects of a prolonged infusion of propofol as a supplement to nitrous oxide anesthesia. Br J Anaesth 1987;59:954–60.
46. Stephan H, Sonntag H, Schenk HD *et al*. Effects of propofol on cardiovascular dynamics, myocardial blood flow and myocardial metabolism in patients with coronary disease. Br J Anesth 1986;58:969–75.
47. Barash P, Kopriva C, Giles R *et al*. Global ventricular function and intubation: radionuclear profiles. Anesthesiology 1980;53:S109.
48. Goldberg AH, Padget CH. Comparative effects of morphine and fentanyl on isolated heart muscle. Anesth Analg 1969;48:978–81.
49. Strauer BE. Contractile responses to morphine, piritramide, meperidine and fentanyl: a comparative study of effects on isolated ventricular myocardium. Anesthesiology 1972;37:304–10.
50. Reitan JA, Stengert KB, Wymore MC *et al*. Central vagal control of fentanyl induced bradycardia during halothane anesthesia, Anesth Analg 1978;57:31–6.
51. Urthaler F, Isobe JH, James TN. Direct and vagally mediated chronotropic effects of morphine studies by selective perfusion of the sinus node of awake dogs. Chest 1975;68:222–8.
52. Philbin DM, Moss J, Akins CW *et al*. The use of H1 and H2 histamine blockers with high dose morphine anesthesia: a double blind study. Anesthesiology 1981;55:292–6.
53. Flacke JW, Flacke WE, Bloor BC *et al*. Histamine release by four narcotics: A double blind study in humans. Anesth Analgl 1987;66:723–30.
54. Lowenstein E, Hallowell P, Levine FH *et al*. Cardiovascular response to large doses of intravenous morphine in man. N Engl J Med 1969;281:1389–93.
55. Lowenstein E, Philbin DM. Narcotic 'anesthesia' in the eighties. Anesthesiology 1981;55:195–7.
56. Hilfiker O, Larsen R, Brockschneider BC *et al*. Morphine 'anesthesia'. Coronary blood flow and oxygen consumption in patients with coronary artery disease. Anaesthetist 1982;31:371–6.
57. Sonntag H, Larsen R, Hilfker O *et al*. Myocardial blood flow and oxygen consumption

during high-dose fentanyl anesthesia in patients with coronary artery disease. Anesthesiology1 1982;56:417–22.

58. Tomichek RC, Rosow CE, Philbin DM et al. Diazepam-fentanyl interaction: hemodynamic and hormonal effects in coronary artery surgery. Anesth Analg 1983;62:881–4.

59. Heikkila H, Jalonen J, Arola M et al. Midazolam as adjunct to high-dose fentanyl anaesthesia for coronary artery bypass grafting operation. Acta Anaesthesiol Scand 1984;28:683–9.

60. Stanley TH, Webster LR. Anesthetic requirements and cardiovascular effects of fentanyl-oxygen and fentanyl-diazepam-oxygen anesthesia in man. Anesth Analg 1978;57:411–6.

61. Tomichek RC, Rosow CE, Schneider RC et al. Cardiovascular effects of diazepam-fentanyl anesthesia in patients with coronary artery disease. Anesth Analg 1982;61:217–8.

62. McDermott RW, Stanley TH. The cardiovascular effects of low concentrations of nitrous oxide during morphine anesthesia. Anesthesiology 1974;41:89–91.

63. Stoetling RK, Creasser CW, Gibbs PS et al. Circulatory effects of halothane added to morphine anesthesia in patients with coronary-artery disease. Anesth Analg 1974;53:449–55.

64. Bennett GM, Stanley TH: Cardiovascular effects of fentanyl during enflurane anesthesia in man. Anesth Analg 1979;58:179–82.

65. Bridenbaugh PO, Moore DC, Bridenbaugh L. Capillary pO_2 as a measure of sympathetic blockade. Anesth Analg 1971;50:26–30.

66. Kennedy WF Jr, Everett GB, Cobb LA et al. Simultaneous systemic and hepatic hemodynamic measurements during high spinal anesthesia in normal man. Anesth Analg 1970;49:1016–24.

67. Greene NM. Physiology of Spinal Anesthesia. 3rd ed. Baltimore: Williams & Wilkins 1981.

68. Hackel DB, Sancetta SM, Kleinerman J. Effect of hypotension due to spinal anesthesia on coronary blood flow and myocardial metabolism. Circulation 1956;13:92–7.

69. McLean APH, Mulligan GW, Otton P et al. Hemodynamic alterations associated with epidural anesthesia. Surgery 1967;62:79.

70. Bonica JJ, Berges PU, Morikawa K. Circulatory effects of peridural block: I. effects of level of analgesia and dose of lidocaine. Anesthesiology 1970;33:619–26.

71. Bonica JJ, Kennedy WF, Akamatsu TJ et al. Circulatory effects of peridural block: III. effects of acute blood loss. Anesthesiology 1972;36:219–27.

72. Baron JF, Decaux-Jaacolot A, Edouard A et al. Influence of venous return on baroreflex control of heart rate during lumbar epidural anesthesia in humans. Anesthesiology 1986;64:188–93.

73. Harrison DC, Sprouse JH, Morrow AG. The antiarrhythmic properties of lidocaine and procaine amide. Clinical and physiologic studies of their cardiovascular effects in man. Circulation 1963;28:486–91.

74. Bonica JJ, Akamatsu TJ, Berges PU et al. Circulatory effects of peridural block: II. effects of epinephrine. Anesthesiology 1971;34:514–22.

75. Ward RJ, Bonica JJ, Freund FG et al. Epidural and subarachnoid anesthesia. Cardiovascular and respiratory effects. J Am Med Assoc 1965;191:275–8.

76. Bromage PR. Epidural Analgesia. Philadelphia: W.B. Saunders, 1978.

77. Stephen GW, Lees MM, Scott DB. Cardiovascular effects of epidural block combined with general anaesthesia. Br J Anaesth 1969;41:933–8.

78. Germann PAS, Roberts JG, Prys-Roberts C. The combination of general anaesthesia and epidural block: I. the effects of sequence of induction on haemodynamic variables and blood gas measurements in healthy patients. Anaesth Intens Care 1979;7:229.

79. Pavek K, Carey JS. Hemodynamics and oxygen availability during isovolemic hemodilution. Am J Physiol 1974;226:1172–7.

80. Chamorro G, Rodriguez JA, Dzindzio B et al. Effect of acute isovolemic anemia on cardiac output and estimated hepatic blood flow in the conscious dog. Circ Res 1973;32:530–5.

81. Hatcher JD, Jennings DB, Parker JO et al. The role of a humoral mechanism in the

cardiovascular adjustments over a prolonged period following the production of acute exchange anaemia. Can J Biochem Physiol 1963;41:1887–99.

82. Fowler NO, Holmes JC. Blood viscosity and cardiac output in acute experimental anemia. J Appl Physiol 1975;39:453–6.

83. Neuhof H, Wolf H. Oxygen uptake during hemodilution. Bibl Haematologica 1975;41:66–75.

84. Prys-Roberts C, Lloyd JW, Fisher A *et al*. Deliberate profound hypotension induced with halothane: studies of haemodynamics and pulmonary gas exchange. Br J Anaesth 1974;46:105–16.

85. Lam AM, Gelb AW. Cardiovascular effects of isoflurane-induced hypotension for cerebral aneurysm surgery. Anesth Analg 1983;62:742–8.

86. Jordan WS, Graves CL, Boyd WA *et al*. Cardiovascular effects of three techniques for inducing hypotension during anesthesia. Anesth Analg Curr Res 1971;50:1059–68.

87. Ivankovich AD. Nitroprusside and other short-acting hypotensive agents. Int Anesthes Clin 1978;16:1–318.

88. Sivarajan M, Amory DW, Everett GB *et al*. Blood pressure, not cardiac output, determines blood loss during induced hypotension. Anesth Analg 1980;59:203–6.

89. Ganz W, Donoso R, Marcus HS *et al*. A new technique for measurement of cardiac output by thermodilution in man. Am J Cardiol 1971;27:392–6.

90. Fischer AP, Benis AM, Jurado RA *et al*. Analysis of errors in measurement of cardiac output by simultaneous dye and thermal dilution in cardiothoracic surgical patients. Cardiovasc Res 1978;12:190–9.

91. Hillis LD, Firth BG, Winniford MD. Comparison of thermodilution and indocyanine green dye in low cardiac output or left-sided regurgitation. Am J Cardiol 1986;57:1201–2.

92. Jansen JRC, Schreuder JJ, Bogaard JM *et al*. Thermodilution technique for measurement of cardiac output during artificial ventilation. J Appl Physiol 1981;51:584–91.

93. Quinones MA, Pickering E, Alexander JK. Percentage of shortening of the echocardiographic left ventricular dimension: Its use in determining ejection fraction and stroke volume. Chest 1978;74:59–65.

94. Benzing G, Stockert J, Nave E *et al*. Evaluation of left ventricular performance: circumferential fiber shortening and tension. Circulation 1974;49:925–32.

95. Feigenbaum H. Echocardiographic examination of the left ventricle. Circulation 1975;51:1–7.

96. Kumar A, Minagoe S, Thangathurai D *et al*. The continuous wave Doppler esophageal probe: a new method for measurement of cardiac output during surgery. J Am Coll Cardiol 1986;7:2A.

97. Rose JS, Nanna M, Rahimtoola SH *et al*. Accuracy of determination of changes in cardiac output by transcutaneous continuous-wave Doppler computer. Am J Cardiol 1984;54:1099–101.

98. Salandin V, Zussa C, Risica G *et al*. Comparison of cardiac output estimation by thoracic electrical bioimpedance, thermodilution and Fick methods. Crit Care Med 1988;16:1157–8.

99. Siegel LC, Shafer SL, Martinez GM *et al*. Simultaneous measurements of cardiac output by thermodilution, esophageal Doppler, and electrical impedance in anaesthetized patients. J Cardiothorac Anesth 1988;2:590–5.

PART SIX

Fetal circulation and cardiac output during pregnancy
and in neonates

24. Maternal cardiac output in normal and complicated pregnancy

KYPROS H. NICOLAIDES and J.GUY THORPE-BEESTON

The importance of hemodynamic changes in pregnancy was first reported in the French literature during the 19th century. Larcher (1859) [1] in a post mortem study of 130 women who died during pregnancy, noted that the left ventricle and atrium were hypertrophied, whilst the right heart was not significantly changed. Since the majority of these women died from 'childbed fever' it was assumed that these changes represented physiological responses to pregnancy.

Hecker and Buhl in 1861 [2] recognised that pregnancy imposed serious risks on patients with valvular heart disease. Indeed, Peter (1874) [3] recommended that women with heart disease should not become pregnant and if they did, then their cardiopulmonary status should be carefully monitored and obstetricians should have a low threshold for intervening if complications develop.

MacDonald (1878) [4] in a review of the existing literature and his own experience, reported that in normal pregnancy there is cardiac hypertrophy and both the circulating blood volume and stroke volume are increased. He also noted that pregnant women with heart disease have a high mortality and particularly so those with mitral stenosis or aortic regurgitation, where the maternal mortality rate was 50%.

This poor prognosis for women with heart disease did not change until the 1920s when antenatal clinics were started to care specifically for such women. Subsequently, there was a dramatic decrease in maternal mortality especially for women with rheumatic fever and valve disease. Patient education and treatment of disease are now considered integral parts of pregnancy management.

Antepartum hemodynamic changes

In normal pregnancy, there are alterations in blood volume, red cell mass, heart rate, stroke volume and systemic vascular resistance. Heart disease may interfere with these physiological changes and adversely affect both the mother and fetus. Furthermore, previously unrecognised heart disease may be unmasked by the increased circulatory burden of pregnancy.

A.-M. Salmasi and A.S. Iskandrian (eds): Cardiac output and regional flow in health and disease, 309–324.
© 1993 Kluwer Academic Publishers. Printed in the Netherlands.

BLOOD VOLUME

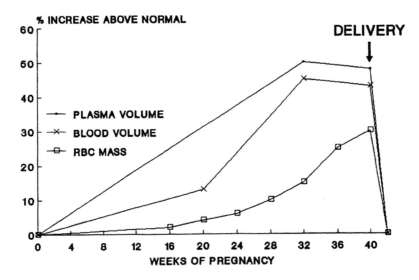

Figure 24.1. Blood volume during pregnancy.

Blood volume

Plasma volume increases in pregnancy from as early as 4–6 weeks' gestation, reaching a plateau at 32–36 weeks, and remaining stable thereafter until delivery [5] (Figure 24.1).

Measurements of plasma volume using either Evan's blue dye or radioactive isotope bound to serum albumin [6–9] have shown considerable individual variation in the degree of volume expansion, ranging from 20% to nearly 100% of non-pregnant values [10]. However, most studies suggest that the increase is approximately 50%.

The increase in maternal blood volume is directly related to the number of fetuses she is carrying [8, 10] and therefore, multiple pregnancies impose a substantially greater burden on the maternal cardio-circulatory system; in the presence of an existing heart disorder, rapid decompensation may occur.

The increase in blood volume during pregnancy is also related to fetal growth and birth weight; indeed this correlation is stronger than between fetal weight and maternal height or weight [11].

The most likely cause of the hypervolemia of pregnancy is estrogen mediated stimulation of plasma renin activity, promoting the hepatic production of angiotensinogen, angiotensin and aldosterone. Evidence for such an estrogenic effect is supported by the finding that bilateral oophorectomy is associated with reduction in blood volume and this is corrected by exogenous estrogen [12]. Furthermore, estrogen taken either as an oral contraceptive or for postmenopausal symptoms causes an increase in blood volume [13, 14].

Other possible mechanisms for the hypervolemia of pregnancy include retention of fluid due to relaxation of the great veins by the increased concentration of progesterone and increased sodium retention due to renin that is produced by the pregnant uterus [15–19].

The role of the fetus in maintaining this hypervolemia is uncertain. Although Longo and Hardesty [20] proposed that the fetal adrenal gland itself may be partly responsible, it has been demonstrated that even in pregnancies with hydatiform moles there is a 50% increase in maternal blood volume [21].

Red cell mass

Maternal red cell mass has been measured by low level radioactive isotopes. Erythropoiesis is stimulated by placental chorionic somatomammotropin, progesterone and possibly prolactin, resulting in a red cell mass which is 20% greater than in non-pregnant women [22]. However, since the increase in plasma volume is greater (50%), the hematocrit decreases (physiological anemia of pregnancy). This hemodilutional effect is maximal at 30–32 weeks' gestation. It has been suggested that hemodilution in pregnancy may have a beneficial effect on uteroplacental circulation by reducing blood viscosity [23]. Supportive evidence is provided by the observation that in pregnant patients with polycythemia vera reduction in hemoglobin concentration has a beneficial effect on fetal outcome [24].

Cardiac output

In 1915, Lindhard used a nitrous oxide technique and demonstrated that during pregnancy there is a 50% increase in cardiac output [25]. Subsequently, several techniques have been employed to measure maternal cardiac output, including the direct Fick principle [26–29], dye dilutional techniques [30, 31], impedance cardiography [32, 33] and echocardiography [34–36].

The increase in cardiac output starts at around the 10th week of gestation and by 30 weeks it reaches the maximum level which is approximately 50% higher than non-pregnant values. It subsequently falls to non-pregnant levels at term.

The maternal heart rate is some 20% greater than the non-pregnant value [31]. Some studies have suggested that the rise in cardiac output in early pregnancy is mainly due to increased stroke volume [37] but with advancing gestation the main contributor is increased heart rate [38, 39]. However, left ventricular function was studied by echocardiography and it has been reported that before 20 weeks gestation the increase in cardiac output was primarily due to maternal tachycardia and after 20 weeks due to increased stroke volume [36].

Cardiac output in pregnancy is greatly influenced by maternal position [34, 35]. Compression of the inferior vena cava by the pregnant uterus in the supine position reduces venous return and cardiac output. Using dye dilution techniques it has been demonstrated that there is a 25–30% reduction in cardiac output in the supine position at 38–40 weeks of pregnancy; this fall was not found before the 24th week [31]. As maternal heart rate in these studies remained unchanged, it was concluded that the postural fall in cardiac output was due to decreased stroke volume.

Kerr suggested that the fall in cardiac output did not lead to a significant change in blood pressure probably due to increased vascular resistance [39]. Subsequent studies have investigated the hemodynamic effects of maternal posture during late pregnancy. Bieniarz and associates using femoral and brachial artery catheterisation techniques confirmed aortic compression by the uterus in women during the late third trimester [40]. Similarly angiographic studies have shown that in 90% of women in the supine position cord blood flow is reduced. The dilated utero-ovarian vessels however provide an excellent collateral return for blood flow, bypassing these obstructions.

Systemic arterial blood pressure

Rubler and colleagues failed to demonstrate significant differences in blood pressure between non-pregnant women and women at different stages of pregnancy [34]. However, most serial studies by brachial sphygmomanometry have shown that both the systolic and diastolic component, but more so the latter, decrease between 10 and 20 weeks by approximately 10 mm Hg. After 34–36 weeks, blood pressure increases to reach pre-pregnancy levels at term [31, 41–44].

Age and parity have a significant influence on blood pressure. Christianson analysed blood pressure readings in white women, dividing the subjects into three age groups, <25 years, 25–34 years, and >35 years [42]. He found that with increasing parity within each group, mean systolic and diastolic blood pressures increased and that within each parity level, mean systolic arterial pressures were similar for the <25 years and 25–34 years groups, but increased in the >35 years old group. Mean diastolic pressure increased with age within each parity group.

Arterial blood pressure is also related to pregnancy outcome. In a prospective study of nearly 15,000 singleton births it was found that if the maternal mean arterial pressure during the second trimester was >90 mm Hg there was a significant increase in the incidence of intrauterine death, intrauterine growth retardation and development of preeclampsia [45].

Systemic vascular resistance

Systemic vascular resistance (SVR) is a measure of the afterload resulting from the left ventricular ejection of blood. During pregnancy, systemic vascular resistance falls, mainly due to a drop in mean arterial pressure and increased cardiac output. This change has been attributed to decreased vascular resistance in the uteroplacental and pulmonary circulation [46]. The likely cause of this drop in SVR is the increased concentration of estrogen and progesterone, since the administration of these hormones to non-pregnant women can significantly lower SVR [13, 47]. Furthermore, it was found that increased levels of circulating prostaglandins PGE_2 and PGI_2 may lead to direct vasodilation and also suggested that prostacyclins may act by reducing the vasoconstrictor effect of angiotensin II during pregnancy [48].

Regional blood flow

Pregnancy causes marked alterations in regional blood flow. Significant increases have been documented in blood flow to the uterus, skin and kidneys.

A. Uterus
A variety of techniques have been used to study uterine blood flow, all documenting an increase during pregnancy. Early studies used electromagnetic flow meters and showed an increase from 50 ml/min at 10 weeks' gestation, to 200 ml/min at 28 weeks' and up to 500 ml/min at term, which is approximately 10% of total cardiac output [49, 50]. Using placental scintography it was thought that the flow may be as great as 1200 ml/min by 37 weeks' gestation [51].

It is likely that the rise in uterine blood flow is facilitated by a progressive fall in vascular resistance. Doppler ultrasound studies of the uterine arteries have documented a decrease in impedance to flow with advancing gestation [52]. As long ago as 1938, it was proposed that the reduced uterine vascular resistance was a consequence of erosion of maternal endometrial vessels by invading placental trophoblast and the formation of arterial-venous fistulae [53].

Direct evidence for arterial-venous communications was provided by Heckel and Tobin who injected 200 μm glass spheres into the uterine arteries of pregnant and non-pregnant women [54]; subsequently they were able to recover the microspheres from the veins of all pregnant women but from only half of the non-pregnant ones. However, since uterine venous blood has a low oxygen content and cardiac output increases rapidly in early pregnancy it is unlikely that the arterio-venous fistulae play the major role in the fall in vascular resistance in pregnancy. It is more likely that hormonal factors play the important role of decreasing vascular resistance in pregnancy. A marked fall in the vascular resistance of the uterine artery in non-pregnant sheep has been demonstrated after infusion of estrogen [55].

B. Kidneys

Renal blood flow increases to 30–80% above non-pregnant values by mid pregnancy and remains stable until term [56–58]. Because of this increase, glomerular filtration increases by 30–50% [56–59].

Renal blood flow is very sensitive to maternal posture, dramatic reductions being observed in pregnant women in the supine position [18, 60] blood flow being preserved in the lateral position.

Changes in renal blood flow are thought to be mediated by steroid hormones [61]. The role of prostacyclin is unclear. Although it may act to decrease vascular resistance [62], contributing to increased renal blood flow, it was demonstrated that prostacyclin has no significant effect on either renal blood flow or glomerular filtration [63].

C. Skin perfusion

Skin perfusion increases slowly until 20 weeks' gestation and then more sharply until 30 weeks [64]. This maximal perfusion is maintained to the end of pregnancy and is thought to serve as a thermoregulatory mechanism, allowing the excess heat of fetal metabolism to dissipate through the maternal circulation. The increased blood flow to the skin is clinically manifested by an increase in skin temperature [65, 66]. Careful examination of the nail beds shows capillary dilatation in most pregnant women and vascular spiders and palmar erythema are common clinical findings.

D. Liver and brain

To date no studies have demonstrated increased blood flow to the liver or brain in pregnancy [67, 68] whilst it is presumed that coronary artery blood flow is increased due to increased cardiac output [41].

Oxygen consumption

Oxygen consumption reflects the rate of body metabolism and is calculated by measurement of the oxygen extracted by the lungs over a given time period. During pregnancy, oxygen consumption increases progressively to a maximum of 20–30% at term [69–71]. This rise reflects the increased metabolic requirements of the developing fetus and its mother. Metcalfe and Ueland pointed out the discrepancy between the steady increase in oxygen consumption throughout gestation and the rapid increase in cardiac output in early pregnancy [46]. They suggested that in early pregnancy the increased cardiac output is proportionally greater than the increase in oxygen consumption, resulting in well oxygenated blood reaching the uterus at a crucial time of organogenesis, before the fetal circulation is fully established.

Invasive hemodynamic measurements

Cardiac catheterisation studies have provided some information about hemodynamic parameters during normal pregnancy [27, 29, 30, 72–74]. These studies suggest that third trimester central venous pressure (CVP), pulmonary capillary wedge pressure (PCWP) and systemic vascular resistance do not differ greatly from non-pregnant subjects.

Central venous pressure

The central venous pressure was studied by cannulation of the external jugular vein in 53 women during the third trimester. The average measurement taken in the supine position was 10 cm of water and this was higher than in non-pregnant subjects. Although antecubital venous pressure did not change with gestation, the femoral venous pressure increased from 8 cm in the first trimester to 24 cm at term [75].

Intra-partum hemodynamics

Significant hemodynamic changes have been observed during labour and delivery, and these have been attributed in a large part to pain and anxiety [76, 77]. However, each uterine contraction expresses approximately 300–500 ml of blood into the central circulation and this may also affect maternal hemodynamics [76, 78]. During uterine contractions, blood flow from the pelvic organs and lower extremities to the heart is improved, as compared with the period between contraction [79].

Cardiac output

Most studies, despite differing methodology, have reported significant increases in cardiac output during labour. In 1956 Hendricks and Quilligan used a pulse pressure method to estimate cardiac output and demonstrated a 31% rise over resting values [76]. The authors suggested that the increased venous return to the heart during uterine contractions was responsible for a transient tachycardia, followed by increase in cardiac output and compensatory bradycardia (Figure 24.2).

The increase in cardiac output during contractions is associated with a rise in blood pressure and pulse rate, and suggests that increased sympathetic tone due to pain, anxiety and muscular activity is the major cause of increased cardiac output [78]. It was felt that the contractile effect of squeezing the blood from the uterus was of less importance.

Kjeldsen used a dye dilution technique to determine cardiac output changes throughout labour and found that during the latent phase cardiac output increased by 1.1 l/min. The increase was 2.46 l/min in the accelerative phase

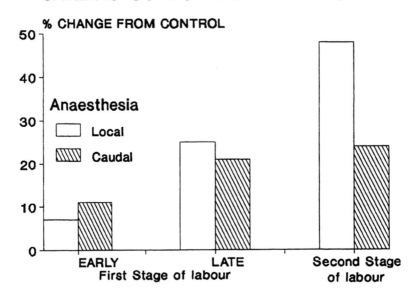

Figure 24.2.

and 2.17 l/min in the decelerative phase [80]. An increase in cardiac output between the early and late stages of labour in supine patients has also been reported [81].

Doppler echocardiographic studies of the pulmonary valve showed that cardiac output increases in labour to 7.88 l/min at a cervical dilatation of 8 cm or more, compared with a pre-labour value of 6.99 l/min. This increase was considered to be the result of augmented stroke volume [82].

Doppler echocardiography was used to study the effects of uterine contractions during early labour in patients who had received epidural analgesia [83]. A small increase in left ventricular diastolic diameter from 4.8–5 cm was reported but there was no significant change in left ventricular ejection fraction. The left ventricular systolic diameter and maternal heart rate were unchanged. Stroke volume and cardiac output increased by 16 and 11% respectively and it was concluded that the increased preload of uteroplacental blood into the maternal circulation was responsible for the increased left ventricular stroke volume via the Frank-Starling principle.

Heart rate

The reported effect of labour on heart rate is variable. Robson and associates found a maternal tachycardia occurred in response to contractions, the increase was 19% at a cervical dilatation of more than 8 cm in the left semi-lateral position [82]. In contrast, Kjeldsen found no significant change in heart rate during labour [80], whilst Ueland and Hansen actually recorded a bradycardia [81]. Winner and Romney believed that this apparent discrepancy was largely due to the different forms of analgesia and posture used during labour [84].

Blood pressure

Both systolic and diastolic blood pressure increase with uterine contraction [76–78, 81, 82, 84, 86, 87]. The systolic blood pressure was found in one study to have a maximal increase of 35 mm Hg during the first stage of labour, with an even greater increase during the second stage. Diastolic blood pressure increased by more than 25 mm Hg and even as much as 65 mm Hg in the second stage. After delivery, blood pressure falls to resting levels. Since there is very little change in peripheral resistance during labour, the increase in blood pressure is largely due to increased cardiac output [78].

Effect of analgesia

The type of analgesia used during labour has, a significant influence on cardiac function. Ueland and associates examined women receiving caudal or para-cervical local anaesthesia and reported that these forms of analgesia did not affect the hemodynamic changes caused by uterine contractions [37, 88, 89]. They concluded that these forms of analgesia were safe in patients with heart disease. The best hemodynamic stability was achieved with epidural anesthesia in the absence of adrenaline.

When local anesthesia is used, tachycardia may develop during the second stage of labour and this can be accentuated during contraction. Furthermore, a small increase in both systolic and diastolic blood pressures has been noted during the first stage, with a larger increase during the second stage. In contrast, caudal anaesthesia is not associated with changes in heart rate or blood pressure, stroke volume is maintained throughout labour, but may increase after delivery.

Ueland and associates also documented the maternal cardiovascular response to cesarean section performed using a variety of anesthetic agents [37, 89, 90]. Following subarachnoid blockade, a marked decrease in stroke volume and cardiac output, associated with a significant increase in heart rate was noted within 10 minutes of administration of the anesthetic. The dose and level of the anesthetic did not correlate with the degree of observed change. Postural change of the mother on to her side completely removed the observed hypotensive effect and no deleterious effects were noted in the newborn. It was concluded that the extent of the cardiovascular changes made this form of analgesia unsuitable for patients with heart disease.

Cardiovascular changes of a much smaller degree were found in patients when cesarean section was performed under thiopentol, nitrous oxide and succinyl choline anesthesia [89]. Although heart rate and diastolic pressure increased, cardiac output was unchanged. Following delivery, heart rate and blood pressure decreased, in association with a small increase in stroke volume and cardiac output. In patients anesthetised using an epidural without adrenaline, stable hemodynamics were recorded [90]. No significant changes were noted in heart rate, cardiac output or stroke volume. Blood pressure declined moderately after induction of anesthesia, but thereafter remained stable. Following delivery, heart rate did not change, but there was a 25% increase in cardiac output above control values.

Thus, maternal hemodynamics may be altered by analgesia at cesarean section, although balanced anesthesia with thiopentol, nitrous oxide and succinyl choline or epidural anesthesia without adrenaline cause minor changes and would be the preferred analgesia in patients with heart disease.

Post-partum hemodynamic changes

Immediately following delivery, there is a transient increase in cardiac output. Cardiac output is 60% and 80% higher than prelabour values when delivery occurred under caudal and local perineal anaesthesia respectively [81] (Figure 24.3). Using Doppler techniques it has been found that the heart rate and cardiac output returned to prelabour values by one hour after delivery [82].

Intrapartum blood volume changes have been shown to be related to the mode of delivery and delivery complications. Pritchard and associates estimated blood loss during vaginal delivery and reported that the loss was <500 ml in 61% of the cases, 500–1000 ml in 32% and 1000–1500 ml in 7% [91]. Thus a normal vaginal delivery, although causing very little change in hematocrit, involves a 20–30% loss in predelivery blood volume. In contrast, the average blood loss in women undergoing cesarean section is approximately 1000 ml (Figure 24.3).

In another study, the blood loss in normal vaginal delivery was estimated to be about 500 ml, as compared with 1000 ml in a group of women undergoing cesarean section [92]. After the third post-partum day, the blood volumes in both groups of patients was 10% lower than predelivery values. Despite similar blood volume losses at this time, a 5.2% rise in hematocrit was noted in patients delivering vaginally in contrast to a 5.8% fall in women delivered surgically. This difference is thought to be due to vaginally delivered women undergoing a diuresis, accounting for the rising hematocrit, whilst the surgically delivered patients, suffering from more extensive blood loss, have a mild compensatory hemodilution.

The high cardiac output immediately following delivery is probably a result of an "autotransfusion" phenomena, whereby blood from the emptied uterus enters the systemic circulation. Furthermore, the reduced caval compression,

CARDIAC OUTPUT POST DELIVERY

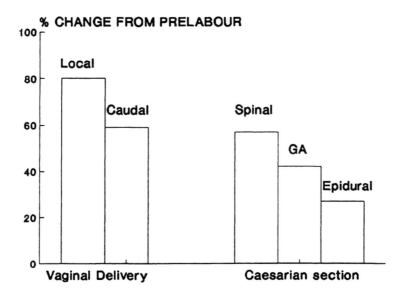

Figure 24.3. Changes in cardiac output following delivery.

allows an increased venous return to the heart [93]. The increase in cardiac output results principally from increased stroke volume [55, 81, 93] and the heart rate decreasing after delivery by 4–17 beats per minute [31, 78, 81, 88]. The arterial blood pressure does not change significantly after delivery [32, 76, 77].

Cardiac output in complicated pregnancy

Hypertension is defined as a systolic rise in pressure >30 mm Hg above baseline values, an absolute systolic value ≥140 mm Hg, a diastolic rise of >15 mm Hg or and absolute diastolic value of ≥90 mm Hg. Such pressures must be observed on two occasions, four or more hours apart. Pregnancy induced hypertension (PIH) is the popular term used to describe the differing categories of pregnancy associated hypertension and includes pre-eclampsia, eclampsia and gestational hypertension [94, 95]. A wide variety of disease severity is observed.

Although the subject of considerable research over a period of many years, the mechanisms underlying the observed changes in PIH are poorly understood. A number of studies have investigated possible changes in cardiac output in such patients, but unfortunately the majority of studies have serious flaws, casting doubt on the usefulness of their findings. Thus, only the most recent studies have used direct methods of assessing cardiac output such as thermodilution, Fick oxygen consumption or Doppler flow techniques. Furthermore, it has been traditional in studies of cardiac output to index measurements to body surface area, however the standard measurements for body surface area in pregnancy do not exist. Some studies have failed to investigate control population [96, 97]. Other confounding variables have not always been excluded, for example the effect of parity and the possibility that concurrent chronic renal pathology, known to be more common in multiparous patients, may be playing a role has not been investigated. Similarly, renal disease is more frequently found in patients with early onset pre-eclampsia, up to two thirds of patients have renal abnormalities other than changes of pre-eclampsia on renal biopsy or intravenous pyelography [98]. These patients may well have differing cardiovascular function than the patient who develops mild pre-eclampsia at term.

Two controlled studies, employing dye dilution or thermodilution techniques have found no significant difference in cardiac output of patients with PIH compared to controls [73, 99]. However, Lim and colleagues studied 25 patients with mild PIH using photoelectric transcutaneous dye dilution and noted that cardiac output increased from 7.8 l/min in the normal population to 8.8 l/min in the study group [100]. Several studies have shown an increase in cardiac output in patients with severe PIH [96, 101–103]. Benedetti has postulated that a rise in cardiac output was an early change in PIH leading to an elevation in BP [104]. When the arterial pressure becomes elevated, cardiac output may vary depending on other variables such as concurrent drug therapy, intravenous infusion or bed rest. Using a pulmonary artery catheter in severely hypertensive pregnant women, Benedetti and colleagues were able to show that pulmonary artery pressures are not increased, whilst pulmonary vascular resistance is low to low-normal for pregnancy [101].

Cardiac output may also be affected by a number of other conditions, including congenital heart disease, rheumatic heart disease, cardiac arrhythmias and cardiomyopathy. Irrespective of the underlying pathology, if the burdens imposed by the pregnancy on an already compromised heart are too great, cardiac failure will develop with consequent reduction in cardiac output. As a general principle, patients with cardiac disease should be carefully evaluated before undertaking pregnancy, and therapy, including surgery should be performed prior to conception.

References

1. Larcher A. Address to the Academy of Science. Archives Generales de Medicine. 1859;XII;291.

2. Hecker C, Buhl L. Einiges über das Wechselverhaltniss zwischen Schwangerschaft rep. Geburt und anderweitigen Krankheiten. Leipzig: Klink der Geburtskundel 1861:172.
3. Peter M. Accidents that may happen to pregnant women suffering from disease of the heart. Br Med J 1874;2:289.
4. MacDonald A. The bearings of chronic disease of the heart upon pregnancy, parturition and childbed: With papers on puerperal-pleuro-pneumonia and eclampsia. London: Churchill, 1878
5. Scott DE. Anemia during pregnancy. Obstet Gynecol Annu 1972;1:219.
6. Caton WL, Roby CC, Reid DE *et al*. Plasma volume and extra vascular fluid volume during pregnancy and the puerperium. Am J Obstet Gynecol 1949;57:471–81.
7. Hytten FE, Paintin DB. Increase in plasma volume during normal pregnancy. J Obstet Gynaecol Br Commonw 1963;70:402–7.
8. Lund CJ, Donovan JC. Blood volume during pregnancy. Am J Obstet Gynecol 1967;98:393.
9. McLennon CE, Thouin LG. Blood volume in pregnancy. Am J Obstet Gynecol 1978;55:1189.
10. Pritchard JA, Rowland RC. Blood volume changes in pregnancy and the puerperium. III. Whole body and large vessel hematocrits in pregnant and non-pregnant women. Am J Obstet Gynecol 1964;88:391–5.
11. Hytten FE, Stewart AM, Palmer JH. The relation of maternal heart size, blood volume, and stature to the birth weight of the baby. J Obstet Gynaecol Br Commonw 1963;70:817–20.
12. Frielander M, Laskey N, Silbert P. Effect of estrogenic substance on blood volume. Endocrinology 1936;20:329–32.
13. Walters WA, Lim YL. Haemodynamic changes in women taking oral contraceptives. J Obstet Gynaecol Br Commonw 1970;77:1007–12.
14. Luotola H, Pyorala T, Lahteenmaki P *et al*. Haemodynamic and hormonal effects of short term oestrodiol treatment in post-menopausal women. Maturitas 1979;1:287–94.
15. Seitchik J. Total body water and total body density of pregnant women. J Obstet Gynecol 1967;29:155–66.
16. Tapia HR, Johnson CE, Strong CG. Effect of oral contraceptive therapy on the renin-angiotensin system in normotensive and hypertensive women. J Obstet Gynecol 1973;41:643–9.
17. Cheek DB, Petrucco OM, Gillespie A *et al*. Muscle growth and the distribution of water and electrolyte in human pregnancy. Early Hum Dev 1985;11:293–305.
18. Lindheimer MC, Katz AI. Renal function in pregnancy. Obstet Gynecol Annu 1972;1:139.
19. Biglier EG, Forsham PH. Studies on the expanded estracellular fluid and the responses to various stimuli in primary aldosteronism. Am J Med 1961;30:564–76.
20. Longo LD, Hardesty JS. Maternal blood volume: measurement, hypothesis of control, and clinical considerations. Rev Perinat Med 1984;5:35.
21. Pritchard JA. Changes in the blood volume during pregnancy and delivery. Anesthesiology 1965; 26: 393–9.
22. Jepson JH. Endocrine control of maternal and fetal erythropoesis. Can Med J 1968;98:844.
23. Koller O. The clinical significance of hemodilution during pregnancy. Obstet Gynecol Surv 1978;72(Suppl):22.
24. Hockman A, Stein JA. Polycythaemia and pregnancy. Obstet Gynecol 1961;18:230.
25. Lindhard J. Über das minutenvolumen des Herzens bei Ruhe und bei Muskelarbeit. Pfluegers Archz 1915;161:233–383.
26. Chesley LC, Duffus GM. Posture and apparent plasma volume in late pregnancy. J Obstet Gynaecol Br Commonw 1971;78:406–12.
27. Palmer AJ, Walter AHC. The maternal circulation in normal pregnancy. J Obstet Gynaecol Br Emp 1949;56:537–47.
28. Zimmerman HA. A preliminary report on intracardiac catheterization studies during pregnancy. J Lab Clin Med 1950: 36: 1007.

29. Bader RA, Bader MG, Rose DJ et al. Hemodynamics at rest and during exercise in normal pregnancy as studied by cardiac catheterization. J Clin Invest 1955;34:1524–36.

30. Walters WA, MacGregor WG, Hills M. Cardiac output at rest during pregnancy and the puerperium. Clin Obstet Gynecol 1966;31:1–11.

31. Ueland K, Novy MJ, Peterson EN et al. Maternal cardiovascular dynamics. IV. The influence of gestational age on maternal cardiovascular response to posture and exercise. Am J Obstet Gynecol 1969;104:856–64.

32. Lees MM, Taylor SH, Scott DB et al. A study of cardiac output at rest throughout pregnancy. J Obstet Gynaecol Br Commonw 1967;74:319–28.

33. Atkins AFJ, Watt JM, Milan P et al. A longitudinal study of cardiovascular dynamics throughout pregnancy. Eur J Obstet Gynaecol Reprod Biol 1981;12:215–24.

34. Rubler S, Prabodhkumar MD, Pinto ER. Cardiac size and performance during pregnancy: Estimates with echocardiography. Clin Obstet Gynecol 1977; 40: 534–40.

35. Katz R, Karliner JS, Resnik R. Effects of a natural volume overload state (pregnancy) on left ventricular performance in a normal human subjects. Circulation 1978:58:434–41.

36. Laird-Meeter K, van de Ley G, Bom TH et al. Cardio-circulatory adjustments during pregnancy – an echocardiographic study. Clin Cardiol 1979;2:328.

37. Ueland K, Metcalfe J. Circulatory changes in pregnancy. Clin Obstet Gynecol 1975;18:41–50.

38. Metcalfe J, Ueland K. Maternal cardiovascular adjustments to pregnancy. Prog Cardiovasc Dis 1974;16:363–74.

39. Kerr MG. Mechanical effects of the gravid uterus in late pregnancy. J Obstet Gynaecol Br Commonw 1965;72:513–20.

40. Bieniarz J, Mapueda E, Caldeyro-Barcia R. Compression of aorta by the uterus in late human pregnancy. I. Variations between femoral and brachial artery pressure with changes from hypertension to hypotension. Am J Obstet Gynecol 1966;95:7950–808.

41. Hytten FE, Leitch I. The Physiology of Human Pregnancy 2nd ed.. Oxford: Blackwell Scientific, 1971:1–111.

42. Christianson RE. Studies on blood pressure during pregnancy. I. Influence of parity and age. Am J Obstet Gynecol 1976;125:509–13.

43. Wilson M, Morganti AA, Zervodakis I et al. Blood pressure, the renin-aldosterone system and sex steroids throughout normal pregnancy. Am J Med 1980:68:97–104.

44. Reis RE, Tizzano TP, O'Shaughnessy RW. The blood pressure course in primiparous pregnancy. A prospective study of 383 women. J Reprod Med 1987;32:523.

45. Page EW, Christianson R. The impact of mean arterial pressure in the middle trimester upon the outcome of pregnancy. Am J Obstet Gynecol 1976;125:740–6.

46. Metcalfe J, Ueland K. The heart and pregnancy. In: Hurst J, Logue RB, Schlant RC et al. (eds.), The heart arteries and veins. New York: McGraw-Hill, 1978: 1721–34.

47. Greiss FC, Anderson SG. Effect of ovarian hormones on the uterine vascular bed. Am J Obstet Gynecol 1970;107:829.

48. Gerber JG, Payne NA, Murphy RC et al. Prostacyclin produced by the pregnancy uterus in the dog may act as a circulating vasodepressor substance. J Clin Invest 1981;67:632–6.

49. Assali NS, Rauramo L, Peltonen T. Measurement of uterine blood flow and uterine metabolism. VIII. Uterine and fetal blood flow and oxygen consumption in early human pregnancy. Am J Obstet Gynecol 1960;79:86–98.

50. Metcalfe J, Romney SL, Ramsey LH et al. Estimation of uterine blood flow in normal human pregnancy at term. J Clin Invest 1955;34:1632–8.

51. Lunell NO, Nylund LE, Lewander R et al. Uteroplacental blood flow in preeclampsia measurements with indium-113m and a computer-linked gamma camera. Clin Exp Hypertens 1982;1:105–17.

52. Campbell S, Bewley S, Cohen-Overbeek T. Investigation of the uteroplacental circulation by Doppler ultrasound. Semin Perinato 1987;11:362–8.

53. Burwell CS, Strayhorn WD, Flickinger D et al. Circulation during pregnancy. Arch Intern Med 1938;62:979–1003.

54. Heckel GP, Tobin CE. Arteriovenous shunts in the myometrium. Am J Obstet Gynecol 1956;71:199-205.
55. Ueland K, Parer JT. Effects of estrogens on the cardiovascular system of the ewe. Am J Obstet Gynecol 1966;96:400-6.
56. Nunlap W. Serial changes in renal hemodynamics during normal human pregnancy. Br J Obstet Gynaecol 1981;88:1-9.
57. Little B. Water and electrolyte balance during pregnancy. Anesthesiology 1965;26:400-8.
58. Chesley LC. Renal functional changes in normal pregnancy. Clin Obstet Gynecol 1960;3:349-63.
59. Simms EAH, Krantz KE. Serial studies of renal function during pregnancy and the puerperium in normal women. J Clin Invest 1958;37:1764-74.
60. Chesley LC, Duffus GM. Preeclampsia, posture and renal function. Obstet Gynecol 1971;38:1-6.
61. Fainstat T. Ureteral dilatation in pregnancy: a review. Obstet Gynecol Surv 1963;18:845-60.
62. Lewis PJ, Boylon P, Freidman L et al. Prostacyclin in pregnancy. Br Med J 1980;280:1581-2.
63. Gallery ED, Ross M, Grigg R et al. Are the renal functional changes in human pregnancy caused by prostacyclin? Prostaglandins 1985;30:1019-29.
64. Katz M, Sokal MM. Skin perfusion in pregnancy. Am J Obstet Gynecol 1980;137:30-3.
65. Herbert CM, Banner EA, Wakim KG. Variations in the peripheral circulation during pregnancy. Am J Obstet Gynecol 1958;76:742-5.
66. Burt CC. Peripheral skin temperature in normal pregnancy. Lancet 1949;2:787-90.
67. Munnell EW, Taylor HC Jr. Liver blood flow in pregnancy: hepatic normal vein catheterization. J Clin Invest 1947;26:952-6.
68. McCall ML. Cerebral blood flow and metabolism in toxemias of pregnancy. Surg Gynecol Obstet 1949;89:715-21.
69. Novy MJ, Edwards MJ. Respiratory problems in pregnancy. Am J Obstet Gynecol 1967;99:1024-45.
70. Prowse CM, Galnslar EA. Respiratory and acid-base changes during pregnancy. Anesthesiology 1965;26:381-92.
71. Pernol ML, Metcalfe J, Schlenker TL et al. Oxygen consumption at rest and during exercise in pregnancy. Respir Physiol 1975;25:285-93.
72. Werko L. Pregnancy and heart disease. Acta Obstet Gynaecol Scand 1954;33:162.
73. Groenendijk R, Trimbos JBMJ, Wallenburg HCS. Heart dynamic measurements in preeclampsia: Preliminary observations. Am J Obstet Gynecol 1984;150:232-6.
74. Hamilton HFH. The cardiac output in normal pregnancy as determined by the Cournard right heart catheterization technique. J Obstet Gynaecol Br Emp 1949;56:548.
75. McLennin CE. Antecubital and femoral venous pressure in normal and toxemic pregnancy. Am J Obstet Gynecol 1943;45:568.
76. Hendricks CH, Quilligan EJ. Cardiac output during labour. Am J obstet Gynecol 1956;71:953-72.
77. Burch GE. Heart disease and pregnancy. Am Heart J 1977;93:104-16.
78. Adams JG, Alexander AM. Alterations in cardiovascular physiology during labour. Am J Obstet Gynecol 1958;12:542-9.
79. Bieniarz J, Crottongini JJ, Curuchet E et al. Aortocaval compression by the uterus in late human pregnancy. II. An angiographic study. Am J Obstet Gynecol 1968;100:203-17.
80. Kjeldsen J. Hemodynamic investigations during labour and delivery. Acta Obstet Gynecol Scand 1979;89(Suppl):10-252.
81. Ueland K, Hansen JM. Maternal cardiovascular dynamics. III. Labour and delivery under local and caudal analgesia. Am J Obstet Gynecol 1969;103:8-18.
82. Robson SC, Dunlop W, Boys R et al. Cardiac output during labour. Br Med J 1987;295:1169-72.

83. Lee W, Miller JF, Cotton DB. The hemodynamic effects of uterine contractions upon maternal cardiac function. Abstract, Eighth Annu Soc Perinat Obstet, Feb 1988.
84. Winner W, Romney SL. Cardiovascular responses to labour and delivery. Am J Obstet Gynecol 1966;95:1104–14.
85. Burg JR, Doder A, Kloster FE *et al*. Alterations of systolic time intervals during pregnancy. Circulation 1974;49:560–4.
86. Rubler S, Hammer N, Schneebaum R. Systolic time intervals in pregnancy and the post partum period. Am Heart J 1973;86:182–68.
87. Hansen JM, Ueland K. The influence of caudal analgesia on cardiovascular dynamics during normal labour and delivery. Acta anaesthesiol Scand Suppl 1966;23:449–52.
88. Ueland K, Gills RE, Hansen JM. Maternal cardiovascular dynamics. I. Cesarean section under subarachnoid block anesthesia. Am J Obstet Gynecol 1968;100:42–54.
89. Ueland K, Hansen J, Eng M *et al*. Maternal cardiovascular dynamics. V. Cesarean section under thiopentol, nitrous oxide, and succinyl choline anesthesia. Am J Obstet Gynecol 1970;108:615–22.
90. Ueland K, Akamatsu TJ, Eng M *et al*. Maternal cardiovascular dynamics. VI. Cesarean section under epidural anesthesia without epinephrine. Am J Obstet Gynecol 1972;114:775–80.
91. Pritchard JA, Baldwin RM, Dickey JC *et al*. Blood volume changes in pregnancy and the puerperium. II. Red blood cell loss and changes during and following vaginal delivery, cesarean section, and cesarean section plus total hysterectomy. Am J Obstet Gynecol 1962;84:1271–82.
92. Ueland K. Maternal cardiovascular dynamics. VII. Intrapartum blood volume changes. Am J Obstet Gynecol 1976;126:671–7.
93. Brigden W, Howarth S, Sharpey-Schafer EP. Posture and peripheral blood flow. Clin Sci 1950;9:79–91.
94. Gant NF, Daley GL, Chand S *et al*. A study of angiotensin II pressor response throughout primigravid pregnancy. J Clin Invest 1973;52:2682–9.
95. Gant NF, Chand S, Worley RJ *et al*. A clinical test useful for predicting the development of acute hypertension of pregnancy. Am J Obstet Gynecol 1974;120:1–7.
96. Graham C, Goldstein A. Epidural anesthesia and cardiac output in severe preeclamptics. Anaesthesia 1980;53:709–12.
97. Cotton DB, Benedetti TJ. Use of the Swan-Ganz catheter in obstetrics and gynecology. Obstet Gynecol 1980;56:641–5.
98. Iule BU, Long P, Oats J. Early onset pre-eclampsia: recognition of underlying renal disease. Br Med J 1987;294:79–81.
99. Assali NS, Holm L, Parker H. Systemic and regional hemodynamic alterations in toxemia. Circulation 1956:29,30(Suppl II):53–99.
100. Lim YL, Walters WA. Hemodynamics of mild hypertension in pregnancy. Br J Obstet Gynaecol 1979;86:198–204.
101. Benedetti TJ, Cotton DB, Read JA *et al*. Hemodynamic observations in severe preeclampsia using a flow directed pulmonary artery catheter. Am J Obstet Gynecol 1980;136:465–70.
102. Rafferty TD, Berkowitz RL. Hemodynamics in patients with severe toxemia during labor and delivery. Am J Obstet Gynecol 1980;138:263–71.
103. Hamilton HF. Cardiac output in pregnancy. Edinburgh Med J 1950;57:1–9.
104. Benedetti TJ. Pregnancy induced hypertension. In: Elkayam U, Gleicher (eds.), Cardiac problems in pregnancy. New York: Alan R. Liss Inc, 1989:323–40.

25. Fetal circulation and cardiac output

J. GUY THORPE-BEESTON and KYPROS H. NICOLAIDES

In the intrauterine life, gas exchange occurs in the placenta. Oxygenated blood returns to the fetus via the umbilical vein and enters the arterial circulation through a series of shunts.

Venous return to the heart

After entering the intra-abdominal portion of the umbilical vein, about half the venous return flows through the ductus venosus, which connects directly the umbilical vein-portal sinus confluence to the inferior vena cava. The remainder of the blood enters the hepatic-portal venous system and flows through the liver [1].

The fetal liver has three sources of blood supply; the portal vein, umbilical vein and hepatic artery which arises from the aorta, contributing 15%, 80% and 5% of the blood flow respectively [1–3]. The left lobe of the liver is almost entirely supplied by umbilical venous blood, which has a hemoglobin oxygen saturation of approximately 80%, while the right lobe receives blood mainly from the portal vein, which has a hemoglobin oxygen saturation of approximately 40% [3, 4].

The thoracic inferior vena cava receives blood of differing oxygen content from the ductus venosus, the left and right hepatic veins and from the inferior vena cava that accepts blood returning from the lower body [1, 5]. Edelstone and Rudolph demonstrated in fetal sheep, using radioactive microspheres, that the highly oxygenated umbilical blood is kept separated from the deoxygenated blood returning from the lower limbs [6]. The better oxygenated blood from the ductus venosus occupies the dorsal and left part of the inferior vena cava and it is thought that this is achieved by the presence of a membrane valve. This functional separation enables ductus venosus blood to be preferentially directed across the foramen ovale to the left atrium, while blood from the distal inferior vena cava, and the right hepatic vein passes across the tricuspid valve to the right ventricle. About two-thirds of cardiac output perfuses the lower body and placenta, returning to the heart via the inferior vena cava [5].

The foramen ovale is situated low in the interatrial septum close to the inferior vena cava. The cephaled margin of the foremen ovale, the crista

A.-M. Salmasi and A.S. Iskandrian (eds): Cardiac output and regional flow in health and disease, 325–347.
© 1993 *Kluwer Academic Publishers. Printed in the Netherlands.*

dividens, overrides the orifice of the inferior vena cava and acts to divide the inferior vena caval return into an anterior and rightward stream (60%) and a posterior and leftward stream (40%). This latter stream is the more highly oxygenated. In spite of this ingenious mechanism, significant mixing of the blood streams still occurs, although the left atrial blood remains more highly saturated than in the right atrium. Blood ejected by the left ventricle passes through the aortic valve to the ascending aortal where it is distributed to the coronary arteries, cerebral circulation, head, neck and upper extremities [6, 7].

Blood returning via the superior vena cava streams preferentially on entering the heart. Apart from that in the coronary sinus, it is the most desaturated blood in the fetus with a pO_2 of 12–14 mm Hg. The blood is directed by the crista interveniens towards the tricuspid valve and right ventricle. Similarly, blood from the coronary sinus is directed to the right ventricle. This streaming therefore preferentially directs the desaturated blood towards the placenta for reoxygenation. Pulmonary venous flow, which represents less than 10% of cardiac output, enters the left atrium and mixes with that part of the inferior vena caval flow that has crossed the foramen ovale. This blood then crosses the mitral valve and becomes the left ventricular output, accounting for 35% of the total cardiac output [8].

During stress the fetus may increase the oxygen delivery to the brain and heart by increasing the oxygen content and total volume of left ventricular output. Preferential streaming in the inferior vena cava is maintained during fetal hypoxemia, and may increase with cord compression [6, 7, 9, 10]. The increase in streaming in the inferior vena cava allows more oxygenated blood from the umbilical vein to reach the left ventricle, relative to the right, with a consequent increase in the volume of umbilical venous blood directed towards the heart and brain.

Cardiac output

Fetal blood flows from the main pulmonary trunk across the ductus arteriosus into the descending aorta, and therefore the lower body receives blood from both the left and right ventricles. Cardiac output in the fetus and newborn is greater per kilogram of body weight than in the adult [11]. The right ventricle ejects approximately two thirds of the cardiac output, the left one-third [5, 8]. Echocardiographic and Doppler ultrasound studies in humans have suggested a similar pattern, although the right ventricle appears to be less dominant [12, 13]. The ventricles eject blood against a similar ventricular resistance and therefore there is little difference in the thickness of their free walls [14].

Left ventricular output enters the ascending aorta, 20% of the cardiac output reaching the brain, upper limbs and thorax, 3% perfuses the myocardium and 10% flows across the ductus arteriosus and perfuses the descending

Table 25.1 Cardiac output and organ blood flows in the fetal lambs.

Cardiac output	450 ml/min/kg
Liver	435 ml/min/100 g
Adrenals	230 ml/min/100 g
Kidneys	220 ml/min/100 g
Heart	200 ml/min/100 g
Brain	130 ml/min/100 g
Lungs	111 ml/min/100 g
Gut	59 ml/min/100 g
Carcass	26 ml/min/100 g

Edelstone *et al.* 1978 [1]; Court *et al.* 1984 [15].

aorta. Two thirds of the combined cardiac output passes to the pulmonary trunk, but only 8% of the total cardiac output reaches the lungs because of the high pulmonary vascular resistance. The regional distribution of cardiac output in the fetal lamb is shown in Table 25.1 [1, 15].

Cardiac output is a function of stroke volume and heart rate. In the fetus cardiac output is related to heart rate, as the fetal heart has only a limited ability to alter stroke volume. Freidman, demonstrated that isolated strips of fetal myocardium were less able to generate tension than equivalent adult tissue [16]. Similarly, in response to a rapid intravenous infusion, the fetal heart increases its output by less than that of an adult given a comparable load. In chronically instrumented fetal lambs there is a direct relationship between heart rate and cardiac output. Changes (spontaneous or induced) in heart rate are associated with corresponding changes in left or right ventricular output [17]. Increasing heart rate from a resting rate of 180 bpm to 250–300 bpm increased cardiac output by only 15–20%. A fall in heart rate to 120 bpm decreased cardiac output by about 25%. The fetal heart rate therefore appears to operate at a high level on its cardiac function curve. The differences between the fetal and adult myocardium may explain partially why preterm infants have such a low threshold for tolerating volume loads and why congestive cardiac failure is the inevitable sequelae in the presence of a large arterial shunt.

Approximately 40% of the combined ventricular output is directed to the placenta. In the sheep fetus, placental flow changes little over a 24–hour period, although the changes that are seen may be associated with changes in fetal arterial and venous pressure and fetal heart rate. Rudolph, demonstrated linear relationships between mean acute blood pressure and umbilical blood flow as well as between heart rate and umbilical blood flow [18].

Blood pressure

Since the fetus is surrounded by amniotic fluid, fetal vascular pressures are recorded in relation to the intra-amniotic pressure. Despite high cardiac output, the fetal blood pressure is low throughout gestation, reflecting the very low resistance of the placental vascular bed. Fetal lambs of 90 days gestation have a systolic pressure of about 40 mm Hg rising to 65–70 mm Hg at term (150 days) [19].

Vascular pressures in the fetus reflect the streaming patterns. Although the ductus venosus is dilated as a result of the high flow through the umbilical veins the mean blood pressure in the fetal lamb umbilical veins (6–8 mm Hg) is 2–3 mm Hg higher than in the inferior vena cava. Right atrial mean pressure (3–4 mm Hg) is slightly higher than left atrial pressure (2–3 mm Hg) because of both the greater flow through the right atrium and streaming into the left atrium from the inferior vena cava. Blood pressure in the main pulmonary trunk and right ventricle is 1–2 mm Hg higher than in the aorta and left ventricle, despite the ductus arteriosus being widely patent.

In the fetus, the low resistance placental circulation is thought to facilitate a high cardiac output. The higher cardiac output in the newborn may reflect an increased metabolic rate (and therefore oxygen consumption) than in the adult (7 ml O_2/kg/min at 10 days compared to 3.9 ml O_2/kg/min in the adult) [11].

Regulation of fetal circulation

Complex neurohumoral and metabolic responses maintain normal fetal blood pressure, heart rate and distribution of blood flow, thus allowing the fetus to meet its oxygen and nutrient requirements and facilitate clearance of its metabolic waste.

Neural regulation

Baroreceptors

Baroreceptors in the aortic arch and carotid sinuses respond to changes in blood pressure; hypertension induces bradycardia and hypotension induces tachycardia. Although Dawes et al suggested that during intrauterine life the threshold for baroreflex response was not reached [20], carotid sinus and vagus nerve activity has been demonstrated synchronous with the arterial pulse, suggesting that in reality there is continuous baroreceptor activity [21, 22].

In chronically instrumented fetal lambs, heart rate slows immediately if there is an increase in systemic arterial pressure [23, 24]. This response becomes progressively more sensitive with advancing gestation [23]. These baroreceptor mediated responses are partially inhibited by denervation of the carotid body and they are abolished by combined carotid and aortic denervation. Atropine administration, acting to block parasympathetic response, also abolishes the reflex.

Chemoreceptors

Stimulation of central (located in the medulla oblongata) or carotid chemoreceptors causes hypertension and mild tachycardia, with increased respiratory activity. In contrast, aortic chemoreceptor activity produces a bradycardia following a small increase in arterial pressure [25], this response precedes the baroreceptor mediated tachycardia [26–28]. Sinoaortic denervation abolishes the responses. Acute fetal hypoxaemia produces bradycardia and hypotension, responses also abolished by sinoaortic denervation. However, carotid sinus denervation alone does not have a major effect on this reflex and it is thought that aortic chemoreceptors play the dominant role in chemoreceptor reflex circulatory activity.

Autonomic nervous system

The effectors of neural regulation are the sympathetic and parasympathetic nervous systems. The sinoatrial and atrioventricular nodes are present in the fetus [29–31] and respond similarly to those in the adult [32, 33]. In the fetal lamb myocardium there is a high concentration of adrenergic receptors but these decrease with gestation and there are very few at term [29]. Cholinergic innervation is fully developed during fetal life.

In the fetal lamb, exogenous cholinergic or adrenergic agonists produce responses as early as 60 days gestation [34, 35]. Sympathetic stimulation results in tachycardia, increased myocardial contractility, and an increased systemic arterial blood pressure. The individual contributions of alpha and beta stimulation have been documented using specific agonists and antagonists. Alpha-adrenergic stimulation results in vasoconstriction of the renal and mesenteric circulations with a resulting increase in systemic blood pressure. Beta-adrenergic stimulation results in tachycardia, increased myocardial contractility and an increase in pulmonary and myocardial blood flow.

The parasympathetic nervous system initiates its action via the vagus nerve, which innervates the sinoatrial and atrioventricular nodes. Parasympathetic input slows the fetal heart rate and this response is more marked with advancing gestation [36, 37]. The vagus nerve is also implicated in fetal heart rate variability [38]. During stress (hypoxia or hemorrhage) beta-adrenergic activity is increased and the administration of propranolol produces a much greater fall in heart rate.

Hormonal regulation

Catecholamines

Hypoxemia or acidemia increase circulatory plasma catecholamine concentrations in fetal sheep [39–41]. Studies in hypoxemic growth-retarded human fetuses have also demonstrated a similar catecholamine response to hypoxemic or anemic stimulation [42]. The adrenal medulla is the main source of circulatory catecholamines and Freidman speculated that these substances have a regulatory function in the fetal cardiovascular system prior to the development of sympathetic innervation [16].

Catecholamines play an increasingly important role in the fetal response to stress with advancing gestation. Thus, Comline *et al.* demonstrated that in early lamb gestation only very low arterial blood oxygen saturations stimulated the fetal adrenal gland, whilst in more mature fetuses, catecholamine secretion is induced by more moderate hypoxemia [39].

Arginine vasopressin

Arginine vasopressin (antidiuretic hormone) is present in fetal blood from early pregnancy and the concentration increases in response to hypoxia, hemorrhage, hypotension and hypernatremia [43, 44]. However, because in normoxic sheep fetuses, concentrations of vasopressin are usually undetectable and maximal antidiuresis in adults occurs with vasopressin concentrations that have no discernable effects on systemic blood pressure, it is thought that vasopressin is unlikely to have a major role in normal homeostatic circulatory regulation.

Nevertheless, Iwamoto and associates demonstrated that infusion of vasopressin, in similar concentrations to those observed during hypoxemia, resulted in decreased cardiac output, increased blood flow to the placenta, heart and brain, and decreased flow to the musculoskeletal system, gut and skin [45]. It was suggested that vasopressin may participate in the redistribution of fetal blood flow in response to stress.

Prostaglandins

Prostaglandins do not usually circulate in adult blood, however in the fetus relatively high concentrations, particularly of prostaglandin E_2 are present in the peripheral circulation. The placenta and fetal blood vessels, including the umbilical vessels, ductus arteriosus, pulmonary arteries and aorta produce significant amounts of PGE_2 [46–49]. In lambs, postaglandins have diverse effects; PGE_1, PGF_{2a} and thromboxane constrict, whereas PGI_2 dilates the umbilical-placental circulation [50, 51], PGE_1 infusions reduced umbilical-placental flow, although no effect was noted on cardiac output or systemic pressure. Blood flow to the myocardium, adrenals and gastro-intestinal tract increased [52].

Prostaglandins have an important role in maintaining relaxation and thereby patency of the ductus arteriosus in the fetus, PGE_2 probably has the major role in relaxing the smooth muscle of this duct [52–56].

Opioids

Naloxone, an endogenous opioid antagonist, has been used to examine the possible role of opioids in modulating autonomic neurotransmission and humoral release in both normoxic and hypoxic lamb fetuses. It has been suggested that endogenous opioids may have a direct vasodilatory effect on the renal and musculoskeletal circulations [57].

Renin-angiotensin

The renal juxtaglomerular apparatus has been shown to be present in lambs in the second half of gestation [58]. This system is involved in controlling the normal fetal circulation and perhaps in its responses to hemorrhage. Plasma renin, circulating angiotensin II and renin substrate have all been demonstrated by 90 days gestation [45, 58–61]. Smith *et al.*, demonstrated that plasma renin is actively increased in response to moderate hemorrhage [58]. Iwamoto and Rudolph, infused angiotensin in fetal lambs and demonstrated a marked increase in arterial blood pressure, heart rate and combined ventricular output [62]. Although renal blood flow decreased, flow to the lungs and myocardium increased.

Inhibition of angiotensin II in unstressed fetuses caused a fall in blood pressure, though cardiac output remained unchanged. Umbilical-placental blood flow also fell, probably due to the fall in systemic arterial blood pressure [60]. Therefore, it appears that angiotensin II has a vasotonic effect on the peripheral circulation of the normal sheep fetus, maintaining systeminc arterial blood pressure and umbilical-placental blood flow. In response to hemorrhage, angiotensin II causes vasoconstriction in the peripheral circulation, thereby maintaining systemic arterial blood pressure.

Fetal oxygenation

Knowledge on fetal oxygenation and metabolism is primarily derived from animal experiments and human studies in labor or at delivery. However, data derived from animal studies may not reflect accurately the undisturbed physiological state of the human fetus because of the large differences in metabolism between species and the difficulty in eliminating stress in the experimental animal. Similarly, the human studies can be criticised because labor is associated with maternal and fetal stress, and even during elective caesarean section maternal fasting and episodes of transient hypotension may affect placental perfusion and the supply of oxygen and nutrients to the fetus.

The first attempt to study human fetal oxygenation was by inspection of the colour of the umbilical cord vessels [63]. Fetuses at 14–18 weeks' gestation were photographed through a telescope introduced transcervically before elective abortion. Westin noted that fetuses were not cyanosed and the cord vessels were much pinker than after delivery. He concluded that the second trimester human fetus was not as hypoxic as suggested by animal or post-delivery studies [63].

With the introduction of cordocentesis, ultrasound guided blood sampling from an umbilical cord vessel [64, 65], it has now become possible to study fetal oxygenation and metabolism under physiological conditions.

Definitions

Oxygenation is the process of transporting molecular oxygen from air to the tissues of the body. In the fetus, this involves: (i) oxygen transfer across the placenta; (ii) reversible binding of oxygen to fetal hemoglobin and fetal blood flow; and (iii) oxygen consumption for growth and metabolism. Energy is derived from the combination of oxygen and glucose to form carbon dioxide and water. Removal of carbon dioxide and protection against acidosis, is by the reverse of the mechanisms for oxygen delivery and is helped by the rapid diffusion, high solubility and volatility of this gas. In the adult, carbon dioxide is excreted in the lungs while bicarbonate and hydrogen ions are removed by the kidney. In the fetus, both these functions are carried out by the placenta. When there is inadequate oxygen supply the Krebs cycle can not operate and the pyruvate is converted to lactic acid. This enters the blood leading to systemic acidosis unless it is either metabolised or excreted.

The amount of oxygen bound to hemoglobin is not linearly related to the pO_2. Each type of hemoglobin has a characteristic oxygen-dissociation curve which can be modified by environmental factors, such as pH and the concentration of 2,3–diphosphoglycerate (2,3–DPG). For example, when 2,3–DPG rises, in response to anemia or hypoxia, it binds to and stabilises the deoxygenated form of hemoglobin, resulting in a shift of the oxygen dissociation curve to the right and therefore release of oxygen to the tissues. Although, *in vitro*, both HbA and HbF have the same oxygen dissociation curves, human adult blood has a lower affinity for oxygen than fetal because of its greater binding of 2,3–DPG. It has been suggested that the higher affinity of fetal blood helps placental transfer of oxygen.

Furthermore, since the greatest amount of oxygen is released for a given fall in pO_2 at the steepest part of the oxygen-dissociation curve, fetal hemoglobin releases more oxygen than adult at low levels of pO_2.

Fetal hypoxia, oxygen deficiency in the tissues, may result from (i) reduced placental perfusion with maternal blood and consequent decrease in fetal arterial blood oxygen content due to low pO_2 (hypoxemic hypoxia); (ii) reduced arterial blood oxygen content due to low fetal hemoglobin concentration (anemic hypoxia); and (iii) reduced blood flow to the fetal tissues (ischemic hypoxia). Hypoxia of any cause leads to a conversion from aerobic to anaerobic metabolism, which produces less energy and more acid. If the oxygen supply is not restored the fetus dies.

Normal fetal oxygenation

Reference ranges of blood gas and acid-base parameters in umbilical venous, umbilical arterial and intervillous blood have been established from analysis of blood obtained by cordocentesis from fetuses investigated for genetic disease and subsequently shown to be unaffected by the condition under investigation.

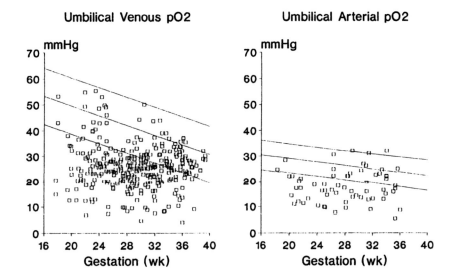

Figure 25.1. Reference ranges with gestation (mean, 5th and 95th centiles) for umbilical venous and arterial blood oxygen tension (mm Hg), and the individual values of small (□) for gestational age fetuses.

In normal fetuses, the blood oxygen tension is much lower than the maternal (Figure 25.1) [66, 67], and it has been suggested that this is due either to incomplete venous equilibration of uterine and umbilical circulations and/or to high placental oxygen consumption. Studies in a variety of animals have also demonstrated that the umbilical venous blood pO_2 is less than half the maternal arterial pO_2 and this observation led to the concept of "Mount Everest in utero". However, the high affinity of fetal hemoglobin for oxygen, together with the high fetal cardiac output in relation to oxygen demand, compensates for the low fetal pO_2 [68]. Furthermore, since the P_{50} of fetal blood is similar to the umbilical arterial pO_2 the fetus operates over the steepest part of the hemoglobin oxygen dissociation curve and therefore a relatively large amount of oxygen is released from the haemoglobin for a given drop in pO_2.

The umbilical venous and arterial pO_2 and pH decrease, while pCO_2 increases, with gestational age [66, 67]. The blood oxygen content does not change with gestational age because of the rise in fetal hemoglobin concentration (Figure 25.2) [69]. Fetal blood lactate concentration does not change with gestation and the values are similar to those in samples obtained at elective cesarean section at term [67]. The umbilical venous concentration is higher than the umbilical arterial suggesting that the normoxemic human fetus is, like the sheep fetus, a net consumer of lactate [70]. Furthermore, the concentration of lactate in umbilical cord blood is higher than in the

Umbilical Venous Oxygen Content   Umbilical Arterial Oxygen Content

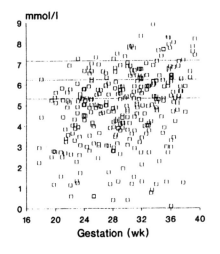
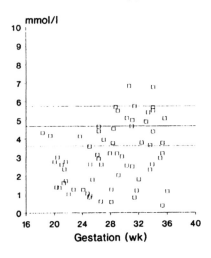

Figure 25.2. Reference ranges with gestation (mean, 5th and 95th centiles) for umbilical venous and arterial oxygen content (mmol/l), and the individual values of small (□) for gestational age fetuses.

maternal blood and the two are correlated significantly. This suggests a common source of lactate, which is likely to be the placenta.

Hypoxemic hypoxia-fetal growth retardation

Small for gestational age fetuses may be constitutionally small, with no increased perinatal death or morbidity, or they may be growth retarded due to either low growth potential, the result of genetic disease or environmental damage, or due to reduced placental perfusion and "utero-placental insufficiency".

Analysis of samples obtained by cordocentesis has demonstrated that some SGA fetuses are hypoxemic, hypercapnic, hyperlacticemic and acidemic (Figures 25.1, 25.2) [67, 71]. Furthermore, both respiratory and metabolic acidemia increase with hypoxemia. In umbilical venous blood mild hypoxemia may be present in the absence of hypercapnia or acidemia. In severe utero-placental insufficiency the fetus can not compensate hemodynamically and hypercapnia and acidemia increase exponentially [67]. The carbon dioxide accumulation is presumably the result of reduced exchange between the utero-placental and fetal circulations due to reduced blood flow. The association between hypoxemia and hyperlacticemia supports the concept of reduced oxidative metabolism of lactate being the cause of hyperlacticemia, and under these circumstances the fetus appears to be a net producer of

Fetal Haemoglobin

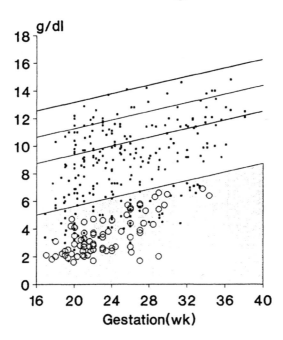

Figure 25.3. Reference range with gestation (mean, 5th and 95th centiles) for fetal blood haemoglobin concentration, and the individual values of hydropic (O) and non-hydropic (■) fetuses from red cell isoimmunised pregnancies.

lactate. These findings demonstrate that asphyxia manifested at birth may not be due to the process of birth itself and provide direct evidence that neonatal hypoxia and its consequences are often wrongly attributed to mismanaged labour [72].

Anemic hypoxia-red cell isoimmunisation

In red cell isoimmunised pregnancies the life span of fetal erythrocytes is reduced, because antibody-coated red cells are destroyed in the reticuloendothelial system. The fetus compensates for moderate degrees of anemia by hemodynamic adjustments until the hemoglobin deficit exceeds 7 g/dl, when the functional reserve of the cardiovascular system is exhausted and hydrops fetalis develops (Figure 25.3) [73].

The fetal blood oxygen content decreases in proportion to the degree of anemia; even in extreme anemia the fetal blood pO_2, pCO_2 and pH, usually remain within the normal ranges. The fetal 2,3–DPG concentration is increased and the consequent decrease in hemoglobin oxygen affinity presumably improves delivery of oxygen to the tissues. In moderate anemia, the umbilical arterial plasma lactate concentration is increased but this is cleared by a single passage through the placenta and normal umbilical venous levels are maintained [74]. Therefore, placental clearance of lactate serves to help repay the fetal oxygen debt [75]. In severe anemia, when the oxygen content is less than 2 mmol/l, the placental capacity for lactate clearance is exceeded and the umbilical venous concentration increases exponentially. These data suggest that in the fetus systemic metabolic acidosis can be prevented, presumably by cardiovascular adjustments, unless the oxygen content decreases below the critical level of 2 mmol/l.

In mild-moderate anemia there is associated reticulocytosis suggesting a compensatory increase in intramedullary erythropoiesis. With severe anemia there is recruitment of extramedullary erythropoietic sites resulting in macrocytosis and erythroblastemia. Finne, sampled umbilical cord blood and amniotic fluid after delivery from red cell isoimmunised pregnancies and found that severe anemia was associated with abrupt increases in plasma and amniotic fluid erythropoietin levels; at lesser degrees of anemia erythropoietin levels increased mildly [76]. It is possible that recruitment of extramedullary erythropoiesis occurs at high concentrations of erythropoietin, whereas the marrow is sensitive to mild elevations in erythropoietin.

Doppler ultrasound investigation of uterine and fetal circulations

Doppler ultrasound provides a non-invasive method for the study of fetal hemodynamics. Investigation of the uterine and umbilical arteries provide information on the perfusion of the utero-placental and feto-placental circulations respectively, while Doppler ultrasound studies of selected fetal organs are valuable in detecting the hemodynamic rearrangements that occur in response to fetal hypoxemia or anemia. Volume flow calculations are fraught with methodological errors and therefore, in Doppler studies the most commonly used indices are those of mean arterial blood velocity and vascular resistance (flow impedance) either by the S/D ratio or the pulsutility index. The latter is preferred because in some pathological conditions, such as fetal acidemia, there is absence of frequencies at the end of diastole in some vessels and therefore the S/D ratio would have the value of infinity.

Normal pregnancy

In normal pregnancy, impedance to flow in the uterine artery decreases with gestation [77, 78] and this presumably reflects the trophoblastic invasion of the spiral arteries and their conversion into low resistance vessels [79]. Similarly, there is a decrease in impedance to flow in the umbilical arteries due to progressive maturation of the placenta and increase in the number of tertiary stem villi. The mean blood velocity in both the descending thoracic aorta and common carotid artery increase with gestation and this may reflect a progressive increase in cardiac output to fulfil the demands of the growing fetus [80]. After 32 weeks' gestation the aortic velocity remains stable, in contrast to the velocity in the common carotid artery which increases linearly with gestation. Furthermore, with advancing gestation there is a decrease in the impedance to flow in the common carotid artery. These findings led to the speculation that in the latter part of pregnancy a proportionally greater fraction of the cardiac output is directed to the fetal brain presumably to compensate for the progressive fall in fetal blood pO_2 and increase in pCO_2.

Hypoxemic hypoxia

Animal studies have demonstrated that in fetal hypoxemia there is a redistribution in blood flow with increased blood supply to the brain, heart and adrenals and a simultaneous reduction in the perfusion of the carcass, gut and kidneys [81]. Doppler ultrasound has enabled the non-invasive confirmation of the brain-sparing effect in human fetuses.

Cross sectional studies in pregnancies with SGA fetuses have shown that increased impedance to flow in the uterine and umbilical arteries is associated with fetal hypoxemia and acidemia [82]. These data support the findings from histopathologic studies that in some pregnancies with SGA fetuses there is firstly, failure of the normal development of maternal placental arteries into low resistance vessels [79] and therefore reduced oxygen and nutrient supply to the intervillous space, and secondly, reduction in the number of placental terminal capillaries and small muscular arteries in the tertiary stem villi [83] and therefore impaired maternal-fetal transfer.

Pulsed Doppler ultrasound studies of the fetal circulation have demonstrated significant associations between the degrees of fetal hypoxemia and acidemia and firstly, increase in the mean blood velocity and decrease in the indices of impedance to flow in the common carotid and middle cerebral arteries [82, 84] and secondly, decrease in blood velocity and increase in impedance in the descending thoracic aorta and renal artery (Figure 25.4) [82, 85]. These findings suggest that in fetal hypoxemia there is an increase in the blood supply to the brain and reduction in the perfusion of the kidneys, gastro-intestinal tract and the lower extremities. Although knowledge of the factors governing circulatory readjustments and their mechanism of action is incomplete, it appears that partial pressures of oxygen and carbon dioxide play a role, presumably through their action on chemoreceptors.

Anemic hypoxia

In red cell isoimmunisation, impedance to flow in the uterine and umbilical arteries is normal. However, fetal anemia is associated with increased cardiac output, increased blood flow in the umbilical vein and increased blood veloc-

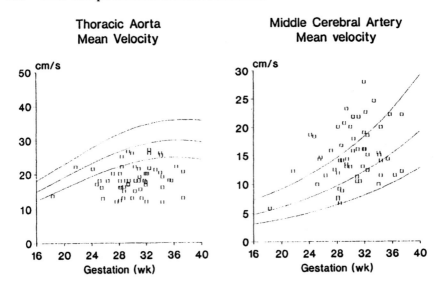

Figure 25.4. Reference ranges with gestation (mean, 5th and 95th centiles) for mean blood velocity in the fetal descending thoracic aorta and middle cerebral artery, and the individual values of small (O) for gestational age fetuses.

ity in the inferior vena cava, in the descending thoracic aorta, and in the common carotid and middle cerebral arteries (Figure 25.5) [86–89].

If it is assumed that in anemia, the cross sectional area of the aorta or other fetal vessels does not change, the increased velocity would reflect an increase in blood flow. These findings presumably reflect the anemia associated increase in cardiac output rather than a chemoreceptor-mediated redistribution in blood flow as seen in hypoxemic growth retarded fetuses. The correlation between anemia and cardiac output may be mediated by an increase in stroke volume due to: first, decreased viscosity leading to increased venous return, second, hypoxic peripheral vasodilation and therefore decreased peripheral resistance; and third, hypoxic stimulation of chemoreceptors leading to improved myocardial contractility.

In hydropic fetuses the aortic mean velocity is decreased. This suggests that in severe anemia there is cardiac decompensation, presumably due to the associated hypoxia and lactic acidosis and to the impaired venous return due to liver infiltration with hemopoietic tissue. Another possible mechanism is increased downstream resistance, due to clogging of placental capillaries with large immature red blood cells. However, this is unlikely because impedance to flow in the umbilical artery is not increased.

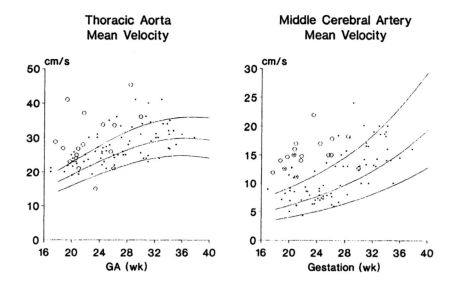

Figure 25.5. Reference ranges with gestation (mean, 5th and 95th centiles) for mean blood velocity in the fetal descending thoracic aorta and middle cerebral artery, and the individual values of fetuses from red cell isoimmunised pregnancies (O).

Cardiovascular changes after birth

At birth there are major cardiovascular changes as gas exchange is transferred from the placenta to the lungs. Pulmonary blood flow increases rapidly, umbilical-placental blood flow ceases and the fetal shunts (ductus arteriosus, ductus venosus and foramen ovale) close. Although the initial phase of this transition occurs within a minute of delivery, its completion may take up to 6 weeks.

Cardiac output

Cardiac output increases postnatally and the individual ventricular output is rapidly redirected. Establishment of pulmonary ventilation and increased pulmonary flow results in disappearance of the disparity between the left and right ventricular outputs. Although the ventricles start to act in series, not parallel, the foramen ovale and ductus arteriosus remain possible sites for left-to-right and right-to-left shunting for some days or even weeks after birth.

Within 24 hours of birth, oxygen consumption increases rapidly, in the newborn lamb it triples [90] and this increase may be due to the decreased ambient temperature. To meet this demand, total cardiac output increases rapidly with the development of a difference in wall thickness between the two ventricles. This major increase in left ventricular output occurs despite an apparent reduced ability of the fetal and neonatal left ventricle to increase stroke volume and cardiac output on demand [16, 91–94]. Cardiac reserve is limited because of the already high resting cardiac output [95]. With advancing postnatal age, the resting cardiac output falls and reserve increases, thereby maintaining maximal cardiac output.

The mechanisms that enable the myocardium to increase its work in the postnatal period when volume loaded are poorly understood. Catecholamines have been implicated, and plasma concentrations of both adrenaline and noradrenaline are elevated on the first day after birth [96, 97]. However, although Teitel *et al.* showed that beta-receptor blockade in the newborn depressed cardiac output [95], other workers have not [93]. Triiodothyronine (T3) and thyroid stimulating hormone (TSH) concentrations also rise rapidly after birth [98, 99], and Breall *et al.* postulated that rising T3 production may help mediate the cardiovascular response [100].

Umbilical circulation

At birth, the smooth muscle of the umbilical arteries constricts in response to several stimuli; traction of the umbilical cord, a fall in ambient temperature and an increase in following pulmonary ventilation. With cessation of umbilical blood flow there is a marked decrease in venous return to the heart and a significant increase in systemic vascular resistance.

Pulmonary circulation

After birth and onset of ventilation, pulmonary vascular resistance falls rapidly and this is associated with a rapid ten fold increase in pulmonary blood flow. Pulmonary vascular resistance falls gradually thereafter for up to 6 weeks postnatally. The changes in pulmonary resistance are induced by local effects and are sustained by humoral changes. The fetal lungs are fluid-filled but after delivery, as the lungs fill with gas, the alveoli expand and as pulmonary vascular resistance falls the pulmonary arterioles dilate [101, 102]. Before birth, the low pO_2 causes vasoconstriction of the precapillary pulmonary arteries, however with increasing fetal oxygenation, the fetal pulmonary vasoconstriction ceases and pulmonary blood flow increases further [103].

Many vasoactive substances have been implicated in contributing to the pulmonary vascular dilation postnatally. In the rhesus monkey, Schwartz and associates demonstrated an increase in lung mast cells [104]. These cells degranulate at birth releasing histamine and PGD_2, both of which are known to cause pulmonary vasodilation [53, 101]. The stimulus for mast cell degranulation is not known.

The physiological role of various prostaglandins is also far from certain.

PGE_2 is a modest pulmonary vasodilator, whilst PGI_2 is a more potent dilator [56, 105, 106]. However, neither substance is specific for the pulmonary circulation. Lung distension or mechanical stimulation of the lungs has been shown to lead to PGI_2 production [107–109] and an increase in bradykinin and angiotensin II levels [110].

Leukotrienes, a further substance derived from arachidonic acid but via the lipoxygenase pathway, have also been implicated because of their contradictory effect on smooth muscle [111]. Leukotriene synthesis is involved in hypoxic pulmonary vasoconstriction [112, 113]. It is likely that the changes in the pulmonary vascular resistance that occurs postnatally represents a balance between increasing vasodilation secondary to PGI_2 and decreasing vasoconstriction due to the leukotrienes, arachadonic acid being the precursor of both substances.

Ductus arteriosus

The ductus arteriosus, unlike the aorta and pulmonary vessels, has smooth muscle lining its medial layer. Closure after birth occurs in two stages; initial functional closure, followed by permanent closure by endothelial destruction and connective tissue formation. The most important stimulus to constriction is the postnatal increase in oxygen concentration [114–117]. Other stimuli implicated have been the release of acetylcholine, bradykinin and catecholamines [115, 117, 118], none of these however appear to be essential under physiological conditions. Concurrent with the release of these vasoconstrictive substances is the reduced availability of PGE_2 as a result of the loss of the placenta (the main production site of PGE_2) and the increased pulmonary metabolism and degradation of PGE_2.

In premature infants, delayed closure of the ductus arteriosus may be related to an ineffective contractile response to the increased oxygen concentration [55, 56, 117]. Rings of ductus arteriosus from immature lamb fetuses have a poorer response to oxygen than those from term animals. The current use of cyclo-oxygenase inhibitors (aspirin and indomethacin) to treat complicated pregnancies needs to be kept under careful review, because of the role of prostaglandins in maintaining the patency of the ductus arteriosus in utero [119].

The second phase of slow anatomic obliteration of the ductus arteriosus occurs by a process of intimal overgrowth following endothelial damage and this may take up to 6 weeks to be completed [120–121].

Foramen ovale

The foramen ovale is a valve able to respond to surrounding pressures. After birth, the left atrial pressure increases, due to the increased pulmonary blood flow, and the right atrial pressure falls, as a result of cessation of umbilical blood flow and the reduced inferior vena caval return. These changes represent a reversal of the fetal circulation. Contributing to the change in pressure difference across the foraminal valve is the reversal of flow in the ductus arteriosus, resulting from the increased left atrial pressure. The foramen is obliterated finally some 6–8 months after delivery by connective tissue growth.

References

1. Edelstone DI, Rudolph AM, Heymann MA. Liver and ductus venosus blood flows in fetal lambs in utero. Circ Res, 1978;42:426–33.
2. Edelstone DI, Rudolph AM, Heymann MA. Effects of hypoxemia and decreasing umbilical flow on liver and ductus venosus blood flows in fetal lambs. Am J Physiol 1980;238:H656–63.
3. Bristow J, Rudolph AM, Itskovitz J et al. Hepatic oxygen and glucose metabolism in the fetal lamb. J Clin Invest 1983;71:1–15.
4. Bristow J, Rudolph AM, Itskovitz J. A preparation for studying liver blood flow, oxygen consumption, and metabolism in the fetal lambs in utero. J Dev Physiol 1981;3:255–66.
5. Rudolph AM, Heymann MA. Circulatory changes during growth in the fetal lamb. Circ Res 1970;26:289–99.
6. Edelstone DI, Rudolph AM. Preferential streaming of ductus venosus blood to the brain and heart of fetal lambs. Am J Physiol 1979;237:H724–9.
7. Reuss ML, Rudolph AM, Heymann MA. Selective distribution of microspheres injected into the umbilical veins and inferior vena cavae of fetal sheep. Am J Obstet Gynecol 1981;141:427–31.
8. Heymann MA, Creasy RK, Rudolph AM. Quantitation of blood flow patterns in the foetal lamb in utero. In: Proceedings of the Sir Joseph Barcroft Centenary Symposium: Foetal and Neonatal Physiology. Cambridge: Cambridge University Press, 1973: 129–35.
9. Rudolph AM. Distribution and regulation of blood flow in the fetal and neonatal lamb. Circ Res 1985;57:811.
10. Itskovitz J, LaGamma EF, Rudolph AM. Effects of cord compression on blood flow and distribution of O_2 delivery. Am J Physiol 1987;252 H100.
11. Dawes GS. Foetal and neonatal physiology. Chicago: Year Book, 1968:141–59.
12. Sahm DJ, Lange LW, Allen HD et al. Quantitative real-time cross-sectional echocardiography in the developing normal human fetus and newborn. Circulation 1980;62:588–97.
13. Reed KL, Meijboom EJ, Sahn DJ et al. Cardiac Doppler flow velocities in human fetuses. Circulation 1986;73:41–6.
14. St John Sutton MG, Raichlen JS, Reichek N et al. Quantitative assessment of right and left ventricular growth in the human fetal heart: pathoanatomic study. Circulation 1984;70:935–41.
15. Court DJ, Parer JT, Block BSB et al. Effects of beta-adrenergic blockade on blood flow distribution during hypoxemia in fetal sheep. J Dev Physiol 1984;6:349–58.
16. Freidman WF. The intrinsic physiological properties of the developing heart. In: Freidman WF, Lesch M, Sonnenblick EM (eds.), Neonatal heart disease. New York: Grune and Stratton, 1973:21–49.
17. Rudolph AM, Heymann MA. Cardiac output in the fetal lamb: the effects of spontaneous and induced changes in heart rate on right and left ventricular output. Am J Obstet Gynecol 1976;124:183–92.
18. Rudolph AM. Factors affecting umbilical blood flow in the lamb in utero. 5th Eur Congr Perinat Med. 1976:159.
19. Rudolph AM. Fetal and neonatal pulmonary circulation. Ann Rev Physiol 1979;41:383–95.

20. Dawes GS, Johnston BM, Walker DW. Relationship of arterial pressure and heart rate in fetal newborn, and adult sheep. J Physiol (Lond)1980;309:405–17.

21. Biscoe TJ, Purves MJ, Sampson SR. Types of nervous activity which may be recorded from the carotid sinus nerve in the sheep foetus. J Physiol (Lond) 1969;202:1–23.

22. Ponte J, Purves MJ. Types of afferent nervous activity which may be measured in the vagus nerve of the sheep foetus. J Physiol (Lond). 1973;229:51–60.

23. Shinebourne EA, Vapaavouri EK, Williams RL *et al*. Development of baroreflex activity in unanesthetized fetal and neonatal lambs. Circ Res 1972;31:710–3.

24. Maloney JE, Cannata JP, Dowling MH *et al*. Baroreflex activity in conscious fetal and newborn lambs. Biol Neonate 1977;31:340–50.

25. Goodlin RC, Rudolph AM. Factors associated with initiation of breathing. In: Hodari AA, Mariona FG (eds.), Proceedings of the International Symposium on Physiological Biochemistry of the Fetus. Springfield IL: Charles C Thomas 1. 1972:294–318.

26. Walker AM, Cannata J, Dowling MH *et al*. Age-dependent pattern of autonomic heart rate control during hypoxia in fetal and newborn lambs. Biol Neonate 1979;35:198–208.

27. Parer JT, Krueger TR, Harris JL. Fetal oxygen consumption and mechanisms of heart rate response during artificially produced late decelerations of the fetal heart rate in sheep. Am J Obstet Gynecol 1980;136:478–82.

28. Itskovitz J, Groetzman BW, Rudolph AM. The mechanism of late decelerations of the heart rate and its relationship to oxygenation in normoxemic and chronically hypoxemic fetal lambs. Am J Obstet Gynecol 1982;142:66–73.

29. Cheng JB, Cornett LE, Goldfein A *et al*. Decreased concentration of myocardial alpha-adrenoreceptors with increasing age in foetal lambs. Br J Pharmocol 1980;70:515–7.

30. Cheng JB, Goldfein A, Cornett LE *et al*. Identification of beta receptors using (3H) dihydroalprenolol in fetal sheep heart: direct evidence of qualitative similarity to the receptors in adult sheep heart. Pediatr Res 1981;15:1083–7.

31. Whitsett JA, Pollinger J, Matz S. Beta-adrenergic receptors and catecholamine sensitive adenylate cyclase in developing rat ventricular myocardium: effect of thyroid status. Pediatr Res 1982;16:463–9.

32. Nuwayhid B, Brinkman Cr III, Su C *et al*. Systemic and pulmonary hemodynamic responses to adrenergic and cholinergic agonists during fetal development. Biol Neonate 1975;26:301–17.

33. Harris WH, Van Patten GR. Development of cardiovascular responses to noradrenaline, normetanephrine and metanephrine in the unanesthetized fetus. Cn J Physiol Pharmacol 1979;57:242–50.

34. Barrett CT, Heymann MA, Rudolph AM. Alpha and beta adrenergic function in fetal sheep. Am J Obstet Gynecol 1972;112:1114–21.

35. Assali NS, Brinkman CR III, Su C *et al*. Development of neurohumoral control of fetal, neonatal, and adult cardiovascular functions. Am J Obstet Gynecol 1977;129:748–59.

36. Vapaavouri EK, Shinebourne EA, Williams RL *et al*. Development of cardiovascular responses to autonomic blockade in intact fetal and neonatal lambs. Biol Neonate 1973;22:177–88.

37. Walker AM, Cannata J, Dowling MH *et al*. Sympathetic and parasympathetic control of heart rate in unanesthetized fetal and newborn lambs Biol Neonate 1978;33:135–43.

38. Parer JT, Laros RK, Keilbron DC *et al*. The roles of parasympathetic and beta-adrenergic activity in beat-to-beat fetal heart rate variability. In: Kovac AGB, Namos E, Rubanyi G (eds.), Cardiovascular physiology. Physiol Sci. Vol 8. New York: Pergamon Press, 1981:327.

39. Comline RS, Silver IA, Silver M. Factors responsible for the stimulation of the adrenal medulla during asphyxia in the foetal lamb. J Physiol (Lond). 1965;178:211–28.

40. Jones CT, Robinson RD. Plasma catecholamines in fetal and adult sheep. J Physiol (Lond) 1975;248:15–28.

41. Lewis AB, Evans WN, Sischo W. Plasma catecholamine responses to hypoxemia in fetal lambs. Biol Neonate 1982;41:115–32.

42. Greenough A, Nicolaides KH, Lagercrantz H. Human fetal sympathoadrenal responsiveness. Ear Hum Dev 1990;23:9–18.
43. Drummond WH, Rudolph AM, Keil LC *et al*. Arginine vasopressin and prolactin after haemorrhage in the fetal lamb. Am J Physiol 1980; 238:H214–9.
44. Rurak DW. Plasma vasopressin levels during hypoxaemia and the cardiovascular effects of exogenous vasopressin in foetal and adult sheep. J Physiol (Lond) 1978;277:341–57.
45. Iwamoto HS, Rudolph AMI Keil LC *et al*. Hemodynamic responses of the sheep fetus to vasopressin infusion. Circ Res 1979; 44: 430–6.
46. Challis JRG, Dilley SRI Robinson JS *et al*. Prostaglandins in the circulation of the fetal iamb. Prostaglandins 1976;11:104–52.
47. Challis JRG, Patrick JE. The production of prostaglandins and thromboxanes in the fetoplacental unit and their effects on the developing fetus. Semin Perinatol. 1980;4:23–33.
48. Mitchell MD I Flint AP I Bibby J *et al*. Plasma concentrations of prostaglandins during late human pregnancy: influence of normal and preterm labor. J Clin Endocrinol Metab 1978;46:947–51.
49. Terragno NAI Terragno Al McGiff JC. Role of prostaglandins blood vessels. Semin Perinatol.11980;4:85–90.
50. Novy MJ, Piasecki G, Jackson BT. Effect of prostaglandins E_2 and F_2 alpha on umbilical blood flow and fetal hemodynamics. Prostaglandins 1974;5:543–55.
51. Berman W Jr, Goodlin RC, Heymann MA *et al*. Effects of pharmocologic agents on umbilical blood flow in fetal lambs in utero. Biol Neonate 1978;33:225–35.
52. Tripp ME, Heymann MA, Rudolph AM. Hemodynamic effects of prostaglandin E_1 on lambs in utero. In: Coceani F, Olley PM (ed.), Prostaglandins and perinatal medicine: advances in prostaglandin and thromboxane research. New York: Raven Press, 1978: 221–9.
53. Cassin S. Role of prostaglandins and thromboxanes in the control of the pulmonary circulation in the fetus and newborn. Semin Perinatol 1980;4:101–7.
54. Olley PM, Bodach E, Heaton J *et al*. Further evidence implicating E-type prostaglandins in the patency of the lamb ductus arteriosus. Eur J Pharmacol 1975;34:247–50.
55. Clyman RI. Ontogeny of the ductus arteriosus response to prostaglandins and inhibitors of their synthesis. Semin Perinatol 1980; 4:115–24.
56. Clyman RI, Heymann MA. Pharmacology of the ductus arteriosus. Pediatr Clin North Am 1981;28:77–93.
57. LaGamma EF, Itskovitz J, Rudolph AM. Effects of naloxone on fetal circulatory responses to hypoxemia. Am J Obstet Gynecol 1980;143:933.
58. Smith FG Jr, Lupu AN, Barajas L *et al*. The renin-angiotensin system in the fetal lamb. Pediatr Res 1974;8:611–20.
59. Broughton-Pipkin F, Lumbers ER, Mott JC. Factors influencing plasma renin and angiotensin II in the conscious pregnant ewe and its foetuses. J Physiol (Lond) 1974;243:619–36.
60. Iwamoto HS, Rudolph AM. Effects of endogenous angiotensin II on the fetal circulation. J Dev Physiol 1979;1:283–93.
61. Carver JG, Mott JC. Renin substrate in plasma of unanesthetized pregnant ewes and their foetal lambs. J Physiol (Lond) 1 1978;276:430–6.
62. Iwamoto HS, Rudolph AM. Effects of angiotensin II on the blood flow and Its distribution in fetal lambs. Circ Res 1980;48:183–8.
63. Westin B. Technique and estimation of oxygenation of the human fetus in utero by means of hystero-photography. Acta Paediatr 1957;46:117–24.
64. Daffos F, Cappela-Pavlovsky M, Forestier F. Fetal blood sampling during pregnancy with use of a needle guided by ultrasound:study of 606 consecutive cases. Am J Obstet Gynaecol 1985;153:655–60.
65. Nicolaides KH, Soothill PW, Rodeck CH1 Campbell S-1 Ultrasound guided sampling of umbilical cord and placental blood to assess fetal wellbeing. Lancet 1986;i:1065–7.
66. Soothill PW, Nicolaides KH, Rodeck CH *et al*. Effect of gestational age on fetal and

intervillous blood gas and acid-base values in human pregnancy. Fetal Therapy 1986;i:168–75.

67. Nicolaides KH, Economides DL, Soothill PW. Blood gases and pH and lactate in appropriate and small for gestational age fetuses. Am J Obstet Gynecol 1989;161:996–1001.
68. Battaglia FC, Meschia G. An introduction to fetal physiology. London: Academic Press, 1986:154–67.
69. Nicolaides KH, Soothill PW, Clewell WH *et al*. Fetal hemoglobin measurement in the assessment of red cell isoimmunization. Lancet 1988;i:1073–5.
70. Burd LI, Jones MD, Simmons MA. Placental production and fetal utilisation of lactate and pyruvate. Nature 1975;254:210–1.
71. Soothill PW, Nicolaides KH, Campbell S. Prenatal asphyxia, hyperlacticaemia, hypoglycaemia and erythroblastosis in growth retarded fetuses. Br Med J 1987;294:1051–3.
72. Illingworth RS. Why blame the obstetrician? A review. Br Med J 1979;1:797–801.
73. Nicolaides KH. Studies on fetal physiology and pathophysiology in rhesus disease. Semin Perinatol 1989;13:328–37.
74. Soothill PW, Nicolaides KH, Rodeck CH. Fetal blood gas and acid-base parameters. In: Rodeck CH (ed.), Fetal medicine. London: Blackwell Scientific Publications,1989:57–89.
75. Huckubee WE, Metcalf J, Prytowsky H et al. Insufficiency of O_2 supply to the pregnant uterus. Am J Physiol 1962;202:198–204.
76. Finne PH. Erythropoietin levels in cord blood as an indicator of intrauterine hypoxia. Acta Paediat Scand 1966;55:478–89.
77. Campbell S, Griffin DR, Pearce JM *et al*. New Doppler technique for assessing uteroplacental blood flow. Lancet 1983;i:675–7.
78. Pearce JM, Campbell S, Cohen-Overbeek TE JM *et al*. Reference ranges and sources of variation for indices used to characterise flow velocity waveforms obtained by duplex, pulsed Doppler ultrasound from the uteroplacental and fetal circulation. Br J Obstet Gynaecol 1988;95:248–56.
79. Brosens I, Dixon HG, Robertson WB. Fetal growth retardation and the arteries of the placental bed. Br J Obstet Gynaecol 1977;84:655–63.
80. Bilardo CM, Campbell S, Nicolaides KH. Mean blood velocities and flow impedance in the fetal descending thoracic aorta and common carotid artery in normal pregnancy. Early Hum Dev 1988;18:213–22.
81. Peeters LLH, Sheldon RF, Jones MD JM *et al*. Blood flow to fetal organs as a function of arterial oxygen content. Am J Obstet Gynecol 1979;135:639–46.
82. Bilardo CM, Nicolaides KH, Campbell S. Doppler measurements of fetal and uteroplacental circulations: relationship with umbilical venous blood gases measured at cordocentesis. Am J Obstet Gynecol 1990; 162:115–20.
83. Giles WB, Trudinger BJ, Baird PJ. Fetal umbilical artery flow velocity waveforms and placental resistance: pathological correlations. Br J Obstet Gynaecol 1985;92:31–8.
84. Vyas S, Nicolaides KH, Bower S JM *et al*. Middle cerebral artery flow velocity waveforms in fetal hypoxaemia. Br J Obstet Gynaecol 1990;162:797–802.
85. Vyas S, Nicolaides KH, Campbell S. Renal artery flow velocity waveforms in normal and hypoxemic fetuses. Am J Obstet Gynecol 1989;161:168–2.
86. Bilardo CM, Nicolaides KH, Campbell S. Doppler studies in red cell isoimmunization. Clin Obstet Gynecol 1989;32:719–27.
87. Vyas S, Nicolaides KH, Campbell S. Doppler examination of the middle cerecral artery in anemic fetuses. Am J Obstet Gynecol 1990;162:1066–8.
88. Rizzo G, Nicolaides KH, Arduini D JM *et al*. Effects of intravascular fetal blood transfusion on fetal intracardiac Doppler velocity waveforms. Am J Obstet Gynecol 1990;163:123–8.
89. Nicolaides KH, Kaminopetros P, Higueras MT JM *et al*. Placental and fetal Doppler in red cell isoimmunization. Fetal Diag Ther. In press.
90. Dawes GS. Changes in the circulation at birth. Br Med Bull 1961;17:148–53.
91. Kirkpatrick SE, Pitlick PT, Naliboff JB *et al*. Frank-Starling relationship as an important determinant of fetal cardiac output. Am J Physiol 1976;231:495–500.

92. Gilbert RD. Control of fetal cardiac output during changes in blood volume. Am J Physiol? 1980;238:H80–6.
93. Klopfenstein HS, Rudolph AM. Postnatal changes in the circulation and responses to loading in sheep. Circ Res 1978;42:839–45.
94. Romero TE, Freidman WF. Limited left ventricular response to volume overload in the neonatal period: a comparative study with the adult animal. Pediatr Res 1979;13:910–15.
95. Teitel D, Sidi D, Chin T et al. Developmental changes in myocardial contractile reserve in the lamb. Pediatr Res 1985; 19: 948–55.
96. Eliot RJ, Lam R, Leake RD et al. Plasma catecholamine concentrations in infants at birth and during the first 48 hours of life. J Pediatr 1980;96:311–5.
97. Padbury JF, Diakomanolis LS, Hobel CJ et al. Neonatal adaptation: sympathoadrenal response to umbilical cord cutting. Pediatr Res. 1981;15:1483–7.
98. Abuid J, Stinson DA, Larsen PR. Serum triiodothyronine and thyroxine in the neonate and the acute increases in these hormones following delivery. J Clin Invest 1973;52:1195–9.
99. Erenberg A, Phelps DL, Lam R et al. Total and free thyroid hormone concentrations in the neonatal period. Pediatrics 1974;53:211–6.
100. Breall JA, Rudolph AM, Heymann MA. Role of thyroid hormone in postnatal circulatory and metabolic adjustments. J Clin Invest 1984;73:1418–24.
101. Cassin S, Dawes GS, Mott JC et al. The vascular resistance of the foetal and newly ventilated lung of the lamb. J Physiol (Lond). 1964;171:61–79.
102. Enhorning G, Adams FH, Norman A. Effect of lung expansion on the fetal lamb circulation. Acta Paediatr Scand 1966;55:441–51.
103. Heymann MA, Hoffman JI. Pulmonary circulation on the perinatal period. In: Thibeault DW, Gregory GA (eds.), Neonatal pulmonary care. Menlo Park: Addison Wesley, 1979:70.
104. Schwartz LW, Osburn BI, Frick OL. An ontogenic study of histamine and mast cells in the fetal rhesus monkey. J Allergy Clin Immunol 1974;56:381.
105. Cassin S, Tod M, Philips JC et al. Effects of prostaglandin D2 in the perinatal circulation. Am J Physiol 1981;240:H755.
106. Tyler TL, Leffler CW, Cassin S. Effects of prostaglandin precursors, prostaglandins, prostaglandin metabolites on pulmonary circulation in perinatal goats. Chest 1977:78:271–3.
107. Edmonds JF, Berry E, Wyllie JH, Release of prostaglandins by distension of the lungs. Br J Surg. 1969;56:622–3.
108. Gryglewski RJ, Korbut T, Ocetkiewicz A. Generation of prostacyclin by lungs in vivo and its release into the arterial circulation. Nature. 1978;273:765–7.
109. Gryglewski RJ. The lung as a generator of prostacylcin. Ciba Found Symp 1980;78:147–64.
110. Dusting GJ. Angiotensin-induced release of a prostacyclin-like substance from the lungs. J Cardiovasc Pharmacol 1981;3:197–206.
111. Samuelsson B. Leukotrienes:tors of immediate hypersensitivity reactions and inflammation. Science? 1983;220:568–75.
112. Ahmed T, Oliver W Jr. Does slow-reacting substance of anaphylaxis mediate hypoxic pulmonary vasoconstriction? Am Rev Resp Dis.) 1983;127:566–71.
113. Morganroth ML, Reeves JT, Murphy RC JM et al. Leukotriene synthesis and receptor blockers block hypoxic pulmonary vasoconstriction. J Appl Physiol 1984;56:1340–6.
114. Kovalcik V. The response of the isolated ductus arteriosus to oxygen and anoxia. J Physiol (Lond)1963;169:185–97.
115. McMurphy DM, Heymann MA, Rudolph AM et al. Developmental changes in constriction of the ductus arteriosus: responses to oxygen and vasoactive substances in the isolated ductus arteriosus of the fetal lamb. Pediatr Res 1972;6:231–8.
116. Oberhansli-Weiss I, Heymann MA, Rudolph AM JM et al. The pattern and mechanisms

of response to oxygen by the ductus arteriosus and umbilical artery. Pediatr Res 1972;6:693–700.

117. Noel S, Cassin S. Maturation of contractile response of ductus arteriosus to oxygen and drugs. Am J Physiol 1976;231:240–3.

118. Heymann MA, Rudolph AM. Control of the ductus arteriosus. Physiol Rev 1975; 55: 62–78.

119. Heymann MA, Rudolph AM. Effects of acetylsalicylic acid on the ductus arteriosus and circulation of fetal lambs in utero. Circ Res 1976;38:418–22.

120. Scammon E, Norris EH. On the time of the post-natal obliteration of the fetal blood passages (foramen ovale, ductus arteriosus, ductus venosus). Anat Rec 1918;15:165.

121. Christie A. Normal closing time of the foramen ovale and ductus arteriosus:anatomic study and statistical study. Am J Dis Child 1930;40:323.

26. Neonatal cardiac output

MARK DRAYTON

Early neonatal circulatory changes

The changes in the circulation that occur during the first 48 hours after birth
are phenomenal and of a greater magnitude than at any other stage in the
organism's development and rival the changes that must also occur in the
respiratory system. To allow a transition from in-utero placental respiration,
the bulk of these changes must be effectively complete within a very small
number of minutes. In utero the two cardiac pumping chambers operate in
parallel with a single circulation supplying all vascular beds including the
placenta. The left and right circulations are placed in parallel by connections
at inflow and outflow from the pumping chambers. Some of the blood returning to the right atrium passes to the left atrium through the patent
foramen ovale while much of the right ventricular output passes into the
systemic circulation through the ductus arteriosus. Flow through the pulmonary vascular bed is limited to about 10% of univentricular cardiac output
by its high vascular resistance. Immediately postnatally, systemic vascular
resistance suddenly increases due to the removal of the low resistance placental vascular bed, while pulmonary vasodilation secondary to lung expansion
and a rise in PaO_2 drops pressure on the right side of the heart. These
pressure changes reverse the gradient across the atrial septum abolishing the
right to left shunt through the foramen ovale, and similarly the shunt through
the ductus arteriosus, which is right to left in utero, changes to a bi-directional
or left to right one. At a slightly more leisurely pace, the ductus arteriosus
constricts in response to elevation in PaO_2, eliminating this shunt entirely.
It is therefore not surprising that problems arise from time to time during
this change. Infants particularly at risk of circulatory difficulty following
delivery are the premature, the asphyxiated, the infected, the anaemic or
polycythemic and infants with congenital malformation, particularly of the
heart or great vessels.

A.-M. Salmasi and A.S. Iskandrian (eds): Cardiac output and regional flow in health and disease, 349–364.
© 1993 *Kluwer Academic Publishers. Printed in the Netherlands.*

Problems of neonatal circulatory adaptation

Circulatory insufficiency
The commonest problem of circulatory adaptation in the sick newborn infant is circulatory insufficiency leading to tissue hypoperfusion, metabolic acidosis, ischaemic damage, systemic hypotension and possibly pulmonary hypertension. This common situation particularly lends itself to the monitoring or measurement of cardiac output to allow therapeutic intervention before the more severe or irreversible complications become established. The causes of this type of circulatory insufficiency are likely to be multiple and sometimes obscure.

Hypovolemia
Hypovolemia would appear to be the immediate antecedent in many neonates, particularly the very preterm, as evidenced by the effectiveness of colloid infusion in correcting metabolic acidosis and hypotension and restoring the peripheral capillary circulation. Hypovolemia may have several etiologies. Clamping of the umbilical cord immediately after delivery and while both systemic and pulmonary circulations are relatively vasoconstricted may leave an excessive proportion of the fetal blood volume within the placental vascular bed, particularly if the midwife or obstetrician holds the newborn infant above or level with the placenta at the time of clamping. The systemic capillary circulation of the preterm newborn infant appears to be leaky, perhaps as a result of free radical damage. This leakiness is particularly manifest in the presence of sepsis, endotoxaemia or severe respiratory disease when prodigious amounts of colloid infusion, sometimes amounting double the normal circulating volume of 70–80 ml/Kg over a 24 hour period, are required to maintain adequate cardiac output, blood pressure and peripheral perfusion. Repeated blood sampling for biochemical and hematological monitoring may further exacerbate the hypovolemia.

Impaired myocardial contractility /
Impaired pump function is not infrequent in the sick neonate and in severe cases the characteristic baggy poorly contractile left ventricle is readily identifiable on echocardiography. Contractility appears to decrease progressively at pH's below 7.20. Perinatal asphyxia and severe sepsis are both important antecedents of impaired myocardial contractility, and neonatal myocardial infarction is probably not uncommon in the former. Patent ductus arteriosus may also contribute to myocardial ischemia (see below). Cardiomyopathy, acute or chronic, may also present in the neonate, the former usually due to acute viral myocarditis, the latter most commonly in infants of diabetic mothers although not infrequently idiopathic. A degree of cardiomyopathy with a predilection for the inter-ventricular septum is almost universal in infants of insulin dependant mothers with poor maternal glycaemic control. The septal hypertrophy may be severe enough to obstruct the left ventricular output tract.

Patent ductus arteriosus

The ductus arteriosus is patent at birth in all normal infants. In term infants however, the ductus arteriosus is usually functionally closed by about 12 hours of age, although a small and haemodynamically insignificant jet may be detectable for a further 48 hours or so [1]. In preterm infants ductal closure is characteristically much slower and as pulmonary vascular resistance falls frequently gives rise to large left to right shunts [2]. The likelihood of delayed closure increases with decreasing gestational age. Previously functionally closed ductuses may also open again following acute hypoxic insults or episodes of sepsis. The left to right shunt 'steals' blood from the systemic circulation and increases flow into the pulmonary circulation. A phase difference between left and right ventricular contraction leads to the maximum systemic steal during diastole when blood flow throughout the systemic arterial system (with the exception of the pre-ductal aorta) tends to reverse and drain into the lungs. During early systole the instantaneous shunt may actually be right to left, but in the absence of pulmonary hypertension, the net shunt is always left to right [3]. The systemic steal tends to produce systemic hypoperfusion, particularly of gut, kidneys and myocardium. The latter is particularly susceptible to ischaemia because it can only be perfused during muscle relaxation in diastole when the shunt is greatest. Moderate left to right shunts are generally readily compensated for by an increase in cardiac output mediated by a combination of both increased stroke volume and heart rate (see below). Larger shunts exceed the heart's ability to compensate. Renal perfusion decreases and blood urea and creatinine levels rise. Gut perfusion decreases, increasing the risk of necrotising enterocolitis. Myocardial perfusion decreases with a resultant impairment of performance leading to the downward spiral of congestive cardiac failure. While the effect of a ductal shunt on the flow velocity waveform within the cerebral circulation is evident, the clinical significance is less certain.

Congenital heart disease

Cardiac output is impaired in a wide variety of congenital heart disease which is revealed when the in utero parallel circulation tries to convert to the ex utero serial left and right circulations. Left ventricular output in particular is characteristically decreased in the hypoplastic left heart syndrome and critical coarctation of the aorta. It is also decreased in intra-cardiac left to right shunts – ventricular and atrio-ventricular septal defects and many more complex anomalies. Presentation of these disorders may be delayed by several days as ductal closure in these infants is often delayed and the systemic circulation may be supported in the meanwhile by the right ventricle.

Persistent fetal circulation

When the pulmonary vascular resistance fails to fall following the establishment of lung ventilation (or it rises again after an initial fall), the gradient from left to right across the atrial septum may remain reversed with a right to left shunt through the foramen ovale. This causes systemic desaturation as oxygen poor blood returning to the right atrium re-enters the systemic circulation without passing through the lungs. An additional but usually smaller right to left shunt occurs through the ductus arteriosus. Persistent fetal circulation is found in both term and preterm infants. In the latter group it frequently complicates the respiratory distress syndrome or congenital pneumonia. In the term infant it is frequently associated with perinatal asphyxia, meconium aspiration pneumonitis or polycythjemia although often no risk factors may be identified. Poor cardiac output due either to hypovolemia or myocardial insufficiency may exacerbate persistent fetal circulation. We may speculate that the vasoconstriction that follows poor cardiac output is not limited to the systemic side of the circulation and that any systemic hypotension may promote a right to left shunt.

Need for circulatory assessment

In the paragraphs above some of the causes of circulatory embarrassment in the newborn are described. The adverse effects on gut, renal and myocardial perfusion have been mentioned. However recent interest in neonatal haemodynamics has to a large extent centred on the cerebral circulation of the preterm infant. Infants of less than 33 weeks gestation have a propensity to develop intracerebral hemorrhage during the first few days of life [4]. The risks increase with decreasing gestational age. These hemorrhages almost invariably originate from the germinal matrix in the subependymal layer below the lateral ventricles. Controversy exists regarding their precise causation but there is increasing evidence for an association with hypotension and poor cardiac output [5, 6]. Some regard the hemorrhages as hemorrhagic infarcts while others relate them to capillary rupture following the transmission of blood pressure transients through a dilated and non-autoregulating arterial vascular tree [7]. Although small hemorrhages do not appear to have any adverse short or long term clinical effects, larger haemorrhages into the cerebral ventricular system may lead to post-hemorrhagic hydrocephalus. Larger hemorrhages extending into the brain parenchyma are associated with adverse neurologic and developmental sequelae [8].

Of even greater longer term significance in the preterm infant are ischaemic cerebral lesions recognised in vivo by periventricular flare-shaped increased echogenicities which may progress to cystic degeneration (cystic periventricular leukomalacia) [9]. These lesions appear in watershed vascular zones between the centripetal and centrifugal arterial blood supplies of the preterm brain. They frequently co-exist with the intracerebral hemorrhages mentioned above, and evidence is strong that these too are hypoperfusion lesions.

The sick and/or preterm newborn infant appears to have limited ability to autoregulate his cerebral perfusion [10, 11] and therefore the maintenance of a steady and sufficient perfusion pressure to avoid dangerous cerebral pathology is extremely important. However, the monitoring of arterial blood pressure alone has serious limitations in this regard as described below.

Methods of circulatory assessment

Cardiac output to most people means left ventricular output. When making comparisons between fetal and neonatal cardiac function, it is important to realise that because of the parallel outputs of the two ventricles, fetal cardiac output is effectively the combined output of both sides of the heart, and is likely to be much higher than post-natal left ventricular output. As described above, large left to right shunts through a patent ductus arteriosus are common in the neonatal period. That portion of the left ventricular output which passes through the ductus arteriosus and into the pulmonary circulation is not available for systemic perfusion. 'Effective' cardiac output may therefore be considered as left ventricular output minus the net ductal shunt.

Tissue oxygen uptake is determined by effective cardiac output, blood hemoglobin concentration and the oxyhaemoglobin dissociation constant for the particular hemoglobin species and tissue biochemical milieu. Hemoglobin concentration is readily measured and if low is amenable to correction by transfusion although it has been suggested that total body red cell mass might be a more appropriate measure of haemoglobin sufficiency [12]. Effective cardiac output then remains the other major determinant of adequate tissue oxygenation and in view of the important pathology that may arise in the newborn infant if it is inadequate, the ability to measure or monitor this parameter in the clinical environment would almost certainly be a major advance in newborn care.

Most methods of direct measurement of cardiac output will actually provide a value for left ventricular output. This may be an important limitation as in the clinical arena it is effective cardiac output that is more likely to be helpful in determining circulatory effectiveness.

Despite the manifest need, to date no method of cardiac output monitoring in the neonatal period has gained clinical acceptability because of the technical skills required and problems of accuracy and validation with the various non-invasive methods. Invasive methods are either very difficult because of the small size of the newborn, especially the preterm infant, or are only applicable to one-off measurements in the cardiac catheterisation laboratory. An ideal method would be simple and non-invasive, would require little or no calibration, would provide values from an individual infant which could be compared with normal data from a healthy population, would measure *effective* cardiac output and would be suitable for continuous monitoring or at least regular intermittent measurement at say quarter hourly intervals. Such a method has yet to be found and therefore clinicians rely on proxy measurements for cardiac output which are more easily obtainable, while non-invasive cardiac output measurement remains a one-off diagnostic measurement or a research tool.

Blood pressure

The most widely used and time honoured method of assessment of circulatory adequacy in the newborn infant is arterial blood pressure measurement. Mean arterial blood pressure may have some value in its own right as it usually approximates to perfusion pressure and tissue perfusion is determined by perfusion pressure and the inverse of peripheral vascular resistance. However in vascular beds which are unable to autoregulate (and this is likely to include the cerebral circulation of the sick newborn infant) a fall in perfusion pressure will produce an immediate fall in perfusion and potentially damage may occur before effective remedial action can be taken. In the newborn infant as in the adult, arterial blood pressure will only fall when all the protective mechanisms which normally maintain an adequate blood pressure have failed. In other words hypotension is a poor measure of circulatory adequacy as it will only provide a late warning of circulatory failure. A discussion of the technical limitations of non-invasive blood pressure monitoring would be out of place here but it should be remembered that the popular oscillometric method tends to overestimate in the presence of hypotension

Capillary Refill

Capillary refill time is the time taken for the blush to return following blanching of the skin in response to gentle thumb pressure. In infants with failing effective cardiac output, skin is one of the first tissues to demonstrate reduced perfusion. Therefore diminished capillary refill time provides an early and sensitive index of cardiac insufficiency and in practice is one of the most useful cot-side techniques currently available. In a well perfused infant capillary refill time is usually less than 1.5 seconds. The limitations of this technique are its lack of specificity and the somewhat subjective nature that makes quantification difficult. Pain, hypothermia, polycythemia and septicemia may all reduce skin perfusion without necessarily implying decreased effective cardiac output while the use of vasodilatory drugs such as Tolazoline may create the impression of good capillary refill while perfusion of organs such as the kidney are reduced.

Toe/core temperature gap

A numeric assessment of skin perfusion may be obtained by measuring the difference between skin temperature at a peripheral site such as the foot or toe and the body core temperature measured at a central site. In a well infant this difference does not usually exceed 2°C. This method of assessing the circulation although semi-quantitative shares most of the limitations of the capillary refill method described above. In addition where very small infants are nursed in closed incubators with very high environmental temperature, the peripheral skin sensor tends to record the ambient rather than the skin temperature.

Laser Doppler skin blood flow has also been used in a similar manner but so far relatively little has been published regarding its neonatal application.

Direct assessment of cardiac output

Limitations
The major limitation of direct measurement of cardiac output in the neonate is that the difference between left ventricular output and effective cardiac output, as described above with reference to patency of the ductus arteriosus, is difficult to quantify. In this circumstance and in the absence of any intra-cardiac shunts, right ventricular output may more accurately reflect the flow of blood which is available for systemic perfusion.

A further but relatively minor limitation of aortic Doppler ultrasound measurement of cardiac output is that myocardial perfusion through the coronary arteries is not included. This has been estimated at 6–7% of left ventricular output.

Invasive methods

Invasive methods of measuring cardiac output include Swan-Ganz pulmonary artery catheterisation with use of the Fick principle, indicator dye dilution, videodensitometry, and radionuclide angiography [13]. At operation Doppler or electromagnetic flowmeters may be placed directly on or around the great arteries. These methods have in the past provided valuable information about normal values for neonatal cardiac output (see below) and even today may be useful in the assessment of complex hemodynamic problems in infants with congenital heart malformations. However, they have no role in the routine management of the sick neonate without primary heart disease.

Doppler ultrasound

Over the last 10 years, Doppler ultrasound has been used in a wide range of studies to measure neonatal cardiac output and is the most popular current methodology. It has the advantages of being safe, portable and non-invasive and although it has not been used successfully in the neonate for continuous monitoring, repeated or sequential measurements may be made. In its simplest form, the equipment required is readily available and need not be expensive. Despite this, its application is fraught with technical difficulties and for reproducible and accurate values to be obtained considerable operator skill is required. A good knowledge of the underlying principles of the application of Doppler ultrasound to volumetric measurement is necessary if unwarranted conclusions are not to be made.

Methodology [14]
Ultrasound which is backscattered from moving blood corpuscles has the properties of changed phase, frequency and power relative to the incident sound beam. These changes follow a well known mathematical relationship dependant on the ultrasound frequency and propagation velocity, the relative

angle between blood corpuscle movement and incident ultrasound beam and the velocity of the corpuscles. The blood corpuscles themselves have a spatial and velocity distribution across the vessel lumen and these distributions are continually changing through the cardiac cycle. The resultant Ultrasound signal is thus highly complex and may be analysed in several different ways to extract information about blood velocity and volume flow. Techniques appropriate to the large vessels of the adult may not scale down well when applied to the preterm neonate whose internal aortic diameter is as small as 4 mm. The Doppler ultrasound technology of neonatal cardiac output measurement is thus more akin to that of adult peripheral vascular volume flow than to adult cardiac output measurement.

The most widely used technique of volumetric Doppler analysis relies on the multiplication of time and spatially averaged blood velocity within an artery by its cross-sectional area. Cross-sectional area is calculated by assuming that the vessel has a circular section and measuring its diameter using M-mode or real time ultrasound imaging. The particular problems that the neonate presents in both aortic velocity and diameter measurement are discussed below.

More recently attenuation compensated Doppler volume flowmeters have been developed that in theory are capable of measuring volume flow independent of Doppler angle, blood vessel dimensions (within a range) and velocity profile. Although there has been some success in the adult and older child, the technique has proved difficult to scale down to the very small aorta and pulmonary artery of the neonate.

Vessel diameter measurement
Although the aortic cross-sectional area may be measured by planimetry from a real-time image, this is inaccurate and the aortic diameter may be measured most accurately using A-or M-mode scanning perpendicular to the vessel wall. As the diameter is squared in the calculation of area, and the diameters in question are so small, the potential for error is very great. A further problem particularly relevant to the neonate is that the aorta and pulmonary artery are distensible, with larger systolic than diastolic diameters [15]. Optimally, a Doppler flowmeter would simultaneously track the vessel diameter and measure instantaneous mean velocity. Its volume flow output would be the instantaneous product of velocity and diameter which could then be integrated with time. In practice, the requirement for a perpendicular ultrasound beam for diameter measurement and an oblique beam to detect the Doppler shift would make such an instrument too bulky and clumsy for use on the neonate. Few studies have addressed this problem.

Several different protocols exist for making M-mode echocardiographic and vascular measurements. That recommended by the American Society of Echocardiography, and in widest use, is the leading edge methodology – from the anterior (most superficial) portion of the anterior vessel wall to the anterior boundary of the posterior vessel wall. These recommendations were chosen to allow the greatest reproducibility between observers [16] but were not selected with accurate internal lumen or Doppler volume flow calculation in mind. Clearly an internal to internal methodology is likely to be more accurate in these latter applications. It is important that minimum ultrasound power output is used to minimise the spread of the image and resulting under-estimation of the lumen diameter.

Mean velocity calculation

In the large aorta of the adult, the velocity profile across the vessel lumen is close to 'plug profile' for most of the cardiac cycle. That is to say all but the most peripheral blood flows at a velocity close to the maximum stream velocity in the centre of the vessel. Thus mean blood velocity across the vessel lumen approximates to the maximum velocity, and mean velocity may be calculated using a relatively simple maximum frequency follower and a small Doppler sample volume placed uncritically centrally within the vessel. In very small vessels such as the neonatal cerebral arteries, the velocity profile is close to parabolic throughout the cardiac cycle. In this instance, mean velocity is close to half the maximum velocity and once more, a simple maximum frequency follower may be used to calculate mean velocity. Unfortunately in intermediate sized vessels which include the great arteries of smaller neonates, the flow profile lies indeterminately between these two extremes and varies considerably in different phases of the cardiac cycle. True volume flow or cardiac output will only be measured if the Doppler sample volume samples evenly right across the lumen and a true power weighted mean frequency analysis is used to extract mean velocity. Many investigators have failed to appreciate this fact and are likely to have made over-estimates of absolute cardiac output.

Accurate calculation of blood flow velocity necessitates accurate measurement of the Doppler angle. The measurement is less critical at small Doppler angles and normal adult practice is to use an approach from the supra-sternal notch when a zero Doppler angle may be assumed without actually making an angle measurement. However, it is more difficult to achieve even insonation across the vessel lumen when the ultrasound beam enters the vessel almost end on and as this is important in the neonate if absolute values are sought, a compromise is probably best. The desired Doppler angle determines the appropriate ultrasound window. A sub-costal 4–chamber approach generally allows an angle between 40 and 50°. If a non-zero angle approach is preferred (i.e. an approach other than from the supra-sternal notch), then a duplex Doppler/imaging system will be needed so that the angle of the ultrasound beam to the vessel wall may be measured.

Accuracy and reproducibility
Our own laboratory studies using a pulsatile flow rig with human donor blood and artificial vessels revealed a coefficient of variation of 2.7% for a

4.3 mm vessel, a 50° Doppler angle and a flow rate of 250 ml/min. In vivo neonatal studies have shown intra-operator variability in the measurement of ascending aortic velocity of 11.7% with little inter observer variability [17]. In the calculation of flow, significant additional variability might be expected from the diameter measurement. Gill tested reproducibility of measurements using the static UI Octoson equipment and a 7 mm fetal umbilical vein and found a Standard Deviations of 0.41 mm (diameter), 3.0° (angle) and 14% (flow) at 45° insonation [18]. Greater error might be expected from most commercially available duplex scanners in the active newborn infant.

Accuracy of neonatal cardiac output measurement has been less stringently assessed. There is really no 'gold standard' against which Doppler methods of measuring cardiac output can be compared as even the invasive techniques carry considerable potential for error. Many of the likely sources of error have been discussed above. Those that are random in distribution may be minimised by taking the mean value of multiple measurements. The major systematic errors are likely to be due to non-uniform insonation of the blood vessel by the ultrasound beam and in some instruments, inaccurate representation of mean velocity. Inappropriate vessel lumen measurement methodology (see above) may also produce systematic error. These systematic errors are likely to be greater in neonatal applications and will in general lead to an over-estimation of cardiac output. Systematic error can be reduced to some extent at the instrument design stage, but it is perhaps more important to calibrate the instrument under laboratory conditions which mirror the physiological situation as closely as possible. As a minimum this probably means using a pulsatile flow generator, vessels with a range of diameters and possibly a range of Doppler angles. Other variables – sample volume size and depth and high-pass filter setting can be standardised both during calibration and in clinical use. Unfortunately such instrument calibration appears to have been carried out only rarely.

Systematic error is less important when comparisons are being made between patients studied using the same apparatus, but may be very important when comparing results from different centres. Similarly in sequential studies, it may not be unreasonable to assume that the diameter of large vessel does not change significantly over a short period and therefore a change in velocity (whose measurement is not subject to such great errors) may be proportional to the change in flow.

Impedance cardiography

Although the technique of impedance cardiography has been known for many years, it is only recently that it has received renewed attention. The great attraction of the technique is that it is non-invasive requiring only the placement of sensing electrodes on the trunk and neck and that it is the only technique allowing continuous monitoring of cardiac output. The method is based on the changes in the electrical conductivity of the thoracic segment

Table 26.1 Cardiac output in healthy infants (ml/Kg/min).

Study	Age (hours)	LVO	RVO	Notes
Prec [22]	2–26	161	161	Indicator injection in umbilical vein – recording ear piece oximeter.
Gessner [23]	0–2	250	161	Indicator injection in left atrium – sampling from aorta.
Burnard [23]	1–28	366	246	Thermodilution. Oxygen consumption values increased.
Arcilla [23]	2–54	215	157	Indicator injection in left atrium – sampling from aorta.
Emmanoulides [23]	6–35	261	199	Indicator injection in left atrium – sampling from aorta.
Walther [24]	24–192	249	–	Pulsed Doppler ultrasound
Alverson [25]	24–168	236	–	Pulsed Doppler ultrasound
Hudson [26]	48–168	231	–	Pulsed Doppler ultrasound
Drayton [15]	1.5	161	–	Pulsed Doppler ultrasound (following laboratory calibration)
Sexson [19]	24–72	205	–	Bioelectric impedance
Belik [20]	48	198	–	Bioelectric impedance

in relation to the aortic blood flow and therefore measures stroke volume on a beat by beat basis. Recent neonatal studies have shown considerable promise with measured values compatible with those obtained using more established techniques although there is still uncertainty as to the optimal algorithm for the calculation of cardiac output in the neonate [19–21]. More studies are awaited.

Normative data

Table 26.1 summarises some of the published data on cardiac output in supposedly healthy newborn infants. Some of the data may not be accurate because of the presence of shunts through the foramen ovale, ductus arteriosus and bronchial vessels and various factors associated with delivery – maternal analgesia/anaesthesia, mode of delivery, amount of placental transfusion and body temperature.

The lower values for right ventricular output (RVO) compared with left ventricular output (LVO) in the invasive studies indicate that there were left to right shunts in the infants studied. It can be argued that if the shunts had no effect on RVO, systemic perfusion – the effective component of LVO, was between 160 and 200 ml/Kg/min, and probably towards the lower end of that range. Although the values from the Doppler studies have become accepted as normal standards, they almost certainly over-estimate flow for all the reasons mentioned above.

Selected clinical studies

Patent ductus arteriosus
The poor tolerance of patent ductus arteriosus (PDA) in the newborn infant, its major effect on neonatal haemodynamics and the availability of methods to close it have made PDA a fertile subject for Doppler studies. Alverson et al. [27] used Doppler ultrasound to measure cardiac output before and after patent ductus closure with indomethacin. Before closure, cardiac output averaged 343 ml/Kg/min; after indomethacin treatment the mean value was 271 ml/Kg/min but after surgical ligation the mean value was 224 ml/Kg/min. These values demonstrate the considerable extra demand that is placed on the left ventricle in the presence of a PDA. Despite these high outputs, the mean velocity in the femoral artery was *decreased* before ductal closure suggesting that the left ventricle was unable fully to compensate for the ductal run-off.

Our own studies [15] have demonstrated that even in term infants at $1\frac{1}{2}$ hours of age, left ventricular output is elevated by 28% compared with the values in the same infants at 48 hours of age. This is likely to be due to the presence of a left to right ductal shunt at $1\frac{1}{2}$ hours which we calculated to be 62 ml/Kg/min. Even with this comparatively modest shunt, effective cardiac output was 21% lower at $1\frac{1}{2}$ hours than at 48 hours.

Walther et al. [28] have also shown that in preterm infants, an elevation of left ventricular output precedes the onset of *symptomatic* patent ductus arteriosus and therefore left ventricular output measurement may be a useful predictive tool.

Stroke volume, heart rate and left ventricular output
Early work largely on the lamb had suggested that the neonate had limited ability to increase its cardiac output when stressed [29]. The recent Doppler studies of human infants with PDA clearly demonstrate that they can respond to this stress by elevating cardiac output although often not adequately to maintain normal systemic perfusion. Linder et al. [30] studying preterm infants with the respiratory distress syndrome showed that they increased their left ventricular output during symptomatic PDA by increasing stroke volume rather than heart rate. Similarly Winberg and Lundell [31] have shown a much closer relationship between stroke volume and cardiac output than heart rate and cardiac output in healthy term infants during the first 72 hours of life. This was different from our own conclusions following a similar study over the first 48 hours of life. Over that period there was a significant reduction in heart rate of 15 beats per minute, the greatest reduction being over the first 12 hours of life as the ductus arteriosus closed. There was also a significant reduction in stroke volume over the 48 hours of 14% but the timing of this decrease did not so closely follow that of ductal closure. We concluded that alterations of both stroke volume and heart rate contributed

to decreased cardiac output. It is likely that changes in pre-and post-load, both affecting cardiac output, may influence heart rate and stroke volume differently. For instance Wallgren and associates reported a reduction in stroke volume and an increase in heart rate following pre-load reduction produced by hemorrhagic hypotension in otherwise healthy term infants.

Prematurity

Walther *et al.* [24] demonstrated that in healthy infants, preterm or term, cardiac output increased linearly with birthweight. In our own studies, we found that patency of the ductus arteriosus was the major determinant of cardiac output and as several of the preterm infants we studied had asymptomatic but significant shunts, the preterm infants as a group had higher left ventricular outputs per Kg than term ones. However, when infants without PDA were compared or effective cardiac output was calculated, we too found no difference in output per Kg between term and preterm infants.

Right ventricular output

Relatively little recent published data exists regarding the measurement of right ventricular output (RVO) although this may correlate better with effective cardiac output (see above). However Walther and his team once more have demonstrated that right ventricular output is readily measured using Doppler ultrasound either by duplex scanning or by a precordial unguided technique [32]. The Doppler measurement of RVO with or without concurrent LVO measurement promises to be useful.

Transient myocardial dysfunction

Walther *et al.* used Doppler ultrasound measurement of cardiac output as a diagnostic aid in transient myocardial dysfunction in neonates, and as a tool to assess the effects of therapy [33]. The infants were selected as having myocardial dysfunction on the basis of M-mode echocardiographic findings – the aetiology in half of them was severe perinatal asphyxia, and in the rest mild asphyxia or unknown. Although hypotension was present in only 8 of the 22 infants studied, cardiac output and stroke volume were low in 20 infants confirming that cardiac output is a more sensitive measure of cardiac dysfunction than is arterial blood pressure.

Six infants with severe asphyxia were given Dopamine (4 to 10 µg/Kg/min). Cardiac output before Dopamine was 114 ± 26 ml/Kg/min and rose to 201 ± 39 ml/Kg/min within an hour of the infusion starting.

Infant of diabetic mother

Walther *et al.* used pulsed Doppler ultrasound to measure cardiac output in infants of diabetic mothers (IDM) who frequently have congenital hypertrophic cardiomyopathy [34]. Cardiac output was depressed in the IDM group and correlated with the degree of interventricular septal hypertrophy. In infants followed sequentially, cardiac function improved over one to two weeks. The cause of the decreased cardiac output was a decreased stroke volume without compensatory increase in heart rate.

Summary

Cardiac output is a vital link in the chain delivering oxygen to the tissues. In the newborn infant, effective cardiac output is frequently impaired and the consequences of such impairment may be severe and long lasting particularly in the brain. Methods of detecting this impairment early and of monitoring the effectiveness of medical intervention are of paramount importance. The widely used 'proxies' for cardiac output measurement are all unsatisfactory for various reasons. The main reason for the limited introduction of routine cardiac output measurement is the technical difficulty and it is noteworthy how many of the published studies emanate from one unit. A further difficulty is that run-off of blood flow through a patent ductus aeriosus will increase cardiac output while decreasing the output actually available for organ perfusion. Wider use of right ventricular output measurement may minimise this last problem but the technical difficulty of Doppler ultrasound volumetric measurements in infants of this size is likely to limit its use to that of a specialist investigation. Current widely accepted Doppler ultrasound derived standards for cardiac output are likely to be an over-estimate of actual flow. Potential error in measuring the aortic diameter make comparisons between infants more problematic than comparisons of sequential measurements in the same infant. In the future bioelectrical impedance monitoring of cardiac output seems to offer great potential.

References

1. Gentile R, Stevenson G, Dodey T et al. Pulsed Doppler echocardiographic determination of time of ductal closure in normal newborn infants. J Pediatr 1981;98:443–8.
2. Dudell GG, Gersony WM. Patent ductus arteriosus in neonates with severe respiratory disease. J Pediatr 1984;104:915–20.
3. Spach M, Serwer GA, Anderson PAW. et al. Pulsatile aortopulmonary pressure-flow dynamics of patent ductus arteriosus in patients with various hemodynamic states. Circulation 1980;61:110–22.
4. Papile L, Burstein J, Burstein H. et al. Incidence and evolution of subependymal and intraventricular haemorrhage: a study of infants with birthweights less than 1,500 gm. J Pediatr 1978;92:529–34.
5. Watkins AMC, West CR, Cooke RW. Blood pressure and cerebral haemorrhage and ischaemia in very low birthweight infants. Early Hum Dev 1989;19:103–10.

6. Bada HS, Korones SB, Perry EH. *et al.* Mean arterial blood pressure changes in premature infants and those at risk for intraventricular haemorrhage. J Pediatr 1990;117:607–14.
7. Drayton MR, Sidmore R. Vasactivity of the major intracranial arteries in newborn infants. Arch Dis Childh 1987;62:236–40.
8. Stewart AL, Thorburn RJ, Hope PL. *et al.* Ultrasound appearance of the brain in very preterm infants and neurodevelopmental outcome at 18 months of age. Arch Dis Childh 1983;58:598–604.
9. Trounce JQ, Rutter N, Leven MI Periventricular leucomalacia and intraventricular haemorrhage in the preterm infant. Arch Dis Childh 1986;61:11961202.
10. Lou HC, Lassen NA, Friis-Hansen B. Impaired autoregulation of cerebral blood flow in the distressed newborn infant. J Pediatr 1979;94:118–21.
11. Kempley ST, Gamsu HR. Autoregulation of cerebral and visceral blood flow velocity in very low birth weight infants. Arch Dis Childh 1992. In press.
12. Hudson I, Cooke A, Holland A. *et al.* Red cell volume and cardiac output in anaemic preterm infants. Arch Dis Childh 1990;65(7 Spec No):672–5
13. Lees MH. Cardiac output determination in the neonate. J Pediatr 1983;102:709–10.
14. Atkinson P Woodcock JP. Doppler ultrasound and its use in clinical measurement. London: Academic Press, 1992.
15. Drayton MR. Neonatal haemodynamics. MD thesis. University of Cambridge, 1987:1–39.
16. Sahn DJ, DeMaria A, Kisslo J. *et al.* Recommendations regarding quantitation in M-mode echocardiography: results of a survey of echocardiographic measurements. Circulation 1978;6:1072–83.
17. Clafin KS, Alverson DC, Pathak D. *et al.* Cardiac output determination in the newborn. Reproducibility of the pulsed Doppler velocity measurement. J Ultrasound Med 1988;7:311–5.
18. Gill RW. Measurement of blood flow by ultrasound: accuracy and sources of error. Ultrasound Med Biol 1985;11:625–41.
19. Sexson WR, Gotshall RW, Miles DS. Cardiothoracic variables measured by bioelectrical impedance in preterm and term neonates. Crit Care Med 1991;19:1054–9.
20. Belik J, Pelech A. Thoracic electric bioimpedance measurement of cardiac output in the newborn infant. J Pediatr 1988;113:890–5.
21. Tibballs J. A comparative study of cardiac output in neonates supported by mechanical ventilation: measurement with thoracic electrical bioimpedance and pulsed Doppler ultrasound. J Pediatr 1989;114:632–5.
22. Prec KJ, Cassels DE. Dye dilution curves and cardiac output in newborn infants. Circulation 1955;11:789–98.
23. Walsh SZ, Lind J. The fetal circulation and its alteration at birth. In: Stavem U, Weech AA (eds.), Perinatal physiology. New York: Plenum Medical Book Company, 1978:129–80.
24. Walther FJ, Siassi B, Ramadan NA. *et al.* Pulsed Doppler determinations of cardiac output in neonates: normal standards for clinical use. Pediatr 1985;76:781–5.
25. Alverson DC, Dykes FD, Lazzara A. *et al.* Noninvasive pulsed Doppler determination of cardiac output in neonates and children. J Pediatr 1983;101:46–50.
26. Hudson I, Houston A, Aitchison T. *et al.* Reproducibility of measurements of cardiac output in newborn infants by Doppler ultrasound. Arch Dis Childh 1990;65:15–19.
27. Alverson DC, Eldridge MW, Johnson JD. *et al.* Effect of patent ductus arteriosus on left ventricular output in premature infants. J Pediatr 1983;102:754–7.
28. Walther FJ, Kim DH, Ebraoimi M. *et al.* Pulsed Doppler measurement of left ventricular output as early predictor of symptomatic patent ductus arteriosus in very preterm infants. Biol Neonate 1989;56:121–8.
29. Dawes GS. Foetal and neonatal physiology. Chicago: Year Book Medical Publishers, 1968.
30. Linder W, Seidel M, Versmold HT. *et al.* Stroke volume and left ventricular output in preterm infants with patent ductus arteriosus. Pediatr Res 1990;27:278–81.

31. Winberg P, Lundell BP. Left ventricular stroke volume and output in healthy term infants. Am J Perinatol 1990;7:223–6.
32. Walther FJ, Van Bel F, Ebrahimi M. Duplex versus unguided pulsed Doppler measurements of right ventricular output in newborn infants. Paediatr Scand 1990;79:41–6.
33. Walther FJ, Siassi B, Ramadan NA. *et al*. Cardiac output in newborn infants with transient myocardial dysfunction. J Pediatr 1985;107:781–5.
34. Walther FJ, Siassi B, King J. *et al*. Cardiac output in newborn infants of insulin-dependent diabetic mothers. J Pediatr 1985;107:109–14.

PART SEVEN

Cardiac output in non-cardiac diseases

27. Cardiac output in pulmonary disease

HOPE BETH HELFELD and BERNARD L. SEGAL

Although the major effect of pulmonary disease upon the heart is on the right ventricle (RV), the left ventricle may also be involved. Significant lung disease through pulmonary vascular obstruction or pulmonary vasoconstriction secondary to hypoxia causes increased pulmonary vascular resistance, pulmonary artery hypertension, and eventually result in cor pulmonale. Etiologies included: recurrent pulmonary embolism, pulmonary vasculitis, fibrosing alveolitis, chronic bronchitis, emphysema, sarcoidosis, cystic fibrosis, increased pressure on the pulmonary arteries from tumor, pulmonary artery aneurysm, fibrosis, radiation, rheumatoid arthritis, systemic lupus erythematosis, mixed connective tissue disease and scleroderma.

The normal right ventricle is a thin-walled, distensible, compliant chamber that accommodates considerable variation in systemic venous return without large changes in filling pressures. Small increments in pulmonary artery pressure are associated with sharp decreases in right ventricular stroke volume and large increases in right ventricular work [1, 2].

A sudden, severe increase in pulmonary artery pressure leads to right ventricular dilatation and acute cor pulmonale. In chronic cor pulmonale, longstanding elevated pulmonary artery pressure leads to dilatation and concentric hypertrophy of the right ventricle. At some stage, the myocardium is unable to function at a high pressure load and fails, leading to RV systolic dysfunction, increased right ventricular end diastolic pressure, tricuspid regurgitation, and right-sided heart failure. This chapter will deal with the different causes of pulmonary disease and their effects on pulmonary vasculature and the heart.

Cystic fibrosis

In cystic fibrosis, pulmonary artery hypertension develops as a consequence of mucous obstruction in airways, recurrent pulmonary infections, progressive multilobar bronchiectasis, and chronic hypoxia. This will eventually leads to cor pulmonale.

Matthay *et al.* studied 22 ambulatory young adults with cystic fibrosis and

A.-M. Salmasi and A.S. Iskandrian (eds): Cardiac output and regional flow in health and disease, 367–381.

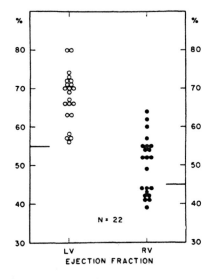

Figure 27.1. Left ventricular (LV) and right ventricular ejection fraction (RVEF) in 22 patients with cystic fibrosis. RVEF is abnormal (45%) in nine, while LVEF is abnormal (<55%) in none. N = number of patients. (From Matthay RA, Berger HJ *et al.* Right and left ventricular performance in ambulatory young adults with cystic fibrosis. Br Heart J 1980;43:474–80; with permission.)

clinically evident pulmonary disease by MUGA scan (Figure 27.1). The RV ejection fraction (EF) was abnormal in 9 patients (6 patients had severe and 3 patients had mild-to-moderate pulmonary disease). Left ventricular ejection fraction (LVEF) were normal in all 22 patients. Patients with an abnormal RVEF had significantly less arterial oxygen tension, forced expiratory volume in one second and forced vital capacity. Within one year of follow-up, 5 of the 9 patients with abnormal RVEF developed respiratory failure, and 4 of the 5 patients died with decompensated cor pulmonale [3]. These findings have been confirmed by other investigators [4].

Panidis *et al.* studied 17 patients with acute exacerbation of cystic fibrosis by echocardiography and Doppler ultrasound. They found no significant difference between patients with cystic fibrosis and normal subjects with regard to RVEF, LVEF, RV systolic and diastolic wall thickness [5].

The majority of investigators have found significant abnormalities in RV wall thickness, RV dimension and systolic function [6–9]. In Panidis' study, most of these patients had mild-to-moderate lung disease. It appears from the most studies [5–9], that systolic RV function is usually maintained in patients with mild-to-moderately severe pulmonary disease and may only be impaired in severe, end-stage disease. Additionally, the studies also showed that the LV function was preserved even with RV dysfunction [5, 6, 10, 11].

Sarcoidosis

Sarcoidosis is a multisystem granulomatous disease which most frequently effects the lungs and causes pulmonary hypertension secondary to fibrotic and/or granulomatous parenchymal disease.

Baughman *et al.* studied patients with restrictive pulmonary disease due to sarcoidosis. First pass radionuclide angiography (RNA) at rest and with supine bicycle stress test were performed in all 14 individuals. All patients had a normal LVEF at rest and 12 of the 14 patients had a normal LVEF response to exercise (Figure 27.2). RVEF was normal in 11 patients at rest but only two patients had a normal response to exercise (Figure 27.3). In this study, a significant correlation was also found between the exercise RVEF and total lung capacity as well as pulmonary artery oxygenation [12]. It also appears that exercise increases the pulmonary artery pressure, and pulmonary vascular resistance. A decrease in cardiac output results secondary to the increased RV afterload.

Adult respiratory distress syndrome

Adult respiratory distress syndrome (ARDS) is a diffuse injury of lung parenchyma resulting from increased pulmonary capillaries and endothelial permeability and fluid leakage into the alveoli. This may be a consequence of sepsis, trauma, pancreatitis, etc.

Zimmerman *et al.* examined 27 patients with severe adult respiratory distress syndrome and found significant elevations in heart rate, pulmonary artery pressure and pulmonary vascular resistance, as well as depressions in LV stroke index and LV stroke work index. Nineteen patients had lower than expected left ventricular stroke index in relation to wedge pressures (Figure 27.4), indicating decreased LV contractility or change in left ventricular pressure relationships. Also 9 of 11 patients had decreased slopes of LV function curves (Figure 27.5). Therefore, LV contractility, compliance, or both are altered in these patients [13]. The etiology of this finding is unclear and it may be secondary to acidosis, hypoxia and anatomic changes in the heart affecting systolic and diastolic function. Improvement in pulmonary function and hemodynamics occurred in survivors [13].

These findings were supported by Zopal and Snider [14] and Unger [15].

Pulmonary emboli

Pulmonary embolus is the impaction of blood clots, air, fat droplets, etc. into the pulmonary artery with resultant obstruction in blood flow. In acute pulmonary embolism, obstruction to flow increases pulmonary artery pressure and resistance causing increased RV.

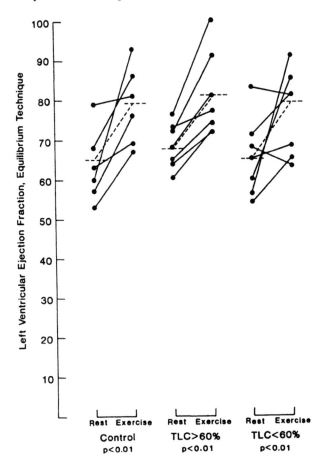

Figure 27.2. Left ventricular ejection fraction (LVEF) at rest and with exercise. In all three groups, there was a significant rise in LVEF with exercise. (From Baughman R, Gerson M, Baken C. Right and left ventricular function at rest and with exercise in patients with sarcoidosis. Chest 1984;85:301–77; with permission.)

McIntyre *et al.* studied 36 patients with pulmonary embolism, 28 of whom had pre-existing underlying heart or lung disease. The extent of pulmonary artery obstruction was determined by pulmonary angiography. In patients with pre-existing heart or lung disease, a relationship could not accurately be measured between the degree of cardiovascular and right ventricular functional impairment and the severity of pulmonary embolic obstruction [16, 17]. In other studies [18] in the absence of pre-existing cardiovascular disease, the degree of cardiovascular impairment was proportional to the extent of embolic obstruction. Among patients free of pre-embolic cardiopulmonary disease, stroke work is directly determined by the extent of angio-

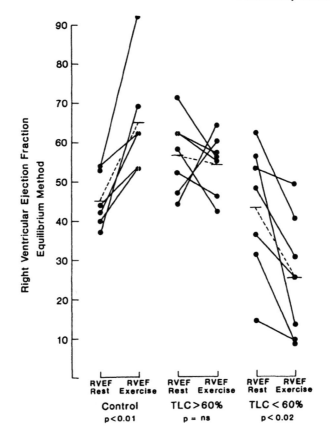

Figure 27.3. Right ventricular ejection fraction (RVEF) at rest and with exercise determined by the equilibrium method. Control group had a significant rise in EF with exercise, while severely affected sarcoid patients (TLC 60% of predicted) all had a fall. (From Baughman R, Gerson M, Baken C. Right and left ventricular function at rest and with exercise in patients with sarcoidosis. Chest 1984;85:301–8; with permission.)

graphic obstruction [18]. In patients with pre-existing heart and lung disease, pulmonary emboli affects the heart and lung according to the pre-existing disease. Albert [19] found that acute right ventricular pressure overload by pulmonary emboli depress cardiac output, left ventricular ejection fraction, stroke work, diastolic and systolic volume.

Bronchitis

Chronic bronchitis is a syndrome manifest by chronic cough and production of mucous for at least three months over two successive years.

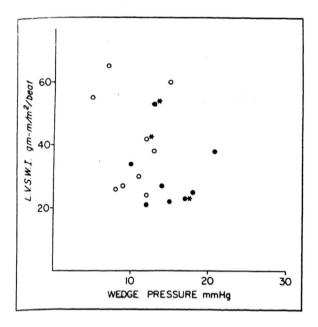

Figure 27.4. Relationship between wedge pressure and left ventricular stroke work index at L time of initial hemodynamic evaluation in patients with ARDS (adult respirator distress syndrome. Open circles indicate data from survivors, and solid circles indicate patients who died. Stars indicate patients receiving intravenous inotropic agents at the time of study. The shaded area indicates the expected relationship between wedge pressure and left ventricular stroke work index. (From Zimmerman G, Morris A, Cengiz M. Cardiovascular alterations in ARDS. AJM 1982; 73:23–34; with permission.)

Fluck and associates studied post-mortem records of patients who had died between the years of 1954–1965 at the Royal Free Hospital, London with the diagnosis of chronic bronchitis. Reports were analyzed for (a) thickness of RV and LV; (b) evidence of ischemic heart disease; (c) presence of nephrosclerosis; (d) evidence of chronic bronchitis; and (e) presence of any condition known to cause LV dysfunction [20]. Those patients with LV hypertrophy were included if systemic hypertension, ischemic heart disease, or significant nephrosclerosis were absent. The upper limit of normal wall thickness for the RV was 5 mm and 15 mm for the LV. a Series of controls were also studied (Table 27.1). In chronic bronchitis a significantly higher incidence of left ventricular hypertrophy was found for the total group ($p < 0.01$), the male patients ($p < 0.05$), but not for the female patients. In chronic bronchitis, 25% of patients had LV hypertrophy where only 7% of controls (normal patients) had LV hypertrophy [20]. This has been supported by other studies [21, 22].

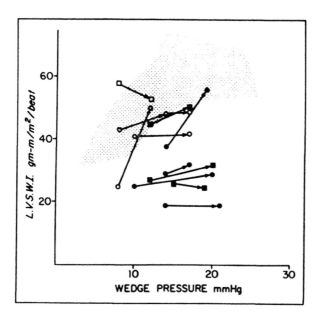

Figure 27.5. Left ventricular (LV) function curves resulting from infusion of blood or colloid in patients with ARDS. The arrows connect valves measured before and after infusion. Circles indicate data from patients receiving no inotropic agent, and squares indicate data from patients receiving dopamine (5–10 μgl/kgl/min) at the time of the study. Open figures indicate patients receiving 0–5 cm H2O of PEEP, and solid figures indicate patients receiving higher levels of PEEP (range 12–30 cm H2O) at the time of the study. The shaded area indicates the expected relationship between wedge pressure and left ventricular stroke work index. (From Zimmerman G, Morris A, Cengiz M. Cardiovascular alterations in ARDS. AJM 1982;73:25–34; with permission.)

Chronic obstructive pulmonary disease

Chronic obstructive pulmonary disease occurs secondary to noxious stimuli with permanent enlargement of airways distal to the terminal bronchioles. This causes reduction in lung elastic recoil, airway collapse with expiration and airway obstruction.

Burrows and associates studied 50 patients with stable chronic obstructive pulmonary disease (COPD) secondary to chronic bronchitis and emphysema. These patients and a normal control group underwent cardiac catheterization and had been followed for over 7 years since their cardiac catheterization. They found that the patients with COPD had a low normal cardiac index, normal pulmonary artery pressures which was high for the level of cardiac output, and elevated peripheral vascular resistance. In patients with COPD, mild exercise in the supine position was associated with a normal increase in cardiac index but an excessive rise in pulmonary artery pressure and

Table 27.1. Incidence of cases with left ventricular wall thickness ≧17 mm in chronic bronchitic and control cases. From Fluck D, Chandrasek R, Gardner F. Left ventricular hypertrophy in chronic bronchitis. (Br Heart J 1966;28:96–7; with permission.)

Left ventricular wall thickness (mm)	Men and women		Men		Women	
	Chronic bronchitics	Controls	Chronic bronchitics	Controls	Chronic bronchitics	Controls
<16	63	77	44	32	19	45
>17	21	6	14	1	7	5
Total	84	83	56	33	26	50

pulmonary vascular resistance. Patients with mild pulmonary disease generally had low normal cardiac output, and normal pulmonary artery pressure at rest, while with exertion all subjects had pulmonary hypertension. With more severe disease cardiac output decreased, pulmonary artery pressure increased, and pulmonary vascular resistance was elevated. With exercise, pulmonary hypertension was observed. In patients with severe chronic hypoxia, pulmonary hypertension develops and cardiac output remains low normal. In the absence of severe hypoxia, reduction in cardiac output is related to the severity of obstructive lung disease [23].

Kahaja and colleagues studied 20 patients with clinical and x-ray evidence of chronic obstructive pulmonary disease; nine of these patients had cor pulmonale. Cardiac catheterization was performed on all patients and cardiac output was measured by green dye during rest and supine bicycle exercise. Fourteen normal patients were used as controls and underwent cardiac catheterization with the same protocol. The mean pulmonary artery pressures were higher in patients with chronic obstructive pulmonary disease than in normal patients. During exercise, patients with COPD developed moderate pulmonary hypertension and abnormal right ventricular filling pressures. Although an increase in heart rate and stroke index during exercise was similar to normal patients, the stroke work index was higher in patients with COPD and this was related to an increase in pressure work. Patients with cor pulmonale exhibited moderate pulmonary hypertension at rest which became severe during exercise and was associated with abnormal RV filling. In normal patients, there was an increase in stroke output with little change in filling pressure. In cor pulmonale, there was little change in stroke output associated with a large increase in right ventricular end diastolic pressure (Figure 27.6). In patients with COPD, there was an intermediate response. LV end diastolic pressure remained normal at rest and with exercise in patients with COPD and in normal controls [24].

Slutskey *et al.* assessed left ventricular response to supine bicycle exercise by gated RNA [25]. They looked at four groups: (a) 10 normal patients; (b) 10 patients with coronary artery disease (CAD); (c) 12 patients with COPD;

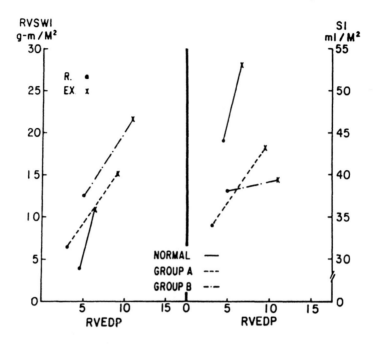

Figure 27.6. Right ventricular (RV) stroke work index is highest in patients with cor pulmonale both at rest (R) and during exercise (EX). All three groups form a single RV function curve, but patients with COPD operate on an extension of this curve with abnormal RV end diastolic pressures (EDP) during exercise. However, when stroke index is related to RVEDP, patients with cor pulmonale show depressed RV function (From Khaja F, Parker J. RV and LV performance in COPD. Am Heart J 1971:82;319–27; with permission.)

and (d) 8 patients with CAD and COPD. With exercise, normal patients had an increase in ejection fraction and stroke volume, decrease in end systolic volume and unchanged end diastolic volume, end systolic volume, stroke work, and pulmonary capillary wedge pressure. In patients with COPD – 6 of the 12 patients had abnormal EF secondary to decreased end diastolic volume, end systolic volume, stroke volume, unchanged pulmonary artery wedge pressure and an increase in pulmonary artery pressure. Patients with CAD and COPD had abnormal EF, as well as increased end diastolic and end systolic volume (Figures 27.7, 27.8, 27.9) They concluded that LVEF response to exercise in patients with COPD is due to a variety of factors including RV pressure overload resulting in a decrease in RV stroke volume, possible interseptal encroachment on LV size and diminished LV preload [25].

Matthay and colleagues studied 30 patients with COPD for RV and LV pump performance during exercise and rest by first pass RNA. Twenty-five untrained normals were used as controls. Patients were exercised by upright

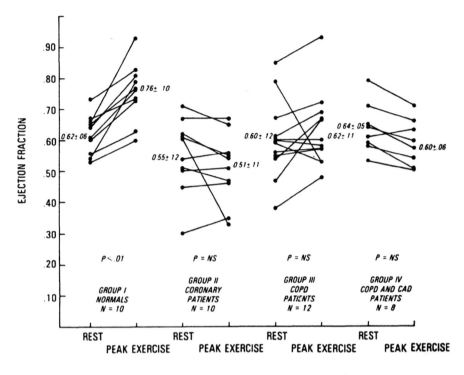

Figure 27.7. Left ventricular ejection fraction (LVEF) at rest and peak response to supine exercise in normal patients (group 1), coronary artery disease (CAD) patterns (group 2), COPD (chronic obstruction pulmonary disease) patients (group 3), and in COPD with CAD patients (group 4). Ns = p > 0.056. (From Slutikey R, Hooper W. Evaluation of LV function in COPD by gated equilibrium RNA. Am Heart J 1981; 101:414–20; with permission.)

bicycle. RVEF was normal in 22 patients at rest and only in 7 patients with submaximal exercise. LVEF was normal in 26 patients at rest and 24 patients with exercise. Patients with abnormal RV exercise reserve had greater resting airway obstruction and arterial hypoxemia [26].

Rao and associates studied 8 patients with COPD and cor pulmonale with LV failure without any recognized cause of LV failure. All patients had pulmonary function tests with moderate-to-severe impairment.

Four of the 8 patients had right heart catheterization which showed mild-to-moderate pulmonary hypertension at rest, two patients had elevated RV end diastolic pressures at rest, three patients had elevated pulmonary capillary wedge pressures; all patients had low resting cardiac output. Five of the 8 patients had necropsy findings with dilated and hypertrophied right and left ventricles. It was concluded that LV failure occurs in a small amount of patients with COPD and is probably multifactorial including hypoxemia, hypercapnia, and infection [27].

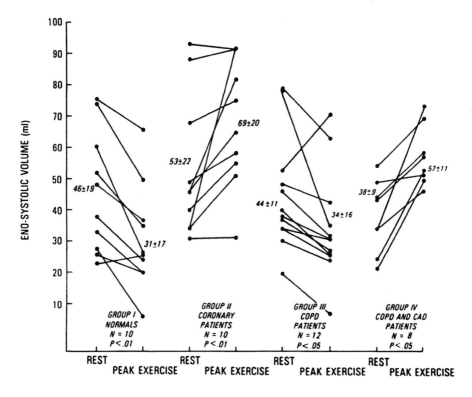

Figure 27.8. Left ventricular (LV) end systolic volume at rest and peak response to supine exercise in four different groups studied. (From Slutikey R, Hooper W. Evaluation of LV function in COPD by gated equilibrium RNA. Am Heart J 1981;101:414–20; with permission.)

Steele *et al.* studied LVEF in 120 patients with severe COPD. Ninety-two of the patients were acutely decompensated and 28 had stable disease. Of the 92 patients with acute respiratory failure, 60 had normal LVEF, 14 had moderate reduction of LVEF, and 19 had severe reduction of LVEF. Of the 19 patients with severely reduced EF, 12 patients had necropsy findings of CAD. Of the 28 stable patients, 12 patients had normal LVEF (>55%), 10 patients had moderately reduced LVEF (41–44%) and 6 patients had severely reduced LVEF (21%). Of the 16 patients with abnormal LVEF, 7 patients had clinical evidence of CAD (angina, history of myocardial infarction, Q-waves on EKG). In conclusion, most patients with severe chronic obstructive pulmonary disease have normal or near normal LVEF, however, some individuals with moderate depression of LVEF had no evidence of CAD [28].

Machee and associates studied right and left ventricular EF in 18 controls, 16 patients with angina, and 45 patients with COPD by first pass RNA.

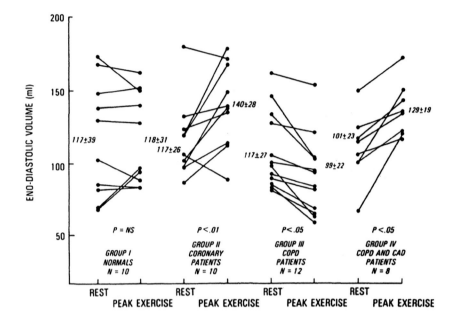

Figure 27.9. Left ventricular (LV) end diastolic volume at rest and peak response to supine exercise in the four different groups studied. (From Slutikey R, Hooper W. Evaluation of LV function in COPD by gated equilibrium (radionuclide angiography) RNA. Am Heart J 1981;101:414–20; with permission.)

Mean RVEF was similar in the control group and the angina group but RVEF was significantly lower in the patients with COPD. LVEF was not significantly different in any group. The patients with COPD who had clinical evidence of cor pulmonale at the time of the study had lower values of RVEF and LVEF than those patients in the COPD group without cor pulmonale (Figure 27.10).

In conclusion, pulmonary hypertension develops secondary to hypoxemia and airway obstruction. With increased pulmonary artery pressure and pulmonary vascular resistance, the right ventricle dilates and hypertrophies to maintain right ventricular cardiac output. Patients with mild COPD generally have normal mean right atrial pressure, and RV end diastolic pressure, normal or low normal cardiac output, and normal or slightly elevated right ventricular pulmonary vascular resistance at rest [23, 30–33]. Right ventricular function tends to be normal [34]. With exercise, pulmonary artery pressure increases, right ventricular stroke work increases, and RVEF falls [1, 2, 35]. As pulmonary disease becomes more severe and pulmonary vascular resistance increases, RV end diastolic pressure increases and RV function

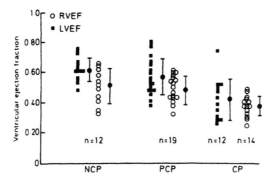

Figure 27.10. Right ventricular ejection fraction (RVEF) and left ventricular ejection fraction (LVEF) in patients with chronic bronchitis and emphysema who had no cor pulmonate (NCP), who had cor pulmonale at the time of the study (CP). The point are individual valves for RVEP (O) and LVEF (≠). The mean values for each group (O ±ISD are shown (NCP v PCP, NS; NCP v CP, p < 0.01). (From Machnee W, Of Xje *et al*. Assessment by RNA of RV and LV function in chronic bronchitis and emphysema. Thorax 1983;38:494–500; with permission.)

becomes abnormal. The latter can be first observed during exercise even when resting function is normal.

Controversy still exists on whether left ventricular function is impaired by pulmonary disease. The right ventricle has been shown to cause left ventricular dysfunction by, (a) interdependence of the ventricles through the intraventricular septum [36–42]; and (b) necropsy findings in which patients with cor pulmonale had unexplained left ventricular hypertrophy [20,27]. It appears that a small group of patients with cor pulmonale develop left ventricular dysfunction and further investigation must be done to explain the etiology.

References

1. Brent BN, Berger HJ, Mattay RA. *et al*. Physiologic correlates of right ventricular ejection fraction in chronic obstructive pulmonary disease:combined radionuclide and hemodynamic study. Am J Cardiol 1982;50:255–62.
2. Burghuber O, Bergmann H. Right ventricular contractility in chronic obstructive pulmonary disease: a combined radionuclide and hemodynamic study. Resp 1988;53:1–22.
3. Matthay RA, Berger HJ, Lake J. *et al*. Right and left ventricular performance in ambulatory young adults with cystic fibrosis. Br Heart J 1980;43:474–80.
4. Chipps BE, Alderson PO, Roland JM. *et al*. Non-invasive evaluation of ventricular function in cystic fibrosis. J Pediatr 1979;95:379–84.
5. Panidis IP, Ren JF, Holsclaw DS. *et al*. Cardiac function in patients with cystic fibrosis: evaluation,, by two-dimensional and Doppler echocardiography. J Am Coll Cardiol 1985;6:701–5.
6. Rosenthal A, Tucker CR, Williams RG. *et al*. Echocardiographic assessment of corpulmonale in cystic fibrosis. Pediatr Clin North Am 1976;23:327–43.

7. Gewitz M, Eshaghpour E, Holsclaw DS. *et al.* Echocardiography in cystic fibrosis. Am J Dis Child 1977;131:275–80.
8. Hirschfeld SS, Fleming DG, Doershuk MD. *et al.* Echocardiographic abnormalities in patients with cystic fibrosis. Chest 1979;75:351–5.
9. Lester SA, Egge AC, Hubbard VS. *et al.* Ventricular interdependence in severe cystic fibrosis. A proposed scoring system. J Pediatr 1980;97:742–8.
10. Jacobstein MD, Hirshfeld SS, Winnie G. *et al.* Non-invasive assessment of left ventricular performance in patients with chronic pulmonary disease. Chest 1981;80:399–404.
11. Kline LE, Crawford MH, MacDonald WJ. *et al.* Non-invasive assessment of left ventricular performance in patients with chronic pulmonary disease. Chest 1977;72:550–64.
12. Baughman R, Gerson M, Bosken C. Right and left ventricular function at rest and with exercise in patients with sarcoidosis. Chest 1984;85:301–7.
13. Zimmerman G, Morris A, Cengiz M. Cardiovascular alterations in adult respiratory distress syndrome. Am J Med 1982;73:25–34.
14. Zapol W, Snider M, Hill J. Extracorporeal membrane oxygenation in severe acute respiratory failure. N Eng J Med 1977;296:476–80.
15. Unger K, Shibel E, Moser K. Detection of left ventricular failure in patients with ARDS. Chest 1975;67:8–13.
16. McIntyre K, Sasahara A: Determinants of right ventricular function and hemodynamics after pulmonary embolism. Chest 1974;65:534–43.
17. Sasahara AA, Canilla JE, Morje RL. *et al.* Clinical and physiologic studies in pulmonary thromboembolism. Am J Cardiol 1967;20:10–20.
18. McIntyre K, Sasahara A. The hemodynamic response to pulmonary embolism in patients without prior cardiopulmonary disease. Am J Cardiol 1971;28:288–94.
19. Albert JS, Rickman FJ, Howe JP. Left ventricular function in massive pulmonary embolism. Chest 1977;71:108–11.
20. Fluck D, Chandraseker R, Gardner F: Left ventricular hypertrophy in chronic bronchitis. Br Heart J 1966;28:92–7.
21. Spain D, Hendler B. Chronic cor pulmonale: sixty cases studied at necropsy. Arch Intern Med 1946;77:37.
22. Kountz W, Alexander H, Prinzmetal M. The heart in emphysema. Am Heart J 1936;11:163.
23. Burrows B, Kettel LJ, Niden AH. *et al.* Patterns of cardiovascular dysfunction in chronic obstructive lung disease. N Eng J Med 1972;286:912–18.
24. Khaja F, Parker J. Right and left ventricular performance in chronic obstructive lung disease. Am Heart J 1971;82:319–27.
25. Slutskey R, Hooper W, Ackerman W. *et al.* Evaluation of left ventricular function in chronic pulmonary disease by exercise gated equilibrium radionuclide angiography. Am Heart J 1981;101:414–20.
26. Matthay RA, Berger HJ, Davies RA. *et al.* Right and left ventricular exercise performance in chronic obstructive pulmonary disease: radionuclide assessment. Ann Int Med 1980;93:234–9.
27. Rao B, Cohen K, Eldridge F. *et al.* Ventricular failure secondary to chronic pulmonary disease. Am J Med 1968;45:229–41.
28. Steele P, Ellis JH, Van Dyke D. *et al.* Left ventricular ejection fraction in severe chronic obstructive airway disease. Am J Med 1975;59:21–8.
29. Macnee W, Xue OF, Hannan WJ. *et al.* Assessment by radionuclide angiography of right and left ventricular function in chronic bronchitis and emphysema. Thorax 1983;38:494–500.
30. Bergofsky EH. Tissue oxygen delivery and cor pulmonale in chronic obstructive pulmonary disease. N Eng J Med 1983;308:1902.
31. Rubin LJ, Handel F, Peter RH. The effect of oral hydralazine on right ventricular end diastolic pressure in patients with right ventricular failure. Circ 1982;65:1369.
32. Sarnoff SJ, Berglund E. Ventricular function. Circ 1954;9:706.

33. Seibold H, Henze E: Right ventricular function in patients with chronic obstructive pulmonary disease. Klin Wochenschr 1985;63:1041.
34. Berger HS, Matthay RA, Lake J. *et al.* Assessment of cardiac performance and quantitative radionuclide angiocardiography: right ventricular ejection fraction with reference to chronic obstructive pulmonary disease. Am J Cardiol 1978;41:897–905.
35. Korr KS, Gandsman EJ, Winkler ML. *et al.* Hemodynamic correlation of right ventricular ejection fraction measured with gated radionuclide angiocardiography. Am J Cardiol 1982;49:71–7.
36. Laks MM, Garner D, Swan HJ. Volumes and compliances measured simultaneously in the right and left ventricle of the dog. Cir Res 1967;20:565.
37. Henderson Y, Prince SA. The relative systolic discharges of the right and left ventricle and their bearing on pulmonary congestion and depletion. Heart 1914;5:217–26.
38. Kounitz WB, Alexander HL, Prinzmetal M: The heart in emphysema. Am Heart J 1936;11:163–72.
39. Parker RL. Pulmonary emphysema: a study of its relation to the heart and the pulmonary arterial system. Ann In Med 1940;14:795–809.
40. Weber KT, Janicki JS, Shroffs. *et al.* Contractile mechanics and interaction of the right and left ventricle. Am J Cardiol 1981;47:686–95.
41. Stool EW, Mullins CB, Leshin SJ. *et al.* Dimensional change of the left ventricle during acute pulmonary arterial hypertension in dogs. Am J Cardiol 1974;33:868–75.
42. Meerson FZ. The myocardium in hypertension, hypertrophy and heart failure. Circ Res 1969;25:1.

28. Variables affecting cardiac output in endocrine disorders

RALPH ABRAHAM

Endocrine disorders present difficult clinical situations in which to understand the etiology of the resulting changes in cardiac function. Apart from the relative low prevalence of these disorders, the presentations are inevitably complicated either by other confounding diseases such as hypertension or hypopituitarism which themselves affect cardiac function or by therapy whose effects are long term (as with radiotherapy for acromegaly). In this chapter, the effects on cardiac function in acromegaly, thyroid disease and phaeochromocytomas will be reviewed.

Acromegaly

Cardiac enlargement in acromegaly is common and has been confirmed at autopsy by many investigators [1–3] ever since its first description by Pierre Marie in 1886 [4]. In "acromegalic" rats bearing growth hormone secreting tumours, heart weight was also found to be increased by 138% above control values with smaller increases being found in skeletal muscle [5]; however, when expressed as the ventricular/body weight ratio, there was no change in one study [6]. In these rats with transplanted growth hormone producing tumours, histology of the heart showed hypertrophy of muscle fibres but none of the additional changes such as interstitial fibrosis and lymphomononuclear infiltrates found in human acromegalic heart [3].

Acromegalic patients studied with echocardiography and systolic time intervals have confirmed the increase in left ventricular mass [7–9]. Mather (1979) found that 14 out of 24 acromegalic patients, without any history of ischaemic heart disease or cardiac failure, had a left ventricular mass greater than 200 g. However, only 4 of these had hypertension and the three highest weights were found in patients with a normal blood pressure suggesting that the cardiac hypertrophy was not secondary to hypertension. Most had been treated with radiotherapy or pituitary surgery and had varying initial growth hormone levels though normal values were present in 13 out of 20 of the patients studied. There was no correlation between the measured left ventricular mass and simultaneous growth hormone levels or the duration of the acromegaly.

Asymmetric interventricular septal hypertrophy has also been noted [5,

A.-M. Salmasi and A.S. Iskandrian (eds): Cardiac output and regional flow in health and disease, 383–393.
© 1993 *Kluwer Academic Publishers. Printed in the Netherlands.*

10]. In 5 out of 24 of Jenkins series, the septum was disproportionately thick but the septum-posterior ventricular wall ratio was increased in only 3 patients. It was felt that this frequency was no greater than that reported for other types of cardiac hypertrophy and was not a special feature of acromegaly.

The cause of the cardiac enlargement in acromegaly is complex. Accompanying hypertension and coronary artery disease complicate most cases while diabetes is also not infrequently present. However, as mentioned above, cardiac enlargement can occur in the absence of these complications and this has led some authors to argue for a specific heart disease of acromegaly [2, 11]. It has been proposed that this might occur as a direct result of the action of growth hormone on locally produced IGF 1 [2, 11].

As always, work on animal models provides greater insight than can be obtained from the study of heterogeneous groups of patients with acromegaly. Recent work [6] in rats bearing growth hormone producing tumours have provided more direct evidence of a direct influence of growth hormone on cardiac function. Maximum isometric force of papillary muscles (normalised per cross-sectional area) increased markedly whereas the maximum unloaded shortening velocity did not change. This occurred despite a marked isomyosin shift towards V3 myosin. The increased curvature of the force-velocity relationship indicated that muscles contracted more economically, again suggesting the involvement of V3 myosin. There was a lack of any change in the Ca^{++} and actin-activated myosin ATPase activities; only the V3 enzymatic sites were involved in total ATPase activity. Chronic growth hormone secretion in these animals leads to a unique pattern of myocardial adaptation which allows the muscle to improve its contractile performance and economy using the mechanism of myosin phenoconversion and the accompanying increase in the number of active enzymatic sites.

Not all investigators agree that there is a direct influence of growth hormone on cardiac muscle fibres or that there exists a specific acromegalic cardiomyopathy [12]. Cardiac failure does occur in acromegaly even when other established causes of heart muscle disease are absent [1, 2, 11–13] and evidence from postmortem studies show an "abnormal" myocardium in 59% of cases and "definite myocarditis" in 26% [3]. These pathological findings may explain the high prevalence of arrhythmias in patients with acromegaly (14 out of 34) in the study reported by Jenkins 1982 [5].

Functional studies in patients have tended to confirm the finding that left ventricular dysfunction does not occur unless other cardiac disease is present. Using systolic time interval measurements, it was found that the preejection period/left ventricular ejection time ratio obtained from phonocardiography, carotid pulse tracing and electrocardiography was abnormal in only 6 out of 10 patients, four of whom also had hypertension and 2 of whom had ischaemic heart disease [14]. Only one of their patients (with Addison's disease) also had an abnormal ejection fraction. Other investigators using both double M-mode echocardiography and radionuclide angiography have come to the same conclusions [7, 8, 15, 16]. Echocardiographic data have to be assessed carefully in acromegaly especially if they are used to assess left ventricular function as the assumptions necessary to calculate ejection fraction can make the technique relatively insensitive. Further errors result from errors in measuring wall thickness and cavity size as these are generally exaggerated when volumes are calculated.

Some authorities feel that there is increasing evidence that radionuclide measurements of diastolic function are more sensitive than measurements of ejection fraction in assessing subclinical cardiac function. Rodrigues and associates used electrocardiography, exercise testing and stress thallium-201 scintigraphy to exclude hypertension and subclinical coronary artery disease in a heterogenous group of 24 patients with acromegaly [17]. Only 7 out of 24 of these patients had a raised growth hormone at the time of study. Left ventricular hypertrophy was found in 12 patients and increased left ventricular mass in 17. There was no correlation between left ventricular wall thickness or left ventricular mass and peak filling rate. However, three patients with no evidence of hypertension or ischaemic heart disease had a dilated left ventricular cavity. As in other studies [7, 9, 14], the finding of a high preejction period/left ventricular ejection time ratio was generally only found in the small proportion of patients with coexisting coronary artery disease. Although no abnormality in systolic function was detected, diastolic indices remained abnormal on exercise even when coronary artery disease and hypertension had been excluded. There was a highly significant difference in resting peak filling rate, the diastolic peak filling rate was reduced and the time to peak filling rate prolonged indicating impaired diastolic relaxation. These findings were more marked in acromegalics with hypertension. As there was no correlation between diastolic filling variables and left ventricular wall thickness or left ventricular mass, it is unlikely that reduced compliance was due to the increased left ventricular mass. It is possible tha the interstitial fibrosis and mononuclear infiltrates first described in human acromegalic heart by Lie and colleagues may underly these functional abnormalities [3].

Treatment of acromegaly is associated with some reversal of the cardiac enlargement as patients with serum growth hormone in the normal range had only moderate or normal left ventricular mass [5]. In patients treated with octreotide (a long-acting somatostatin analogue), heart rate and blood pressure decreased after one year so once again indirect effects on the change in left ventricular mass are relevant [18].

Phaechromocytomas

Phaechromocytomas, especially when more commonly secreting noradrenaline, lead to intermittent or persistent hypertension. Predominantly adrenaline-secreting tumours are suspected in patients who are predominantly normotensive with intermittent or persistent tachycardia. Control of the hypertension is usually satisfactorily achieved with alpha adrenergic receptor antagonists with the subsequent addition of β receptor antagonists in many cases [19]. Heart failure is unusual though in one series of six patients 5 died in pulmonary oedema within 24 hours of onset of symptoms; all had normal sized hearts but focal myocardial necrosis was present at necropsy [20].

Concentric left hypertrophy is an expected result of the hypertension if it has been present long enough [21] but asymmetric septal hypertrophy [22], systolic anterior motion of the mitral apparatus [21, 22] and dilated cardiomyopathy [23–25] have also been described. Many of these changes appear reversible and marked improvement of left ventricular function with alpha and beta blockade has been shown with two-dimensional echocardiography and radionuclide angiography in a patient with catecholamine induced cardiomyopathy [26].

Captopril has also been shown to improve the hypertension caused by catecholamine secreting tumours in rats with implanted phaeochromocytomas [27–30]. The blood pressure reduction occurred despite continuing high levels of catecholamines and the histological changes of catecholamine-induced cardiomyopathy were considerably improved. These animals did not have raised renins even though catecholamine-induced activation of β-adrenergic receptors in the kidney is a well known stimulus for renin release. Similar improvements in these experimental models of phaeochromocytoma also occur after clonidine therapy [31]. The mechanism by which ACE inhibitors lower blood pressure in phaeochromocytomas is not known. An effect on catecholamine sensitivity possibly directly via catecholamine receptors seems likely as phenylephrine-induced contractions in aortic ring segments is markedly desensitised by captopril.

Van Vliet (1966) first showed the distinct histological features (distinct foci of mixed inflammatory cells, myofibrillar degeneration and interstitial and replacement fibrosis) in 15 out of 26 patients with phaeochromocytomas defining the histological nature of the cardiomyopathy caused by excess catecholamines [32]. The focal "contraction band" myocardial necrosis with associated chronic mononuclear cell inflammatory reaction leads to focal myocardial fibrosis [33, 34].

Thyroid heart disease

Thyroid hormones act on every cell in the body acting primarily to increase O_2 consumption and substrate utilisation. This shows itself as an increased basal metabolic rate, for long one of the standard methods of measuring thyroid status in man. The increased basal metabolic rate is accompanied by an increase in cardiac output. The heart has been thought for many years to be a major target organ for thyroid hormones and thyrotoxicosis was first thought to be a disease of the heart.

Heart failure in thyrotoxicosis may be complicated by intrinsic heart disease with decompensation produced by peripheral vasodilatation or rate and rhythm induced impairments of ventricular filling. Clinical thyrotoxic heart disease is often complicated by rhythm disturbances. In one series, as many as 43% of 150 thyrotoxic patients had atrial arrhythmias with only 5% having cardiac failure without an accompanying arrhythmia [35]. Heart failure in thyrotoxicosis is therefore commonly a consequence of a supraventricular tachycardia [36–38] and this is much more likely after exercise in thyrotoxics [38]. However, there have been reports of heart failure related only to thyrotoxicosis and reversible after control of the thyrotoxicosis [39]. Forfar demonstrated progressive impairment of myocardial contractility with exertion arguing that a specific reversible cardiomyopathy was the cause [40]. A similar impairment of myocardial contractility has been found by Goto in isolated left ventricles of thyrotoxic rabbits [41]. The O2 consumption per beat (VO2)/the systolic pressure-volume area (PVA) and the VO2/force-time integral (FTI) and end-systolic pressure-volume relations were assessed in cross circulated isovolumically beating hearts and used to measure the chemomechanical energy transduction efficiency of the contractile machinery and the energy cost of excitation-contraction coupling. Goto found that the thyrotoxic left ventricle has a decreased contractile efficiency and increased energy cost of excitation-contraction coupling and the decreased contractile efficiency in hyperthyroid hearts is probably due to the increased V1/V3 ratio of the myosin isoform component [41].

Recently there have been considerable developments in the understanding of the biochemical basis of thyroid hormone action in the heart [42]. Thyroid hormones lead to an increase in myosin-mediated ATP hydrolysis in the heart and this is regulated by other myofibrillar proteins and by the cytosolic concentration of Ca^{++} [43–46]. Increased myosin ATPase activity leads to increased muscle fibre shortening [47]. In addition less ATP goes into providing energy for the contractile purpose and more of it goes toward heat production which causes a decrease in the efficiency of the contractile process. Both extranuclear and nuclear mechanisms are involved. Nuclear T3 effects work by binding of T3 to specific nuclear receptor.proteins resulting in the increased transcription of T3 responsive cardiac genes especially that of the myosin heavy chain alpha gene. In thyrotoxic myocardial hypertrophy, the isozymic shift from V3 to V1 myosins is progressive, region specific and directly correlated with duration of the hyperthyroidism [48].

Experimentally induced hyperthyroidism in rats is associated with cardiac hypertrophy, increased heart rate and increased myocardial contractility *in vivo* [49–51]. The hypertrophy almost certainly results from the increased heart rate and contractility as these two factors are major determinants of myocardial oxygen demand which in turn is a powerful stimulus to cardiac muscle growth. Thyroid hormones can be shown to have a direct effect on the heart increasing chronotropism and inotropism of cardiac muscle fibres. At the cellular level there is an increaed rate of diastolic depolarisation and decreased duration of the action potential of sino-atrial node cells [52, 53].

There is also increased spontaneous sarcoplasmic reticulum Ca^{++} release with depletion of sarcoplasmic reticulum Ca stores and reduction of subsequent twitch amplitude [54]. This is the basis for the increased prevalence of atrial premature contractions, paroxysmal atrial tachycardia and atrial fibrillation in thyrotoxicosis. Atrial fibrillation occurs in 10–22% of patients [55, 56] and this percentage increases in patients over the age of 65 years. These arrhythmias are frequently the cause of high output cardiac failure. Ventricular muscle from hyperthyroid rats are more prone to develop triggered activity under conditions believed to cause myoplasmic Ca^{++} overload; the severity of reperfusion arrhythmias are also enhanced in hyperthyroid cardiac muscle preparations [57].

Left ventricular contractile force is increased more than would be expected from a consideration of Starling's law; the preejection phase of the systolic time intervals decreases together with shortened or unaltered duration of electromechanical systole with an increase in stroke volume as well as heart rate [58]. Heart rate increases 40% together with an increase in stroke volume and cardiac work and a doubling of left ventricular work [43, 44, 59–61]. Other contractile properties such as the rate of ventricular pressure development and the velocity of contraction are also uniformly increased [38, 62–64]. Tseng has shown that hyperthyroidism is associated with a significantly shortened mean isovolumetric contraction time, preejection period (PEP), and PEP/left ventricular ejection time (LVET) [65]. Even subclinical hyperthyroidism (normal free T4 and T3 but suppressed TSH) had isovolumetric contraction time, PEP and PEP/LVET significantly shortened.

Not all investigators have found abnormal cardiac contractility when patients are studied. Smallridge found normal cardiac responses though exercise time was increased once patients became euthyroid again. 2D M-mode echocardiograms showed all measures of diastolic flow velocity, deceleration and compliance to be enhanced in thyrotoxicosis [63, 66]. Some of these parameters improved with betablockade and all were reversible when the patients became euthyroid again.

Despite the evidence that thyroid hormones have a direct effect on the heart, Klein has presented much evidence that the changes in cardiac output in thyrotoxicosis are more a response to the direct effects of thyroid hormones on the peripheral vascular system [67]. It is known that one of the earliest responses to an increase in circulating thyroid hormones is a decrease in peripheral resistance with an increase in blood flow to the skin, kidneys, heart and muscles [37, 38, 44, 68–72]. There is also an increase in blood volume and this increase is closely correlated with the increase in the BMR and changes in direct relation with changes in thyroid status [73]. The mechanism of this seems to be through erythropoiesis and erythropoietin [45]. This increase in blood volume contributes to the rise in right atrial pressure and the increase in cardiac preload and cardiac output [44, 74]. The changes in afterload, preload and heart rate in hyperthyroidism all vary in a way which enhances noninvasive measures of cardiac contractility [62–64, 72, 75].

The decrease in peripheral resistance is reversible with beta adrenergic blockers though atropine also has a partial effect [76]. This occurs despite the fact that there is no increase in circulating catecholamines in hyperthyroidism [77]. The ability to block the elevated cardiac output in thyrotoxicosis by pharmacologically reversing the changes in systemic vascular resistance is evidence that the altered cardiovascular haemodynamics of hyperthyroidism occur as a result of changes in the peripheral tissues. It was shown that a significant decrease in cardiac output after phenylephrine raised peripheral resistance in hyperthyroid subjects [70]. The mechanism by which thyroid hormones affects peripheral resistance is not fully understood. There is probably a direct effect on Na and K flux in smooth muscle cells [78, 79] which leads to a decrease in smooth muscle contractility and vascular resistance [71].

Factors related to cardiac growth include workload, pressure and volume work, nutritional status and hormones including GH and catecholamines as well as thyroxine. The administration of excess thyroxine leads to an increase in left ventricular weight [80–82]. Klein has argued that thyroxine induced cardiac hypertrophy is mediated by increased cardiac work – firstly propranolol inhibits thyroxine induced hypertrophy and secondly, in experiments with heterotopic cardiac transplants (not connected to the circulation but beating normally and perfused by identical blood) there are no changes of hypertrophy and there was a lack of a direct effect of T4 on amino acid incorporation into myocardial contractile protein synthesis in the heterotopically transplanted heart [80].

Hypothyroidism

The cardiovascular clinical manifestations of hypothyroidism, particularly when severe and longstanding, are overt and often important clues to diagnosis. Bradycardia is usual and the peripheries are cool with a subnormal temperature often recordable. The heart sounds may be distant and the jugular venous pulse raised particularly if there is a small pericardial effusion present (these effusions rarely compromise cardiac function as they are seldom large enough to impair diastolic filling and develop slowly). They can be shown to be present by echocardiography in 30% of cases subclinically [83, 84].

The characteristic haemodynamic changes in hypothyroidism are diametrically opposite to those of hyperthyroidism [37, 59] with a low cardiac index decreased stroke volume, decreased vascular volume and increased systemic vascular resistance [37, 62]. The decline in cardiac output seems appropriate for the decrease in total body oxygen consumption [37].

There does not appear to be any evidence for cardiac failure in myxoedema [85]. The electrocardiogram shows minor repolarisation changes but occasionally gross T wave inversion occurs which is reversible with T4 replacement. Further the haemodynamic responses obtained using radionuclide ventriculography with simultaneous R heart catheterisation (cardiac output, heart rate, stroke volume and left ventricular ejection fraction) in 9 hypothyroid patients to exercise were almost normal (90% of predicted normal value) [86]. In all patients peak filling rate was lower but time to peak filling was not affected by the thyroid state. The authors concluded that the rate of active diastolic relaxation is decreased in short duration hypothyroidism.

When heart failure occurs in hypothyroidism, it generally represents an exacerbation of preexisting intrinsic cardiac disease by the superimposed haemodynamic effects of thyroid hormone deficiency: namely bradycardia, diminished myocardial contractility and markedly increased peripheral cardiovascular resistance [85]. Numerous noninvasive [62, 87] and invasive [85] studies have demonstrated the reversibility of reduced myocardial contractility after treatment. Systolic time interval measurements have confirmed the significantly lengthened isovolumetric contraction time, the preejection period (PEP) and the PEP/left ventricular ejection time though only in overt hypothyroidism and not in subclinical hypothyroidism [65].

Replacement therapy with thyroxine is always cautious as left ventricular failure or angina with infarction may occur. In fact angina oftens improves with increasing doses of thyroxine and there is rarely need for invasive intervention before a euthyroid state is achieved.

References

1. Hejtmaneik MR, Bradfield JY, Hermann GR. Acromegaly and the heart: a clinical and pathological study. Ann Int Med 1951;34:1445–56.
2. Courville CB, Mason VR. The heart in acromegaly. Arch Int Med 1938;61:704–13.
3. Lie JT, Grossman SJ. Pathology of the heart in acromegaly: anatomic findings in 27 autopsied patients. Am Heart J 1980;100:41–52.
4. Huchard H. Anatomie pathologique, lesions et troubles cardio-vasculaires de l'acromegalie. J Practiciens 1895;9:249.
5. JS Jenkins. Acromegalic heart disease. In Evans T, Mitchell AG (eds): Specific heart muscle disease. Bristol: John Wright & Sons, Ltd. 1983;62–74.
6. Timsit J, Riou B, Bertheral J et al. Effects of chronic growth hormone hypersecretion on intrinsic contractility, energetics, isomyosin pattern and myosin adenosine triphosphatase activity of rat left ventricle. J Clin Invest 1990;86(2):507–15.
7. Martins JB, Kerber RE, Sherman BM et al. Cardiac size and function in acromegaly. Circulation 1977;56:863–9.
8. Savage DD, Henry WL, Eastman RC et al. Echocardiographic assessment of cardiac anatomy and function in acromegalic patients. Am J Med 1979;67:823–9.
9. Mather HM, Boyd MJ, Jenkins JS. Heart size and function in acromegaly. B Heart J 1979;41:697–701.
10. Hearne MJ, Sherber HS, de Leon AC. Asymmetric septal hypertrophy in acromegaly – an echocardiographic study [abstract]. Circulation 1975;51(52 suppl II):35.
11. Pepine CJ, Aloia J. Heart muscle disease in acromegaly. Am J Med 1970;48:530–4.
12. McGuffin WL, Sherman BM, Roth J et al. Acromegaly and cardiovascular disorders. Ann Intern Med 1974;81:11–8.

13. Rossi L, Thiene G, Caregaro L *et al*. Dysrhythmias and sudden death in acromegalic heart disease. A clinico pathologic study. Chest 1977;72:495–8.
14. Jonas EA, Aloia JF, Lane FJ. Evidence of subclinical heart muscle dysfunction in acromegaly. Chest 1975;67:190–4.
15. O'Keefe JC, Grant SJ, Wiseman JC *et al*. Acromegaly and the heart – echocardiographic and nuclear imaging studies. Aust NZ J Med 1982;12:603–7.
16. Griebenow R, Kramer L, Frangenberg U *et al*. Cardiac function in endocrine diseases. I Acromegaly. Klin Wochenschr. 1989;67(22):1126–31.
17. Rodrigues EA, Caruana MP, Lahiri A *et al*. Subclinical cardiac dysfunction in acromegaly: evidence for a specific disease of heart muscle. Br Heart J 1989;62:185–94.
18. Thuesen L, Christensen SE, Weeke J *et al*. The cardiovascular effects of octreotide treatment in acromegaly: an echocardiographic study. Clin Endocrin 1989;30(6):619–25.
19. Manger WM, Gifford RW, Hoffman BB. Phaeochromocytoma: a clinical and experimental overview. Curr Prob Cancer 1985;9:5–89.
20. Sardesai SH, Mourant AJ, Sivathandon Y *et al*. Phaeochromocytoma and catecholamine induced cardiomyopathy presenting as heart failure. Br Heart J 1990;63(4):234–7.
21. Cueto L, Arriaga J, Zinser J. Echocardiographic changes in phaeochromocytoma. Chest 1979;76:600–1.
22. Mardini MK. Echocardiographic findings in phaeochromocytoma. Chest 1982;81:394–5.
23. Schaffer MS, Zuberbuhler P, Wilson G *et al*. Catecholamine cardiomyopathy: an unusual presentation of phaeochromocytoma in children. J Paediat 1981;99:276–9.
24. Lam JB, Shub C, Sheps SG. Reversible dilatation of hypertrophied left ventricle in pheochromocytoma: serial two-dimensional echocardiographic observations. Am J Heart 1985,109:613–5.
25. Imperato-McGinley J, Gautier T, Ehlers K *et al*. Reversibility of catecholamine-induced dilated cardiomyopathy in a child with phaechromocytoma. N Engl J Med 1987;316:793–7.
26. Sadowski D, Cujec B, McMeekin JD *et al*. Reversibility of catecholamine-induced cardiomyopathy in a woman with pheochromocytoma; Can Med AJ 1989;141:923–4.
27. Hu Z, Billingham M, Tuck M *et al*. Captopril improves hypertension and cardiomyopathy in rats with phaeochromocytoma. Hypertension 1990;15:210–5.
28. Loute G, Guffens P, Waucquez J-L *et al*. Effect of captopril on hypertension due to pheochromocytoma. Lancet 1984;2:175.
29. Israeli A, Gottehrer N, Gavish D *et al*. Captopril and phaeochromocytoma. Lancet 1985;1:278–9.
30. Blam R. Enalapril in pheochromocytoma. Ann Intem Med 1987;106:326–7.
31. Hoffman BB. Observations in New England Deaconess Hospital rats harboring phaeochromocytoma. Clin Invest Med 1987;10:555–60.
32. Van Vliet PT, Burchell HB, Titus JL. Focal myocarditis associated with phaeochromocytoma. N Engl J Med 1966;274:1102–8.
33. Silver MD. Myocardial lesions in pheochromocytoma. Can Med Ass J 1990;142(2):99.
34. Kline IK. Myocardial alterations associated with pheochromocytomas. Am J Pathol 1961;38:539–51.
35. Sandler G, Wilson GM. The nature and prognosis of heart disease in thyrotoxicosis. Q J Med 1959;28:347–69.
36. Forfar JC, Caldwell GC. Hyperthyroid heart disease. Clin Endocrinol Metab 1985;14:491–509.
37. Graettinger JS, Muenster JJ, Selverstone LA *et al*. A correlation of clinical and haemodynamic in patients with hyperthyroidism with and without congestive heart failure. J Clin Invest 1959;38:1316–27.
38. Ikram H. The nature and prognosis of thyrotoxic heart disease. Q J Med 1985;54:19–28.
39. Likoff WB, Levine SA. Thyrotoxicosis as the sole cause of heart failure. Am J Med Sci 1943;206:425–34.

40. Forfar JC, Muir AL, Sawers SA *et al*. Abnormal left ventricular function in hyperthyroidism: evidence for a possible reversible cardiomyopathy. New Eng J Med 1982;307:1165–70.
41. Goto Y, Slinker BK, LeWinter MM. Decreased contractile efficiency and increased nonmechanical energy cost in hyperthyroid rabbit heart. Relation between O2 consumption and systolic pressure-volume area or force-time integral. Circ Res 1990;66(4):999–1011.
42. Dillmann WH. Biochemical basis of thyroid hormone action in the heart. Am J Med 1990;88:626–30.
43. Klein I, Levey GS. New perspectives on thyroid hormone, catecholamines and the heart. Am J Med 1981;76:167–71.
44. Morkin E, Flink IL, Goldman S. Biochemical and physiologic effects of thyroid hormone on cardiac performance. Prog Cardiovasc Dis 1983;25:435–64.
45. Klein I, Levey GS. Unusual manifestahons of hypothyroidism. Arch Int Med 1984;144:123–8.
46. Suko J. Alterations of Ca^{++} uptake and Ca^{++} activated ATPase of cardiac sarcoplasmic reticulum in hyper- and hypothyroidism. Biochem Biophys Acta 1971;252:324–7.
47. Schwartz K, Lecarpentier Y, Martin JL *et al*. Myosin isoenzyme distribution correlates with speed of myocardial contraction. J Moll Cell Cardiol 1981;13:1071–5.
48. Seiden D, Srivatsan M, Navidad PA. Changes in myosin isozyme expression during cardiac hypertrophy in hyperthyroid rabbits. Acta Anat Basel. 1989;135(3):222–30.
49. Taylor RG, Covell JW, Ross J Jr. Influence of the thyroid state on left ventricular tension-velocity relations in the intact sedate dog. J Clin Invest 1969;48:775–84.
50. Strauer BE, Scherpe A. Experimental hyperthyroidism 1: Haemodynamics and contractility *in situ*. Basic Res Cardiol 1975;70:115–29.
51. Goldman S, Olajos M, Griedman H *et al*. Left ventricular performance in conscious thyrotoxic calves. Am J Physiol 1982;242:H113–21.
52. Johnson PN, Freedberg AS, Marshall JM. Action of thyroid hormone on the transmembrane potential from sino-atrial cells and atrial muscle cells in isolated atria of rabbits. Cardiology 1973;58:273.
53. Arnsdorf MF, Childers RW. Atrial electrophysiology in experimental hyperthyroidism in rabbits. Circ Res 1970;26:575.
54. Josephson RA, Spurgeon HA, Lakatta EG. The hyperthyroid heart. An analysis of systolic and diastolic properties in single rat ventricular myocytes. Circ Res 1990;66(3):773–81.
55. Sandler G, Wilson GM. The nature and prognosis of heart disease in thyrotoxicosis. Q J Med 1959;28:347–69.
56. Agner T, Abundal T, Thorsteinzson B *et al*. A reevaluation of atrial fibrillation in thyrotoxicosis. Dan Med Bull 1984;31:157–9.
57. Miyazawa K, Hashimoto H, Uematsu T *et al*. Electrophysiological abnormalities and enhanced reperfusion arrhythmias in the isolated hearts of hyperthyroid rats. Br J Pharm 1989;97(4):1093–100.
58. DeGroot EJ, Leonard JJ. Hyperthyroidism as a high cardiac output state. Am Heart J 1970;79:265.
59. Smallridge RC, Goldman MH, Rianes K *et al*. Rest and exercise left ventricular ejection fraction before and after therapy in young adults with hyperthyroidism and hypothyroidism. Am J Cardiol 1987;60:929–31.
60. DeGroot LJ. Thyroid and the heart. Mayo Clin Proc 1972;47:864–71.
61. Grossman W, Rubin NL, Johnson LW *et al*. The enhanced myocardial contractility of thyrotoxicosis. Ann Inter Med 1971;74:869–74.
62. Amidi M, Leon DF, DeGroot WJ *et al*. Effect of the thyroid state on myocardial contractility and ventricular ejection rate in man. Circulation 1968;38:229–39.
63. Friedman MJ, Okada RD, Ewy GA *et al*. Left ventricular systole and diastolic function in hyperthyroidism Am Heart J 1982;104:1303–8.
64. Nixon JV, Anderson RJ, Cohen ML. Alterations in left ventricular mass and performance in patients treated effectively for hyperthyroidism. Am J Med 1979;67:268–76.
65. Tseng KH, Walfish PG, Persaud JA *et al*. Concurrent aortic and mitral valve echocardiogra-

phy permits measurement of systolic time intervals as an index of peripheral tissue thyroid functional status. J Clin End Metab 1989;69(3):633–8.

66. Mintz G, Pizzarello R, Goldman M *et al.* Cardiac diastolic function in hyperthyroidism: response to therapy. Clin Res 1989:37:520A.
67. Klein I. Thyroid hormone and the cardiovascular system. Am J Med 1990;88:631–7.
68. Kapitola J, Vilimovska D. Inhibition of the early circulatory effects of triiodothyronine in rats by propranolol. Physiol Bohemoslov 1981;30:347–52.
69. Klein I. Thyroid hormone and high blood pressure. In: Laragh JH, Brenner BM, Kaplan NM (eds), Endocrine mechanisms in hypertension. Vol 2, New York: Raven Press, 1989:61–80.
70. Theilen EO, Wilson WR. Haemodynamic effects of peripheral vasoconstriction in normal and thyrotoxic subjects. J Appl Physiol 1967;22:207–10.
71. Klein I. Thyroid hormone and high blood pressure. In: Laragh JH, Brenner BM, Kaplan NM (eds), Endocrine mechanisms in hypertension. Vol. 2, New York: Raven Press, 1989:1661–74.
72. Merillon JP, Passa PH, Chastre J *et al.* Left ventricular function and hyperthyroidism. Br Heart J 1981;46:137–43.
73. Gibson JG, Harris AW. Clinical studies of the blood volume. V. Hyperthyroidism and myxedema. J Clin Invest 1938;18:59–65.
74. Guyton AC. The relationship of cardiac output and arterial pressure control. Circulation 1981;64:1079–88.
75. Feldman T, Borow KM, Sarne D *et al.* Myocardial mechanics in hyperthyroidism: importance of left ventricular loading conditions, heart rate and contractile state. J Am Coll Cardiol 1986;7:967–74.
76. Kontos HA, Shapiro W, Mauck P Jr *et al.* Mechanisms of certain abnormalities of the circulation to the limbs in thyrotoxicosis. J Clin Invest 1965;41:947–56.
77. Coulombe P, Dussault JH, Walker P. Plasma catecholamine concentrations in hyperthyroidism and hypothyroidism. Metabolism 1976;25:973.
78. Haber RS, Loeb JN. Effect of 3,5,3'triiodothyronine treatment on potassium efflux from isolated rat diaphragm: role of increased permeability in the thermogenic response. Endocrinology 1982;3:1217–23.
79. Ismail-Beigi F, Haber RS, Loeb JN. Stimulation of active Na and K transport by thyroid hormone in a rat liver cell line: role of enhanced Na entry. Endocrinology 1986;119:2527–36.
80. Klein I, Hong C. Effects of thyroid hormone on the myosin content and myosin isoenzymes of the heterotopically transplanted heart. J Clin Invest 1986;77:1694–80.
81. Sanford CF, Griffin EE, Wildenthal K. Synthesis and degradation of myocardial protein during the development and regression of thyroxine-induced cardiac hypertrophy in rats. Circ Res 1978;43:688–94.
82. Klein I. Thyroxine-induced cardiac hypertrophy: time course of development and inhibition by propranolol. Endocrinology 1988;123:203–10.
83. Hardisty CA, Naik DR, Munro DS. Pericardial effusion in hypothyroidism. Clin Endoc 1980;13:349–54.
84. Kerber RE, Sherman B. Echocardiographic evaluation of pericardial effusion in myxoedema, incidence and biochemical and clinical correlation. Circulation 1975;52:823–7.
85. Graettinger JS, Muenster JJ, Checchia CS *et al.* Correlation of clinical and haemodynamic studies of patients with hypothyroidism. J Clin Invest 1958;37:502–10.
86. Wieshammer S, Keck FS, Waltzinger K *et al.* Left ventricular function at rest and during exercise in acute hypothyroidism. Br Heart J 1988;60:204–11.
87. Santos AD, Miller RP, Mathew PK *et al.* Echocardiographic characterization of the reversible cardiomyopathy of hypothyroidism. Am J Med 1980;68:675.

29. Variables affecting cardiac output in obesity and diabetes

RALPH ABRAHAM

In 1933, Smith and Willius first showed that mean weight of the heart was greater in obese subjects than in normal hearts (376 g versus 272 g) and in those patients that were both obese and hypertensive, the mean weight was even greater at 467 g [1]. The increased heart size associated with human obesity has been attributed to both an increased adiposity of the heart and ventricular hypertrophy [2–4]. In humans, two distinct patterns of fatty heart have been described. Lipid can accumulate in the cytoplasm [1] and fatty infiltration also occurs with accumulation of adipose tissue in the subepicardium and interstitially in the myocardium [1], particularly in the right ventricle and atrioventricular sulci [1, 5].

Any increase in body mass – whether predominantly of adipose or muscular tissue requires a higher cardiac output and expanded intravascular volume in order to meet higher metabolic demands [6, 7]. Provided that arterial blood pressure does not change, the increase in cardiac output is associated with a decrease in vascular resistance. Body Mass Index correlates inversely with left ventricular ejection fraction (LVEF) and directly with cardiac output and total blood volume [7, 8]. The increase in cardiac output in obesity (for an unchanged heart rate) occurs by means of an increased stroke volume and stroke work [2,6,7,9,10], though the LVEF may remain normal [10] or reduced in some morbidly obese patients [11]. Left ventricular filling pressure and volume increase, shifting left ventricular function to the left on the Frank-Starling curve leading to chamber dilatation. Left ventricular end-diastolic volume is increased [7, 12], a thicker interventricular septum and a larger thickness of the left ventricular posterior wall in systole have also been reported [12]. Nakajima (1985) also found increases in end-diastolic left ventricular dimension and stroke volume as absolute values [13, 14]. The left ventricular hypertrophy results in an increase in diastolic left ventricular dimension index (end diastolic dimension/cube root of body surface area) and stroke index, normalising the increase in wall stress and maintaining unchanged left ventricular function. Thus myocardial mass increases and left ventricular hypertrophy of the eccentric type (i.e. a parallel increase in wall thickening and chamber dilatation) follows [14]. Left ventricular dilatation and hypertrophy however, increase diastolic stiffness and this loss of compliance results in a higher filling pressure [20].

In left ventricular dysfunction of all types, the preejection period (PEP)

A.-M. Salmasi and A.S. Iskandrian (eds): Cardiac output and regional flow in health and disease, 395–407.
© 1993 *Kluwer Academic Publishers. Printed in the Netherlands.*

obtained by measuring systolic time intervals (reflecting a reduced rate of contraction of myocardial fibres during the isovolumic contraction time from mitral valve closure to onset of ejection into the aorta), tends to increase while the left ventricular ejection time (LVET) decreases with an increase in the PEP/LVET ratio (after rate correction). The increase in PEP/LVET has been correlated with varying degrees of left ventricular hypertrophy and it represents a means of detecting early left ventricular dysfunction secondary to hypertrophy [15].

A number of important variables confound measurements of cardiac function in obesity. Abnormalities shown to occur in morbidly obese patients (>200% ideal body weight) may not be seen in milder more commonly seen obesity. Also abdominal or visceral obesity (usually characterised clinically by an increased waist : hip ratio or, as in the study of Nakajima and associates by computerised tomography of fat deposits in the abdomen) was found to be associated with a higher diastolic dimension and stroke indices than patients with more subcutaneous fat [16]. The duration of obesity at the time of study is also important and is an independent factor affecting cardiac function even in mild obesity [13]. Measurements of end diastolic dimension index, stroke index and radius/wall thickness ratio of the left ventricle were all positively correlated with the duration of obesity while ejection fraction is inversely correlated with the duration of obesity [17].

The most important confounding factor is the fact that obesity and hypertension are often present in the same patient. The high afterload of arterial hypertension leads to concentric hypertrophy space increase in muscle mass at the expense of chamber volume) while the high volume overload of obesity [6, 7] leads to increased preload and eccentric hypertrophy with parallel increases in left ventricular wall thickness and cavity dimensions [8, 17, 18]. This double burden often leads to early left ventricular dysfunction, left ventricular enlargement and premature congestive heart failure even if systemic arterial blood pressure is not elevated [2, 3, 19]. However, even in the absence of hypertension, alterations in left ventricular structure in extreme obesity are seen [4, 14, 17, 19, 21–23]. In between 32–56% of obese patients, an increase in left ventricular internal diastolic dimension, right ventricular internal dimension, left atrial dimension, ventricular septal and left ventricular posterior wall thickness was shown [14]. When hypertension and angiographically demonstrable coronary artery disease are excluded, Carabello and associates found the preload (end-diastolic stress) greater and the afterload (end-systolic stress) also greater in obese patients [24] but despite these abnormalities in loading conditions, the ejection fraction, the mean velocity of circumferential fiber shortening, the ratio of end-systolic stress/end-systolic volume index and the stress velocity of fiber shortening relations were all normal implying unchanged contractile function. Both concentric and eccentric left ventricular hypertrophy (with longstanding arterial hypertension) are associated with more premature ventricular contractions and higher grade arrythmias and are risk factors for mortality and morbidity independent of arterial pressure [25, 26].

Clinical assessment of left ventricular contractile function is often difficult and fraught with assumptions which depend partly on the method used and partly on the accompanying loading conditions. Fractional shortening can be obtained as the per cent change in left ventricular internal dimensions made at end-diastole and end-systole. Myocardial contractility, when evaluated using isovolumic or ejection phase indices of LV function is highly dependent on cardiac loading conditions [6, 13, 14, 17, 27]. De Divitis (1981) showed that the left ventricular contractile element velocity at zero load (VMax) was inversely correlated with body weight in 10 obese subjects [6]. Using the ratio of end-systolic wall stress/volume index, a load independent sensitive indicator of ventricular inotropic state, Garavaglia and associates (1988) found it to be reduced even in mild obesity and it also correlated with BMI and left ventricular mass index inversely [28]; load dependent indices (ejection fraction, fractional fibre shortening and velocity of circumferential fibre shortening) were found to be unchanged though M-mode echocardiographic studies have revealed a greater fractional shortening in the obese subject [11, 12]. The conclusion made by Garavaglia *et al.* that some obese patients have depressed myocardial contractility despite well preserved pump function seems reasonable in the light of all the available evidence.

In order to further analyse the mechanism behind the cardiac hypertrophy in obesity, we need to look at work done in animals. Wall thickening and concentric hypertrophy are usually observed in pressure overload conditions, whereas chronic volume overload results in a chamber enlargement and eccentric hypertrophy [29]. Where direct measurements of pressure-volume curves were obtained in lean and obese rat ventricles using a distensible fluid filled balloon placed in the left ventricle, obese and lean end-diastolic pressure-volume curves were not different implying no change in left ventricular chamber compliance [30]. The diminished ability to develop the same peak systolic stress from the same end-diastolic volume suggested that, in the obese rat, the hypertrophied left ventricle of the heart is dilated or that its contractility is depressed or both. Wall thickness to internal radius ratio of obese rat heart was also increased when values were compared at intraventricular volumes that yielded equal peak systolic stresses and this is consistent with hypertrophy resulting from a modest pressure overload though a component due to volume overload as well is not excluded.

Using radionuclide ventriculography and echocardiography, Alpert reported that obese patients with increased left ventricular mass commonly have abnormal left ventricular exercise responses even when resting left ventricular systolic function is normal [31]. Exercise produced no change in those with an increased left ventricular mass (10 out of 23 of the patients). Other investigators have also shown a strong positive correlation between left ventricular mass and the impaired LVEF response to exercise (r = 0.83)

[32]. The results suggest that an increased left ventricular mass predisposes morbidly obese patients to impairment of left ventricular systolic function during exercise.

Abnormalities have also been shown in left atrium emptying indices. The left atrial emptying index is thought to be an indicator of early diastolic abnormalities in the left ventricle [33]. Using electrocardiogrphy and M-mode echocardiography, the left atrium has been shown to be larger in obesity [14] and the left atrial emptying index was reduced especially if the obese subjects were also hypertensive [34].

It is well established that complications of morbid obesity such as hypoxia may produce pulmonary hypertension and clinical manifestations compatible with right ventricular dysfunction. Alpert et al. [31] showed that a significant negative correlation was also found between %IBW (r = 0.86) and internal dimensions of the right ventricle and the right ventricular exercise response. It was suggested that right ventricular dilatation may predispose to right and left ventricular systolic dysfunction.

Although cardiomegaly regresses during weight reduction [35], a review by Alexander concluded that cardiac hypertrophy was not reversible with weight loss [36] and more recent work on only 10 patients also showed nonsignificant reductions in interventricular septal thickness, left ventricular wall thickness and left ventricular volume [37]. However, other more recent studies have shown significant reduction in left ventricular mass after weight loss. In the study of MacMahon and associates in 1986, patients with a body mass index of >26 losing only 8 kg showed a small but significant decrease in left ventricular mass (20%), septal (14%) and posterior-wall thickness (11%) even though the hearts were of normal size before weight loss [38]. They concluded that changes in weight, independent of changes in blood pressure were directly associated with changes in left ventricular mass. The decrease in left ventricular mass was greater though than the decrease from surface area alone which could only account for 25% of the reduction in left ventricular mass. The remaining 75% change in left ventricular mass may be accounted for by sympathetic mechanisms (reduced heart rate) or through the reduction in plasma renin and aldosterone in hypertensive subjects after weight loss [39]. In spontaneously obese rats the major component of the weight loss from heart muscle is water [40]. It was reported that a weight loss of 55 kg reduced left ventricular chamber enlargement and improved systolic function with an increase in mean left ventricular fractional shortening in a subgroup with low preoperative LV fractional shortening [14]. However, in contrast to MacMahon's study, there was no reduction in septal or posterior wall thickness [14, 32] and this discrepancy remains unexplained and could be accounted for by patient selection and the presence of mild hypertension. Ramhamadany and associates (1989) showed that the resting left ventricular ejection fraction fell significantly only in obese patients who were hypertensive [32]. In this study, the impaired LVEF response to exercise returned to normal after weight loss in patients without coronary artery disease. Also Kinner (1985) showed that, after dieting, hypertensive but not normotensive obese patients had a significant decrease in systolic time intervals such as left ventricular ejection time and total electromechanical systole, myocardial oxygen consumption and cardiac output; there was no change in preejection index and stroke volume [41]. Rate corrected PEP and PEP/LVET were found to be lowered after dieting [42].

Diabetes

There is an increased mortality and morbidity from all cardiovascular causes in diabetes, especially in women, even when other risk factors are taken into account [43, 44]. Diabetic "cardiopathy" was a term coined to describe the large vessel coronary artery disease, diabetic cardiac autonomic neuropathy and small coronary arteriolar disease in diabetes [45]. Angina in patients with normal coronary arteries is commonly found in diabetes and was postulated to be caused by microvessel disease [46]. Conversely painless myocardial infarction has been noted in diabetes [47]. The term specific heart disease of diabetes has been recommended as a more accurate description of the pathology and functional abnormalities [48, 49].

Histological studies of the heart in diabetes have shown focal areas of fibrosis [50] or micro infarction of the myocardium [51]. Most postmortem studies included patients who had died from coronary artery disease. Specific myocardial hypertophy and interstitial fibrosis has often been noted in patients with diabetes and coronary artery disease [52–54], but also in patients without hypertension or coronary artery disease [55] where subendothelial proliferation in small intramural arteries has also been noted [56, 57]. The proliferative lesions and thickening of the walls of the intramural blood vessels are not common and it has therefore been suggested that myocardial fibrosis is of greater importance [58, 59]. Severe myocardial interstitial fibrosis is found in diabetes particularly when hypertension is present [60], but it is a non specific sequelae of any disease where there is dilatation or hypertrophy of the ventricle (e.g. hypertensive heart disease) and is found in non diabetic hypertensive heart disease as well [61, 62]. When endomyocardial biopsy specimens have been examined, no small vessel changes were seen [63] though there is an accumulation of collagen, often PAS positive, in the interstitium [55, 56, 58, 60, 64, 65]. This may be the cause of the intraventricular conduction disturbances present in some patients with diabetes [66]. Sutherland and associates showed histological changes including thickening of the arteriolar wall and prominent interstitial fibrosis of the myocardium but no myocardial capillary basal lamina thickening in normotensive patients without coronary artery disease [67].

There is no difference between diabetic and control subjects in resting cardiac output [68]. Resting work product was greatest in diabetic patients with autonomic neuropathy because of the increase in both resting heart rate and systolic blood pressure in these patients. Invasive studies of stroke volume and cardiac output in diabetic subjects showed that the increase in cardiac output was significantly reduced compared to control subjects due to both a smaller increase in stroke volume (starting from lower resting values) and a greater increase in systemic vascular resistance [69]. Few of these studies attempted to exclude underlying asymptomatic and silent coronary artery disease and this would particularly confound any measurements made after exercise. When this is done, there is abundant evidence supporting the concept of myocardial dysfunction separate from epicardial coronary artery disease in diabetes [70]. In the studies from Pfeifer's laboratory for example, the presence of autonomic neuropathy had a marked effect in reducing the increase in cardiac output at matched % maximum oxygen uptake; the maximum increase in work product was impaired in diabetes but not affected by autonomic neuropathy [68].

The interstitial fibrosis found in the myocardium in diabetes manifests itself by abnormal systolic time intervals – a shorter left ventricular ejection time (LVET), a longer preejection period (PEP) and a higher PEP/LVET ratio in the absence of coronary artery disease or cardiac failure in some studies [71–82]. Interpretation in some of the studies is confounded by concomitant hypertension and for the proper exclusion of silent coronary artery disease, a number of ancillary methods must be used in the same patients. However, in studies where attention to these caveats have been made, impaired left ventricular function as manifested by an increased PEP/LVET ratio does occur early in diabetes.

There has been a suggestion that cardiac abnormalities occur more commonly in patients with microangiopathic complications (retinopathy, nephropathy) [74, 77, 89–91]. Metabolic changes may be relevant in some parameters as, for example, the increase in the PEP/LVET ratio in gestational diabetes returns to normal after pregnancy, but only in type 2 patients and not in Type 1 patients [72]. In type 2 patients, dietary therapy normalises abnormal systolic time intervals in some patients [78, 92] though not in those whose initial PEP/LVET was higher [92]. Myocardial lactate and amino acid uptake at rest is impaired in insulin-dependent patients without coronary artery disease and this is related to a relative hypoinsulinaemia and hyperglycaemia [93]. The importance of metabolic control in maintaining the contractile properties of cardiac muscle is revealed strikingly by the normalisation of relaxation rates by an aldose reductase inhibitor which reduced elevated sorbitol levels in left ventricular papillary muscles of streptozotocin rats with diabetes for only 13 weeks [94].

Results from echocardiographic investigations in diabetes have not been consistent possibly because different diabetic groups were selected for study without rigorous exclusion of hypertension (ventricular wall thickness increases and left atrial hypertrophy is usually associated with hypertension in diabetes [78, 79, 89, 90] or because different echocardiographic techniques were used. However, in a recent study where patients were grouped according to microalbuminuria and hypertension, left ventricular mass and mean septal thickness correlated with systolic blood pressure [95]. In 8/12 patients without evidence of coronary artery disease, Regan showed abnormal diastolic filling with increased resting left ventricular end-diastolic pressure; end-diastolic volume was reduced and the end-diastolic pressure/volume ratio increased, suggesting increased stiffness of the left ventricle wall. Systolic function was abnormal with diffuse hypokinesis of the left ventricle wall and a reduced ejection fraction [58]. A more recent study has shown that aortic pulse wave velocity and the wall thickness to radius ratio were significantly increased in diabetes with early peak velocities (E) reduced and parameters related to the atrial (late) contribution to left ventricular filling and the isovolumic relaxation time significantly increased in young type 1 patients [96]. These studies confirm work on papillary muscle in rabbits which indicate that chronic diabetes diminishes contractility and prolongs the duration of contraction [97, 98].

Left ventricular dimensions and volume [78–82, 91, 99–102] and measurements of the thickness of the left ventricular posterior wall and the intraventricular septum [79, 81, 100, 102, 103] have usually been found to be normal though slight ventricular dilatation [82, 103–105] and reduced ventricular size [106–108] have also been noted in some studies. Measurements of left ventricular systolic function including fractional shortening, mean velocity of circumferential shortening and ejection fraction were also found to be normal in many studies [78–81, 83, 99–104]. When patients with advanced complications are studied, systolic function has been found to be depressed [77, 82, 89, 108]. Where increased systolic function has been shown to occur in patients with microvascular disease [107, 109] it returns to normal when blood glucose control is improved [110].

Where digitization of the echocardiographic tracing is used, there is a prolonged isovolumic relaxation of the left ventricle and an increase in the time from the minimal dimensions of the left ventricle to the opening of the mitral valve – the late atrial filling which is thought to reflect changes in ventricular compliance [90, 91, 102, 104, 106–108, 111, 112]. There is an increase in this time also after exercise (Danielsen R 1988). Diastolic abnormalities have now been shown to occur in insulin dependent patients without evidence of ischaemic heart disease and with normal systolic function when pulsed Doppler ultrasound techniques are used [113, 114]. The ratio of peak mitral valve flow rates during the early rapid filling phase and the late atrial filling phase was lower in diabetic subjects especially if they had cardiac autonomic neuropathy [113].

Another measure of myocardial contractility, LVEF, is normal at rest in Type 1 diabetic patients [48, 115–121] except in patients with autonomic neuropathy [122] who also have depressed diastolic filling both at rest and after exercise [123]. There is no reduction in ejection fraction responses to exercise when younger diabetic patients are studied [116–118, 121], but a reduced fraction is found in older patients when coronary artery disease has been carefully excluded [48, 120]. This may be related to the increased prevalence of complications in older patients as Margonato showed that reduced ejection fraction responses to exercise were more reduced in patients with severe retinopathy compared to those without retinopathy [124] though no such difference was observed in the work reported by Pauwels et al. [125]. From work done in non-insulin-dependent rats with reduced rates of contractility and relaxation, the diastolic ventricular stiffness is related to impaired handling of calcium with a rise in total tissue calcium content resulting from reduced sarcoplasmic reticular calcium uptake [98]. In younger diabetic patients without autonomic neuropathy or microangiopathy, radio-nuclide ventriculography showed increased peak ejection and peak filling rates in diabetic subjects [126] and wall motion abnormalities (abnormal amplitude and phase shift) of the left ventricle were seen in all the 14 young type 1 patients without echocardiographic evidence of cardiac disease studied by Pauwels and associates (1985) [125].

There have been few well controlled studies which address the reversibility of some of the reported abnormalities of cardiac function after restoration of normoglycaemia. After continuous subcutaneous insulin infusion for one week there was no change in the resting ejection fraction but the rise in LVEF after exercise was reduced [118]. Abnormal systolic time intervals returned to normal in type 2 patients after dietary treatment [92, 127] and oral therapy [78] and after institution of insulin therapy [128] but in general, when other non invasive measures are used, there is little consistent evidence for reversibility after improved glycaemic control [117, 118].

References

1. Smith HL, Willius FA. Adiposity of the heart: a clinical and pathologic study of one hundred and thirty-six obese patients. Arch Intern Med 1933;52:910–31.
2. Alexander JK. Obesity and cardiac performance. Am J Cardiol 1964;14:864–5.
3. Alexander JK. The heart and obesity. In Hurst, JW, Logue RB, Schlant RC et al. The Heart (4th Ed) New York: McGraw-Hill, 1978; 1701–6.
4. Warnes CA, Roberts WC. The heart in massive (more than 300 pounds or 136 kg) obesity: analysis of 12 patients studied at necropsy. Am J Cardiol 1984;54:1087–91.
5. Roberts WC, Roberts JD. The floating heart or the heart too fat to sink; an analysis of 55 necropsy patients. Am J Cardiol 1983;52;1286–9.
6. De Divitis O, Fazio S, Petitto M et al. Obesity and cardiac function. Circulation 1981;64:477–82.
7. Licata G, Scaglione R, Barbagallo M et al. Effect of obesity on left ventricular function studied by radionuclide angiocardiography. Int J Obes 1991;15:295–302.
8. Messerli FH, Sundgaard-Riise K, Reisin ED et al. Dimorphic cardiac adaptation to obesity and arterial hypertension. Ann Int Med 1983;99:757–61.
9. Kaltman AJ, Goldring RM. Role of circulatory congestion in the cardiorespiratory failure of obesity. Am J Med 1976;60:645–53.
10. Iskandrian AS. Radionuclide evaluation of cardiac function in obesity. Am Heart J 1986;111(5):1003.

11. Alpert MA, Singh A, Terry BE *et al*. Effect of exercise on left ventricular systolic function and reserve in morbid obesity. Am J Cardiol 1989;63(20):1478–82.
12. Kinner B, Goos H, Ewers P *et al*. The relation of anthropometric parameters and echocardiography findings in the evaluation of left ventricular form and function in extreme obesity. Z Gesamte Inn Med 1989;44(5):152–7.
13. Nakajima T, Fujioka S, Tokunaga K *et al*. Noninvasive study of left ventricular performance in obese patients: influence of duration of obesity. Circulation 1985;71:481–6.
14. Alpert MA, Terry BE, Kelly DL. Effect of weight loss on cardiac chamber size, wall thickness and left ventricular function in morbid obesity. Am J Cardiol 1985;55:783–6.
15. Romano M, Carella G, Cotecchia MR *et al*. Am Heart J 1986;112:356.
16. Nakajima T, Fujioka S, Tokunaga K *et al*. Correlation of intraabdominal fat accumulation and left ventricular performance in obesity. Am J Cardiol 1989;64(5):369–73.
17. Messerli FH, Sundgaard-Riise K, Dreslinski GR *et al*. Disparate cardiovascular effects of obesity and hypertension. Am J Med 1983;74:808–12.
18. Messerli FH, Christie B, DeCarvalho JGR *et al*. Obesity and essential hypertension: haemodynamics, intravascular volume, sodium excretion and plasma renin activity. Arch Intern Med 1981;141:81–5.
19. Amad KH, Brennan JC, Alexander JK. The cardiac pathology of chronic exogenous obesity. Circulation 1965;32:740–5.
20. Wilcken DE. Left ventricular volume in man; the relation to heart rate and to end-diastolic pressure. Australas Ann Med 1968;17(3):195–205.
21. Alexander JK. The cardiomyopathy of obesity. Prog Cardiovasc Dis 1985;27:325–33.
22. Alexander JK. Obesity and the heart. Curr Prob Cardiol 1980;5:6–41.
23. Messerli FH. Cardiovascular effects of obesity and hypertension. Lancet 1982;1:1165–8.
24. Carabello BA, Gittens L. Cardiac mechanics and function in obese normotensive persons with normal coronary arteries. Am J Cardiol 1987;59(5):469–73.
25. Messerli FH. Cardiopathy of obesity – a not-so-Victorian Disease. New Eng J Med 1986;314(6):378–80.
26. Messerli FH, Ventura HO, Elizardi DJ *et al*. Hypertension and sudden death: increased ventricular ectopic activity in left ventricular hypertrophy. Am J Med 1984;77;18–22.
27. Alexander JK, Pettigrove JR. Obesity and congestive heart failure. Geriatrics 1967;22:101–6.
28. Garavaglia GE, Messerli FH, Nunez BD *et al*. Myocardial contractility and left ventricular function in obese patients with essential hypertension. Am J Cardiol 1988;62(9):594–7.
29. Mirsky I. Elastic properties of the myocardium: a quantitative approach with physiological and clinical applications. In: Handbook of physiology. The cardiovascular system, Bethesda, MD: Am Physiol Soc, 1979, Sect 2, Vol 1, Ch 14:497–531.
30. Paradise NF, Pilati CF, Payne WR, *et al*. Left ventricular function of the isolated genetically obese rat's heart. Am J Physiol 1985; 248: H438–44.
31. Alpert MA, Singh A, Terry BE *et al*. Effect of exercise and cavity size on right ventricular function in morbid obesity. Am J Cardiol 1989;64:1361–5.
32. Ramhamadany E, Dasgupta P, Brigden G *et al*. Cardiovascular changes in obese subjects on very low calorie diet. Int J Obes 1989;13(Suppl 2):95–9.
33. Dreslinski GR, Frolich ED, Dunn FG *et al*. Echocardiographic diastolic ventricular abnormality in hypertensive heart disease: atrial emptying index. Am J Cardiol 1981;47:1087–90.
34. Lavie CJ, Amodeo C, Ventura HO *et al*. Left atrial abnormalities indicating diastolic ventricular dysfunction in cardiopathy of obesity. Chest 1987;92(6);1042–6.
35. Alexander JK, Peterson KL. Cardiovascular effects of weight reduction. Circulation 1972;45:310–8.
36. Alexander JK. The cardiomyopathy of obesity. Prog Cardiov Dis 1985;27:325–34.
37. Archibald EH, Stallings VA, Pencharz PB *et al*. Changes in intraventricular septal thickness left ventricle wall thickness and left ventricular volume in obese adolescents on a high protein weight reducing diet. Int J Obes 1989;13(3):265–9.

38. MacMahon SW, Wilcken DEL, MacDonald GJ. The effect of weight reduction on left ventricular mass: a randomized controlled trial in young, overweight mildly hypertensive patients. New Eng J Med 1986;314:334–9.
39. Tuck ML, Sowers J, Dornfeld L et al. The effect of weight reduction on blood pressure, plasma renin activity and plasma aldosterone levels in obese patients. N Engl J Med 1981;304:930–3.
40. Crandall DL, Lizzo FH, Cervoni P. Alterations in cardiac composition with weight reduction in the obese rat. Metabolism 1985;34(5):405–7.
41. Kinner B, Ries W, Sauer I et al. Changes in noninvasive cardiovascular parameters by inpatient weight reduction. Z Gesamte Inn Med 1985;40(12):369–72.
42. Caviezel F, Margonato A, Slaviero G. et al. Early improvement of left ventricular function during caloric restriction in obesity. Int J Obes 1986;10:421–6.
43. Garcia MJ, McNamara PM, Gordon T et al. Morbidity and mortality in diabetics in the Framingham population. Sixteen year follow-up study. Diabetes 1974;23:105–11.
44. Reckless JPD. The epidemiology of heart disease in diabetes mellitus. In: Taylor KG (ed.), Diabetes and the Heart. Castle House Publications Ltd, 1987:1–18.
45. Lundbaek K. Diabetic angiopathy. A specific vascular disease. Lancet 1954;i:377–9.
46. Zoneraich S. Angina pectons in diabetic patients with normal coronary arteries. [letter] J Am Med Assoc 1979;241:2311.
47. Selvester RH, Rubin HB, Hamlin JA et al. New quantitative vectorcardiographic criteria for the detection of unsuspected myocardial infarction in diabetics. Am Heart J 1968;75:335–48.
48. Fisher BM, Gillen G, Lindop GBM et al. Cardiac function and coronary arteriography in asymptomatic type 1 (insulin-dependent) diabetic patients: evidence for a specific diabetic heart disease. Diabetologia 1986;29:706–12.
49. Watson RDS, Waldron S. Heart disease and diabetes mellitus. In: Taylor KG (ed), Diabetes and the heart. Castle House Publications Ltd, 1987:19–41.
50. Vitolo E, Madoi S, Sponzilli C et al. Vectorcardiographic evaluation of diabetic cardiomyopathy and of its contributing factors. Acta Diabetol Lat 1988;25:227–34.
51. Riff ER, Riff KM. Abnormalities of myocardial depolarization in overt, subclinical and prediabetes. A vectorcardiographic study. Diabetes 1974;23:572–8.
52. Fischer VW, Barner HB, Leskiw ML. Capillary basal laminar thickness in diabetic human myocardium Diabetes 1979;28:713–9.
53. Fischer VW, Barner HB, LaRose LS. Quadriceps and myocardial capillary basal laminae. Their comparison in diabetic patients. Arch Pathol Lab Med 1982;106:336–41.
54. Fischer VW, Barner HB, LaRose LS. Pathomorphologic aspects of muscular tissue in diabetes mellitus. Hum Pathol 1984;15:1127–1236.
55. Rubler S, Dlugash J, Yuceoglu YZ et al. New type of cardiomyopathy associated with diabetic glomerulosclerosis. Am J Cardiol 1972;30:595–602.
56. Hamby RI, Zoneraich S, Sherman L. Diabetic cardiomyopathy. J Am Med Assoc 1974;229:1749–54.
57. Zoneraich S, Silverman G, Zoneraich O. Primary myocardial disease, diabetes mellitus and small vessel disease. Am Heart J 1980;100:754–5.
58. Regan TJ, Lyons MM, Ahmed SS et al. Evidence for cardiomyopathy in familial diabetes mellitus. J Clin Invest 1977;60:884–99.
59. Crall FV Jr, Roberts WC. The extramural and intramural coronary arteries in juvenile diabetes mellitus: analysis of nine necropsy patients aged 19 to 38 years with onset of diabetes before age 15 years. Am J Med 1978;64:221–30.
60. van Hoeven KH, Factor SM. A comparison of the pathological spectrum of hypertensive, diabetic and hypertensive-diabetic heart disease. Circulation 1990;82(3):848–55.
61. Factor SM, Minase T, Sonnenblick EH. Clinical and morphological features of human hypertensive-diabetic cardiomyopathy. Am Heart J 1980;99:446–58.
62. Factor SM. Intramural pathology in the diabetic heart: interstitial and microvascular alterations. Mt Sinai J Med 1982;49:208–14.

63. Shirey EK, Proudfit WL, Hawk WA. Primary myocardial disease. Correlation with clinical findings, angiographic and biopsy diagnosis. Follow-up of 139 patients. Am Heart J 1980;99:198-207.
64. Ledet T. Diabetic cardiopathy: quantitative histological studies of the heart from young juvenile diabetics. Acta Pathol Microbiol 1976;84(sect A):421-8.
65. Nunoda S, Genda A, Sugihara N *et al*. Quantitative approach to the histopathology of the biopsied right ventricular myocardium in patients with diabetes mellitus. Heart Vessels 1985;1(1):43-7.
66. Yang Q, Kiyoshige K, Fujimoto T *et al*. Signal-averaging electrocardiogram in patients with diabetes mellitus. Jpn Heart J 1990;31(1):25-33.
67. Sutherland CG, Fisher BM, Frier BM *et al*. Endomyocardial biopsy pathology in insulin-dependent diabetic patients with abnormal ventricular function. Histopathology 1989;14(6):593-602.
68. Roy TM, Peterson HR, Snider HL *et al*. Autonomic influence on cardiovascular performance in diabetic subjects. Am J Med 1989;87(4):382-8.
69. Karlefors T. Circulatory studies during exercise with particular reference to diabetics. Acta Med Scand 1966;180(Suppl):449.
70. Zarick SW, Nesto RW. Diabetic cardiomyopathy. Am Heart J 1989;118(5 Pt 1):1000-12.
71. Ahmed SS, Jaferi GA, Narang RM *et al*. Preclinical abnormality of left ventricular function in diabetes mellitus. Am Heart J 1975;89:153-8.
72. Cellina G, Lo Cicero G, Brina A *et al*. Reversible alteration of myocardial function in gestational diabetes. Eur Heart J 1983;4:59-63.
73. Dai RH, Zhong XL, Zhu BQ *et al*. Diabetic cardiopathy. Chin Med J. 1982;95:71-5.
74. Jermendy G, Kammerer L, Koltai ZM *et al*. Preclinical abnormality of left ventricular performance in patients with insulin-dependent diabetes mellitus. Acta Diabetol Lat 1983;20:311-20.
75. Jermendy G, Koltai ZM, Kammerer L *et al*. Myocardial systolic alterations of insulin-dependent diabetes mellitus in rest. Acta Cardiol 1984;39:185-90.
76. Rynkiewicz A, Semetkowska-Jurkiewicz E, Wyrzykowski B. Systolic and diastolic time intervals in young diabetics. Br Heart J 1980;44:280-3.
77. Seneviratne BI. Cardiac cardiomyopathy: the preclinical phase. Br Med J 1977;i:1444-6.
78. Shapiro LM, Leatherdale BA, Coyne ME *et al*. Prospective study of heart disease in untreated maturity onset diabetics. Br Heart J 1980;44:342-8.
79. Shapiro LM, Howat AP, Calter MM. Left ventricular function in diabetes mellitus. I: methodology and prevalence and spectrum of abnormalities. Br Heart J 1981;45:122-8.
80. Zoneraich S, Zoneraich O, Rhee JJ. Left ventricular performance in diabetic patients without clinical heart disease. Evaluation by systolic time intervals and echocardiography. Chest 1977;72:748-51.
81. Atalli JR, Sachs RN, Valensi P *et al*. Asymptomatic diabetic cardiomyopathy: a noninvasive study. Diabetes Res Clin Pract 1988;4:183-90.
82. Uusitupa M, Sitonen O, Pyorala K *et al*. Left ventricular function in newly diagnosed non-insulin-dependent type 2 diabetics evaluated by systolic time intervals and echocardiography. Acta Med Scand 1985;217:379-88.
83. Airaksinen K, Ikaheimo M, Kaila J *et al*. Systolic time intervals and the QT-QS2 interval in young female diabetics. Ann Clin Res 1984;16:188-91.
84. dei Cas L, Zuliani U, Manca C *et al*. Noninvasive evaluation of left ventricular performance in 294 diabetic patients without clinical heart disease. Acta Diabetol Lat 1980;17:145-52.
85. Pillsbury HC, Hung W, Kyle MC *et al*. Arterial pulse waves and velocity and systolic time intervals in diabetic children. Am Heart J 1974;87:783-90.
86. Posner J, Ilya R, Wanderman K *et al*. Systolic time intervals in diabetes. Diabetologia 1983;24:249-52.
87. Rubler S, Sajadi MR, Araoye MA *et al*. Noninvasive estimation of myocardial performance in patients with diabetes. Effect of alcohol administration. Diabetes, 1978;27:127-34.

88. Northcote RJ, Semple C, Kesson CM *et al.* Systolic time intervals in adolescents with insulin-dependent diabetes mellitus. Diabetic Med 1985;2:465–7.
89. Shapiro LM, Leatherdale BA, MacKinnon J *et al.* Left ventricular function in diabetes mellitus II. Relation between clinical features and left ventricular function. Br Heart J 1981;45:129–32.
90. Shapiro LM. Echocardiographic features of impaired ventricular function in diabetes mellitus. Br Heart J 1982;47:439–44.
91. Sanderson JE, Brown DJ, Rivellese A *et al.* Diabetic cardiomyopathy? An echocardiographic study of young diabetics. Br Med J 1978;i:404–7.
92. Uusitupa M, Sitonen O, Aro A *et al.* Effect of correction of hyperglycemia on left ventricular function in non-insulin-dependent (type 2) diabetics. Acta Med Scand 1983;213:363–8.
93. Avogaro A, Nosadini R, Doria A *et al.* Myocardial metabolism in insulin-deficient diabetic humans without coronary artery disease. Am J Physiol 1990;258(4 Pt 1):E606–18.
94. Cameron NE, Cotter MA, Robertson S. Contractile properties of cardiac papillary muscle in streptozotocin-diabetic rats and the effects of aldose reductase inhibition. Diabetologia 1989;32(6):365–70.
95. Sampson MJ, Chambers J, Springings D *et al.* Intraventricular septal hypertrophy in type 1 diabetic patients with microalbuminuria or early proteinuria. Diabetic Med 1990;7(2):126–31.
96. Paillole C, Dahan M, Paycha F *et al.* Prevalence and significance of left ventricular filling abnormalities determined by Doppler echocardiography in young type I (insulin-dependent) diabetic patients. Am J Cardiol 1989;64(16):1010–6.
97. Fein FS, Miller-Green B, Sonnenblick EH. Altered myocardial mechanics in diabetic rabbits. Am J Physiol 1985;248(5 Pt 2):H729–36.
98. Schaffer SW, Mozaffari MS, Artman M *et al.* Basis for myocardial mechanical defects associated with non-insulin-dependent diabetes. Am J Physiol 1989;256:(1 Pt 1):E25–30.
99. Friedman HS, Sacerdote A, Bandu I *et al.* Abnormalities of the cardiovascular response to cold pressor test in type I diabetes. Correlation with blood glucose control. Arch Int Med 1984;144:43–7.
100. Fisher BM, Cleland JGF, Dargie HJ *et al.* Noninvasive evaluation of cardiac function in young patients with Type 1 diabetes. Diabetic Med 1989;6:677–81.
101. Gregor P, Widimsky P, Rostlapil J *et al.* Echocardiographic picture in diabetes mellitus. Jpn Heart J 1984;25:969–77.
102. Hausdorf G, Rieger U, Koepp P. Cardiomyopathy in childhood diabetes mellitus: incidence, time of onset and relation to metabolic control. Int J Cardiol 1988;19:225–36.
103. Lababidi ZA, Goldstein DE. High prevalence of echocardiographic abnormalities in diabetic youths. Diabetes Care 1983;6:18–22.
104. Pozzoli G, Vitolo E, Collini P *et al.* Assessment of left ventricular function with M-mode echocardiography in a selected group of diabetic patients. Acta Diabetol Lat 1984;21:71–84.
105. Rubler S, Sajadi MRM, Araoye MA *et al.* Noninvasive estimation of myocardial performance in patients with diabetes. Effect of alcohol administration. Diabetes 1978;27:127–34.
106. Airaksinen K, Ikaheimo M, Kaila J *et al.* Impaired left ventricular filling in young female diabetics. An echocardiographic study. Acta Med Scand 1984;216:509–16.
107. Airaksinen K, Ikaheimo M, Linnaluoto M *et al.* Increased left atrial size in young women with insulin-dependent diabetes: a pre-clinical sign of the specific heart disease of diabetes? Diabetes Res 1987;6:37–41.
108. Danielson R, Nordrehaug JE, Lien E *et al.* Subclinical left ventricular abnormalities in young subjects with long-term Type 1 diabetes mellitus detected by digitized M-mode echocardiography. Am J Cardiol 1987;60:143–6.
109. Thuesen L, Christiansen JS, Mogensen CE *et al.* Cardiac hyperfunction in insulin-dependent diabetic patients developing microvascular complications. Diabetes 1988;37:851–6.

110. Thuesen L, Christiansen JS, Falstie-Jensen N *et al.* Increased myocardial contractility in short-term type 1 diabetic patients: an echocardiographic study. Diabetologia 1985;28:822–6.

111. Uusitupa M, Mustonen J, Laakso M *et al.* Impairment of diastolic function in middle-aged type 1 diabetic patients free of cardiovascular disease. Diabetologia 1988;31:783–91.

112. Danielsen R, Nordrehaug JE, Vik-Mo H. Left ventricular diastolic function in young long-term type 1 (insulin-dependent) diabetic men during exercise assessed by digitized echocardiography. Eur Heart J 1988;9:395–402.

113. Airaksinen K, Koistenen MJ, Ikaheimo M *et al.* Augmentation of atrial contribution to left ventricular filling in IDDM subjects as assessed by Doppler echocardiography. Diabetes Care 1989;12:159–61.

114. Zarich SW, Arbuckle BE, Cohen LR *et al.* Diastolic abnormalities in young asymptomatic diabetic patients assessed by pulsed doppler echocardiography. J Am Coll Cardiol 1988;12:114–20.

115. Arvan S, Singal K, Knapp R *et al.* Subclinical left ventricular abnormalities in young diabetics. Chest 1988;93:1031–4.

116. Harrower AD, McFarlane G, Parekh P *et al.* Cardiac function during stress testing in long-standing insulin-dependent diabetics. Acta Diabetol Lat 1983;20:179–83.

117. Goldweit RS, Borer JS, Jovanovic LG *et al.* Relation of haemoglobin A1 and blood glucose to cardiac function in diabetes mellitus. Am J Cardiol 1985;56(10):642–6.

118. Larsen S, Brynjolf I, Birch K *et al.* The effect of continuous subcutaneous insulin on cardiac performance during exercise in insulin-dependent diabetics. Scand J Clin Invest 1984;44:683–91.

119. Mildenberger RR, BarScholomo B, Druck MN *et al.* Clinically unrecognized ventricular dysfunction in young diabetic patients. J Am Coll Cardiol 1984;4:234–8.

120. Vered Z, Battler A, Segal P *et al.* Exercise-induced left ventricular dysfunction in young men with asymptomatic diabetes mellitus (diabetic cardiomyopathy). Am J Cardiol 1984;54:633–7.

121. Fisher BM, Gillen G, Ong-Tone L *et al.* Cardiac function and insulin-dependent diabetes: radionuclide ventriculography in young diabetics. Diabetic Med 1985;2:251–6.

122. Zola B, Kahn JK, Juni JE *et al.* Abnormal cardiac function in diabetic patients with autonomic neuropathy in the absence of ischaemic heart disease. J Clin Endocrin Metab 1986;63:208–14.

123. Kahn JK, Zola B, Juni JE *et al.* Radionuclide assessment of left ventricular diastolic filling in diabetes mellitus with and without cardiac autonomic neuropathy. J Am Coll Cardiol 1986;7:1303–9.

124. Margonato A, Gerundini P, Vicedomini G *et al.* Abnormal cardiovascular response to exercise in young asymptomatic diabetic patients with retinopathy. Am Heart J 1986;112:554–60.

125. Pauwels EK, Lemkes HH, Gonsalves S *et al.* Scintigraphic evidence of asymptomatic impaired left ventricular function in type 1 diabetics. Clin Nucl Med 1985;10(12):861–4.

126. Ferraro S, Fazio S, Santomauro M *et al.* Cardiac function and sympathetic activity in young diabetics. Diab Res Clin Pract 1990;8(2):91–9.

127. Sykes CA, Wright AD, Malins JM *et al.* Changes in systolic time intervals during treatment of diabetes mellitus. Br Heart J 1977;39:255–9.

128. Mustonen J, Laakso M, Uusitupa M *et al.* Improvement of left ventricular function after starting insulin treatment in patients with non-insulin-dependent diabetes. Diabetes Res 1988;9:27–30.

PART EIGHT

Regional circulation

30. The coronary circulation

WILLIAM P. SANTAMORE and WILLIAM CORIN[1]

Balance between myocardial oxygen demand and supply

The primary function of the coronary circulation is to supply the heart's metabolic needs. Thus, any discussion of the physiology of the coronary circulation must begin by emphasizing the unusually close relationship between myocardial metabolism and perfusion. Figure 30.1 schematically illustrates this relationship. Because the heart has a limited and short-lived capacity for anaerobic metabolism, its steady-state metabolic needs can be considered solely in terms of oxidative metabolism. Myocardial oxygen uptake can be expressed as the product of coronary blood flow and the coronary arterial-venous oxygen difference. One unique feature of the coronary circulation is its high degree of oxygen extraction under basal conditions. Normally, about 65% of the oxygen in coronary arterial blood is removed in its passage through the myocardial capillary bed; little additional oxygen can be removed from this blood. Accordingly, changes in myocardial oxygen demand require changes in coronary flow that are quantitatively similar.

Factors governing demand

Although the determinants of myocardial oxygen demand are complex, three factors predominate: contractility, heart rate, and ventricular wall stress [1]. Substantial changes in myocardial oxygen uptake can result from changes in contractility (inotropic state) caused by hemodynamic metabolic interventions, such as altered cardiac sympathetic neural activity or administration of calcium or an inotropic agent. Heart rate primarily affects myocardial oxygen demand by the number of contractions per minute, although the positive inotropic effects of increased rate are also involved. Ventricular wall stress, expressed as force per unit area (g/cm^2), is directly proportional to ventricular systolic pressure and radius of curvature and inversely proportional to ventricular wall thickness. Because of the ease with which it can be measured, the "double product" of systemic arterial systolic pressure and

1. The authors thank April L. Jackson for careful preparation in this manuscript.

A.-M. Salmasi and A.S. Iskandrian (eds): Cardiac output and regional flow in health and disease, 411–431.
© 1993 Kluwer Academic Publishers. Printed in the Netherlands.

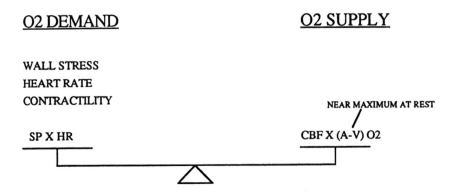

Figure 30.1. Schematic representation of the normal balance between myocardial oxygen demand and supply. (SP, systolic arterial pressure; HR, heart rate; CBF, coronary blood flow; A − V)O₂, coronary arteriovenous oxygen difference.)

heart rate is often used clinically as an index of total left ventricular oxygen consumption [2].

Other factors affecting myocardial oxygen uptake are somewhat minor. Under basal conditions, approximately 80% of the heart's total oxygen requirements can be related to the above three parameters. Although the heart's stroke volume can vary considerably with interventions, the independent effect of stroke volume on myocardial oxygen uptake is limited. Several minor determinants, include left ventricular fiber shortening, myocardial fiber activation, and basal metabolic myocardial requirements. The relative contribution of each determinant is dependent on the type of cardiac stress. Most physiologic perturbations affect several determinants simultaneously. The interactions of heart rate, pressure, and other variables, are complex. Thus, it is difficult to predict the effect of various therapeutic interventions on myocardial oxygen consumption and coronary blood flow. In general, the greatest increases in myocardial oxygen consumption occur, in decreasing magnitude, with increases in contractility, heart rate, left ventricular wall stress, ventricular muscle shortening, activation, and basal metabolic rate.

Factors governing coronary flow

Physiologic factors governing coronary flow can be considered in terms of aortic blood pressure and impedance. Aortic pressure is the primary force for coronary blood flow. Unlike all the other circulatory beds, myocardial oxygen demands are directly related to its perfusion pressure: the heart requires extra oxygen to generate higher aortic perfusion pressure. The physical properties of the blood and the cross-sectional area of the vasculat-

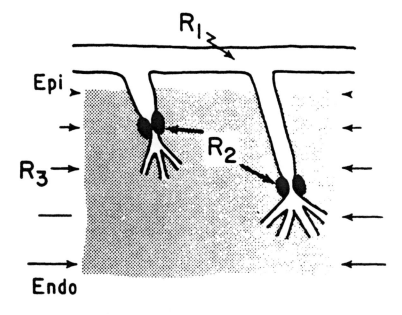

Figure 30.2. Schematic diagram of the coronary arterial circulation in the normal heart, illustrating the three components of coronary resistance. (Epi, subepicardium; Endo, subendocardium; R_1, epicardial, R_2 – precapillary arteriolar, and R_3 – compressive components of coronary resistance). Precapillary arteriolar resistance can change greatly in magnitude but requires several cardiac cycles to do so. Compressive forces are especially important during systole and cause substantial variations in resistance during a single cardiac cycle. Arrows indicate magnitude of intramyocardial pressure during systole. Klocke [45] reproduced with permission.

ure determine the impedance (Figure 30.2). The physical properties of the blood that affect oxygen delivery include its resistance to flow, or viscosity, and the oxygen content of the blood, which depends upon hematocrit, hemoglobin, and pH.

Aortic blood pressure is somewhat constant and blood properties change only slowly with time. Thus, on a moment-to-moment basis and on a quantitative basis, the cross-sectional area of the coronary vasculature remains the single most important factor controlling coronary flow. The coronary vascular resistance can be viewed as three components: the large epicardial vessels (R_1), the precapillary arterioles (R_2) and the intramyocardial resistance capillaries (R_3) (Figure 30.2) [2]. Normally, large epicardial vessel resistance is small and has only a minimal effect on coronary blood flow.

The precapillary arteriolar resistance primarily controls coronary flow by changing the vasomotor tone at the precapillary sphincter. Flow resistance is inversely proportional to the fourth power of radius. Thus, small changes in luminal dimension can profoundly affect resistance. Under basal conditions, this vasomotor tone is high. The vasomotor tone can change over a

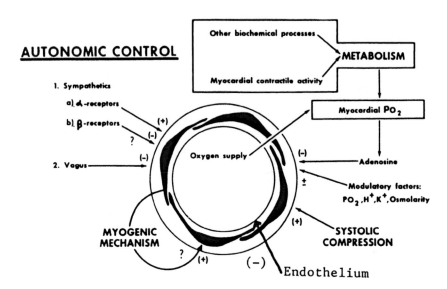

Figure 30.3. Principal factors influencing coronary blood flow. (+) = factors that reduce arteriolar lumen by compression or by contraction of vascular smooth muscle (ring of four overlapping cells). (−) = factors that relax vascular smooth muscle. Note that metabolic factors can act either via adenosine or other metabolites or by some direct effect on the vessel wall. Modified from Berne [46] with permission.

few cardiac cycles in response to metabolic demand, increasing blood flow for increased metabolic demand by decreasing resistance and vice versa. The ability of the resistance to decrease in response to increased myocardial oxygen demand or decreased coronary arterial pressure is commonly called "coronary reserve." The magnitude of coronary reserve is sufficient to allow coronary flow to increase by factor of 4 to 6 at normal levels of arterial pressure [3]. This reserve capacity for vasodilation is of pivotal importance in pathologic states and during stressful interventions. Coronary reserve also plays a pivotal role in myocardial reactive hyperemia, that is, the increase in blood flow that follows period of coronary arterial occlusion or in relative ischemia as during an exercise stress test.

Control of autoregulatory resistance

As pointed out above, the control of precapillary arteriolar resistance is of primary importance in the regulation of coronary blood flow. Mechanisms for adjusting vasomotor tone can be classified under these headings (see Figure 30.3).

Metabolic factors

Among the various mechanisms, metabolic factors probably play the largest role. This conclusion is based on the close relationship between myocardial oxygen consumption and coronary flow. Anaerobic myocardial metabolic byproducts act directly and indirectly to reduce smooth muscle contraction. The metabolic regulators of resistance are adenosine, oxygen tension, carbon dioxide tension, pH, lactic acid, potassium, and phosphate. The precise mediators controlling autoregulation have not been identified. Besides myocardial metabolism, the vascular smooth muscle cellular milieu is altered by changes in osmolality, prostaglandin generation and inhibition, regional acidosis or hypoxia. These can all contribute to modulation of vasomotor contraction or relaxation.

It is possible that some vasoactive agents exert their influence indirectly by modulating local release of adrenergic transmitters. It is also possible that more than one vasoactive agent is operative at any given time [4].

Neurohumoral factors

The role of the autonomic nervous system in the regulation of coronary blood flow is minor compared to that of the metabolic modulators. Coronary vascular smooth muscle is subject to neurohumoral influences through direct autonomic innovation and in response to vasoactive agents introduced via the coronary circulation. Neurohumoral adjustments in coronary vascular tone are often reduced reflexively. Sympathetic fibers act directly to constrict the vessels, and parasympathetic fibers to dilate the vessels.

Myogenic

According to the myogenic hypothesis, resistance vessels respond intrinsically to changes in transmural pressure. An increase in transmural pressure stimulates contraction of vascular smooth muscle, whereas a decrease in transmural pressure results in vasodilation [5]. Thus, myogenic factors remain a possible element in the control of coronary resistance but definitive information about their role is not currently available.

Endothelium

The role of the endothelium in mediating vasomotion in resistance vessels, which are responsible for control of perfusion, has not yet been well established. This is because of the difficulty in functionally inhibiting or destroying the endothelium without causing simultaneous damage to the adjacent tissue. The problems caused by increasing overlap with concurrent metabolically induced vasomotion in the microcirculation renders such a quantitative evaluation extremely difficult. Evidence is accumulating, however, that endothelium – mediated vasomotion plays a significant role in the microcirculation of various beds [6].

Large vessel pathophysiology

Except for extreme exercise, certain angina syndrome [7], and extensive hypertrophy [8–10], the coronary circulation can increase blood flow to meet the oxygen demands. Clinically, the primary factor preventing adequate blood flow is atherosclerotic lesions in the large epicardial coronary arteries. These atherosclerotic lesions obstruct flow by decreasing the luminal area of the artery, thereby increasing flow resistance at the stenosis. Under resting conditions, these obstructions may have little effect on flow, but with exercise, these stenoses can restrict maximal flow.

Figure 30.4a presents how these reductions in luminal area can affect physical activity. Figure 30.4a plots the percent area reduction on the X-axis versus the myocardial blood flow on the Y-axis. Additionally, Figure 30.4a presents the level of physical activity corresponding to the blood flow. Given the many factors that influence the relationship between myocardial blood flow and particular level of exercise [11], Figure 30.4a should only be considered qualitative for the physical activity lines. Under resting or sedentary conditions, blood flow needs are relatively low and are not influenced until the area reduction is greater than 90%. Even high levels of physical activity that require high blood flow are not influenced until the percent luminal area reduction has exceeded 60%. After that, further increases in percent area reduction begin to significantly affect the maximum blood flow. This restricts the maximal level of physical activity that can be achieved without an imbalance between oxygen supply and demand. Figure 30.4a highlights the steepness of the luminal area-flow relations. Once the luminal area decrease begins to restrict maximal coronary blood flow, further luminal area decreases lead to large decreases in maximal flow. Going from an 80 to an 85% stenoses causes only a 5% decrease in luminal area, but results in 20% decrease in maximal flow.

Figure 30.4a also shows the underlying principle of a stress test. Coronary blood flow may be adequate under resting conditions. When the patient begins the treadmill stress test, their level of physical activity increases resulting in an increase in myocardial oxygen demand. In the presence of severe coronary disease, coronary blood flow will be unable to increase adequately to meet the higher myocardial oxygen demands. A relative ischemia or imbalance between myocardial oxygen supply-demand occurs. This results in local abnormalities in the electrocardiogram and wall motion and a maldistribution of the coronary blood flow. Figure 30.4a also shows some potential limitations of the exercise stress test. A very high underlying percent stenosis is required before blood flow is influenced. For the elderly population, many of whom limit their physical activity, fatigue will restrict their maximal levels

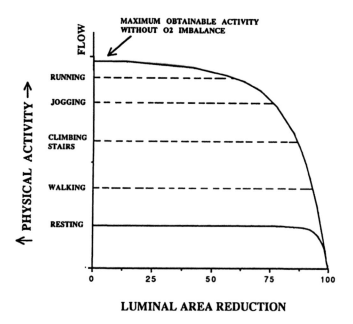

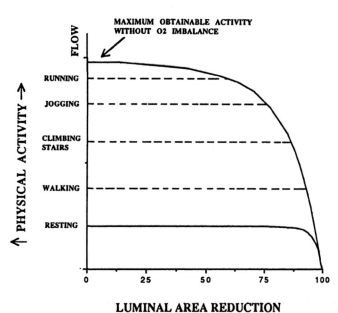

Figure 30.4. (a) Plots the resting and maximal coronary blood flow through an artery versus the percent luminal area reduction. Superimposed on the graph are levels of physical exercise associated with different levels of blood flow. (b) Plots the resting and maximal coronary blood flow through an artery versus the percent luminal area reduction. This graph shows the effects of training on the obtainable levels of physical exercise.

of physical activity. Thus, only critical or severe lesions will be detected at these low exercise levels.

The other factor influencing this curve (Figure 30.4a) is the physical condition of the patient. There is not a fixed relationship between coronary blood flow and physical activity. Myocardial oxygen requirements for a given level of exercise can be reduced by physical training. The reduction in oxygen demand is due mainly to the diminished heart rate during exercise in the conditioned individual. With increases in physical conditioning, higher levels of physical activity can be obtained with the same or smaller increases in coronary blood flow [11]. For a person with poor physical conditioning, their maximum obtainable level of physical activity may be severely reduced, even with only minimal coronary artery disease. With severe underlying coronary disease, even minimal levels of physical activity can result in angina pectoris. With exercise training (physical therapy or cardiac rehabilitation), a higher physical level of activity can be obtained for the same level of blood flow. Thus, for the same underlying percent stenosis, the patient can now achieve a much higher level of physical activity (Figure 30.4b). Thus, there would be an improvement in the signs and symptoms of the disease without any significant changes in the underlying severity of the stenosis.

Dynamic coronary artery stenosis

If coronary lesions were hard and geometrically fixed, then Figure 30.4a would explain most of the signs and symptoms of coronary artery disease. Yet anatomical studies indicate that most human coronary stenosis contain at least some normal wall segment [12, 13].

Figure 30.5 graphically depicts different types of stenoses and their responses to a 10% shortening of the normal portions of the arterial wall [14]. For a normal epicardial coronary artery vasoconstriction will decrease the luminal area, but this will have no significant effects on either flow or pressure across the vessel. For a truly circumferential stenosis, unable to change its size and shape, vasoconstriction will have no influence on its cross sectional area or stenotic hemodynamic severity. For diffuse smooth muscle stenosis and eccentric stenosis, alterations in smooth muscle tone will have significant, physiologically important effects on the cross sectional areas, possibly causing rest or exertional angina.

Factors influence large vessel size

Since most coronary artery stenoses can vasoconstrict and since small changes in stenotic luminal area can cause large changes in coronary artery blood flow, interventions that modify stenotic vessel size will have a major effect on myocardial blood flow. There are three primary mechanisms that control

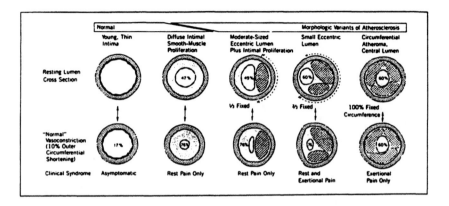

Figure 30.5 Morphologic spectrum of normal and diseased coronary artery cross sections. In regions where smooth-muscle viability and flexibility are retained, 10% isovolumetric outer circumferential shortening causes dramatic changes in lumen caliber. Size of resting and constricted lumen in each section determines associated anginal syndrome. Brown [14], reproduced with permission.

or regulate large vessel size: neural, humoral, or drugs; endothelium; and intraluminal pressure.

Neural, humoral or drugs

Serotonin and thromboxane A_2 are probably the most potent, naturally occurring, constrictor of the large coronary arteries [15]. Large coronary arteries also can constrict with neural stimulation or circulating alpha-adrenoceptor agonists. The epicardial coronary vessels are densely innervated with sympathetic adrenergic nerve fibers [4]. Still the magnitude of alpha-adrenergic vasoconstriction is not that large. In the intact, closed-chest dog [16] showed angiographically, a 42% reduction in left anterior descending coronary artery cross-sectional area following serotonin infusion. Yet, a similar phenylephrine infusion decreased left anterior descending coronary artery cross-sectional area by only [11]. These constriction responses can be augmented by high cholesterol levels, which directly effect the vascular smooth muscle [17]. Cholesterol also indirectly augment constriction by disrupting endothelial function [18] and by accentuating platelet aggregation [19].

It was only recognized in 1980 that the endothelium plays a major role in control arterial size [20]. An intact endothelium is required for many compounds, such as acetylcholine, ADP, ATP, bradykinin, and histamine, to elicit a vasodilator response in the coronary arteries. These vasodilators thus do not act directly on vascular smooth muscle. In the absence of endothelium, several of these substances-particularly acetylcholine-cause constriction of the coronary (and other) arteries. The endothelium of muscular arteries appears to have receptors for these vasodilators. When they are bound to the receptors, these vasodilators cause release from endothelial cells of a potent vasodilator, endothelium-derived relaxation factor (EDRF which is probably nitric oxide). EDRF activates guanylate cyclase in vascular smooth muscle, resulting in an increase in intracellular cyclic guanosine monophosphate (cyclic GMP), which presumably is responsible for the vascular relaxation [21].

The endothelium also senses the shear stresses within the artery. Increases in blood flow or shear stress cause the endothelium to release EDRF, which in effect matches the vessel size to the blood flow requirements [22]. The implications of endothelial function in controlling vascular responses are still evolving. At presence, it appears that endothelial function is abnormal with even minimal coronary artery disease [23]. Experimentally produced atherosclerosis in primates impairs the endothelial-dependent vascular relaxation to acetylcholine. Acetylcholine infused into normal coronary arteries of patients undergoing coronary arteriography causes a dose-dependent dilatation. In contrast, when infused into stenotic coronary vessels, acetylcholine causes marked constriction (Figure 30.6). Thus, the potential protective effects of the endothelium might not occur in patients with coronary artery disease.

Although often overlooked, intraluminal arterial pressure is a major determinate of vessel size. Further, the effects of neural, humoral, and drug interventions are strongly influenced by arterial pressure. High arterial pressures inhibit the effects of vasoconstrictors, while low arterial pressures decrease the efficacy of vasodilators. In one study that made use of a uniform vasoconstriction stimulus [24] there was a 30% decrease in coronary artery diameter at an intraluminal pressure of 20 mm Hg, whereas no effective vessel shortening occurred above an intraluminal pressure of 140 mm Hg. Lastly, for a coronary stenosis, distal coronary arteriolar resistance by modifying intraluminal pressure will influence vessel size. As blood flows through a stenosis, the high blood flow velocity causes a decrease in intraluminal pressure: the potential pressure energy is converted to kinetic energy. Decreasing distal resistance will further decrease the intraluminal pressure within a stenosis, which may decrease the stenotic luminal area [25].

Large versus small coronary arteries

Figure 30.7 and Tables 30.1 and 30.2 highlight difference between large and small coronary arteries and show that these arteries can respond differently to the same vasoactive substances. In whole-animal and isolated-heart preparations, the small-vessel vasodilatation with nitroglycerin was found to last only 20 to 30 seconds, whereas the larger coronary arteries remained dilated for up to 10 minutes [26]. Except for calcium-channel blocking agents, most nonnitrate vasodilators dilate the small coronary arteries and have minimal

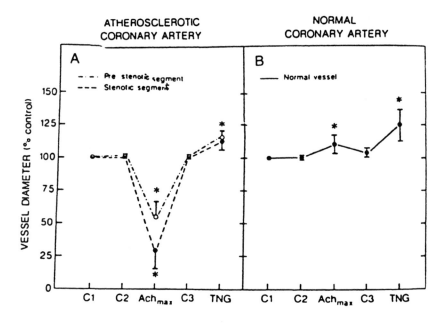

Figure 30.6 Responses of coronary arteries to intracoronary administration of an endothelium-dependent vasodilator (acetylcholine) and a direct smooth-muscle vasodilator (nitroglycerin (TNG) in eight atherosclerotic coronary arteries (A) and four normal coronary arteries (B). C1 = control; C2 = vehicle control; Ach$_{max}$ = response to maximal dose of acetylcholine; C3 = repeated control; asterisks = p < 0.01 for the comparison with C1. (From Ludmer [23]. Reproduced by permission.)

effect on the large coronary arteries. Adenosine and dipyridamole, for example, primarily produce vasodilatation of the small coronary arteries. Table 30.1 list some common vasodilators and compares their effects on large conduit coronary arteries (large artery resistance) versus the small coronary arteries.

The difference in response to vasoconstrictors between the large and the small coronary arteries has not been extensively studied. *In vitro*, α-receptor stimulation with norepinephrine was shown to be more effective on large than on small vessels [27, 28] observed that norepinephrine at low concentrations constricted large coronary arteries. Higher concentrations of norepinephrine relaxed the large coronary arteries. In contrast, norepinephrine always caused relaxation of the small coronary arteries. In a closed-chest animal preparation, Brum and associates used quantitative coronary angiography to document the effects of ergonovine and angiotensin on the coronary arteries. Both ergonovine and angiotensin constricted the proximal coronary arteries and increased total coronary resistance [29]. High concentrations of angioten-

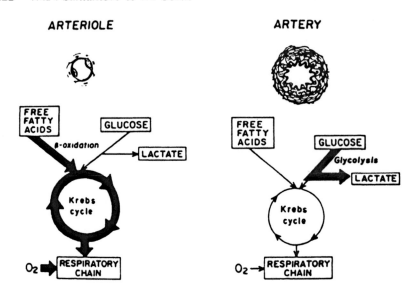

Figure 30.7 Metabolic pathways in coronary arterioles and arteries. The arterioles (left panel) posses high aerobic capacity and weak glycolytic potential. By contrast, the artery (right panel) exhibits high glycolytic capacity and weak aerobic potential. Cook [47], reproduced by permission.)

sin may, however, cause dilation if systemic pressure rises sufficiently to distend the artery.

There are several reasons for the differences in response between large and small coronary arteries. In vivo, the small arteries are surrounded by the medium they perfuse and are affected by local metabolites. In addition,

Table 30.1. Physiological and biochemical characteristics.

Characteristics	Large	Small
Autoregulation	No	Yes
Reactive hyperemia	Slight Constriction	Dilation
Ischemia	Constriction	Dilation
Passive distension	Yes	Yes then autoregulation
Total resistance (%)	5–20	95–80
Adenosine	Constriction	Dilation
Hypoxia	NoΔ	Dilation
KCN	NoΔ	Dilation
Mitochondria	10/unit	23/unit
Succinic dehydrogenase	1	2.6

From Winbury [44] reproduced by permission.

Table 30.2. Effects of coronary drugs.

Coronary drugs	RL and RT ABP	Q	RL	RT	RL/RT
TNG	0	0	−	+	−
DIP	−	+ + +	+	−	+ + +
PAP	0	+	+	−	+
CHR	0	+ + +	+ +	--	+ + +
PREN	−	+ +	+	−	+
LIDO	−	+	+	−	+ +
VER	−	+	+	−	+ +
NIF	−	+ +	0+	−	+ +
AMINO	−	+	+	−	+

Key: TNG, nitroglycerin; DIP, dipyridamole; PAP, papaverine; CHR, Chromonar; PREN, prenylamine; LIDO, lidoflazine; VER, verapamil; NIF, nifedipine; AMINO, aminophylline; ABP, blood pressure; Q, coronary blood flow; RL, large artery resistance; RT, total coronary resistance-decrease; +, increase.
Winbury [44], reproduced by permission.

the smooth muscle cells of small coronary arteries have a greater concentration of mitochondria and a higher succinylcholine activity than do large coronary arteries. Resting membrane potential and electrical impedance are similar in the cells of both large and small arteries. But, as with the mechanical responses of these vessels, nitroglycerin blocks the action potentials in the larger coronary arteries and not in the small coronary arteries, whereas adenosine blocks the action potentials in the small and not in the large arteries [30].

Effects of modulating vessel size

Figure 30.8 show how changing large vessel size can influence myocardial blood flow. Similar to Figure 30.4, the resting flow-luminal area and maximum flow-luminal area relationships are presented in Figures 30.8a and 30.8b. Figure 30.8a is basically Figure 30.4a with two different stenotic percentages highlighted. Point A represents an initial luminal area reduction of 60%, while point B represents a severe stenosis with an initial luminal area reduction of 90%. In a geometrically fixed stenosis, (Figure 30.8b) the arterial wall is rigid, and the luminal area cannot change. Regardless of the degree of stenosis, decreasing distal resistance always increases flow, while increasing distal resistance always decreases flow. Figure 30.8a shows these relationships. With a mild underlying stenosis (point A), decreasing distal resistance leads to a large flow increase. With a severe stenosis (point B), decreasing distal resistance results in a greatly attenuated flow increase. As depicted in Figure 30.8a, a patient with A lesion can perform substantial physical exercise, such as, running. A patient with lesion B, can only perform light work, such as climbing stairs.

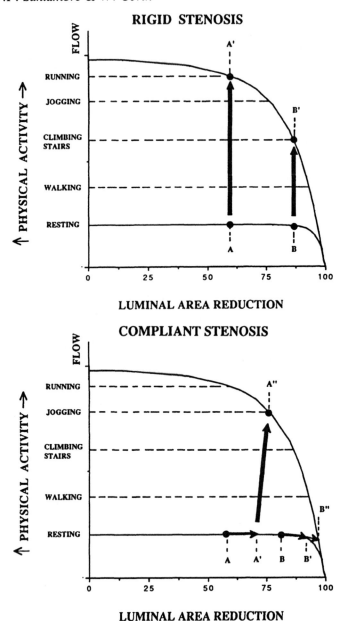

Figure 30.8 (a) Plots flow versus the percent luminal area reduction for a rigid coronary artery stenosis. Resting and maximal flow curves are presented. Point A represents and initial mild stenosis of 60%. Point B represents an initial severs stenosis of 90%. A^1 and B^1 represent the luminal area following a reduction in the distal coronary arteriolar resistance. (b) Plots flow versus the percent luminal area reduction for a dynamic stenosis. A^1 and B^1 represent the luminal area reduction caused by proximal coronary artery constriction. A_{11} and B_{11} represent the further luminal are reduction caused a reduction in distal coronary arteriolar resistance. Compared to Figure 30.8a, significantly less work can be achieved without an oxygen imbalance for a dynamic stenosis.

In contrast, Figure 30.8b depicts the response for a stenosis capable of vasomotion. For dynamic stenoses, because vasoconstriction, perfusion pressure and distal resistance can each alter luminal area, interactions among vasoconstriction, perfusion pressure and distal resistance can occur. Altering distal resistance changes the luminal area: decreasing distal resistance decreases the luminal area, while increasing distal resistance increases the luminal area. Also, proximal coronary artery vasoconstriction can decrease the vessel size. For example, for a mild underlying stenosis (point A), proximal coronary artery vasoconstriction would decrease the luminal area (A^1). Decreasing distal resistance would further decrease the luminal area (A^{11}). Because of this further decrease in luminal area, the coronary blood flow increase would be less than the response observed for fixed stenoses (Figure 30.8a). As indicated on Figure 30.8b, this will decrease the maximum level of physical activity achievable: This patient will only achieve a light to moderate work level such as jogging. For severe stenoses (point B, Figure 30.8b), proximal coronary artery vasoconstriction would decrease the luminal area (B^1) Decreasing distal resistance would further decrease luminal area (B^{11}), which might cause paradoxically a small flow decrease as compared to the fixed stenosis response. As compared to Figure 30.8a, maximum physical activity will be severely decreased and an imbalance between myocardial oxygen demand and coronary blood flow will occur at rest. This patient will experience rest angina without any physical exertion.

Coronary artery steal

Two potential types of coronary artery steal can occur. Both require stenoses in the proximal large coronary arteries. One type involves only one coronary artery and is caused by a redistribution of flow between the endocardium and the epicardium. As described before subendocardium is subjected to greater stress and thus needs a higher blood flow. In the presence of a proximal stenoses, the epicardial vessels may be maximally vasodilated even under resting flow conditions. Distal coronary arteriolar vasodilation results in a greater pressure decrease across the stenosis, resulting in a decrease in distal coronary pressure. This pressure decrease can cause a decrease in flow to the subendocardium. This partially explains why ST-segment elevation is observed on stress test.

The second type of steal involves a decrease in collateral blood flow. With the gradual obstruction of a coronary vessel, collateral vessels develop from the other (donor) coronary vessels. Collaterals are thin-walled anastomotic connections that exist between coronary arteries without an intervening capillary bed. They are anatomically present from early life, but enlarge only if need for additional coronary flow exists in some region of the heart. These collateral vessels supply blood flow to the myocardium normally perfused by the diseased (recipient) vessel. The collateral blood flow may be adequate to maintain the resting energy requirements of the myocardium. However, the collateral circulation is insufficient to meet the needs of the myocardium during periods of physiologic stress. In this setting, distal coronary arteriolar vasodilation has been reported to shunt blood flow away from the diseased vessel (coronary artery steal). Consequently, these vessels do not prevent the development of ischemic changes in the exercise electrocardiogram or abnormalities of ventricular contraction and performance.

Coronary artery steal probably only occurs in the presence of proximal resistance in the donor circulation. Steal does not occur without stenosis in the proximal recipient artery. For a proximal rigid stenosis in the recipient circulation, coronary steal is due solely to a decrease in collateral blood flow. For a rigid stenosis, the magnitude of the flow reduction is directly related to the decrease in collateral blood flow. In contrast, for a compliant stenosis in the recipient circulation, coronary steal is due primarily to a decrease in flow through the diseased vessel. One the other hand, for dynamic stenosis, the largest decrease in flow occurred through the native coronary vessel a-self- steal phenomenon.

Measurement of coronary blood flow

Despite the importance of coronary blood flow, its measurements is difficult and rarely performed on a routine basis. The problems in measuring coronary blood flow are complex and relate in part to the temporal and spatial distribution of coronary blood flow, movement of epicardial vessels as the heart contracts, "tortuosity" of coronaries with multiple branches, and coronary artery disease. The reader is directed to several recent reviews of blood flow measurement techniques [31, 32].

Coronary blood flow normally varies both transmurally (spatially) and temporally. During systole, intramyocardial pressure is near ventricular pressure in the subendocardium and decreases monotonically toward the epicardium [33], Compressive resistance, designated R_3 in Figure 30.2, presents the actions on coronary blood vessels of local forces produced by intramyocardial tissue pressure. Compressive resistance varies during the cardiac cycle. During systole, compressive resistance is especially large and can reduce instantaneous flow to a small fraction of that occurring during diastole. This compression during systole causes most of the normal temporal and transmural variations in blood flow. Although compressive resistance is small in magnitude in diastole, it becomes increasingly important when ventricular diastolic pressure (preload) is elevated. An inner-to-outer diastolic gradient for compressive resistance also seems likely [34].

Transmural variation in blood flow also occur because of the higher myocardial oxygen demands of the subendocardium. The oxygen consumption per gram of tissue is normally greater in the inner (subendocardium) than in the outer (subepicardium) layers of the heart. An inherently greater oxygen demand in the subendocardium is consistent with transmural variations in developed stress [35] and diastolic sarcomere length [36]. The greater oxygen consumption results in transmural flow heterogeneity, that is, by a larger flow per gram in the subendocardium than in the subepicardium [33] and by a larger subendocardial oxygen extraction [37]. Despite the greater oxygen requirements, flow to the inner layers of the heart is minimal during systole because of the "throttling" effect of systolic compressive resistance in the subendocardium. To compensate for these factors, flow to the inner layers of the heart during diastole must exceed that to the outer layers [38, 39]. Thus, the basic resistance is normally less in the inner portion of the myocardial wall than the outer due to the inherent transmural gradient of capillary density favoring the subendocardium [40]. This reduction in resistance is not by itself adequate, and some available subendocardial coronary reserve must be used. The degree to which subendocardial autoregulatory reserve is used under both normal and abnormal conditions varies considerably with heart rate.

Inert gas clearance techniques

Inert gas clearance methods are derived from the work of Kety and Schmidt [41]. When the heart is fully saturated with an inert gas and tracer input ceases, the arterial concentration will fall more rapidly than the venous concentration, since the indicator in the heart will continue to diffuse back into the coronary venous system. The integrated difference in gas concentration between the arterial and coronary sinus concentrations is proportional to coronary flow per unit weight.

These techniques have proved useful measurements in hypertrophied ventricles, and in defining patients with angiographically normal vessels with limited vasodilator reserve (syndrome X). Only radioactive gasses can be used to determine myocardial blood flow in patients with coronary atherosclerosis since regional localization of flow with nonradioactive gasses is impossible. In addition to poor spatial resolution, the time required for measurement is long, and variations in venous drainage patterns, make comparisons between patients difficult.

Thermodilution techniques

The coronary sinus thermodilution method is at present the most widely used clinical technique for the estimation of myocardial blood flow. Introduced by Ganz *et al.* in 1971 [42] the principle of this technique is simple. A miscible fluid indicator (saline) with a known temperature lower than that of blood is infused into the coronary sinus or great cardiac vein. The change in temperature of the downstream fluid-blood mixture is proportional to blood flow.

The coronary sinus thermodilution technique is limited by very crude spatial resolution and only modest temporal resolution. Because of wide variations in coronary venous drainage patterns, it can only be used to estimate regional flow in the left anterior descending distribution when placed in the coronary sinus at the termination of the great cardiac vein. Phasic flow also cannot be assessed with this technique, since phasic venous flow (primarily systolic) is different from phasic arterial flow (primarily diastolic).

Doppler ultrasound

The Doppler principle uses the fact that when sound waves are reflected from a moving structure, the frequency of the reflected wave is shifted to a higher or lower frequency. The frequency shift is proportional to the velocity of the moving structure. To measure velocity in coronary arteries, transmitted frequencies of 20 Mhz are needed to produce a Doppler shift that is readily detectable. Their temporal resolution is ideal, thus allowing for continuous on-line measurements of changes in velocity following interventions. The principle disadvantages are that velocity rather than flow is actually measured. Methods, such as quantitative coronary angiography are required to determine vessel size, and thus flow. Hence, relative rather than absolute measurements are generally obtained. Diseased vessels with certain types of anatomy (very proximal obstructions, large branches prior to an obstruction) cannot be studied. Also, in diffusely stenosed small vessels, the presence of the catheter may change the caliber of the vessel, producing inaccuracy due to the artifact of the catheter in the narrowed area. Furthermore, only one vessel at a time can be examined, the technique is not completely safe, (i.e., a catheter must be placed in the coronary artery) and the transmural distribution of perfusion cannot be assessed.

Videodensitometry – digital subtraction angiography

This approach uses a measurements of contrast density at two sequential locations in the vessel to determine the transit time of the bolus between the two points. The volume of the arterial segment between the points is determined and flow through the segment is then calculated. This technique works best on vessels that are large in caliber and have a long straight course free of branches, i.e., coronary artery by-pass graphs. Measuring flow in native coronary vessels, with small caliber, complex three-dimensional course, short length, and multiple branch points is tenuous, especially at high flow rates.

These approaches have been enhanced by digital angiography [43]. Regional flow is determined by the mean time required for the contrast bolus to travel from the coronary ostium to the distal perfusion field. Using color-coded images, relative coronary flow ratios in various regions of interest are determined by comparing images obtained at rest and during the hyperemic flow state induced by the previous contrast injection. This approach is more qualitative than quantitative.

Advantages of the videodensitometric method are its safety and its ability to study all portions of the coronary tree in a given patient. Its disadvantages relate to poor temporal resolution, importance of major confounding variables influencing flow measurements (injection techniques, etc.), and dependence on flow ratios rather than absolute flow.

Positron emission tomography

Unsolved by all of the previously described methods, tomographic technique can assess transmural differences in myocardial perfusion. This is especially true for patients with coronary disease in whom subendocardial perfusion abnormalities are the initial manifestation of decreases in coronary perfusion. This theoretically ideal situation, however, has not yet reached fruition.

Perfusion measurements with positron emission tomography have been hampered by several methodologic problems, including limited resolution of the positron cameras (8 mm x 1 cm), motion artifacts (cardiac, respiratory, or skeletal muscle), partial volume effects, spill over count rate recovery, and assumptions regarding left ventricular thickness. Many of these problems, however, are presently being resolved.

References

1. Parmley WW, Tyberg JV. Determination of good myocardial oxygen demand. Prog Cardiol 1976;5:19–36.
2. Klocke FJ, Ellis AK. Control of coronary blood flow. Ann Rev Med 1980;31:489–508.
3. Marcus ML. The coronary circulation in health and disease. New York: McGraw-Hill, 1983.
4. Feigl EO. Coronary physiology. Physiol Rev 1983;63:1–205.
5. Folkow B. Description of the myogenic hypothesis. Circ Res 1964;15:1–279.
6. Bassenge E, Busse R. Endothelial modulation of coronary tone. Prog Cardiovasc Dis 1988;30:349–80.
7. Cannon RO, Epstein SE. Microvascular angina as a cause of chest pain with angiographically normal coronary arteries. Am J Cardiol 1988;61:1338–43.
8. Wicker P, Tarazi RC. Coronary blood flow in left ventricular hypertrophy: a review flow in left ventricular hypertrophy: a review of experimental data. Eur Heart J 1982;3(Suppl A):111–18.
9. Weiss MB, Ellis K, Sciacca RR. Myocardial blood flow in congestive and hypertrophic cardiomyopathy: relationship to peak wall stress and mean velocity of circumferential fiber shortening. Circulation 1976;54:484–94.
10. Nitenberg A, Foult JM, Antony I. *et al.* Coronary flow and resistance reserve in patients with chronic aortic regurgitation, angina pectoris and normal coronary arteries. J Am Coll Cardiol 1988;11:478–86.
11. Bove AA, Lowenthal DT. Exercise medicine. Physiological principles and clinical applications. Orlando: Academic Press, 1983.
12. Freudenberg H, Lichtlen PR. The normal wall segment in coronary stenosis. A postmortem study. Z Kardiol 1981;70:863–9.
13. Vladover Z, Edwards JE. Pathology coronary atherosclerosis. Prog Cardiovasc Dis 1971;114:256–74.
14. Brown BG. Coronary vasospasm: observations linking the clinical spectrum of ischemic

heart disease to the dynamic pathology of coronary atherosclerosis. Arch Inter Med 1981;41:716–22.

15. Young MA, Vetner SF. Regulation of large coronary arteries. Circ Res 1986;:579–96.
16. Bove AA, Dewey JD. Effects of serotonin and histamine on proximal distal coronary vasculature in dogs: comparison with alpha – adrenergic stimulation. Am J Cardiol 1983;52:133–9.
17. Yokoyama M, Henry PD. Sensitization of isolated canine coronary arteries to calcium ions after exposure to cholesterol. Circ Res 1979;45:479–86.
18. Tomita T, Ezaki M, Miwa M. *et al*. Rapid and reversible inhibition by low density lipoprotein of the endothelium-dependent relaxation to hemostatic substances in porcine coronary arteries. Circ Res 1990;66:18–27.
19. Shattil SJ, Bennett J, Coleman RW. *et al*. Platelet hypersensitivity induced by cholesterol. J Clin Invest 1975;55:636.
20. Furchgott RF, Zawadzki JV The obligatory role of endothelial cells in the relaxation of arterial smooth muscle by acetylcholine. Nature 1980;288:373–6.
21. Furchgott RF, Vanhoutte PM. Endothelium-derived relaxing and contracting factors. FASEB J 1989;3:2007–18.
22. Langille BL, O'Donnell F. Reductions in arterial diameter produced by chronic decreases in blood f,low are endothelium-dependent. Science 1986;231:405–7.
23. Ludmer PL, Selwyn AP, Shook TL. *et al*. Paradoxical acetylcholine – induced coronary artery constriction in patients with coronary artery disease. N Engl J Med 1986;308:1046–51.
24. Cox RH. Mechanical aspects of larger coronary arteries. In: Santamore WP, Bove AA (eds.), Coronary artery disease: etiology; hemodynamic consequences; drug therapy; clinical implications. Baltimore: Urban and Schwarzenberg, 1982:19–38.
25. Brown BG, Josephson MA, Petersen RB. *et al*. Intravenous dipyridamole combined with isometric handgrip for near-maximal acute increase in coronary flow in patients with coronary artery disease. Am J Cardiol 1981;48:1077–85.
26. Cohen MV, Kirk ES. Differential response of large and small coronary arteries to nitroglycerin and angiotensin: autoregulation and tachyphylaxis-Circ Res 1973;33:445–53.
27. Toda N. Response of isolated monkey coronary arteries to catecholamines and to transmural electrical stimulation. Circ 1981;49:1228–36.
28. Zuberbuhler RC, Bohr DF. Responses of coronary smooth muscle to catecholamines. Circ Res 1965;16:431–40.
29. Brum JM, Sufan Q, Dewey J *et al*. Effects of angiotensin and ergonovine on large and small coronary arteries in the intact dog. Basic Res Cardiol 1985;80:333–42.
30. Winbury MM, Howe BB, Hefner MA. Effect of nitrates and other coronary dilators on large and small coronary vessels: an hypothesis for the mechanism of action of nitrates. J Pharmacol Exp Ther 1065; 168:70–95.
31. Klocke FJ. Coronary blood flow in man. Prog Cardiovasc Dis 1976;19:117–66.
32. White CW, Wilson RF, Marcus ML. Methods of measuring myocardial blood flow in humans. Prog Cardiovasc Dis 1988;31:79–94.
33. Hoffman JIE, Buckberg GD. Transmural variations in myocardial perfusion. Prog Cardiol 1976;5:37–86.
34. Rouleau J, Boerboom LE, Surjadhana A *et al*. The role of autoregulation and tissue diastolic pressures in the transmural distribution of left ventricular blood flow in anesthetized dogs. Circ Res 1979;45:804–15.
35. Mirsky I. Left ventricular stresses in the intact human heart. Biophys J 1969;9:189.
36. Yoran C, Covell JW, Ross J Jr. Structural basis for the ascending limb of left ventricular function. Circ Res 1973;32:297.
37. Monroe RG, Gamble WJ, LaFarge CG. Transmural coronary venous O_2 saturations in normal and isolated hearts. Am J Physiol 1975;228:318.
38. Rovai D, L'Abbate A, Lombardi M. *et al*. Nonuniformity of the transmural distribution of

coronary blood flow during the cardiac cycle. *In vivo* documentation by contrast echocardiography. Circulation 1989;79:179–87.

39. Chilian WM, Eastham CL, Layne SM. *et al.* Small vessel phenomena in the coronary microcirculation: phasic intramyocardial perfusion and coronary microvascular dynamics. Prog Cardiovasc Dis 1988;29:17–38.
40. Wusten B, Buss DD, Deist H. Dilatory capacity of the coronary circulation and its correlation to the arterial vasculature in the canine left ventricle. Basic Res Cardiol 1977;72:636.
41. Kety SS, Schmidt CF. The determination of cerebral blood in man by the use of nitrous oxide in low concentration. Am J Physiol 1945;143:53–66.
42. Gantz W, Tamura K, Marcus HS. Measurement of coronary sinus blood flow by continuous thermodilution in man. Circ 1971;44:181–95.
43. Vogel RA, Bates ER, O'Neill WW *et al.* Coronary flow reserve measurement. During cardiac catheterization. Arch Intern Med 1984;144:1773–6.
44. Winbury MM. Proximal and distal coronary arteries. In: Santamore WP, Bove AA (eds.), Coronary artery disease: etiology; hemodynamic consequences; drug therapy; clinical implications. Baltimore Urban and Schwarzenberg, 1982;63–77.
45. Klocke FJ, Ellis AK. Physiology of the coronary circulation. In: Parmley WW, Chatterjee K (ed.), Cardiology, Volume 1, Physiology, pharmacology, diagnosis. Philadelphia: J,B. Lippincott Company, 1988: Chapter 7.
46. Rubio R, Berne RM. Regulation of coronary blood flow. Prog Cardiovasc Dis 1975;18:105–26.
47. Cook BH, Granger HJ, Taylor AE. Metabolism of coronary arteries and arterioles. A histochemical study. Microvasc Res 1977;14:145–59.

General references

Berne RM, Rubio R. Coronary circulation. In: Berne RM (ed.), Handbook of physiology, section 2, the cardiovascular system. Bethesda: American Physiological Society, 1979:873.
Feigl EO. Coronary physiology. Physiol Rev 1983;63:1.
Marcus ML. The coronary circulation in health and disease. New York: McGraw-Hill, 1983.

31. Dynamics of blood circulation

IBRAHIM SUKKAR

The interest in studying blood flow dynamics lies in the range of diseases in which malfunctions in the circulatory system are directly implicated. One of the major causes of abnormal circulation is the formation of atheroma. Among the factors contributing to atherosclerosis are haemodynamic factors such as extreme shear stresses and wave reflections [1–4], eddy currents or vortices [5], flow turbulence and vessel wall vibrations [6, 7]. Vascular dynamics relates the effects of hydraulic forces to the biological response of blood vessels. There are several inter-dependent dynamic properties of the arterial system. These include the transmission and cushioning of cardiac pulsations and, arterial wall distensibility and viscosity. Understanding the dynamic and rheologic behaviour of blood flow could well improve the diagnosis and treatment of atherosclerotic disease [8–23]. The subject of haemodynamics in health and disease is dealt with in several basic and advanced textbooks [24–40].

Physics of the arterial wall

The arterial system is a branching network of visco-elastic vessels with distinctive mechanical properties. The most elaborate feature of the system is spatial non-uniformity and temporal non-linearity, particularly with regard to distensibility or compliance [41–43]. Central or proximal vessels are more compliant than peripheral or distal vessels. The wall of large arteries behave, under physiologic conditions of pressure and flow, like a two-phase material (elastin + collagen) with composite mechanical properties differing from those of the interacting components [44]. For instance, at very low intra-arterial pressures [<75 mm Hg], the arterial wall acts as a vessel of pure elastin. This means that, the extent of deformation is proportional to the amount of force (or pressure) applied, and such that when the force is removed the wall will regain its original size and shape (Hooke's law of a perfectly elastic material). As the pressure increases (>75 mm Hg), more collagen fibres will be recruited (in the lamellar unit structure) to bear some of the stress already carried by the elastin fibres. At this stage, the elastic behavior of the arterial wall is becoming increasingly non-linear i.e. not obeying Hooke's law. At very high pressures (>200 mm Hg), a major part

A.-M. Salmasi and A.S. Iskandrian (eds): Cardiac output and regional flow in health and disease, 433–467.
© 1993 *Kluwer Academic Publishers. Printed in the Netherlands.*

of the wall elasticity is lost, and the artery has now become very stiff behaving like a tube of pure collagen [45]. This two-phase behavior of the arterial wall (media) makes vascular dilatation a gradually less satisfactory response to increasing intra-lumenal pressure. This is to say, the arterial wall becomes less and less distensible with increasing circumference under pressure. This gradual loss of distensibility is determined by more collagen loading, which makes the Young's modulus of elasticity non-constant for the arterial wall (see later). In addition, thickening of the wall of an artery (assuming no changes occur in the physico-chemical pattern of the wall constituents) will result in a decrease in strain i.e. increase in (structural) stiffness.

The presence of a central highly-compliant reservoir[1] (aorta) provides the physiologic benefit of reducing the oscillatory component of cardiac work, by allowing the heart to function at a rate and stroke volume optimal for a given cardiac output. Also, this high aortic compliance helps dampening the sudden and sharp pressure pulse produced by cardiac action, thereby sparing the peripheral (less compliant and small) vessels some appreciable damage to their walls. The fall in arterial compliance which takes palce as we move towards the periphery lessens an intrinsic problem of distensible systems. This is the tendency for oscillations to appear between various parts of the system resulting in diminished efficiency. Nevertheless, this type of behavior is likely to happen in diseased arteries with the establishment of standing waves that may damage the intima even further [45, 46]. The changes that occur with pathological alterations (and with age) in vessels reduce the stress-bearing proportion of collagen fibres. It has been found (contrary to common belief) that hypertensive vessels are more distensible than normal ones at high pressures (150–200 mm Hg), and *large* arteries in human hypertensives have increased arterial diameter and decreased shear conditions at the ar-terial wall in comparison to normotensives [47]. On the other hand, arterial aneurysms appear to form at sites marked by an unbalanced elastin-collagen activity [45]. Furthermore, compliance may be important to the ability of the vessel wall to resist atherosclerosis. For instance, the pulmonary artery is the most compliant artery in the body. It has been found that in hyper-cholesterolemic dogs, the pulmonary artery will remain plaque-free when exchanged in site with the abdominal aorta, whereas the aorta in the pulmon-ary circulation will develop plaques [48].

Compliance is a mechanical property of the arterial wall chiefly residing in the ealstin fibres (but also is contributed to by smooth muscle cells). Compliance is the ability of some (large) arteries e.g. aorta (high elastin/col-

---

1. The *Windkessel* model of the aorta is used in reference to the cushioning function of arteries. It was first used by the English clergyman *Stephen Hales in* 1769 in describing his measurements of arterial pressures in dogs and horses, and in his calculations of peripheral resistance. Later, it was described in more hydraulic terminology by *Otto Frank in* 1899. *Windkessel* is German translation for an (inverted) air-filled dome. This was used in old fire engines to convert or smooth out the intermittent spurts or injections of water from a water pump into a steady stream of water from a fireman hose nozzle.

lagen content ratio) to expand passively under pressure and take up a certain volume of blood during systole, and to shrink passively during diastole discharging the volume of blood smoothly along distal vessels. These vessels contain a higher proportion of collagen fibres md smooth muscle cells, which they need to control the flow by altering their lumen diameter. Compliance of a circular arterial segment is measured from the change in its radius, diameter, or circumference induced by a given change in intra-lumenal (lateral) pressure. Expressed in terms of diameter [49–51] (d = 2 radius r):

$$\text{Compliance} = \frac{\text{relative change in diameter } (\Delta d/d)}{\text{change in presure } (\Delta p)}$$

$$= \frac{\Delta r/r}{\Delta p} \text{ (Stiffness = 1/compliance).}$$

$$\text{Distensibility} = \frac{\text{relative change in volume } (\Delta v/v)}{\text{change in pressure } (\Delta p)}$$

$$\approx \frac{2\,\Delta r/r}{\Delta p}\ (\Delta v \ll v, v = \pi r^2 x l, l = \text{length}).$$

Elasticity of a material is, however, best expressed in terms of the *Young's modulus of elasticity* E, the standard term for compliance or distensibility in the physical sciences. E is a theoretical concept and refers to the stress that must be applied on a given material to induce 100% elongation. Since no material has uniform elastic properties, E is measured from small changes in stress (force *per* unit area) and strain [38] (tensile or compressive deformation). Strictly speaking, E applies only to homogeneous materials with a constant relationship between stress and strain i.e that obeys Hooke's law. Arteries do not conform to this law (over the whole range of physiological pressures), being more distensible (less elastic[2]) at low pressures and less distensible (more elastic) at high pressures. The implication is that E is not constant for the arterial wall, and it should be calculated at different stress and strain changes. Since arteries are cylindrical structures, it is more convenient to express arterial elasticity in terms of pressure and diameter changes. The most popular such index is *Peterson's pressure-strain modulus* Ep [52]. This modulus describes the pressure change required for (theoretic) 100% increase in diameter:

$$\textbf{Ep (dyne/cm}^2) = \Delta p / \frac{\Delta d}{d},$$

---

2. The biologist is apt to consider 'increased elasticity' to mean 'increased distensibility', but the 'increased elasticity' really means 'increased rigidity' for the physicist, so that a 'more elastic' material has a higher Young's modulus i.e. the material is less distensible or deformable.

Table 31.1. Young's modulus (E), Peterson modulus (Ep), and Pulse Wave Velocity (PWVc) in experimental animals and young human subjects. Summarised by McDonald [26] from a variety of sources.

	$E(dyne/cm^2) \times 10^6$	$Ep(dyne/cm^2) \times 10^6$	PWVc(cm/sec)
Ascending aorta		0.34–1.47	400–500
Descending aorta	3.0–9.4	0.40–1.55	400–700
Abdominal aorta	9.8–14.2	1.54–2.40	550–850
Iliac artery	11.0–35.0	2.76–9.62	700–800
Femoral artery	12.3–55.0	1.60–3.26	800–1300

where Δp = pressure change (dyne/cm^2) d = initial diameter (cm), and Δd = diameter change (cm).

Resistance of the arterial wall to deformation is also due to its viscosity. All components of the arterial wall contribute to this viscosity, and mostly the smooth muscle cells because of their bulk and, the mucoproteins because of their gelatinous consistency. Arterial wall viscosity is that property of the wall which is responsible for the (small but definite) delay between applied pressure and resulting diameter change. The major effect of wall viscosity is to dampen the arterial pulse wave. This effect is similar in magnitude to that caused by blood viscosity within the vessel. Detailed discussions of arterial wall viscosity can be found in Bergel [53–55] and Gow [56, 57].

Owing to the non-uniform elastic behaviour of the arterial system (wall becomes more elastic or stiffer as we proceed distally away from the heart), the cardiac pressure pulse travels towards the peripheral arteries at an increasing velocity (Table 31.1). This velocity (PWVc) may be calculated using the Moens–Korteweg equation [26, 38]:

$$PWV_c = \sqrt{\frac{E.h}{2.r.\rho}} = \sqrt{\frac{Ep}{2.\rho}},$$

where E = Young's modulus of elasticity, Ep = Peterson's modulus of elasticity h = arterial wall thickness, r = arterial lumen radius, ρ = blood density.

Thomas Young, a London physician (1773–1829), was the first to explore (around 1808) the relationship between arterial elasticity and pulse wave velocity [58]. He calculated the characteristic pulse wave velocity (PWVc) along an arterial segment as follows:

$$PWVc = \sqrt{\frac{\Delta p}{\rho \Delta v/v}} = \sqrt{\frac{\Delta p}{2\rho \Delta r/r}}$$

where Δp = change in pressure, Δv = change in volume, v = initial volume, Δr = change in radius, r = initial radius, ρ = blood density $\approx$ 1055 kg/m^3.

Pulse wave velocity can also be derived non-invasively from the time difference between the foot of two pulse velocity waveforms recorded simultaneously at a known distance apart along an arterial segment [49]. On the other hand, arterial compliance (C) is related to PWVc by the following equation:

$$C = \frac{1}{2\rho PWVc^2}.$$

Arterial compliance (C), conveniently defined by Gosling [49] as the percentage change in lumen diameter per 10 mm Hg change in pressure[3] ($\equiv 1334.16 \, N/m^2$), is given by [51]:

$$\%\,C/10 \text{ mm Hg} = \frac{100 \times 1334.16}{2 \times 1055 \times PWVc^2}$$

$$= 63.23/PWVc^2 \; (PWVc^2 = \text{length(m)/transit time (sec)}).$$

The above equations show that, PWV increases with increasing distending pressure and with an increase in E towards the periphery (while r decreases[4]). PWV also increases with age and in arterial disease because of reduced arterial compliance [61–67]. An adequate PWV in the arterial system will alleviate the effect of overloading on the heart due to fast arterial wave reflections (when PWV is very high) and the effect of arterial billowing due to high arterial distensibility [68] (when PWV is very low).

During its downstream journey, the arterial pulse wave is continuously modulated and amplified. This is known to be critical for the efficient functioning of certain organs e.g. lungs, kidneys [45]. These modifications in the pulse shape and amplitude are the result of wave reflections occuring at arterial junctions and branching sites due to alterations in elasticity and to impedance discontinuities. More importantly, these reflections are very frequent at the pre-capillary sphincters near the arterial terminations or arterioles [26, 30, 69–71]. Pulse reflections at bifurcations increase the amplitude of antegrade pressure wave, thus impeding the antegrade flow [72]. This is because reflected pressure waves are in phase with incident pressure waves, whereas retrograde flow waves are out of phase with antegrade flow waves [26, 30]. In order for flow to remain unchanged through the bifurcation (i.e. with minimal reflections, or maximal pulse transmission), the total cross-sectional area of the two daugther vessels must increase by a factor of $\sqrt{2}$ (= 1.414) relative to the cross section of the mother vessel. Normally, the area ratio at an arterial bifurcation is lower than $\sqrt{2}$, which introduces more resistance to flow [73]. However, it was shown that minimum reflection at the aorto-iliac bifurcation occurred at an area ratio of 1.15 [1, 74]. Li [75]

---

3. Measuring C in humans and animals using $1/2\rho PWVc^2$ gave a mean value of $\approx 0.001 \, s^2 \, cm/g$. Thus, it was convenient to express C as %C per 10 mm Hg pulse pressure, so that the value usually appears as one order of magnitude (Gosling 1990, Milan workshop abstract).
4. Tapering of the arterial system occurs basically at branching points. Between 2 consecutive branching sites, the diameter of the artery remains essentially constant [26, 59]. Where very slight tapering has been observed, it is more likely to be due to small branches [60].

has shown that local reflection at the normal aorto-iliac (in dogs) is only a few percent (6%) for the antegrade pulse wave, and 17% when iliac artery is 50% stenosed. Increased or decreased area ratio (and arterial stiffness) from optimal could impair adequate pulse transmission to organ vascular beds [76].

The term vascular impedance or input impedance (similar to electrical, acoustical, and hydraulic impedance) represents the *total* vascular opposition to oscillatory (pulsatile) and non-oscillatory (steady) blood flow through a vascular bed. In the normal circulatory system, arterioles account for 72% of the total flow resistance, capillaries for 16%, veins for 10% and, major arteries for 2% [77]. Input impedance describes the relationship between the sinusoidal components of input pressure wave and associated flow wave harmonics at the input of a vascular bed. Input impedance is expressed as impedance modulus (amplitude of pressure/amplitude of flow) and as impedance phase (delay of flow after pressure), both as a function of frequency of the pressure and flow harmonics [78, 79]. Values of vascular input impedance of common femoral artery related directly to the severity of atherosclerotic lesions [80–83]. However, a large impedance variation was shown in human subjects regardless of the presence or absence of atherosclerosis [84] and, it was unable to predict accurately the result of bypass operations for occlusion of the superficial femoral artery [78]. On the other hand, it was shown that, the reflection coefficient R at a branching junction (in a tubular model) could be calculated as follows [85]:

$$R = \frac{Zt - Zo}{Zt + Zo},$$

where Zt = modulus of terminal impedance of the mother vessel (i.e. characteristic impedance of the daugther vessel) (Zt at zero frequency is the peripheral resistance) Zo = modulus of characteristic impedance of the mother vessel (i.e. without wave reflections).

Characteristic impedance depends on local geometric and elastic vessel wall properties, and the fluid contained in the vessel [82]. It does not depend on the state of the (bed) vasculature, contrary to input impedance [89].

Zo is related to PWV through the 'Water-Hammer' formula [68]:

Zo (dyne sec. cm^{-3}) = ρ . PWV

where ρ = blood density (g/cm^3), PWV = pulse wave velocity (cm/sec).

Pressure-flow relations

In attempting to understand the dynamics of blood flow in the animal or human circulatory system, one has to consider the physical laws which apply to fluids at rest and in motion. Clearly, numerous additional complications

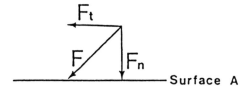

Figure 31.1. The tangential (Ft) and normal (Fn) components of a force F acting on a surface area A. Ft/A is called shear stress and, Fn/A is called normal stress or pressure.

are introduced over classical *in-vitro* fluid mechanics when dealing with the *in-vivo* situation. These are mainly due to (a) elasticity of blood vessels; (b) heterogeneity of blood as a fluid[5]; (c) anomalous properties of blood viscosity; and (d) pulsatility and complex pattern of blood flow.

Stress, strain and viscosity

In order to flow, a fluid must be subjected to imbalanced mechanical forces capable of inducing fluid deformation that increases or decreases continuously with time. The extent of deformation or strain is proportional to the applied force per unit area i.e. stress. Since a force F acting on a surface A may have components parallel and perpendicular to that surface, the stress components are also so identified (Figure 31.1). A parallel or tangential stress vector to the surface is called *shear stress* τ and is defined as:

$$\tau = \frac{Ft}{A},$$

where Ft (dyne) is the tangential force acting on a surface with area A (cm^2).

A perpendicular or normal stress vector to the surface can be either tensile or compressive. Pressure represents the normal compressive stress vector in a fluid, and it is given by:

$$\text{pressure} = \frac{Fn}{A},$$

where Fn is the normal for acting at riht angles on a surface with area A.

At rest, a fluid element has no shear stress, but it can have both shear and pressure stresses while in motion. With respect to arterial blood flow, most of the pressure is absorbed by the elastic, collagenous and smooth muscle cells in the sub-endothelium, while the endothelium is principally subjected to all of the shear stress. In large arteries e.g. thoracic aorta,

---

5. Blood may be considered as a viscoelastic liquid composed of a viscous liquid phase (colloid), and an elastic suspended phase whicll is neither liquid (as to form a true emulsion) nor solid (as to form a true suspension). This suspended phase is a collection of liquid droplets each enclosed in a solid elastic lipo-protein envelope i.e. cells.

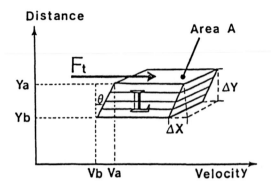

Figure 31.2. Schematic diagram showing the viscous displacement Δx undergone by the top fluid layer (with area A) at position Ya relative to the bottom fluid layer at position Yb under the effect of a shear force Ft. Va and Vb are the velocities of the top and bottom fluids layers respectively. Shear strain = Δx/(Ya − Yb). Velocity gradient = (Va − Vb)/(Ya − Xb) = tangent θ.

laminar shear stresses up to 30 dyn/cm^2 are typical [86]. In arterioles (20–40 μm internal diameter), shear stresses range from 5–25 dyn/cm^2. The degree and nature of deformation the flowing element experiences depends on the type of acting stress: A *shear* stress produces a *shear* strain. A *compressive* stress produces a *compressional* strain. A *tensile* stress produces an *extensional* strain.

Shear stress and shear strain are of greatest interest in hemorheology [87]. If we imagine a viscous fluid element L made up of infinitesimally thin layers of fluid sliding past each other in parallel planes (Figure 31.2) under the effect of a shear stress τ, then, the induced *shear strain*[6] γ will be defined as:

$$\gamma = \frac{\Delta x}{\Delta y},$$

where Δx is the horizontal distance the topmost fluid layer has moved forward relative to the bottom layer, and Δy is the (constant) height of the fluid element.

The fluid laminae moving with increasing velocities (horizontal axis) from bottom (stationary plate) to top (moving plate) establish a velocity gradient which is given by the tangent of the angle θ (Figure 31.2):

---

6. Shear stress and shear strain are usually linearly related by a constant [87]: Shear stress (τ) =Shear strain (γ) × Shear modulus of elasticity G, Normal stress = Normal strain × - Normal modulus of elasticity E. These two equations briefly describe the elastic component of blood viscoelastic behaviour. Normal stress and normal strain are either compressional or extensional. E is the Young's modulus of elasticity. E and G are constants with E > G.

$$\text{velocity gradient} = \text{tangent } \theta = \frac{v_a - v_b}{y_a - y_b} = \frac{\Delta v}{\Delta y} \, (\text{sec}^{-1}),$$

where v_a = top layer velocity, v_b = bottom layer velocity, $y_a y_b$ are top and bottom layer positions respectively relative to some reference.

In the context of a homogeneous fluid moving steadily through a cylindrical tube, the shear stress τ is highest at the tube wall, and decreasing linearly towards the tube centre where it becomes zero. Also, the shear stress is acting in a direction parallel and opposite to that of flow velocity. This causes the flow velocity to be vanishingly small at the wall (stationary plate) and maximum at the tube centre. The shear stress τ at a given radial distance r' from the tube axis is given by [22, 87]:

$$\tau_{r'} = \frac{\Delta P \cdot r'}{2.1},$$

where ΔP = pressure difference between two points a distance l apart along a tube of radius r ($\Delta P/l$ = pressure gradient). At the tube centre, $r' = 0 \Rightarrow \tau_{r'} = 0$. At the tube wall, $r' = r \Rightarrow \tau_{r'}$ is maximum. The above expression for $\tau_{r'}$ is vlaid for a steady flow in a cylindrical tube, and whether flow is laminar or turbulent.

Since flow is a continuous deformation in time, the shear strain will be a function of time. The *shear strain rate* D describes the shear strain γ per unit of time:

$$D = \lim_{\Delta t \to 0} \frac{\Delta \gamma}{\Delta t} = \frac{d\gamma}{dt} = \frac{d(\Delta x/\Delta y)}{dt} = \frac{d(\Delta v \cdot t/\Delta y)}{dt} = \frac{\Delta v}{\Delta y} = \text{velocity gradient},$$

where $\Delta \gamma$ is the change in shear strain which occurs in a time interval Δt, and $(d\gamma/dt)$ is the time differential of γ i.e. the infinitesimal limit of $(\Delta \gamma / \Delta t)$ as $\Delta t \to$ zero.

A fluid in which the rate of shear strain D is a function of shear stress τ is termed a viscous fluid. In contrast with an elastic material, a viscous material will not recover its initial shape when the stress is removed, and the energy imparted to cause deformation will be dissipated as heat due to internal friction. A viscous fluid is called *Newtonian* when τ and D are linearly related as follows[7].

$$\tau(\text{dyne/cm}^2) = D(\text{sec}^{-1}) \times \mu,$$

where μ = Coefficient of viscosity (dyne sec/cm^2 = poise).

---

7. The shear rate D at a given radial position r' from the tube axis is given by:

$$D_{r'} = \frac{\tau_{r'}}{\mu},$$

where $\tau_{r'}$ = shear stress at radial position r' and μ = fluid viscosity. $D_{r'} = 0$ at the tube axis, and maximum at the tube wall.

In other words, μ is constant for a newtonian fluid i.e. it is independent of τ and D (water, blood serum and plasma are examples of newtonian fluids[8]). A non-newtonian fluid does not exhibit this linear behaviour of viscosity i.e. μ varies with τ (in different ways) and thus, it cannot be characterised by a single coefficient of viscosity[9]. Regarding the viscosity of whole blood, some studies have suggested that blood behaves like a newtonian fluid at high shear stresses [88–90] and, others have shown that blood behaves like a non-newtonian fluid at low shear stresses [91–93]. This means that, blood viscosity is high and variable at low shear stresses (non-linear behaviour of viscosity) and, low and quasi-constant at high shear stresses [38, 87] (linear behaviour of viscosity, blood viscosity: 0.035–0.05 poise). Nevertheless, blood exhibits a Newtonian behavior (pressure-flow curves are essentially linear) in the physiological range of flows and pressures [94]. The presence of the plasma protein *fibrinogen* and red blood cells causes blood to exhibit this non-newtonian pseudo-plastic behaviour of viscosity i.e. the blood at rest could resist a low shear stress up to some characteristic value (the yield stress[10]) before starting to flow slowly at first, and later more quickly at higher shear stresses [95]. This is due to red blood cells aggregating into *rouleaux* at very low shear stress or flow rate favoured by the presence of fibrinogen [96]. At a higher shear stress, the red cell aggregations begin to loosen up and disperse, thus enabling the blood to flow faster. On the other hand, at any given shear rate, blood viscosity is a function of the concentration and deformability of the red cells, and the nature and concentration of the plasma proteins [97, 98]. It appears, however, that cell aggregation and consequent increase in blood viscosity are not seen in arteries where flow is pulsatile [38]. The behavior of blood viscosity is further complicated by the *Fahraeus-Lindqvist* effect [99]. These investigators found that blood viscosity was lower in capillary tubes (<300 microns in diameter) than would have been expected from measurements in wider tubes. They attributed this effect to the axial streaming or accumulation of red blood cells, leaving a cell-free zone of plasma close to the wall of the capillary tube. The equation $\tau = D . \mu$ represents the viscous component of the viscoelastic behavior of blood. The elastic component (structural viscosity) may be due to the formation of rouleaux of red cells. Briefly, blood exhibits non-linear viscoelasti city and/or thixotropy (timependent properties) [87, 100, 101]. Finally, blood viscosity is termed *apparent*[11] because it is affected by several factors including shear stress [102–106]. These are (a) temperature

---

8. Water viscosity [20] ≈ 0.01 poise (at 20°C) (≈ 0.007 at 37°C), blood plasma viscosity ≈ 0.018 poise (at 20°C) (≈ 0.011 at 37°C).

9. $\tau = D . \mu$ is still valid for a non-Newtonian fluid, but giving different μ values for different τ or D values.

10 A non-newtonian plastic fluid has a yield stress > 0. A non-newtonian pseudo-plastic fluid has a yield stress ≈ 0.

11. The apparent viscosity of a non-newtonian fluid is equal to the viscosity of a newtonian fluid which would have the same flow rate when flowing under the same pressure head.

(viscosity increases if temperature decreases and vice versa); (b) hematocrit (viscosity increases with hematocrit); and (c) red cell deformability (viscosity increases if deformability decreases).

Laminar and turbulent flow

Flow is said to be *laminar* when the fluid particles move in parallel planes or sheets i.e. there is no interchange of fluid between laminae. If flow conditions change slightly e.g. an increase in flow velocity or a decrease in fluid viscosity, the stable laminar flow starts to become disturbed in the sense that the flow laminae now exhibit a certain wavy and undulating pattern. In this case, the flow is termed *transitional*. With dramatic changes in flow conditions, the ensuing flow disturbance is so severe that turbulence sets in [107]. Turbulent flow is unstable and chaotic; it is characterised by random velocity vectors and disordered pressure fluctuations occuring in all directions and with varying magnitudes.

In laminar flow, the pressure head loss (to overcome fluid viscosity) along a straight cylindrical tube is proportional to the speed of flow, as in *Poiseuille's* experiments [108]. The pressureflow equation for Poiseuille-type of flow is given by:

$$Q = \frac{\Delta P}{R},$$

where Q = mean flow through the tube (flow velocity × tube cross-section), ΔP = mean pressure drop along the tube, and R = resistance to flow.

Resistance to flow arises mainly from viscous or frictional forces between adjacent layers in the flowing liquid. Using the Hagenbach-Poiseuille equation, R is given by [26]:

$$R = \frac{8 . \mu . l}{\pi . r^4} \left(= \frac{128 . \mu . l}{\pi . d^4} \right)$$

where μ = viscosity of liquid, l = length of tube, r = radius of tube, d = diameter of tube = 2r.

Substituting R in the pressure-flow equation above gives:

$$\Delta P = Q . R = v . \pi . r^2 . \frac{8 . \mu . l}{\pi . r^4} = \frac{8 . \mu . l . v}{r^2},$$

where v = spatial average flow velocity, πr^2 = tube cross-sectional area.

Since flow Q is proportional to r^2, small changes in r will result in large changes in flow. For example, a 10% decrease in radius r would decrease flow by about 19%, and a 50% decrease in r would decrease flow by about 75% (provided other flow factors remain constant).

The conditions which are implicit in the derivation of Poiseuille's law are:

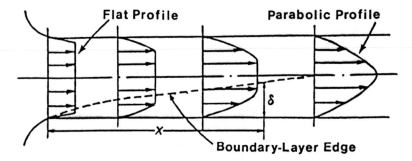

Figure 31.3. The change in velocity profile that occurs in (steady flow) as the fluid moves away from the tube inlet (left), where the profile is flat, towards the right where the profile becomes gradually more parabolic. Note the growing thickness δ of the boundary layer (where a velocity gradient is present) with distance x from the inlet. This is due to viscous effects at the tube wall spreading towards the tube axis, causing retardation of adjacent fluid layers through shearing forces. The thickness of the boundary layer increases with an increase in fluid viscosity. Were the fluid non-viscous, the velocity profile would remain flat all along the tube, and proceed with its original inertia. A radially symmetric velocity profile for a laminar flow can be expressed as follows [22]:

$$\frac{V'}{V_{max}} = 1 - \left(\frac{r'}{r}\right)^n,$$

where V' = veocity of a fluid layer at a radial location r' from the tube axis ($r' = 0$ at the tube axis, $r' = r$ at the tube wall), r = tube radius, V_{max} = maximum axis velocity of fluid, n = integer number. For a parabolic profile:

$$\frac{V'}{V_{max}} = 1 - \left(\frac{r'}{r}\right)^2 \text{ and } V_{average} = \frac{V_{max}}{2}.$$

The larger the vlaue of n, the flatter the proflie. For a purely flat profile, $n \rightarrow \infty$: $V_{average} = V_{max}$. (Figure from Caro *et al.* Mechanics of circulation. Oxford University Press. Reproduced with permission.)

1. The fluid is newtonian i.e. viscosity is constant at all shear stress or rates.
2. The flow is laminar and steady i.e. with no accelerations or decelerations.
3. The flow is fully developed i.e. with established parabolic velocity profile across the tube (Figure 31.3).
4. The tube is rigid i.e. diameter does not vary with distending pressure.
5. The tube is straight and diameter is constant along the length of the tube.

Clearly, Poiseuille's assumptions do not hold for the arterial circulation for the following reasons: (a) blood is heterogeneous and non-newtonian; (b) blood flow is pulsatile and occasionally non-laminar; (c) blood velocity profile is variable during the cardiac cycle; and (d) arteries are non-rigid structures with curvatures and varying diameter at junctions and branching sites.[12]

---

12. At a branch point, the fluid enters with a relatively flat (plug) velocity profile, and it takes a distance of several vessel diameters from the branch inlet before the profile can become

In an *in-vitro* experiment, Byar and associates [113] applied the Poiseuille's equation to the study of stenoses, and found that the effects (on flow) of the stenosis radius, stenosis length, fluid viscosity, and differential pressure were considerably overestimated using the equation.

In turbulent flow (as it happens downstream of a stenosis), the pressure drop is mainly used to provide kinetic energy for whirlpools and is proportional to the square of the flow velocity (ΔP is proportional to v^2). In fact, the viscous resistance to flow (and hence ΔP) is augmented by inertial energy losses due to changes in flow velocity and direction [114]. These inertial effects are proportional to the square of the flow velocity ($K \cdot \frac{1}{2} \cdot \rho \cdot v^2$, where k = constant and ρ = fluid density), and are dependent on the surface roughness of the tube. At low flow rates, viscous forces predominate and the flow is laminar. As the flow velocity (v) increases, the viscous forces become less able to dampen out random inertial forces, because these increase as v^2, whereas the viscous forces increase only as v. Under these circumstances, the inertial forces predominate, and the flow become turbulent [20]. Once turbulence has occurred, it becomes almost impossible to predict the exact relationship between pressure and flow. All one can say is that flow will be less than predicted from pressure-flow relations at lower flow rates. This means that, a considerably greater pressure head is required to force a given flow of fluid through the same tube under conditions of turbulence, compared with the pressure required for laminar flow. This is due to dissipation of pressure energy to provide the kinetic energy of turbulence. Professor Osborne Reynolds (English engineer) defined a criterion as to when a flow would be laminar or turbulent. He demonstrated that flow, in a long smooth tube, would be laminar provided a parameter **Re** (after Rey-

---

fully developed (Figure 31.3). Since arterial branchng is so frequent in the circulatory system, the velocity profile is usually not fully developed [109, 110]. Theoretical values for the entrance length, i.e. flow development region, required for entrance effects to dissipate [111]: 10 cm for common carotid artery, 19 cm for renal arteries, 8 cm for external iliac and common femoral arteries, 5 cm for superficial femoral artery, 2–9 mm for posterior tibial and dorsalis pedis arteries.

$$\text{Entrance length [112]} = \frac{0.2 \times (\text{tube diameter})^2 \times \text{fluid maximum velocity}}{4 \times \text{fluid viscosity}}$$

Entrance length for laminar flow in a straight tube [30]:

$$\frac{0.03 \times (\text{tube diameter})^2 \times \text{fluid density} \times \text{fluid average velocity}}{\text{fluid viscosity}}$$

$$= 0.03 \times \text{tube diameter} \times \text{Reynolds number}.$$

Entrance length for turbulent flow in a straight tube [30]:

$$0.693 \times \text{tube diameter} \times \sqrt[4]{\text{Reynolds number}}.$$

nolds) did not exceed a certain critical value, otherwis turbulence would start. Re, a dimensionless parameter called Reynolds number[13], is given by:

$$\mathbf{Re} = \frac{\rho.v \cdot 2r}{\mu} \left(= \frac{2 \cdot \rho \cdot Q}{\pi \cdot r \cdot \mu} \right),$$

where ρ = fluid density (g/cm^3), v = average flow velocity (cm/sec), r = tube radius (cm), μ = fluid viscosity (poise) Kinematic viscosity $v = (\mu/\rho)$ (cm^2/sec)), and Q = flow volume (cm^3/sec).

Re equation can be modified to apply to tubes of any shape and size [26]. When Re of a steady flow, in a straight rigid cylindrical and non-branching pipe, is > 2000 (dominant inertial forces), turbulent flow usually results [115]. Re < 100 (dominant viscous forces) represents a flow which is strictly laminar and undisturbed [87]. 100 < Re < 2000 indicates the presence of some disturbance in laminar flow (transitional). Depending on flow entrance conditions, unsteadiness, curvatures, branching, constrictions and other specifications of the flow system, the critical Re value ($\simeq$ 2000) will either increase or decrease, making the onset of turbulence more difficult or easier [116]. For instance, in pulsatile (unsteady) flow experiments [24], initiation of turbulence occurs at a critical Re $\simeq$ 1200 and is therefore less retarded as compared to steady flow [117, 118]. Under normal physiological conditions of blood flow, turbulence occurs only in large vessels and only during a short period of the cardiac cycle (systolic deceleration phase) when Re values become high [26]. However, with high pulsatility of flow, there may not be enough time for turbulence to develop, even with the deceleration period. This means, a highly pulsatile flow exerts a stabilising effect on the flow field [22]. Anemia, on the other hand, predisposes to turbulence because of diminished hematocrit (resulting in decreased blood viscosity), and increased cardiac output (resulting in increased flow velocity). The Re values in the micro-circulation (where the resistance vessels are located) are so low that it is extremely unlikely for turbulence to develop [36, 110]. Typical physiologic transition or critical Re values (Rec) in humans are [119, 120]:

Rec $\simeq$ 200 in coronary arteries, Rec $\simeq$ 400 in carotid arteries,

Rec $\simeq$ 1500 in abdominal aorta, Rec $\simeq$ 1000 in femoral arteries.

Example. Suppose the common femoral artery has a 1-cm diameter, a peak-systole flow velocity at rest of 20 cm/sec under normal conditions (30 cm/sec with hyperaemia), blood density of 1.05 g/cm^3 and blood viscosity of 0.04 poise (dyne sec/cm^2), therefore: Re = (1.05 × 20 × (2 × 0.5))/0.04 $\simeq$ 525 at peak systole at rest ($\simeq$787 at peak systole with hyperaemia). These figures are well below the critical value of 1000.

Flow turbulence gives rise to vessel wall vibrations which are recognized as murmurs and thrills [107, 121–124] and can be an initiating factor in localized

---

13. Re is expressed by the ratio of inertial forces ($\propto$ ($\rho \cdot v^2/2r$)) to viscous forces ($\propto$ ($\mu \cdot v/4r^2$), and is used to characterise the flow field as laminar, transitional or, turbulent [20].

deposition of atheroma leading to further encroachment on the arterial lumen by atherosclerotic plaques [73, 125]. In fact, it has been demonstrated that flow turbulence contributes to thrombus formation [126]. The mechanism may include the modification of platelet function by abnormal hemodynamic stresses and, the increased likelihood that red cells and platelets will intensely collide with each other and with the vessel wall leading to endothelial cell damage [11, 127, 128]. Turbulence may also contribute to the progressive increase in the size of an aneurysm[14] and to the post-stenotic dilatation occasionally seen, for example, in the sub-clavian artery in thoracic outlet syndrome [129]. With unsteady flow, the non-dimensional Womersley frequency parameter α is also used, with critical Re, to indicate the tendency to flow turbulence. In pulsatile flow, α describes the shape of the velocity profile as compared to the parabolic profile usually seen in steady laminar flow, and it is given by [26, 36]:

$$\alpha = r \sqrt{\frac{\omega}{\nu}},$$

where, r = tube radius, ω = angular frequency of the pulse rate (= 2π . heart rate), ν = kinematic viscosity = (fluid viscosity/fluid density).

Example. Suppose the common femoral radius = 0.5 cm, heart rate = 70 beats/mn

$$\left(\omega = 2\pi . \frac{70}{60} = 7.33 \text{ radians/sec}\right), \nu_{blood} = \frac{\text{viscosity}}{\text{density}}$$

$$= \frac{0.04 \text{ poise}}{1.05 \text{ g/cm}^3} = 0.038 \text{ cm}^2/\text{sec, therefore } \alpha = 0.5\sqrt{\frac{7.33}{0.038}} \simeq 7.$$

Small α values reflect quasi-parabolic velocity profiles ($\alpha = 0 \leftrightarrow$ true parabolic profile), while large α values e.g. with high heart rates relate to less parabolic i.e. flatter profiles. If critical Re number is plotted against Womersley number c for flow in the major arteries of several species including man, the points fall close to the boundary which marks the transition from laminar to turbulent flow [130]. This means, it would take only minor geometric or hemodynamic changes to create turbulence. Finally, the effects of a stenosis in terms of energy losses can be quantitated as a dimensionless parameter, the Strouhal number S [131, 132]:

$$S = \frac{2\alpha^2}{\pi . \text{Re}},$$

where α = Womersley frequency parameter, Re = Reynolds number. Duncan and associates [133] explored the use of the Strouhal number in the

---

14. It has been shown experimentally that arterial wall vibration at low frequency (due to turbulent flow) can be highly destructive to the wall structural components, especially the elastin fibre [129].

spectral analysis of arterial bruits from carotid stenoses (carotid phonoangio-graphy). They found that the product of the 'break' frequency[15] (Fb) of the bruit spectrum and the residual lumen diameter (d, in mm) of the stenosis to be constant for the human carotid bifurcation in different patients: Fb . d = S . V ≈ 500 where S = Strouhal number, and V = blood flow velocity (mm/sec). On the other hand, Chapman and Charlesworth [124] found that the bruit frequencies at which peak spectral amplitudes occurred remained fairly constant (for a given tube) and were independent of the type or degree of stenosis and the Reynolds number. Also, these resonant frequencies were higher for stiffer tubes, and it followed that an arteriosclerotic artery was less likely to vibrate/resonate than a normal one, and that after endarterec-tomy noise may still be heard despite the fact that a stenosis has been corrected [124].

Bernoulli theorem

Introduced by Daniel Bernoulli [134] in 1726, a swiss mathematician (1700–1782), and clarified by his friend Leonard Euler, the theorem explains the interconversion of potential and kinetic energy of a steady laminar flow when an ideal (i.e. non-viscous) liquid flows in streamlines through a series of tubes of different diameters (Figure 31.4). Since the liquid is assumed to be inviscid, there are no energy losses due to viscous forces along the tube system, and so the theorem states that, the sum of potential and kinetic energy components of a *steady, laminar, and frictionless flow* is the same at all points along the tube system (more precisely along a streamline). The total energy of a flowing liquid consists of [16, 135, 136]:

Potential energy + Kinetic energy + Gravitational energy.

Potential energy includes static pressure (a form of potential energy/unit of volume) which represents the fluid lateral pressure in a tube. Pressure due to cal diac pumping is also a form of potential energy/unit of volume. Gravitational energy (Eg) is that part of potential energy due to changes in height of the flowing liquid (Eg = 0 in a horizontal tube), and reflects the ability of the liquid to perform work by gravity. Kinetic energy represents the dynamic energy of flow i.e. when the fluid is in motion, and is proportional to the square of the flow velocity (dynamic pressure is a form of kinetic en-ergy/unit of volume). Consider Figure 31.4 where two tubes A and C of equal diameters (2ra = 2rc) are connected via a 3rd. tube B of a smaller diameter (2rb). Since the cross-section of tube B (πrb^2) is smaller than that of tube A (πra^2), the flow velocity in B (Vb) must consequently be larger than in A (Va) in order to obtain the same flow volume through the (fric-tionless) tube system (principle of conservation of mass).

---

15. The 'break' frequency is the spectral frequency at which the amplitude falls off sharply for the higher frequencies.

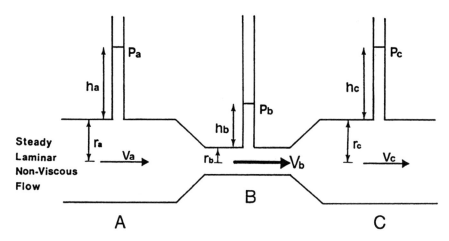

Figure 31.4. Shematic diagram to demonstrate the Bernoulli principle as applied to a nonviscous fluid flowing steadily through a series of rigid tubes (A, B, C) with different diameters. The effect of the constriction (B) is to increase the flow velocity (V) and decrease the lateral pressure (P) in comparison to those in tube A in order to preserve the flow volume. Furthermore, due to absence of fluid energy losses in terms of viscosity and inertia, the flow velocity and pressure are restored in C and are equal to those in tube A. h = height of fluid column = lateral pressure, r = tube radius.

According to Bernoulli energy-balance principle, the total liquid energy per unit of volume (erg/cm^3) in A is equal to that in B (and indeed that in C) (principle of conservation of energy):

Potential energy (A) + Kinetic energy (A) = Potential energy (B) + Kinetic energy (B) $\Rightarrow$

$Pa + \frac{1}{2} . \rho . Va^2 = Pb + \frac{1}{2} . \rho . Vb^2 (= Pc + \frac{1}{2} . \rho . Vc) \Rightarrow$

$\rho . g . ha + \frac{1}{2} . \rho . Va^2 = \rho . g . hb + \frac{1}{2} . \rho . Vb^2 (= \rho . g . hc + \frac{1}{2} . \rho . Vc^2)$,

where Pa, Pb, and Pc are the liquid lateral pressures in tubes A, B, and C respectively; ρ = liquid density (g/cm^3); Va, Vb, and Vc are the spatial average flow velocities (cm/sec) in tubes A, B, and C; ha, hb, and hc are the heights of liquid (cm) in tubes A, B, and C due to lateral pressure, and g = acceleration due to gravity = 980 cm/sec^2.

As the flow moves from tube A to tube B ($\equiv$ to a stenosis), it will undertake a transfer of potential energy towards kinetic energy: Pb becomes lower than Pa, while $\frac{1}{2} . \rho . Vb^2$ becomes higher than $\frac{1}{2} . \rho . Va^2$. By leaving tube B to tube C, the flow experiences a *reversed* transfer of energy i.e. kinetic to potential: Pc becomes higher than Pb, and $\frac{1}{2} . \rho . Vc^2$ becomes lower than $\frac{1}{2} . \rho . Vb^2$. In the case of an *ideal*, i.e. non-viscous, fluid, and no energy losses occuring, there will be a complete recovery of potential energy in tube C: Pc = Pa (also $\frac{1}{2} . \rho . Vc^2 = \frac{1}{2} . \rho . Va^2$ by virtue of the Bernoulli principle).

If $ra \geqslant rb$ i.e. $Va \leqslant Vb$, therefore the pressure difference between A and B expressed in centimeters of liquid will be:

$$ha - hb \simeq \frac{1}{2} \cdot \frac{Vb^2}{g}.$$

Similarly, the pressure difference between B and C is given by:

$$hb - hc \simeq -\frac{1}{2} \cdot \frac{Vb^2}{g}.$$

This means that, pressure difference does not always determine flow. In fact, liquid is flowing against a pressure gradient from $B \rightarrow C$ (minus sign). Strictly speaking, it is the *energy gradient* that forces the liquid to flow from $A \rightarrow B \rightarrow C$ (at inlet of tube A, energy due to pumping must also be considered) [38]. The other implication of Bernoulli principle is that, the lateral pressure measured side-on to the direction of flow is lower than that measured end-on to the direction of flow. This is because end-on pressure measurement converts kinetic energy into potential energy, so that the total liquid energy will be mostly expressed in terms of pressure only:

static/radial/lateral pressure + dynamic/axial/head-on/impact pressure.

The application of Bernoulli theorem to blood circulation in arteries is valid if the effects of blood viscosity are negligible. This is so in relatively wide arteries, over short distances, with high Reynolds number (Re), and where laminar flow is retained [38, 117, 118, 137, 138]. Looking back at Figure 31.4 and assuming tube B represents an arterial stenosis, the pre-stenotic-trans-stenotic pressure drop (i.e. from $A \rightarrow B$) in mm Hg can be derived as follows:

$$\rho_{Hg} \cdot g \cdot ha + \tfrac{1}{2} \cdot \rho_{blood} \cdot Va^2 = \rho_{Hg} \cdot g \cdot hb + \tfrac{1}{2} \cdot \rho_{blood} \cdot Vb^2 \Rightarrow$$

$$ha - hb = \frac{1}{2 \cdot g} \cdot \frac{\rho_{blood}}{\rho_{Hg}} \cdot (Vb^2 - Va^2), \tag{31.1}$$

where ρ_{Hg} = density of mercury ($= 13.6 \text{ g/cm}^3$), ρ_{blood} = density of blood ($= 1.05 \text{ g/cm}^3$).

If $Vb^2 \gg Va^2$, then:

$$ha - hb \simeq \frac{1}{2 \cdot g} \cdot \frac{\rho_{blood}}{\rho_{Hg}} \cdot Vb^2 = \frac{1}{2 \times 980} \times \frac{1.05}{13.6} \times Vb^2 \Rightarrow$$

$$ha - hb \text{ (cm Hg)} \simeq 0.0000394 \times Vb^2 \text{ (cm/sec)}.$$

Expressing the pressure drop in mm Hg and flow velocity in m/sec gives:

$$ha - hb \text{ (mm Hg)} \simeq 0.0000394 \times Vb^2 \text{ (m/sec)} \times 10 \times (10^2)^2 \Rightarrow$$

$$ha - hb \text{ (mm Hg)} \simeq 3.94 \, Vb^2 \simeq 4 Vb^2. \tag{31.2}$$

This is the *simplified Bernoulli* equation[16] frequently used to approximate the pressure drop across an arterial stenosis. If the velocity profile in the stenosis is flat, the spatial average flow velocity Vb ≃ Vmax = maximum flow velocity. On the other hand, the pressure drop is highest at the *vena contracta*[17] i.e. where the streamlines are maximally constricted or flow velocity is highest. The modified Bernoulli equation should not be confused with the similar *orifice formula of Gorlin and Gorlin* [140] (also known as Torricelli's law) which applies to flow of a viscous fluid through an orifice (as in incompetent or regurgitant mitral and tricuspid cardiac valves, ventricular septal defects) and out in a (free) jet[18], and where potential energy of flow is lost within the orifice due to viscous resistance, and beyond the orifice to provide the kinetic energy required for downstream turbulence and vortices. The maximal pressure drop P1 − P2 (mm Hg) across the orifice is given by [141–143]:

$$P1 - P2 \, (\text{mm Hg}) = \frac{1}{2g} \frac{\rho_{blood}}{\rho_{Hg}} V_{jet}^2 \cdot 10^5 \approx 4V_{jet}^2 \, (\text{m/sec}), \qquad (31.3)$$

where V_{jet} = jet maximum velocity (m/sec), g = 980 cm/sec^2.
The orifice area Ao is given by:

$$Ao(\text{m}^2) = Q \, (\text{m}^3/\text{sec}) \sqrt{\frac{10^5 \times \rho_{blood}}{2 \times g \times \rho_{Hg} \times (P1 - P2)}} \Rightarrow$$

---

16. A denominator constant α is introduced by some workers depending on the state of flow:

$$ha - hb \approx \frac{4vb^2}{\alpha},$$

where $\alpha = \frac{1}{2}$ in laminar flow, and $\alpha = 1$ in turbulent flow [138].

17. The *vena contracta* is a jet flow region with minimal cross-section occuring just beyond a constriction with a sharp-edged entrance, and causing the subsequent jet crosssection (Ac) to be smaller than that of the constriction (Ao). With a smooth-edged constriction entrance, the cross-sectional area of the *vena contracta* will be that of the constriction or very close that. The location of the *vena contracta* is related to the geometry of the constriction, provided the flow rate is above a given threshold. The ratio (Ac/Ao) defines the contraction coefficient of the constriction [22, 139].

18. An orifice jet is termed *free* when it flows into a relatively stagnant environment e.g. left or right atrium, and where the cross-sectional area of the jet is $<\frac{1}{5}$-th. of that of the chamber into which it is flowing. A free jet develops free from influence of chamber boundaries i.e. no wall or viscous effects. On the other hand, a *confined or bounded* jet is influenced by upstream flow, severity of constriction, and distal expansion of constriction. Stenotic aortic and pulmonary valves and other peripheral stenotic arterial lesions produce confined flow jets. With sudden stenosis expansion, the jet expands more slowly in the radial direction. A recirculation region of flow (vortices) develop near the vessel wall (outer fringes of the jet) due to interactions between jet inertia, viscous effects and adverse axial pressure gradients. Further downstream, the jet re-attaches itself to the wall and the flow reconstitutes [22].

$$\text{Ao (cm}^2) \simeq \frac{Q \text{ (ml/sec)}}{50\sqrt{P1 - P2} \text{ (mm Hg)}},$$

Invasive pressure measurements downstream from the *vena contracta* will under-estimate the maximal pressure drop at the *vena contracta* (due to downstream pressure recovery). If this maximal pressure drop is estimated non-invasively using ultrasound Doppler (say) from the jet velocity at the *vena contracta* ($4V_{jet}^2$), an incorrect impression can be produced: that the orifice formula (or the modified Bernoulli equation) is over-estimating the pressure drop. Other contributory factors to this false impression are those of catheter placement outside the central jet in the turbulence zone and/or orientation of the pressure port into the streamlines of flow, with conversion of kinetic energy into sensed pressure by the measuring device [22, 144]. Ideally, the pressure port must lie sidewise with respect to the flow streamlines, and within the *vena contracta* of the jet [139].

For orifices of diameter >3.5 mm, and jet velocity >3 m/sec, the estimation of pressure drop (>70 mm Hg) from velocity alone (using $P1 - P2 \simeq 4V_{jet}^2$) was shown to be reasonably accurate [142, 143]. Holen and associates [145], demonstrated the validity (*in-vitro*) of Torricelli's law for orifice diameters >1.6 mm (pressure differences 3–100 mm Hg, Re 400–2500, $\mu = 0.01$–0.05 poise). Faccenda et al. [146] obtained a high correlation coefficient ($r > 0.9$) between Doppler-derived pressure drop estimations and intra-arterial pressure measurements in the thoracic aorta of dogs. These results encouraged the clinical application of the simplified Bernoulli equation in the non-invasive ultrasound Doppler evaluation of lower-limb atherosclerotic disease in vascular patients. Using ultrasound duplex imaging, Langsfeld et al. [147] achieved a correlation coefficient $r = 0.9$ ($n = 11$ cases) between the Doppler-estimated pressures (on one hand) and invasively-measured pressures during arteriography (on the other hand), for moderate and severe aorto-iliac stenoses (>50% diameter reduction). Kohler et al. [148] tested equation (31.1) i.e. pressure drop $\simeq$ 4(trans-stenotic velocity^2-pre-stenotic velocity^2), in the evaluation of aorto-iliac stenotic disease. Theoretically, the exclusion of the pre-stenotic velocity term (Va), as in equation (31.2), leads to over-estimating the pressure drop. Despite including this term in the equation, the pressure drop was surprisingly over-estimated for mild stenoses (i.e. <20 mm Hg measured pressure drop, $r = 0.54$), and in despite of using the maximum pre-stenotic velocity at peak systole (instead of the spatial average velocity at peak systole). It may be that, they had measured the pressure (invasively) in the post-stenotic arterial region, when they should have made the measurements at the *vena contracta* just beyond the stenosis, where the pressure drop is highest by comparison with that beyond the mild stenosis (where little kinetic energy is lost into heat and for turbulence, and the rest is converted back into potential energy or pressure). For severe stenoses (i.e. >40 mm Hg), however, the equation under-estimated the pressure drop (as would be expected), mainly because of not taking into account the viscous effects of blood flow (see below) which became important in severe cases [145, 149–151].

Equations (31.2) and (31.3) appear to be exactly the same, the difference is that, the modified Bernoulli equation (31.2) will provide a very accurate estimation of pressure drop if some conditions are satisfied i.e. flow is steady, laminar, and frictionless. In practice, however, blood flow in arteries is pulsatile, subjected to a viscous drag, and can become turbulent e.g. beyond a stenosis. Under these circumstances, a more complete expression for pressure drop across an arterial (or valvular) stenosis must further include a term for viscous losses of flow (potential) energy due to friction, and another term for inertial losses of energy due to changing flow rate[19] (because of flow pulsatility or time-varying pressure head) [143]:

| Loss in flow potential energy, equivalent to pressure drop. | = gain in kinetic energy, due to flow convective or spatial acceleration through the stenosis. | + gain in viscous energy, due to fluid friction against the wall of the stenosis, and is manifested as heat. | + gain in inertial energy, due to flow local acceleration and deceleration i.e. temporal unsteadiness. |

Therefore, using equation (31.2) or (31.3) (which neglects the viscosity and inertia terms) will inevitably result in under-estimation of the pressure drop. However, the neglect of the pre-stenotic velocity (Va) compensates for this error [139]. The extent of such an error (mostly due to ignoring the viscosity term increases with progressively smaller orifices and longer[20] stenoses [138, 139, 152, 153]. In an *in-vitro* study, Requarth et al. [154] demonstrated that as the stenosis became more severe, the *full* energy-balance equation) showed a slight systematic under-estimation of the pressure drop, while the modified Bernoulli equation produced a marked under-estimation. With mild discrete (short-segment) stenoses, however, the full equation over-estimated the pressure drop by as much as or more than the modified equation underestimated it.

The clinical use of the full equation in studying arterial stenotic disease is not straightforward. The difficulty arises when attempting to calculate the frictional losses of pressure, which themselves depend on the *in-situ* stenosis

---

19. Pressure drop due to inertance of the mass of blood $= L(dq/dt)$, where L = blood inertance, and (dq/dt) = rate of change of flow over time. (dq/dt) is negligible when flow is changing slowly e.g. at mid-systole or mid-diastole [137].
20. *In-vitro* data suggest that a long-segment stenosis exists when the stenosis length is greater than twice the stenosis diameter [138] i.e. (stenosis length/stenosis diameter $> 2 \Rightarrow$ dominant viscous losses of energy.

geometry[21]. This is even more stressed for turbulence losses of energy in the post-stenotic region, and where turbulence contributes most to the total pressure drop across the stenosis [117, 118, 155]. Using a formula for pressure drop which incorporated a term for turbulence losses of energy, in addition to viscous and inertial losses, Flanigan et al. [156] could accurately reproduce pressure measurements in a canine model. Valid application of the simplified Bernoulli equation to clinical situations (with the exception of the coronary arteries) is possible if, the viscous and inertial effects can be neglected [22]. This is true at peak of systole during the cardiac cycle, when flow is quasi-steady and blood viscosity is low (since velocity is high). Consequently, the simplified Bernoulli equation becomes:

$$\Delta P_{peak} = (P_1 - P_2)_{peak} \simeq 4(V_2^2 - V_1^2)_{peak},$$

where ΔP_{peak} = pressure drop at peak of systole, P_1 = pressure at peak of systole proximal to the stenosis, P_2 = pressure at peak of systole within the stenosis, V_1 = spatial average flow velocity at peak of systole proximal to the stenosis, V_2 = spatial average flow velocity at peak of systole within the stenosis.

If the velocity profile can be assumed to be flat, then, the spatial average flow velocity at peak of systole the maximum flow velocity at peak of systole. Also, if $V_1^2 \ll V_2^2 \Rightarrow \Delta P_{peak} \simeq 4V_{2(peak)}^2$. Provided invasive catheter pressure measurements are made at peak of systole and within the *vena contracta*, and the pressure port of the sensing catheter is placed sidewise along the streamlines of flow (and not facing them), then, the non-invasive estimation of the pressure drop using $\Delta P_{peak} \simeq 4V_{2(peak)}^2$ should be very accurate [22].

Finally, other factors that are important in clinical studies include the effects of arterial branching, tortuosity, and wave reflection, which makes the clinical application of the Bernoulli principle somewhat critical.

Haemodynamic modeling and significance of arterial stenoses

In terms of energy, blood flow experiences several energy losses by entering, moving through, and leaving an arterial stenosis [149, 157–159]:

1. *Contraction loss*: it occurs at the converging part or entrance of the stenosis, where potential energy is transferred to kinetic energy in order to accelerate flow through the stenosis. The amount of energy lost during this transfer accounts for 30–40% of the total energy loss [138].

---

21. The pressure drop caused by frictional effects within a stenosis may be estimated using Poiseuille equation (for steady, laminar and developed flow:

$\Delta P = 8 . \mu . l . v/r^2,$

where μ = fluid viscosity, l = length of stenosis, r = radius of stenosis, v = mean flow velocity in the stenosis [139].

2. *Friction loss*: it results from the (increased) frictional or viscous forces that develop between the moving blood in the stenosis and the wall boundary of the stenosis. This kind of energy loss is proportional to (stenosis length/stenosis diameter) × flow kinetic energy through the stenosis [160] (Darey-Weisbach formula), and it accounts for 4–20% of the total energy loss [138]. With progressively tighter stenoses (up to some critical level), the kinetic energy of stenotic flow will gradually increase, and so will the proportion of friction loss of energy.

3. *Expansion loss*: it occurs at the diverging part or exit of the stenosis, where kinetic energy is transferred *back* to potential energy. The amount of energy lost during this transfer accounts for 50–60% of the total energy loss [139]. This is because the high-speed stenotic jet discharges into a slow-moving blood mass in the post-stenotic site (sudden flow deceleration), resulting in the formation and maintenance of vortices/eddies and turbulence. Consequently, the post-stenotic potential energy does not regain the prestenotic energy level. Hence, a pressure drop is established across the stenosis, which increases with the extent of arterial narrowing, and is a reflection of non-recoverable loss of energy through and at the outlet of the stenosis. Whether a near-complete or incomplete recovery of potential energy occurs beyond the stenosis will depend on the degree of severity of the stenosis i.e. non-severe (mild to moderate) versus severe, and the type of expansion of the stenosis i.e. gradual versus abrupt expansion [22]. Berguer and Hwang [159] found that, in non-elastic tubes with severe stenoses, the potential energy in the post-stenotic region approximated that in the stenosis itself, but it was much lower than that in the pre-stenotic region.

The development of a pressure drop explains why, for instance, femoral pulses are sometimes very weak or even unperceptible in the presence of severe proximal aorto-iliac atheromatous disease. The changes seen in femoral pulse are related not only to the degree of arterial narrowing in the proximal segment but also to the velocity of flow through the stenosis [161]. This is primarily controlled by the peripheral resistance of the terminal vascular bed. The clinical phenomenon of "disappearing' femoral and pedal pressure pulses noticed following exercise or peripheral vasodilatation has been well documented [157, 162–165]. This is because diminished peripheral resistance (induced by exercise) causes flow enhancement which, in turn, is responsible for a further drop in post-stenotic pressure leading to the disappearance of palpable femoral and pedal pulses. Distal occlusions or a cuff wrapped around the thigh and inflated to a supra-systolic pressure level should result in a stronger femoral pulse. If it does not, one might believe the particular patient to have a good collateral circulation (profunda femoris artery) [166]. In summary:

In the case of a constant peripheral resistance

An increase in stenotic resistance $\Rightarrow$

   a) A decrease in flow rate

   b) An increase in pressure drop
      (i.e. a decrease in post-stenotic pressure)

In the case of a constant stenotic resistance

An increase in peripheral resistance $\Rightarrow$

   a) A decrease in flow rate

   b) A decrease in pressure drop
      (i.e. an increase in post-stenotic pressure)

Flow regimes in stenotic vessels

When the flow enters the converging part of a stenosis, the velocity profile is of an entrance type i.e. flat, and the pressure drops acutely with a minimum occuring slightly downstream from the 'throat' of the stenosis (i.e. at the *vena contracta*) [116]. Within the stenosis, the increased viscous forces close to the stenosis wall cause the fluid layers near the wall to be retarded. Consequently, a boundary layer will occur i.e. the velocity profile will become less flat and more parabolic [139]. At the diverging part, the flow near the wall may stagnate (flow separation) and even may reverse direction (flow reversal/recirculation) if pressure recovery is too high or peripheral resistance is increased [167–169]. Further downstream, forward flow is re-established (re-attachment point). Experimental observations have shown 3 basic flow regimes for a given stenosis [15, 117, 118, 170]:

1. At a low Reynolds number (Re), uni-directional laminar flow exists before, within, and after the stenosis.
2. At a moderate Re number e.g. mild to moderate stenosis, the flow remains laminar, but a thin separation layer is seen in the diverging downstream segment. This separation layer predisposes to flow instability and turbulence at high Re numbers.
3. At a high Re number e.g. severe stenosis, the flow beyond the stenosis is unstable and turbulent. As Re increases, the separation zone, originally thin and just downstream from the stenosis, becomes thicker and moves upstream, and the laminar re-attachment point is displaced further downstream.

Regarding the spatial propagation of turbulence beyond the stenosis, it appears that the length of propagation relative to the dimensions of the vessel and stenosis may be linear within the biological range, with more severe stenoses giving rise to greater flow disturbances and turbulence [171, 172]. Stroke volume also seems to take part in the extent of propagation, and is relatively independent of whether or not the narrowing is axisymetric [173–177]. Usually, turbulence disappears at a distance of 4–5 multiples of vessel diameter from the stenosis [178]. Felix et al. [179] provided evidence of disturbed flow up to 15 cm beyond an arterial stenosis. Therefore, it is important to know the spatial . relationship between the stenosis site (e.g. aorto-iliac) and the recording site (e.g. femoral), otherwise the assessment of the stenosis may be unreliable [180].

Significance of arterial stenoses

In order to explain the behaviour of blood flow in increasingly stenosed arteries, Weale [121] visualized this flow in two concentric zones:

1. *The axial flow* is that central fraction of the flow in which the major job of transport is carried out, and where the flow velocity is usually greatest.
2. *The resistance flow* is that relatively stagnant fraction of the flow surrounding the axial stream, and where there is a velocity gradient (boundary layer).

The relative proportions of the axial and resistance streams are determined by the total resistance of the flow system. The greater this resistance, the less important is the axial stream, and hence the flow rate. If the vessel lumen is narrowed until the vessel wall impinges on the axial stream, or if the flow rate is increased until the contour of the axial stream touches the vessel wall, the flow will be severely compromised for any further similar changes, due to the steep velocity gradient developing between the axial flow and the stationary wall leading to the onset of turbulence distal to the stenosis (or at the end of the tube *in-vitro*). This introduces the term *critical stenosis* defined as the size of stenosis in which relatively small increments in its degree of severity (e.g. small decrements in stenosis area) will cause precipitous fall in (post-stenotic) flow and pressure. Other variants of this definition included '... that constriction which would produce a 5% fall in distal mean pressure, or a 10% decrease in distal mean flow' [181], '... that cross-sectional area at which 80% of the pressure gradient, obtainable on total occlusion, occurs' [121]. Most investigators, however, produced evidence that about 80% lumenal area reduction ($\equiv$ to 55% diameter reduction[22]) must take place before abrupt changes in flow and pressure can be noted [149, 156, 159, 182–185]. Others presented data suggesting that the lumen area of a major artery must be reduced by at least 90% ($\equiv$ to 68% diameter reduction) in order to produce impairement of blood flow behind the ischemic symptoms [186, 187]. May et al. [188] found that the critical stenosis for human femoral artery was 95% area reduction, and for iliac artery 94% area reduction ($\equiv$ to 78% and 76% diameter reduction respectively). Similarly, Kupper et al. [189] used 75% diameter reduction as the size of the critical stenosis in lower limb arteries. The discrepancies seen in the size of the critical stenosis can be explained by the fact that, this critical size depends on such factors as (1)

---

22. Equations for conversion between % area reduction (AR) and % diameter reduction (DR): $\%DR = (1 - \sqrt{1 - AR}) \times 100$, $\%AR = \{1 - (1 - DR)^2\} \times 100$, example: $\%AR = 75\% = 0.75$ is equivalent to $\%DR = (1 - \sqrt{1 - 0.75}) \times 100 = 50\%$.

the peripheral resistance of the terminal vascular bed; (2) the flow volume in the vessel; (3) the length and diameter of the stenosis; (4) the geometry of the stenosis; and (5) the lumen area of the normal unstenosed vessel [184, 190, 191]. This means that each arterial segment would have its proper level of critical stenosis under well defined conditions. For instance, it was shown that, at flow rates comparable to the resting level in human aorto-iliac arteries, no significant pressure drops were apparent with <80% area reduction stenoses [192, 193]. Ahmed and Giddens [194] studied axisymmetric stenoses wlth pulsatile flow at a physiologic Reynolds number of 600 *in-vitro*, and found that turbulence occurred only with stenoses greater than 50% diameter reduction. Also, asymmetrical stenoses with rough surfaces produced greater pressure drops than equivalent axisymmetric stenoses with rounded and smooth lumenal surface [195, 196]. Furthermore, as flow rates increased and/or peripheral resistance decreased (e.g. with exercise, drug-induced vaso-dilation, sympathectomy), significant pressure drops did develop even with less severe stenoses i.e. the magnitude of the critical stenosis shifted towards lower (% area reduction) values [149, 155, 184, 188, 197, 198]. This is because the fraction of the total energy of flow allocated to the kinetic energy component is significantly bigger in the case of high flow rate than in low flow rate. This means that, the flow kinetic energy in the stenosis will reach some critical upper limit (just sufficient to maintain a constant flow) more quickly in high-flow condition than in low-flow condition [159].

Regarding the effect of multiple stenoses on flow and pressure, Weale [199] examined the series and parallel relationships, drawn from electrical circuitry, to see if analogies based on Ohm's law (voltage = resistance × current) were applicable to blood flow. It was found that the parallel-resistance relationship $(1/R_t = 1/R_1 + 1/R_2 + 1/R_3, \ldots$, where R_t = total resistance, R_1; R_2; R_3 are resistances in parallel) did apply except when one of the resistances was too high. The series-resistance relationship $(R_t = R_1 + R_2 + R_3 + \ldots$ where R_1; R_2; R_3 are resistances in series) did not describe blood flow under all conditions. Instead R_t approximated to the value of the maximum (stenotic) resistance. This was later confirmed by Robbins and Bentou [190]. Flanigan *et al.* [156] studied the effect of multiple sub-critical stenoses on flow and pressure and found it to be additive (both in steady and pulsatile flow conditions), but in a non-linear fashion[23]. This means, each newly introduced stenosis produced less of a pressure drop (across the entire series) than the previous one. As a result of this additive effect, a series of sub-critical stenoses may well become hemodynamically significant or critical and, thus, produce symptoms of arterial insufficiency. The cumulative effect was equally valid for serial critical stenoses [201]. Distance between the stenoses did not considerably alter the results [200], with the pressure drop *marginally* increasing with larger spacing due to flow

---

23. Karayannacos *et al.* [200] found the pressure drop across a series of non-critical stenoses to be linearly additive.

Table 31.2. See text for details.

	Lower abdominal aorta	Common iliac artery	Coronary artery
Normal internal diameter (mm)	15	8	3
Critical residual diameter (mm)	4	3	1
Critical % diameter reduction	73%	63%	67%
Critical % area reduction	93%	86%	89%

re-attachment (to the vessel wall) before the next stenosis is reached[24]. On the other hand, when a non-critical stenosis exists in series with another critical stenosis, the total effect on flow and pressure is governed entirely by the more severe critical stenosis [199, 201].

Regarding the question of *how the stenosis might be quantified*, most investigators have used the *percent reduction in lumen area or diameter*, whereas others have suggested the use of the *actual or absolute value of the lumen residual area or diameter*; while claiming that the area of the un-stenosed segment of the vessel bears (under some circumstances) little re-lation to the hemodynamic response of the stenosis. This is because the resistance to flow offered by the stenosis and the peripheral vascular bed is much greater than that offered by the internal viscous forces in the un-obstructed part of the vessel. The latter position was adopted by Fiddian and co-workers [184], who found that under the same conditions of proximal pressure, peripheral resistance, and fluid viscosity, the absolute size of the critical stenosis in three differing-diameter tubes was the same. Clearly, the % diameter reduction of the critical stenosis was different for the 3 tubes. It would, therefore, be misleading to judge the severity of each stenosis on the basis of one common % value e.g. 50% diameter reduction. In practice, however, the error introduced by using % values is somehow lessened. This is because larger arteries tend to have lower peripheral resistance and, thus, bigger critical stenosis residual diameter than do smaller arteries. Fiddian *et al.* [184] gave approximate figures for the critical stenosis residual diameters as they occurred in some human arteries (with ≠ peripheral resistances) (Table 31.2). According to these figures, there is a difference of up to 10% diameter reduction (73%–63%). On the other hand, considering 50% (as it is frequent) as the threshold between non-critical and critical stenoses will obviously *over-estimate* the severity of such stenosis with, say, 58% diameter reduction in any of the above vessels.

---

24. Most of the pressure drop per stenosis, associated with increased spacing, is attained before the distance between two stenoses exceeds twice the intact vessel diameter [200].

References

1. Lallemand RC, Gosling RG, Newman DL. Role of the bifurcation in atheromatosis of the abdominal aorta. Surg Gynecol Obstet 1973;137:987.
2. Zamir M. The role of shear forces in arterial branching. J Gen Physiol 1976;67:213.
3. Dewey CF, Bussolari SR, Gimbrone MA *et al.* The dynamic response of endothelial cells to fluid shear stress. J Biomech Eng 1981;3:171.
4. Levesque MJ, Nerem RM. Elongation and Orientation of cultured endothelial cells in response to shear. J Biomech Eng 1985;7:341.
5. Meisner JE, Rushmer RF. Eddy formation and turbulence in flowing liquids. Circ Res 1963;12:455.
6. Texon M. The hemodyamic concept of atherosclerosis. Bull NY Acad Med 1960;36:263.
7. Wesolowski SA, Fries CC, Sobini AM *et al.* Significance of turbulence in hemic systems and the distribution of atherosclerotic lesions. Surgery 1965;57:155.
8. Copley AL. The rheology of blood. A survey. J Colloid Sci 1952;7:323.
9. Texon M. The hemodynamic concept of atherosclerosis. Bull NY Acad Med 1960;36:263.
10. Fry DL. Acute vascular endothelial changes associated with increased blood velocity gradients. Circ Res 1968;22:165.
11. Fry DL. Certain histological and chemical responses of the vascular interface to acutely induced mechanical stress in the aorta of the dog. Circ Res 1969;24:93.
12. Whitmore RL. Rheology of the circulation. Oxford; Pergamon Press, 1968.
13. Gessner FB. Hemodynamic theories of atherogenesis. Circ Res 1973;33(3):259.
14. Anadere I, Chmiel H, Hess H *et al.* Clinical blood rheology. Biorheology 1979;16:171.
Young DF. Fluid mechanics of arterial stenoses. J Biomech Eng 1979; 101:157.
16. Barnes RW. Hemodynamics for the vascular surgeon. Arch Surg 1980;115:216.
17. Carter SA. Hemodynamic considerations in peripheral and cerebrovascular disease. Sem Ultrasound 1981;2(4):254.
18. Caro CG. Arterial fluid mechanics and atherogenesis Recent Adv Cardiovasc Dis 1981;2(Suppl):6.
19. Chien S. Hemorheology in clinical medicine. Clin Hemorheol 1982;2:137.
20. McGrath MA. Dynamics of the peripheral circulation. Inter Angio 1984;3(1):3.
21. Chien S, Dormandy J, Ernst E, Matrai A. Clinical hemorheology. Boston: Martinus Nijhoff Pub., 1987.
22. Yoganathan AP, Cape EG, Sung HW *et al.* Review of hydrodynamic principles for the cardiologist: applications to the study of blood flow and jets by imaging techniques. J Am Coll Cardiol 1988;12(5):1344.
23. Hell KMD, Balzereit A, Diebold U *et al.* Importance of blood viscoelasticity in arteriosclerosis. Angiology 1989;40(6):539.
24. Attinger EO. Pulsatile blood flow. New York: McGraw Hill, 1964.
25. Bergel DH. Cardiovascular fluid dynamics. New York: Academic Press; 1972.
26. McDonald DA. Blood flow in arteries. 2nd ed. London: Arnold, 1974.
27. Strandness DE, Sumner DS. Hemodynamics for surgeons. New York: Grune and Stratton, 1975.
28. Rushmer RF. Cardiovascular dynamics. London: Saunders, 1976.
29. Hwang WHC, Normann WA. Cardiovascular flow dynamics and measurements. Baltimore: University Park Press, 1977.
30. Caro CG, Pedley RC, Schroter RC *et al.* The mechanics of the circulation. Oxford: Oxford University Press, 1978.
31. Shepherd JT, Vanhoutte PM. The human cardiovascular system. New York: Raven Press, 1980:222.
32. Stehbens WE. Hemodynamics the blood vessel wall. Illinois: Thomas Springfield, 1979.
33. Patel DJ, Vaishnav RN. Basic haemodynamics and its role in disease processes. Baltimore: University Park Press, 1980.

34. Pedley TJ. The fluid mechanics of large blood vessels. Cambridge University Press, 1980.
35. Schwartz CJ, Wethessen NT, Wolf S. Structure and function of the circulation. New York: Plenum Press, 1980.
36. Texon M. Haemodynamic basis of atherosclerosis. New York, London: McGraw Hill, 1980.
37. Milnor WR. Hemodynamics, Baltimore: William and Wilkins, 1982.
38. O'Rourke MF. Arterial function in health and disease. Edinburgh: Churchill Livingstone, 1982.
39. Fung YC. Biodynamics: Circulation. New York: Springer-Verlag, 1984.
40. Nichols WW, O'Rourke MF. McDonald's blood flow in arteries. Theoretical, experimental and clinical applications. 3rd ed. London: Edward Arnold, 1990.
41. Bergel DH. The viscoelastic properties of the arterial wall. PhD thesis. University of London, 1960.
42. Cleary E. A correlative and comparative study of the non-uniform arterial wall. MD thesis, University of Sydney.
43. Taylor MG. The elastic properties of arteries in relation to the physiological functions of the arterial system. Gastroenterology 1967;52:358.
44. Wolinsky H, Glagov S. Structural basis for the static mechanical properties of the aortic media. Circ Res 1964;14:400.
45. Berry C. Changes in large artery function in disease. Top Circ 1989;3(3):7.
46. Newman DL, Batten JR, Bowden NLR. Partial standing wave formation above an abdominal aortic stenosis. Cardiovasc Res 1977;11:160.
47. Simon A, Flaud P, Levenson J. Non-invasive evaluation of segmental pressure drop and resistance in large arteries in humans based on a poiseuille model of intra-arterial velocity distribution. Cardiovasc Res 1990;24:623.
48. Woyda WC, Berkas EM, Ferguson DJ. The atherosclerosis of aortic and pulmonary artery exchange autografts. Surgical Forum 1960;11:174.
49. Gosling RG. Extraction of physiological information from spectrum-analysed doppler-shifted continuous wave ultrasound signals obtained non-invasively from the arterial system. In: Hill WD, Watson BW. IEEE medical electronics monograph (21). Stevenage: Peter Peregrinus, 1976;4(2):73.
50. Laogun AA, Gosling RG. In vivo arterial compliance in man. Clin Phys Physiol Meas 1982;3(3):201.
51. Wright JS, Cruickshank JK, Kontis S, Doré C, Gosling RG. Aortic compliance measured by non-invasive Doppler ultrasound: description of a method and its reproductibility. Clin Sci 1990;78(5):463.
52. Peterson LH, Jensen RE, Parnell J. Mechanical properties of arteries *in-vivo*. Circ Res 1960;8:622.
53. Bergel DH. The static elastic properties of the arterial wall. J Physiol 1961;156:445.
54. Bergel DH, Schultz DL. Arterial elasticity and fluid dynamics. Prog Biophys Molc Biol 1971;22:1.
55. Bergel DH. Mechanics of the arterial wall in health and disease. In: Bauer RD, Busse R (eds), The arterial system. Berlin: Springer Verlag, 1978.
56. Gow BS. Influence of vascular smooth muscle on the visco-elastic properties of blood vessels. In: Bergel DH (ed). Cardiovascular fluid dynamics. New York: Academic Press, 1972:65.
57. Gow BS. Circulatory correlates: impedance, resistance and capacity. In: Bohr DF, Somlyo AP, Handbook of physiology, Section 2. The cardiovascular system, Vol. 2 Vascular smooth muscle. Maryland: American Physiological Society, 1980.
58. Laird JD, Thomas Young MD. (1773–1829). Am Heart J 1980;100:1.
59. Milnor WR, Bertram CD. The relation between arterial viscoelasticity and wave propagation in the canine femoral artery *in-vivo*. Circ Res 1978;43:870.
60. Milnor WR, Nichols WW. A new method of measuring propagation coefficients and characteristic impedance in blood vessels. Circ Res 1975;36:631.

61. Learyod BM, Taylor MG. Alterations with age in the viscoelastic properties of human arterial walls. Circ Res 1966;18:278.
62. O'Rourke MF, Blazek JV, Morreels CL *et al.* Pressure wave transmission along the human aorta. Changes with age and in arterial degenerative disease. Circ Res 1968;23:567.
63. O'Rourke MF. The arterial pulse in health and disease. Am Heart J 1971;82:687.
64. Mozersky DJ, Sumner DS, Hokanson DE *et al.* Transcutaneous measurement of the elastic properties of the human femoral artery. Circ 1972;46:948.
65. Carter SA. Role of pressure measurements in vascular disease. In: Bernstein EF (ed.), Noninvasive diagnostic techniques in vascular disease. St. Louis: C.V. Mosby, 1978:261.
66. Levenson JA, Simon AC, Safar ME *et al.* Systolic hypertension in arteriosclerosis obliterans of the lower limbs. Clin Exp Hypert 1982;41:1059.
67. Lo CS, Relf IRN, Myers KA *et al.* Doppler ultrasound recognition of preclinical changes in arterial wall in diabetic subjects: compliance and pulse-wave damping. Diabetes Care 1986;9:27.
68. Taylor MG. Wave travel in a non-uniform transmission line, in relation to pulses in arteries. Physics Med Biol 1965;10:539.
69. O'Rourke MF, Taylor MG. Vascular impedance of the femoral bed. Circ Res 1966;18:126.
70. Westerhof N, Spikema P, Van Den Bos GC *et al.* Forward and backward waves in the arterial system. Cardiovasc Res 1972;6:648.
71. Papageorgiou GL, Jones NB. Arterial system configuration and wave reflection. J Biomed Eng 1987;9:299.
72. Newman DL, Gosling RG, Bowden NLR *et al.* Pressure amplitude increase on unmatching the aorto-iliac junction of the dog. Cardiovasc Res 1973;7:6.
73. Barker WF. Peripheral arterial disease. London: Saunders, 1966.
74. Gosling RG, Newman DL, Bowden NLR *et al.* The area ratio of normal aortic junctions. Br J Radiol 1971;44:850.
75. Li JKJ. Pulse wave reflections at the aorto-iliac junction. Angiology 1985;36:516.
76. Papageorgiou GL, Jones BN, Redding VJ *et al.* The area ratio of normal arterial junctions and its implications in pulse wave reflections. Cardiovasc Res 1990;24:478.
77. Green HD. In: Glasser D (ed.), Medical physics. Chicago: Year Book Publishers, Vol 2, 1952:531.
78. Cave FD, Walker A, Naylor GP *et al.* The hydraulic impedance of the lower limb: Its relevance to the success of bypass operations for occlusion of the superficial femoral artery. Br J Surg 1976;63:408.
79. Farrar DJ. Large artery hemodynamics and vascular impedance in graded arterial stenosis and in human peripheral atherosclerosis. PhD dissertation, University of North Carolina, Chapel Hill, 1976.
80. Patel DJ, Greenfield JC, Austen WG *et al.* Pressure-flow relationships in the ascending aorta and femoral artery of man. J Appl Physiol 1965;20:459.
81. Mills CJ, Gabe IT, Gault JH *et al.* Pressure-flow relationships and vascular impedance in man. Cardiovasc Res 1970;4:405.
82. Farrar DJ, Malindzak GS, Johnson G. Large vessel resistance and characteristic vascular impedance in experimental stenosis. Fed Proc 1976;35:448.
83. Farrar DJ, Green HD, Peterson DW. Noninvasively and invasively measured pulsatile haemodynamics with graded arterial stenosis. Cardiovasc Res 1979;13:45.
84. Farrar DJ, Malindzak GS, Johnson G. Large vessel impedance in peripheral atherosclerosis. Circ 1977;56(Suppl 2):171.
85. Taylor MG. An approach to an analysis of the arterial pulse wave. 1. Oscillations in an attenuating line. Physics Med Biol 1957;1:258–69.
86. Davies PF. How do vascular endothelial cells respond to flow? News in Physiol Sci 1989;4:22.
87. Matrai A, Wittington RB, Skalak R. Biophysics. In: Chien S, Dormandy J, Ernst E *et al.* (eds.), Clinical hemorheology. Boston: Martinus Nijhoff Pub, 1987:9.

88. Young DF. Effects of a time-dependent stenosis on flow through a tube. J Eng Ind Trans ASME 1968;90:248.
89. Deshpande MD, Giddens DP, Mabon RF. Study of laminar flow through modelled vascular stenoses. J Biomechanics 1976;9:165.
90. McDonald DA. On steady flow through model vascular stenoses. J Biomechanics 1979;12:13.
91. Iida N, Murata T. Theoretical analysis of pulsatile blood flow in small vessels. Biorheology 1980;17:377.
92. Shukla JB, Parihar RS, Rao BRP. Effects of stenosis on non-newtonian flow of blood in an artery. Bull Math Biology 1980;42:283.
93. Inglis TCM, Carson PJ, Stuart J. Clinical measurement of whole-blood viscosity at low shear rates. Clin Hemorheol 1981;1:167.
94. Haynes RH, Burton AC. Role of the non-newtonian behavior of blood in hemodynamics. Am J Physiol 1959;197:943.
95. Merrill EW, Benis AM, Gilliland ER et al. Pressure-flow relations of human blood in hollow fibers at low flow rates. J Appl Physiol 1965;20:954.
96. Stoltz JF, Donner M. Erythrocyte aggregation: Experimental approaches and clinical implications. Inter Angio 1987;6:193.
97. McGrath MA, Penny R. Paraproteinemia. Blood viscosity and clinical manifestations. J Clin Investigations 1976;58:1155.
98. McGrath MA. Blood viscosity in macroglobulinemia, multiple myeloma and polycythemia. In: Dintenfass L, Seaman GVF, Blood viscosity factors in heart disease, thrombombolism and cancer, 1981.
99. Fahraeus R, Lindqvist T. Viscosity of blood in narrow capillary tubes. Am J Physiol 1931;96:562.
100. Thurston GB. Viscoelasticity of human blood. Biophys J 1972;12:1205.
101. Darby R. Viscoelastic fluids. New York: Marcel-Dekker Inc, 1976.
102. Wells RE, Merrill EW. Influence of flow properties of blood upon viscosity-hematocrit relationships. J Clin Invest 1962;41:1591.
103. Merrill EW, Gilliland ER, Cokelet GR et al. Rheology of human blood near and at zero flow. Effects of temperature and hematocrit level. Biophys J 1963;3:199.
104. Whittington RB, Harkness J. Viscosity-temperature variations in human blood and plasma. Biorheology 1968;5:252.
105. Dormandy JA, Chien S. Blood viscosity and cell deformability. In. Verstraete M (ed), Methods in angiology. Amsterdam: Martinus Nijhoff, 1980.
106. Rieger H. The role of hemorheology in the patho-physiology and treatment of arterial occlusive disease. Inter Angiol 1986;5:161.
107. Coulter NA, Pappenheimer JR. Development of turbulence in flowing blood. Am J Physiol 1949;152:401.
108. Poiseuille JLM. Recherches experimentales sur le mouvement des liquides dans les tubes de tres petit diametre. Comptes Rendus Hebdomadaires des Seances de L'Academie des Sciences 1842;11:961.
109. Schultz DL. Pressure and flow in large arteries. In: Bergel DH. Cardiovascular fluid dynamics, London: Academic Press.
110. Fung YC. Biodynamics: Circulation. New York: Springer-Verlag, 1984.
111. Evans DH. On the measurement of the mean velocity of blood flow over the cardiac cycle using Doppler ultrasound. Ultrasound Med Biol 1985;11:735.
112. Harris PL. The role of ultrasound in the assessment of peripheral arterial disease. MD thesis. University of Manchester, 1975.
113. Byar D, Fiddian RV, Quereau M et al. The fallacy of applying the poiseuille equation to segmental arterial stenosis. Am Heart J 1965;70:216.
114. Benis AM, Usami S, Chien S. Evaluation of viscous and inertial pressure losses in isolated tissue with a simple mathematical model. Microvasc Res 1972;4:81.

115. Bird RD, Stewart WE, Lightfoot EN. Transport phenomena. New York: John Wiley and Sons, 1960:71.
116. Kandarpa K, Davis N, Gardiner GA et al. Hemodynamic evaluation of arterial stenoses by computer simulation. Invest Radiol 1987;22:393.
117. Young DF, Tsai FY. Flow characteristics in models of arterial stenosis. I. Steady flow. J Biomech 1973;6:395.
118. Young DF, Tsai FY. Flow characteristics in models of arterial stenosis. II. Unsteady flow. J Biomech 1973;6:547.
119. Davids N, Kandarpa K. Analysis of hemodynamic factors in atherogenesis of branching sites. Progress Report, NHLI PHS Grant No. IR-01-HL-11289–05. Department of Engineering Science and Mechanics, the Pennsylvania State University. Pennsylvania: University Park, 1975.
120. Mates RE, Gupta RL, Bell AC et al. Fluid dynamics of coronary artery stenosis. Circulation Res 1978;42:152.
121. Weale FE. Haemodynamics of incomplete arterial obstruction (with observations of the generation of turbulence). Br J Surg 1964b;51:689.
122. Fredberg JJ. The origin and character of vascular murmurs: model studies. J Acoust Soc Am 1977;61:1077.
123. Carter SA. Arterial auscultation in peripheral vascular disease. J Am Med Assoc 1981;246(15):1682.
124. Chapman B, Charlesworth D. Analysis of the factors influencing the production of sound in tubes. Vasc Diag Therapy 1981;2:23.
125. Charlesworth D, Gerrard JH. Atherosclerosis and disturbances in flow. Ann Vasc Surg 1988;2:57.
126. Smith RL, Blick EF, Coalson J et al. Thrombus production by turbulence. J Appl Physiol 1972;32:261.
127. Flaherty JT, Pierce JE, Ferrans VJ et al. Endothelial nuclear patters in the canine arterial tree with particular reference to hemodynamic evetns. Circ Res 1972;30:23.
128. Carew TE, Patel DJ. Effect of tensile and shear stress on intimal permeability of the left coronary artery in dogs. Atherosclerosis 1973;18:179.
129. Roach PJ. Computational fluid mechanics. Albuquerque: Harmosa Publishers, 1972.
130. Nerem RM, Seed WA. An in-vivo study of aortic flow disturbances. Cardiovasc Res 1972;6:1.
131. Reul H, Schoenmackers J, Starke W. Loss of pressure, energy and performance at simulated stenoses in pulsatile quasiphysiological flow. Med Biol eng 1972;10:711.
132. Charlesworth D. Relationship of blood rheology to blood flow. In: Low GDO (ed.), Clinical aspects of blood viscosity and cell deformability. Berlin: Springer-Verlag, 1981:91.
133. Duncan GW, Gruber JO, Dewey FC et al. Evaluation of carotid stenosis by phoangiography. N Engl J Med 1975;293:1124.
134. Bernoulli D. In: The general properties of matter. Newman and Searle. London: Edward Arnold, 1957.
135. Burton A. Physiology and biophysics of the circulation. Chicago: Year Book Medical Publishers Inc, 1972.
136. Badeer HS. Elementary hemodynamic principles based on modified Bernoulli's equation. The Physiologist 1985;28:41.
137. Spencer MP, Arts T. Some hemodynamical aspects of large arteries. In: Doppler ultrasound in the diagnosis of cerebro-vascular disease. Research Studies Press, 1982:59.
138. Goldberg SJ. The principles of pressure drop in long segment stenosis. Herz 1986;11:291.
139. Popp RL, Teplitsky I. Lessons from in vitro models of small, irregular, multiple and tunnel-like stenoses relevant to clinical stenoses of valves and small vessels. J Am Coll Cardiol 1989;13:716.
140. Gorlin R, Gorlin SG. Hydraulic formula for calculation of the area of the stenotic mitral valve, other cardiac valves, and central circulatory shunts. Am Heart J 1951;41:1.

141. Holen J. Determination of pressure gradient in mitral stenosis with a noninvasive ultrasound Doppler technique. Acta Med Scand 1976;199:455.

142. Holen J, Aaslid R, Landmark K *et al*. Determination of effective orifice area in mitral stenosis from non-invasive ultrasound Doppler data and mitral flow rate. Acta Med Scand 1977;201:83.

143. Hatle L. Noninvasive assessment of mpressure drop in mitral stenosis by Doppler ultrasound. Br Heart J 1978;40:131.

144. Levine RA, Jimoh A, Cape EG *et al*. Pressure recovery distal to a stenosis: potential cause of gradient 'overestimation' by Doppler echocardiography. J Am Coll Cardiol 1989;13:706.

145. Holen J, Waag RC, Gramiak R *et al*. Doppler ultrasound in orifice flow. *In vitro* studies of the relationship between pressure difference and fluid velocity. Ultrasound Med Biol 1985;11:261.

146. Faccenda F, Usui Y, Spencer MP. Doppler measurement of the pressure drop caused by arterial stenosis: an experimental study: a case repoort. Angiology 1985;36:899.

147. Langsfeld M, Nepute J, Hershey FB *et al*. The use of deep duplex scanning to predict hemodynamically significant aortoiliac stenoses. J Vasc Surg 1988;7:395.

148. Kohler TR, Nicholls SC, Zierler RE *et al*. Assessment of pressure gradient by Doppler ultrasound: experimental and clinical observations. J Vasc Surg 1987;6(6):460.

149. May AG, DeWeese JA, Rob CG. Hemodynamic effects of arterial stenosis. Surgery 1963;53:513.

150. Vasko SD, Goldberg SJ, Requarth JA *et al*. Factors affecting accuracy of *in vitro* valvular pressure gradient estimates by Doppler ultrasound. Am J Cardiol 1984;54:893.

151. Wong M, Vijayaraghavan G, Bae JH *et al*. *In vitro* study of the pressure-velocity relation across stenotic orifices. Am J Cardiol 1985;56:465.

152. Hatle L, Angelsen B. Doppler ultrasound in cardiology: physical principles and clinical applications. 2nd ed. Philadelphia: Lea & Febiger, 1985.

153. Teirstein PS, Yock PG, Popp RL. The accuracy of Doppler ultrasound measurement of pressure gradients across irregular, dual, and tunnel-like obstructions to blood flow. Circulation 1985;72:577.

154. Requarth JA, Marx GR, Goldberg SJ *et al*. Is the modified Bernouilli equation accurate for estimating pressure drop in long segment stenosis? Circulation 1985;79:435.

155. Young DF, Cholvin NR, Robth AC. Pressure drop across artifically induced stenosis in the femoral arteries in dogs. Circ Res 1975;36:735.

156. Flanigan DP, Tullis, JP, Streeter VL *et al*. Multiple subcritical arterial stenoses: effect on post-stenotic pressure and flow. Ann Surg 1977;186:663.

157. Keitzer WE, Fry WJ, Kraft RO *et al*. Hemodynamic mechanism for pulse changes seen in occlusive vascular disease. Surgery 1965;57:163.

158. O'Rourke MF. Steady and pulsatile energy losses in the systemic circulation under normal conditions and in simulated arterial disease. Cardiovasc Res 1967;1:313.

159. Berguer R, Hwang NHC. Critical arterial stenosis: a theoretical and experimental solution. Ann Surg 1974;180:39.

160. Rouse H. Elementary fluid mechanics. New York: John Wiley & Sons, 1946;201.

161. Young DF, Cholvin NR, Kirkeeide RE *et al*. Hemodynamics of arterial stenoses at elevated flow rates. Circ Res 1977;41:99.

162. McDonald L, Semple R. Exercise test in intermittent claudication. Br Heart J 1952;14:91.

163. Kroeker EJ, Wood EH. Comparison of simultaneously recorded central and peripheral arterial pressure pulses during rest, exercise and tilted position in man. Circ Res 1955;3:623.

164. DeWeese JA. Pedal pulses disappearing with exercise: a test for intermittent claudication. N Engl J Med 1960;262:1214.

165. Barner HB, Kaiser GC, William VL *et al*. Clinical documentation of the hemodynamics of the disappearing pulse. Arch Surg 1968;97:341.

166. Blaisdell FW, Gauder PJ. Paradoxical variation of the femoral pulse in occlusion of the iliac artery. Surgery 1961;50:529.

167. Pritchard WH, Gregg DE, Shipley RE *et al*. A study of flow pattern responses in peripheral arteries to the injection of vasomotor drug. Am J Physiol 1943;138:731.
168. Lee BY, Castillo HT, Madden JL. Quantification of the arterial pulsatile blood flow waveform in peripheral vascular disease. Angiology 1970;21:595.
169. Hutchison KJ, Karpinski E. Stability of flow patterns in the *in-vivo* post-stenotic velocity field. Ultrasound Med Biol 1988;14:269.
170. Roschke EJ, Back LH. The influence of upstream conditions on flow re-attachment lengths downstream of an abrupt circular channel expansion. J Biomechanics 1976;9:481.
171. Yongchareon W, Young DF. Initiation of turbulence in models of arterial stenoses. J Biomech 1979;12:185.
172. Campbell JD, Hutchison KJ, Karpinski E. Variation of Doppler ultrasound spectral width in the post-stenotic velocity field. Ultrasound Med Biol 1989;15:611.
173. Clark C. The propagation of turbulence produced by a stenosis. J Biomechanics 1980;13:591.
174. Clark C. The propagation of turbulence produced by a stenosis. In: Taylor DEM, Stevens AL (eds.), Blood flow. Theory and practice. London: Academic Press, 1983:39.
175. Wille SO, Walloe L. Pulsatile pressure and flow in arterial stenoses simulated in a mathematical model. J Biomed Eng 1981;3:17.
176. Evans DH, MacPherson DS, Asher MJ *et al*. Changes in Doppler ultrasound sonograms at varying distances from stenoses. Cardiovasc Res 1982;16:631.
177. Buss GY. Transition to turbulence in a model of the human superficial femoral artery. In: Taylor DEM, Stevens Al (eds.), Blood flow. Theory and practice. London: Academic Press, 1983:7.
178. Tamura T, Fronek A. Ratio of simultaneous reverse and forward velocity components as an index of degree of stenosis. Fed Proc 1982;41:1672.
179. Felix WR, Sigel B, Gibson RJ *et al*. Pulsed Doppler ultrasound detection of flow disturbances in arteriosclerosis. J Clin Ultras 1976;4:275.
180. Ojha M, Johnston KW, Cobbold RSC *et al*. Potential limitations of center-line pulsed doppler recordings: an *in vitro* flow visualization study. J Vasc Surg 1989;9:515.
181. Brice JG, Dowsett DJ, Lowe RD. Haemodynamic effects of carotid artery stenosis. Br Med J 1964;2:1363.
182. Mann FC, Herrick JF. The effect on the blood flow of decreasing the lumen of a blood vessel. Surgery 1938;4:249.
183. Haimovici H, Escher DJW. Aortoiliac stenosis: diagnostic significance of vascular hemodynamics. Arch Surg 1956;72:107.
184. Fiddian RV, Byar D, Edwards EA. Factors affecting flow through a stenosed vessel. Arch Surg 1964;88:83.
185. Delin NA, Ekestrom S, Telenius R. Relation of degree of internal carotid artery stenosis to blood flow and pressure gradient. Invest Radiol 1968;3:337.
186. Wylie EJ, McGuinness JS. The recognition and treatment of arteriosclerotic stenoses of major arteries. Surg Gynecol Obstet 1953;97:425.
187. Udoff EJ, Barth KH, Harrington DP *et al*. Hemodynamic significance of iliac artery stenosis: pressure measurements during angiography. Radiology 1979;132:289.
188. May AG, Van DeBerg L, DeWeese JA *et al*. Critical arterial stenosis. Surgery 1963;54(1):250.
189. Kupper CA, Young L, Keagy BA *et al*. Spectral analysis o the femoral artery for idenification of iliac artery lesions. Bruit 1984;8:157.
190. Robbins SL, Bentov I. The kinetics of viscous flow in a model vessel. Effect of stenoses of varying size, shape, and length. Lab Invest 1967;16:864.
191. Kindt GW, Youmans JR. The effect of stricture length on critical arterial stenosis. Surg Gynecol Obstet 1969;128:729.
192. Schultz RD, Hokanson DE, Strandness DE. Pressure-flow and stress-strain measurements of normal and diseased aortoiliac segments. Surg Gynecol Obstet 1967;124:1267.

193. Thiele BL, Bandyk DF, Zierler RE *et al.* A systematic approach to the assessement of aorto-iliac disease. Arch Surg 1983;118:477.
194. Ahmed SA, Giddens DP. Pulsatile poststenotic flow studies with laser Doppler anemometry. J Biomechan 1984;17:695.
195. Young DF, Tsai FY, Morgan BE. Influence of geometry on flow in models of arterial stenoses. ACEMB Proc 1971;24:325.
196. Solzbach U, Wollschlager H, Zeiher A *et al.* Effect of stenotic geometry on flow behaviour across stenotic models. Med Biol Eng Comput 1987;25:543.
197. Shipley RE, Gregg DE. The effect of external constriction of a blood vessel on blood flow. Am J Physiol 1944;141:289.
198. Moore WS, Malone JM. Effect of flow rate and vessel calibre on critical arterial stenosis. J Surg Res 1979;26:1.
199. Weale FE. The values of series and parallel resistances in steady blood-flow. Br J Surg 1964;51:623.
200. Karayannacos PE, Talukder N, Nerem RM *et al.* The role of multiple non-critical arterial stenoses in the pathogenesis of ischemia. J Thor Cardiovasc Surg 1977;73:458.
201. Beckmann CF, Levin DC, Kubicka RA *et al.* The effect of sequential arterial stenoses on flow and pressure. Radiology 1981;140:655.

32. Skeletal muscle blood flow

THIERRY H. LEJEMTEL and STUART D. KATZ

The ability of the skeletal muscle vasculature to meet the high metabolic requirements of the active skeletal muscle probably represents the most striking adaptation of the cardiovascular system to heavy exercise. Indeed, up to 90% of the increased cardiac output, which can reach 25–30 L/min, is distributed to the lower limbs during maximal treadmill or bicycle exercise [1]. Thus, while the cardiac output increases from rest by a factor of 4 to 5, blood flow to the skeletal muscle involved in exercise increases by a factor ranging from 15 to 20. In normal and diseased states, blood flow to skeletal muscle involved in exercise closely correlates with peak aerobic capacity. Moreover, measurement of skeletal muscle blood flow (SMBF) is critical to study the metabolism of the skeletal muscles [2]. However, studies of SMBF in man are few and only a handful of laboratories have been active in this area over the years [3–9]. This, by far, does not stem from a lack of interest in the skeletal muscle vasculature, but reflects the difficulties in measuring SMBF in normal subjects and in patients with cardiac disease. In addition, determination of SMBF during exercise has been hampered by our inability to quantify the amount of skeletal muscle mass actively participating in exercise. If 50% of the total muscle mass is active, the flow per 100 g or per kg is considerably lower than if only 30% of the total muscle is active. Thus, prior to reviewing the data currently available on SMBF in man, the advantages and limitations of the techniques used to measure SMBF will be briefly discussed.

Thermodilution technique

Several laboratories have elected to measure SMBF by determining lower limb blood flow using the thermodilution technique with single bolus injection [10–16]. This technique requires a thorough mixing of injectate and blood to ensure accurate measurements. The inability to measure SMBF at rest with the single bolus injection technique suggests that mixing may be inadequate when the blood flow is low. When blood flow increases, mixing becomes complete and reliable measurements of SMBF can be obtained during exercise. The nature of the flow measured depends on the location of the catheter. When the catheter is positioned in the deep femoral vein, the flow

A.-M. Salmasi and A.S. Iskandrian (eds): *Cardiac output and regional flow in health and disease*, 469–478.
© 1993 *Kluwer Academic Publishers. Printed in the Netherlands.*

is equivalent to SMBF, as the deep femoral vein almost exclusively contains blood from skeletal muscles [17]. If the catheter is advanced in the iliac vein, the flow is a mixture of the lower limbs, skeletal muscle, anterior abdominal wall, and cutaneous tissues drained by the great saphenous vein. An important concern when using the thermodilution technique with single bolus injection is the thermistor response time, which in commercially available catheters, is quite long when compared to the transit time of the wave carrying the temperature changes. The continuous thermodilution technique with constant infusion of injectate and dual thermistor catheters avoids the issue of the long thermistor response time [18–22]. Moreover, when the injectate is infused at a constant rate, ranging from 40 to 60 ml/min, excellent mixing conditions of injectate and blood are obtained even at low flow. The continuous thermodilution technique with constant infusion appears particularly suited to measure SMBF at rest and during low level exercise. Thermoconductivity within the catheter may falsely lower measurements of blood flow during heavy or maximal exercise.

Local [133]xenon washout technique

The local [133]xenon clearance method is the only technique which allows direct determination of SMBF during exercise in man [23, 24]. 100 μCi of [133]xenon is dissolved into 0.1 ml of normal 9% saline solution and injected into the skeletal muscle. A small cadmium telluride semiconductor detector (RMD) is affixed over the injection depot with adhesive tape [25]. Activity is determined every 5 seconds and data acquired into the IBM PC microcomputer which stores, displays and analyzes the data count [26]. SMBF is derived from the formula SMBF = λ (slope) 100 ml (100 g/min^{-1}). A value of 0.7 is used for λ, the partition coefficient of [133]xenon between muscle tissue and blood. The slope is calculated by the computer from a least-square line fitted through the data points.

The initial washout rate after the intramuscular injection of [133]xenon leads to an overestimation of SMBF due to the trauma of injection. Thus, the first 15 minutes of the washout should be disregarded. In addition, the late portion of the washout curve is influenced by recirculation of the [133]xenon due to venous arteriolar shunting by diffusion and accumulation of [133]xenon in the fat tissue lining the veins, which both lead to an under-estimation of the SMBF by as much as 200% [27]. Underestimation can be attenuated by peeling off the terminal portion of the washout curve. A limitation of the [133]xenon washout technique is repeating the intramuscular injection at exactly the same site in the muscle during serial determinations. The presence of a dual circulation in the skeletal muscle and the uneven perfusion of the different skeletal muscle fibers probably contributes to the substantial variability of baseline determination of SMBF [28]. However, during conditions of high flow, i.e. exercise, the skeletal muscle appears to be more evenly perfused and the slight variation in the site of injection does not matter as much as during resting conditions.

Indocyanine green dilution technique

This technique was applied by Jorfeldt and Wahren to measure limb blood flow [29]. It requires insertion of catheters into the femoral artery and femoral vein on each side. Indocyanine green solution is infused through the femoral artery catheter and samples are taken from the femoral venous catheters. Three or four pairs of samples are drawn, and the concentrations are determined spectrophotometrically against a calibration curve. The lower limb blood flow (LLBF) is calculated from the concentration of the infusion dye solution (C_i) the dye concentration in the femoral vein of the infused leg (C_v) and the opposite leg (C_2), the rate of infusion (F_i) and the hemotocrit (Hct) according to the formula:

$$\text{LLBF} = \frac{F_i(C_i - C_v)}{(C_v - C_2)(1 - \text{Hct})}.$$

The reproducibility of the indocyanine green dilution technique is acceptable with a coefficient variation of 3–6%. The major limitation of this method is the need for an intra-arterial catheter to inject dye. Although the catheter may be extremely thin and flexible, bleeding can occur and a large inguinal hematoma can develop during maximal exercise on the bicycle ergometer. In addition, this technique requires complete mixing of dye and blood with a stable dye concentration in the femoral vein of the infused leg. A variability in the dye concentration of the femoral venous blood has been noted at rest but has not been observed during exercise when lower limb blood flow is elevated.

Plethysmography

Limb blood flow can be measured noninvasively by venous occlusion plethysmography. The changes in limb circumference are obtained by using a mercury-in-rubber strain gauge [30]. Changes in limb circumference are assumed to be linearly related to limb blood flow [31]. The limb blood flow measured by venous occlusion plethysmography is nonspecific, and includes flows from cutaneous and subcutaneous tissues, skeletal muscles, bones and tendons. The major limitation of the plethysmography technique is that blood flow cannot be measured during exercise, as the motion artefacts introduced by exercise prevent reliable readings. Nevertheless, hyperemic response to ischemia following arterial occlusion for 5 to 10 minutes or immediately after exercise can be measured, and provides indirect information on the vasodilatory response of the limb skeletal muscle vasculature to exercise.

Skeletal muscle blood flow during exercise

Blood flow to the lower limb skeletal muscles increases linearly with the work performed during graded maximal bicycle or treadmill exercise. Even though maximal cardiac output response is reached and maximal aerobic capacity attained, SMBF does not reach a plateau. In a seminal study of the SMBF during isolated graded work involving exclusively the quadricep femoris muscle group of one leg, Andersen and Saltin showed that, in man, blood flow steadily increases with the workload, to an average value of 5.7 L/min^{-1} [20]. Since SMBF of the quadricep femoris muscles was estimated to range between 0.15 and 0.40 L/min^{-1} at rest, the increase of SMBF was 20 fold or more during maximal exercise [32]. The data of Andersen and Saltin for maximal SMBF during exercise are far superior to that previously reported in man, but are in agreement with maximal SMBF measured in animals with similar degree of capillarization of skeletal muscles to that of man. With a mean estimated weight of the quadricep femoris muscle of 2.3 kg, the perfusion of maximally exercising skeletal muscle of man is in the order of 2.5 L/min^{-1}.

If 20 kg of muscle were exercising and able to reach a similar peak SMBF as the quadricep femoris muscle did, a cardiac output of 50 L/min^{-1} would be required, which far exceeds the capacity of the cardiac pump [22]. Thus, when the mass of active skeletal muscle is large, the relatively limited ability of the heart to pump blood requires that vasoconstriction takes place in the vasculature of the exercising skeletal muscle in order to maintain an adequate blood pressure. Sinoway and Prophet have recently provided evidence that metaboreceptor-mediated vasoconstriction is the predominant and crucial mechanism for preventing cardiac output from being outstripped during heavy exercise [33]. Stimulation of the skeletal muscle metaboreceptor caused a vasoconstriction capable of significantly limiting extreme peripheral vasodilatation.

The linear elevation of SMBF with work demonstrated by Andersen and Saltin differs from the initial reports of SMBF measurements during graded maximal exercise involving the lower limbs. Using the [133]xenon washout technique, Grimby et al showed that during maximal two legged bicycle exercise, SMBF in the lateral portion of the quadriceps gradually rose with increasing work levels, but when approaching maximal work level, the rate of flow increase tended to decline [34]. Clausen and Lassen, also using the [133]xenon washout technique, demonstrated a levelling off of SMBF in the *m. vastus lateralis* at about 70% of maximal workload performed on the bicycle ergometer [24]. These investigators cautioned that the rate of working of *m. vastus lateralis* may not be proportional to the rate of working of the subject as a whole on the bicycle ergometer. The levelling off of the blood flow in the *m. vastus lateralis* was observed during bicycling performed with both legs, as well as with one leg. Wahren *et al.* measured lower limb blood flow at rest and during bicycle exercise at workloads that increased in steps to near maximal level of work intensity in well-trained 52–59 year old men and in younger subjects of 25–30 years of age [35]. Lower limb blood flow was measured using a constant rate intra-arterial indicator diffusion technique. As previously mentioned, this technique requires uniform dispersion of the indicator before blood reaches the sampling site in the vein. Wahren et al demonstrated that this was indeed the case by sampling femoral vein blood at two sites which were 1–2 cm apart and recorded the same indicator concentration. Lower limb blood flow rose linearly with systemic oxygen uptake at submaximal workloads, but tended to level off at the heaviest workload. The rise in lower limb blood flow during exercise was less in the middle-aged group. Accordingly, Wahren *et al.* concluded that lower limb blood flow rises in a curvilinear manner in response to exercise of increasing intensity in middle-aged men and that lower limb circulation during exercise becomes relatively hypokinetic with age [35]. The decrease in lower limb blood flow during maximal bicycle exercise in middle-aged men, when compared to that of younger subjects, has to be put in the context of a reduction in cardiac output response to exercise which gradually occurs with age [36]. A close correlation between lower limb blood flow and systemic oxygen uptake during graded exercise on a bicycle ergometer was also reported by Jorfeldt *et al.* who assessed flow by the thermodilution technique with a single bolus injection [3]. At workloads ranging from 25–150 watts,a linear relationship was found between lower limb blood flow and systemic oxygen uptake. Whether lower limb blood flow would have leveled off at higher workloads is unclear.

Despite the apparent disparity between the data of Andersen and Saltin [20] who studied the response to maximal exercise of an isolated group of muscles, i.e. knee extensors, and the findings of Grimby *et al.* [34], Clausen and Lassen [24], Wahren *et al.* [35], and Jorfeldt *et al.* [3], who examined the response to maximal exercise of the lower limb skeletal muscle vasculature, it is well recognized that SMBF can increase tremendously during exercise. When the mass of exercising skeletal muscles is large, the increase in SMBF is limited by a reflex-mediated increase in resistances in the active skeletal muscles vasculature, which is aimed at maintaining adequate systemic arterial perfusion pressure. In normal subjects, the capacity of the skeletal muscles to accept blood far exceeds the capacity of the heart to supply it when a large fraction of the muscle is actively engaged in exercise.

The situation appears different in patients with congestive heart failure (CHF). At the early stages of the syndrome of CHF, left ventricular performance is depressed, and this is most apparent during exercise. The peripheral circulation is normal, as evidenced by a hyperemic response after arterial occlusion for five minutes identical to that of normal subjects of similar age.

The predominant factor which limits peak aerobic capacity in patients at the early stages of CHF is the central circulation. When compared to normal subjects of similar age, peak aerobic capacity is reduced since cardiac output response to exercise in patients with CHF is abnormal. At a more advanced stage of the syndrome of CHF, patients develop abnormalities in the peripheral circulation which, in the skeletal muscle vasculature, are characterized by a limited and fixed capacity vasodilatory response to exercise [37, 38]. Enhancement of ventricular performance with inotropic drugs does not acutely improve peak aerobic capacity in patients with severe CHF, as the abnormalities of the peripheral circulation are not immediately affected by acute therapy [39]. In contrast to normal subjects and patients with mild to moderate CHF, peak aerobic capacity is not primarily limited by depressed cardiac performance in patients with severe CHF, but is directly related to the inability of the peripheral circulation to dilate in response to exercise [21, 40]. With long-term therapy with angiotensin converting enzyme inhibitors, the abnormalities of the peripheral circulation are ameliorated and peak aerobic capacity increases [25].

Hemodynamic determinants of skeletal muscle blood flow increase during exercise

In normal subjects, the increase in SMBF of a well-defined group of muscles, such as knee extensors, is mediated by two mechanisms [20]. A decrease in resistance of the skeletal muscle vasculature is responsible for the increase in SMBF at workloads which correspond to <70% of the peak oxygen uptake for this group of muscles. This decrease in vascular resistance reaches a plateau at approximately 70% of peak oxygen uptake, and thereafter a rise in blood pressure is entirely responsible for the further increase in SMBF. However, one must stress that the blood pressure response to exercise is heavily dependent on the amount of active muscle mass. As demonstrated by Martin and associates, all blood pressure expressed as a function of oxygen uptake remains inversely related to active muscle mass during exercise [41]. When exercising a small muscle mass, local vasodilatation has less effect on total systemic vascular resistances, and the concomitant increase in cardiac output is associated with a pronounced elevation in blood pressure [42]. In contrast, when exercising a large muscle mass, more extensive dilatation lowers systemic vascular resistances and the increase in cardiac output is accompanied by less elevation in blood pressure. If one accepts that maximal vasodilation is reached in the skeletal muscle vasculature at approximately 70% of the relevant peak oxygen uptake, one understands why the continuous increase in SMBF, up to 100% of peak oxygen uptake, is greater when exercise involves a small active muscle mass than when a large muscle mass is engaged in exercise. Exercise with a small active muscle mass is associated with a pronounced rise in blood pressure which, from submaximal to maximal

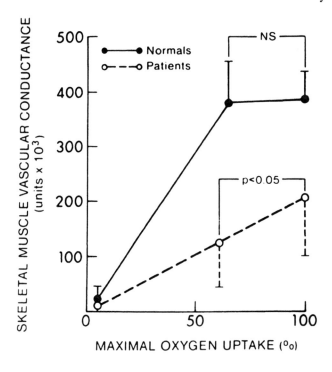

Figure 32.1. Mean skeletal muscle vascular conductance as a function of relative work intensity, i.e. percentage of maximal oxygen uptake, in 9 patients with severe CHF and 5 normal subjects of similar age. Vascular conductance reached a plateau in normal subjects, while it did not in patients with severe congestive heart failure.

exercise, substantially increases SMBF, while exercise with a much larger muscle mass is accompanied by less increase in blood pressure which, in turn, produces less increase in SMBF.

In view of the abnormalities of the peripheral circulation which are characteristically present at an advanced stage of the syndrome of CHF, we assessed the hemodynamic determinants of SMBF increase during exercise in patients with severe CHF and normal subjects of similar age. Upright exercise was performed on an electronically-braked bicycle ergometer at a submaximal workload, which corresponded to two-thirds of maximal oxygen uptake, and at maximal workloads. Expired gas was continuously monitored using a metabolic cart (Beckman Instruments), and maximal oxygen uptake was derived from standard formulae. Systemic arterial pressure was directly monitored via a radial artery catheter, and SMBF was determined by the [133]xenon washout technique after injection of 100 μCi of [133]xenon in the lateral aspect of the quadricep muscle at a depth of 2.5 cm, 1.5 cm above the superior aspect of the patella and 2 cm lateral to midline. SMBF was calculated

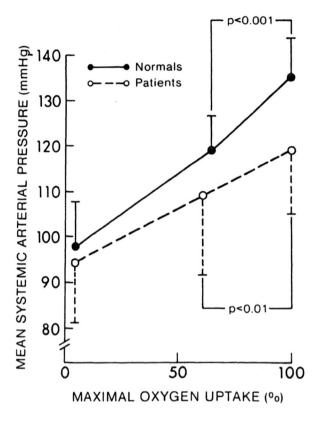

Figure 32.2. Group average of mean systemic arterial pressure as a function of work intensity in 9 patients with severe CHF and 5 normal subjects of similar age. The increase in mean systemic arterial pressure from submaximal to maximal exercise was more pronounced in normal subjects than patients with severe congestive heart failure.

assuming a coefficient of partition of [133]xenon between muscle tissue and blood of 0.7. Systemic vascular conductance, expressed in units $\times 10^3$, was calculated as SMBF divided by mean systemic arterial pressure which was electronically derived. Skeletal muscle vascular conductance increased from rest to submaximal exercise to a much greater extent in normal subjects than in patients with CHF (Figure 32.1). However, while skeletal muscle vascular conductance did not increase from submaximal to maximal exercise in normal subjects, it further increased in patients with severe CHF. The increase in mean systemic arterial pressure from rest to submaximal exercise tended to be less in patients with severe CHF than in normal subjects (Figure 32.2). Moreover, mean systemic arterial pressure substantially increased from submaximal to maximal exercise in normal subjects, while the increase was less pronounced in patients with severe CHF. Thus, the vasodilatory response of the skeletal muscle vasculature is not only reduced in patients with severe CHF, but in contrast to normal subjects, the vasodilatory response does not reach a plateau at submaximal exercise.

References

1. Folkow B, Neil E. Muscle circulation. In: Folkow B, Neil E (eds.), New York, London, Toronto: Oxford University Press, 1971:399–416.
2. Pernow B, Wahren JK, Zelterquist S. Studies on the peripheral circulation and metabolism in man. IV. Oxygen utilization and lactate formation in the legs of healthy young men during strenuous exercise. Acta Physiol Scand 1965;64:289–98.
3. Jordfeldt L, Juhlin-Dannfelt A, Pernow B. *et al*. Determination of human leg blood flow: a thermodilution technique based on femoral venous bolus injection. Clin Sci Molec Med 1978;54:517–23.
4. Tonnesen KH, Sejrsen P. Washout of [133]xenon after intravascular injection and direct measurement of blood flow in skeletal muscle. Scand J Clin Lab Invest 1970;25:71–81.
5. Henriksen O, Amtorp O, Faris I. *et al*. Evidence for a local sympathetic venoarteriolar "reflex" in the dog hind leg. Circ Res 1983;52:534–42.
6. Sejrsen P, Tonnesen KH. Shunting by diffusion of inert gas in skeletal muscle. Acta Physiol Scand 1972;86:82–91.
7. Lingdbjerg IF, Andersen AM, Munck O. *et al*. The fat content of leg muscles and its influence on the [133]xenon clearance method of blood flow measurement. Scand J Clin Lab Invest 1966;18:525–34.
8. Lassen NA, Lindbjerg I, Munck O. Measurement of blood flow through skeletal muscle by intramuscular injection of xenon[133]. Lancet 1984;1:686–9.
9. Kjellmer I, Lindbjerg I, Prerovsky I. *et al*. The relation between blood flow in an isolated muscle measured with the xenon[133] clearance and a direct recording technique. Acta Physiol Scand 1967;69:69–78.
10. Fronek A, Ganz V. Measurement of flow in single blood vessels including cardiac output by local thermodilution. Circ Res 1960;8:175–82.
11. Ganz V, Hlavova A, Fronek A. *et al*. Measurement of blood flow in the femoral artery in man at rest and during exercise by local thermodilution. Circulation 1964;30:86–9.
12. Sorlie D, Myhre K. Determination of leg blood flow in man by thermodilution. Scand J Clin Lab Invest 1977;37:117–24.
13. Wilson JR, Martin JL, Ferraro N. *et al*. Effect of hydralazine on perfusion and metabolism in leg during upright bicycle exercise in patients with heart failure. Circulation 1983;68:425–32.
14. Sullivan MJ, Beckley PD, Hanson KM. *et al. In vivo* validation of a thermodilution system designed to measure peripheral blood flow. Med Instrument 1987;19:38–40.
15. Sullivan MJ, Knight DJ, Higginbotham MB. *et al*. Relation between central and peripheral hemodynamics during exercise in patients with chronic heart failure. Muscle blood flow is reduced with maintenance of arterial perfusion pressure. Circulation 1979;80:769–81.
16. Drexler H, Banhardt U, Meinertz T. *et al*. Contrasting peripheral short-term and long-term effects of converting enzyme inhibition in patients with congestive heart failure. A double-blind, placebo-controlled trial. Circulation 1989;79:491–502.
17. Pernow B, Zelterquist S. A metabolic approach to the evaluation of the nutritive blood flow. Scand J Clin Lab Invest 1967;99(Suppl)90–4.
18. Ganz W, Tamura K, Marcus HS. *et al*. Measurement of coronary sinus blood flow by continuous thermodilution in man. Circulation 1971;54:181–95.

19. Haggmark S, Biber B, Sjodin JG. *et al*. The continuous thermodilution method for measuring high blood flows. Scand J Clin Lab Invest 1982;42:315–32.
20. Andersen P, Saltin B. Maximal perfusion of skeletal muscle in man. J Physiol 1985;366:233–49.
21. LeJemtel TH, Maskin CS, Lucido D. *et al*. Failure to augment maximal limb blood flow in response to one-leg versus two-leg exercise in patients with severe heart failure. Circulation 1986;74:245–51.
22. Rowell LB, Saltin B, Kiens B. *et al*. Is peak quadriceps blood flow in humans even higher during exercise with hypoxemia? Am J Physiol 1986;251:H1038–44.
23. Tonnesen KH. Blood flow through muscle during rhythmic contraction measured by [133]xenon. Scand J Clin Lab Invest 1963;16:646–54.
24. Clausen JP, Lassen NA. Muscle blood flow during exercise in normal man studied by the [133]xenon clearance method. Cardiovasc Res 1971;5:245–54.
25. Mancini DM, Davis L, Wexler JP *et al*. Dependence of enhanced maximal exercise performance on increased peak skeletal muscle perfusion during long-term captopril therapy in heart failure. J Am Coll Cardiol 1987;10:845–50.
26. Davis L, Wexler JP, Rabinowitz A *et al*. Data acquisition using a scintillation detector interfaced to a personal microcomputer. J Nucl Med 1985;26:85–7.
27. Cerretelli P, Marconi C, Pendergast D *et al*. Blood flow in exercising muscles by [133]xenon clearance and microsphere trapping. J Appl Physiol 1984;56:24–30.
28. Barlow TE, Haigh AL, Walder DN. Evidence for two vascular pathways in skeletal muscle. Clin Sci 1961;20:367–85.
29. Jorfeldt L, Wahren J. Leg blood flow during exercise in man. Clin Sci 1971;41:459–73.
30. Corbally MT, Brennan MF. Non-invasive measurement of regional blood flow in man. Am J Surgery 1990;160:313–21.
31. Greenfield ADM, Whitney RJ, Mowbray JF. Methods for the investigation of peripheral blood flow. Br Med Bull 1963;19:101–9.
32. Saltin B. Hemodynamic adaptations to exercise. Am J Cardiol 1985;55:42D-7D.
33. Sinoway L, Prophet S. Skeletal muscle metaboreceptor stimulation opposes peak metabolic vasodilation in humans. Circ Res 1990;66:1576–84.
34. Grimby G, Haggendal E, Saltin B Local xenon[133] clearance from the quadriceps muscle during exercise. J Appl Physiol 1967;22:305–10.
35. Wahren J, Saltin B, Jorfeldt L *et al*. Influence of age on the local circulatory adaptation to leg exercise. Scand J Clin Lab Invest 1974;33:79–86.
36. Granath A, Johnson B, Strandell T. Circulation in healthy old men studied by right heart catheterization at rest and during exercise in supine and sitting positions. Acta Med Scand 1964;176:425–37.
37. Zelis R, Longhurst J, Capone RJ *et al*. A comparison of regional blood flow and oxygen utilization during dynamic forearm exercise in normal subjects and patients with congestive heart failure. Circulation 1974;50:137–43.
38. Mancini DM, LeJemtel TH, Factor S *et al*. Central and peripheral components of cardiac failure. Am J Med 1986;80(Suppl 2B):2–13.
39. Maskin CS, Forman R, Sonnenblick EH *et al*. Failure of dobutamine to increase exercise capacity despite hemodynamic improvement in severe chronic heart failure. Am J Cardiol 1983;51:177–82.
40. Wilson JR, Martin JL, Schwartz D *et al*. Exercise intolerance in patients with chronic heart failure: role of impaired nutritive flow. Circulation 1984;69:1079–87.
41. Martin WH, Berman WI, Buckey JC *et al*. Effects of active muscle mass size in cardiopulmonary responses to exercise in congestive heart failure. J Am Coll Cardiol 1989;14:683–94.
42. Lewis SF, Taylor FW, Graham KM *et al*. Cardiovascular responses to exercise as functions of absolute and relative workload. J Appl Physiol 1983;54:1314–23.

33. The splanchnic circulation

RICHARD E. LEE and MUNTHER I. ALDOORI[1]

The splanchnic circulatory system contains a fifth of the total blood volume
[1] and receives a quarter of the cardiac output at rest [2]. The mesenteric
circulation conveys over two thirds of this to the intestines. This vast blood
supply is out of proportion to the relatively small mass of tissue it supplies.
The intestine has a low oxygen extraction reflecting its generous blood supply,
the fasting arterioportal oxygen difference being only 1.9 volumes per cent
[3]. This arrangement enables the viscera to meet increased oxygen requirements by increasing oxygen uptake as well as by increasing blood flow, and
serves to protect against intestinal mucosal hypoxia, the consequences of
which are so severe [4].

The intestinal blood flow is regulated by locally acting intrinsic mechanisms
and controlled extrinically by neural and hormonal mechanisms, of which
the sympathetic nervous system and circulating catecholamines seem to be
most important. Postprandial mesenteric hyperaemia has been widely studied
in man and animals. The stimulus for this seems to be mucosal absorption
of the products of digestion; the mechanism remains unclear, but seems
to involve gut hormones and other circulating agents in addition to local
mechanisms [5].

Most of our knowledge about intestinal blood flow is derived from animal
studies, supplemented by a small number of studies using invasive techniques
in man. ecent advances in ultrasonic technology have permitted noninvasive
measurement of blood flow in healthy and diseased subects, including neonates, both at rest and in response to physiological and pharmacological
stress [6, 7]. The superior mesenteric artery, portal vein and, to a lesser
extent, the branches of the coeliac artery have been most widely studied.
Few, if any data, however, are available concerning the inferior mesenteric
artery blood flow and the relation of blood flow to colonic function.

---

1. Dedicated to the memory of our friend, Mohammed Qamar MD, PhD, MRCP. His
   tragically early death in 1989 cut short the pioneering work in noninvasive measurement
   of the intestinal blood flow which forms the basis of this chapter.

A.-M. Salmasi and A.S. Iskandrian (eds): Cardiac output and regional flow in health and disease, 479–504.
© 1993 *Kluwer Academic Publishers. Printed in the Netherlands.*

Anatomical factors

The splanchnic circulation is via the derivatives of the three primitive gut arteries. The foregut derivatives, stomach, proximal duodenum, liver and spleen, all receive blood from the coeliac artery. The midgut, consisting of the remainder of the duodenum, the small intestine and the colon almost as far distally as its splenic flexure, is supplied via the superior mesenteric artery, while the remainder of the colon, the primitive hindgut, is supplied via the inferior mesenteric artery. Whereas the coeliac and inferior mesenteric arteries anastomose with extracoelomic collaterals around the lower oesophagus and rectum, the superior mesenteric is functionally an end artery; consequently, the usual effect of occluding it suddenly is intestinal infarction, although asymptomatic gradual occlusion is not uncommon [4].

The arteries form arcades on the mesenteric border of the viscera which anastomose before penetrating the muscularis and forming an extensive vascular network in the submucosa. The mucosal villi are each supplied by a single arteriole which, passing to the tip of the villus, breaks up into a fountain of capillaries. These reunite to form a venule which originates just below the tip of the villus. The "hairpin" formed by the parallel arteriole and venule enable a countercurrent multiplier exchange mechanism to function in each villus [8]. About 75% of the total resting intestinal blood flow is distributed to the mucosa/submucosa and the remainder to the muscularis/serosa. Intestinal venous blood enters the portal vein via mesenteric veins accompanying the arteries and passes through the liver.

The regulation of splachnic blood flow

The intestinal blood flow is determined by changing demands: it is subject to regulation by local metabolic and myogenic mechanisms independent of neural control, and to extrinsic regulation by the autonomic nervous system and by the effect of circulatin vasoactive substances [5, 9].

Local regulatory mechanisms (Intrinsic regulation)

Moment by moment control of blood flow requirements are met by local regulatory mechanisms. Two theories, metabolic and myogenic, have been advanced as mechanisms to explain observed phenomena such as auto-regulation, reactive hyperaemia, autoregulatory escape and functional hyperaemia. The metabolic theory proposes that local blood flow changes in response to any stress causing an imbalance between oxygen supply and demand. This results in an outpouring of metabolites (for example, K^+, H^+ adenosine, adenine nucleotides) which, by local diffusion, cause relaxation of arterioles and/or precapillary sphincters. The myogenic theory proposes that arteriolar tension receptors modulate vascular smooth muscular tone in response to changes in transmural pressure.

The mechanism of *pressure-flow autoregulation* maintains a steady state blood flow to a vascular bed despite fluctuations in arterial pressure. Althouh not as refined as in the renal or cerebral circulations, this occurs within the mesenteric microcirculation, especially in mucosal villi. An increase in venous pressure results in a redistribution of blood away from the mucosa, which normally receives over 80% of total flow.

Reactive hyperaemia is the period of increased flow following transient occlusion of arterial supply. This phenomenon occurs in the visceral blood vessels, as in all circulations, and affects predominantly the circulation to the muscularis.

Autoregulatory escape is the intrinsic ability of the intestinal vascular bed to escape from the continuous vasoconstriction resulting from sympathetic stimulation, or from circulating catecholamines or angiotensin. It is a process independent from autoregulation, and seems to involve metabolic and myogenic mechanisms operating concurrently; in autoregulation and reactive hyperaemia the mechanisms seem to operate as sequential modulators [5].

Functional hyperaemia is the increase occuring in intestinal blood flow to meet the needs arising from absorption, digestion and bowel motility. During anticipation or hunger the superior mesenteric artery resistance increases, probably as a result of increased sympathetic tone. During digestion and absorption hyperaemia occurs. There is evidence from animal models using whole intestine and isolated jejunal segments that regional vasodilatation occurs in reponse to where in the intestine food actually is [10], and microsphere distribution studies demonstrate that the hyperaemia is concentrated in the mucosa [11]. These observations are not universally accepted, however.

In the regulation of postprandial hyperaemia, metabolic (hypoxic) and myogenic responses seem to be relatively unimportant [5]. Mechanical stimulation of the mucosa alone results in increased blood flow [12], and the physical presence of chyme within the lumen of the intestine might be expected to produce the same effect, but it is generally agreed that the presence of products of digestion is the most potent stimulus. Although intraluminal injection of undigested food produces no change in mesenteric blood flow, the same food when injected in digested form increases flow markedly [13]. In animal experiments [14] and some human studies [15], the products of lipid metabolism were found to be the most potent stimulators of blood flow, and protein metabolites and glucose less so. Brandt found protein metabolites produced most pronounced hyperaemia [16], but Qamar demonstrated that carbohydrate, fat and protein meals produce comparable hyperaemic responses in normal subects, the peak flow being reached at varying times after the different meals [17]. The osmolality and pH of luminal contents seem not to be important physioloical stimuli of blood flow.

Intestinal chyme produces vasodilatation by both neural and hormonal mechanisms. The response is abolished by local anaesthetic, suggesting a local reflex thought to be cholinergic [18]. Cross perfusion experiments demonstrate the involvement of a hormonal agent [19], and although many hormones have been shown to increase blood flow, this is enerally in resonse to a pharmacological dose only. Cholecystokinin (CCK-PZ) probably increases mesenteric blood flow in physiological concentration, however, using 5-hydroxytryptamine as a transmitter [20].

Extrinsic regulation of intestinal blood flow

Neural factors
Extrinsic neural control of the intestinal vasculature is essentially via its sympathetic innervation. The study of the influence of central nervous stimulation on intestinal blood flow has been confined to animal experiments. Defensive behaviour or electrical stimulation of the "defense" area of the feline hypothalamus reduces intestinal blood flow [21], whereas electrical stimulation of lateral hypothalamus an area associated with control of appetite) increases blood flow [22], perhaps as a result of increasing intestinal motility. Intestinal blood flow rises during sleep [23].

Adrenergic nerves innervate the mesenteric arteries, arterioles and the larger veins, but not the precapillary sphincters, capillaries, venules or small veins [24]. Sympathetic nerve activation results in mesenteric vasoconstriction and a fall in intestinal blood flow through the action of noradrenaline [25]. This catecholamine, which constricts vascular smooth muscle by α adrenergic stimulation, is considered to be a physiological regulator of the mesenteric circulation, whether released from the adrenal medulla or from postsynaptic terminals. Adrenaline infused at low dose is a mesenteric vasodilator via a β effect, but acts as a pressor at higher dose [26]. Although it has vasoactive properties [27], dopamine does not seem to be of relevance in the physiology of intestinal blood flow regulation.

No direct cholinergic innervation of the mesenteric vasculature has been demonstrated, and although sinus nerve stimulation and acetyl choline injection increase intestinal blood flow, this may occur secondarily to baroceptor stimulation and increased intestinal motility.

Circulating stimuli
Many hormones and gastrointestinal peptides have vasoactive properties when administered intra-arterially in pharmacological doses, but few if any of these substances fulfil criteria to establish that the observed response is due to hormone mediated physiological mechanism [5]. The action of high dose gastrin, CCK, and glucagon in increasing intestinal blood flow is inhibited by atropine, suggesting they act via acetyl choline [28]. Intrinsic

nerves release a variety of peptides which have vasoactive properties which may act as circulatory regulators. Only VIP seems to be released during postprandial hyperaemia [29].

Although less powerful than vasopressin, which reduces human superior mesenteric blood flow by 50% [30], the angiotensins are potent intestinal vasoconstrictors, acting directly on the vascular cell membrane via prostacyclin. The feline mesenteric circulation is one one the major sites for the conversion of angiotensin I into the more potent vasoconstrictor angiotensin II, suggesting the latter has a physiological role, perhaps in reducing the splanchnic blood volume in shock states [31].

Local regulators

Histamine is present in most tissues and affects the circulation in most vascular beds. In the canine mesenteric vessels both H_1 and H_2 receptors are present. Infusion of histamine produces a large and brisk increase in intestinal blood flow followed by a smaller sustained increase [32]. The former is thought to be due to stimulation via H_1 receptors and the latter to H_2. The mesenteric endothelium contains histamine and histidine decarboxylase suggesting a physiological role for histamine as a local regulator, but the nature of this is unclear. Perhaps it is necessary for pressure autoregulation, as in the renal circulation [33].

Prostaglandins of the E, A, B, and I series dilate rat and dog mesenteric arteries, whereas those of the F and D series decrease intestinal blood flow. The vascular role of prostaglandins is not well established, however; vasoactive agents probably use them as mediators [34].

5-HT has potent effects on mesenteric blood vessels. These are not affected by or B adrenergic blockers, atropine or H_1 or H_2 blockers [35], and perhaps act using inositol triphosphate as a second messenger. Although the existense of specific receptors for 5-HT is established, its varied actions make its precise role as a regulator unclear; for example, in low dose vasodilatation is observed, in higher dose constriction.

The measurement of splanchnic blood flow

Our understanding of the pathophysiology of the splanchnic circulation relies heavily on data extrapolated from animal studies. Since different mammalian species have evolved different digestive systems to cope with widely diverse diets and behaviour, animal studies are of necessity limited in value in elucidating human mechanisms. Before the advent of ultrasonic techniques, the only methods for intestinal blood flow measurement available for use in man were invasive, and not suitable for routine clinical application. Nevertheless, the importance of studies using these techniques in establishing the fundamentals of intestinal blood flow should not be underestimated. Modern

Doppler ultrasonographic techniques represent a major advance, enabling the measurement of blood flow noninvasively in a conscious subject and the monitoring of flow changes in reponse to physiological and pathological stresses, and avoiding the adverse effects of anaesthesia and instrumentation.

Invasive measurment of splanchnic and mesenteric blood flow in man

Bromsulphalein (BSP) clearance by the liver provides a method of measuring total liver blood flow (it is discussed more fully below under *Liver blood flow measurement*); since this is also total splanchnic flow, BSP clearance enables changes in intestinal blood flow to be studied. The technique has been used to measure resting fasted total splanchnic blood flow [2], to study postprandial changes [2, 16] and measure the effects of exercise [1, 2], pyrexial reaction [2] and cirrhosis [2, 16].

Lantz *et al.* used a *video-dilution technique* to estmate coeliac blood flow as 13–19% and superior mesenteric blood flow 11–20% of the resting cardiac output [36].

Norryd *et al.* measured superior mesenteric artery blood flow using a dye *dilution technique*, injecting indocyanine green dye into the superior mesenteric artery and sampling blood from the superior mesenteric vein. He measured resting flow [37] and the effects of meals of different composition [38], including a model for dumping syndrome [39], and vasoactive substances [30]. Other invasive methods used to measure superior mesenteric artery blood flow include spill-over angiographic reflux [40] and inert gas wash-out [41].

Doppler ultrasonic blood flow measurement in the visceral arteries

The principle of blood flow measurement using Doppler ultrasound is the calculation of the instantaneous mean blood flow velocity over the cardiac cycle using analysis of the waveform of Doppler-shifted ultrasound reflected from the cellular elements of the moving blood within the blood vessel under study. The volume of blood flow is the product of the mean velocity and the cross sectional area of the blood vessel. A duplex ultrasonic scanner, combining a real-time imaging system with a range-gated pulsed Doppler system, provides a convenient method of measuring both. Qamar used an ATL 500 duplex scanner (Squibb Medical Systems) [6, 17, 42–47], but scanners of this early type have been superceded by more refined systems which provide on-line analysis of ultrasonic waveforms and instantaneous display of velocity and flow data.

Measurement of the volume of blood flow depends upon clear visualisation of the blood vessel under study in order to measure accurately the luminal cross-sectional area and also to place the sample volume of the pulsed Doppler ultrasonic beam so that ultrasound is reflected from all parts of the vessel cross-section, both from slowly and rapidly moving blood cells.

Table 33.1. Resting blood flow in the superior mesenteric artery.

Blood flow (ml/min)	Method	Author
705 ± 106[a]	dye dilution	Norryd, 1974 [37]
500 – 600[b]	inert gas washout	Hulten, 1976 [41]
456 ± 94[a]	spillover angiographic reflux	Clark, 1980 [40]
250 – 890 (502)[b]	duplex Doppler	Qamar, 1986 [45]
383 ± 90[a]	duplex Doppler	Sato, 1987 [53]
478 ± 166[a]	duplex Doppler	Nakamura, 1989 [54]

[a] Mean ± standard deviation.
[b] Range (median).

Inadequate visualisation of upper abdominal blood vessels is frequently the result of interference by bowel gas; the effects of this may be minimised by performing studies after an over-night fast. The angle at which ultrasound interrogates the blood vessel should be kept as acute as possible; inaccuracies in the measurement of this angle are disproportionately high when it exceeds 60° [48]. Errors arise in the calculation of blood vessel cross-sectional area, and are proportionately greater for small vessels. Some authors claim that blood flow velocity, and especially the end-diastolic velocity, provides as much information as volume blood flow, but can be measured more accurately in that a calculation of blood vessel cross-sectional area is not required [15, 49–51].

Qamar found his technique acceptably reproducible in the long and short term, and accurate when tested *in vitro* (validated against a calibrated electromagnetic flow meter in a flow rig) [52]. Other authors have validated their duplex ultrasonic techniques *in vivo* using anaesthetised dogs [53, 54].

Qamar was the first to measure coeliac axis blood flow noninvasively in man [44]. In 42 healthy, fasted subjects resting flow was 703 ± 24 ml/min, without age or sex variation. Immediately after a liquid meal a transient 38% increase in blood flow was observed. This resting flow measurement accords with the estimate of 13 to 19% of the cardiac output using a video-dilution technique [36]. Qamar measured the resting superior mesenteric artery blood flow in 70 subects as 250–890 ml/min (median 517) [45]. The flow values, which did not vary with age or sex, are in accordance with measurements made using invasive techniques and by other authors using Doppler ultrasound [37, 40, 41, 53, 54] (see Table 33.1).

Post-prandial blood flow

Numerous studies have demonstrated an increase in the blood flow to the stomach and small intestine after digestion in animals [55]. Total splanchnic blood flow increased by 35% after a protein meal but not after a glucose meal in three normal subjects studied using bromsulphalein clearance [16]. Using dye dilution, Norryd and colleagues demonstrated an increase in superior mesenteric blood flow averaging 113% [38], and a threefold rise after instillation of hypertonic glucose into the jejunum [39].

Qamar [44] demonstrated a 38% increase in coeliac blood flow rapidly following a liquid meal, and a return to normal within 30–60 minutes. Blood flow in the superior mesenteric artery increased by more than 100% after a solid meal and by 63% after a liquid meal [6].

Lilly and associates [51] found that peak systolic and diastolic blood flow both increased significantly in coeliac and superior mesenteric arteries after a 710 kcal liquid meal; changes were maximal in the coeliac artery at 40 minutes and had returned to normal at 60 minutes, whereas superior mesenteric artery hyperaemia persisted beyond 60 minutes. Other workers have not confirmed a postprandial rise in coeliac blood flow, perhaps performing measurements too late after the meal [15].

Jager and associates [50] found the SMA blood flow increased within 15 minutes of 1000 Kcal meal, with a doubling of peak systolic flow velocity at 45 minutes and a return to resting values by 90 minutes. The end-diastolic flow velocity increased threefold at maximal hyperaemia and the authors proposed this parameter as the most easily measured index of the peripheral vasodilatation of functional hyperaemia.

The effect of different foods on intestinal blood flow

Qamar [17] measured the effects of carbohydrate, fat and protein isocaloric, isovolumetric liquid meals on the superior mesenteric blood flow in 12 healthy subjects. The maximum blood flow in each case was about 160% of the fasting, but the peaks occured at different times: for carbohydrate after 15 minutes, for fat at 30 minutes and for protein at 45 minutes. An equal volume of water produced no increase in flow, demonstrating that the content and not the volume of the meal determines the hyperaemic response. He proposed that the rapid digestion and absorption of carbohydrate led to an early rise in blood flow, but that the protein and fat required a longer and more complicated hydrolysis and produced a later hyperaemic response. This would suggest that absorption of the products of digestion is the principal determinant of postprandial functional hyperaemia. In another experiment adding weight to this view, Qamar found that SMA flow increased after ingestion of isotonic glucose but not after isotonic lactulose which is not absorbed significantly [46]. This is supported by animal experiments [56, 57].

Moneta *et al.* [15] measured SMA blood flow following ingestion of a variety of meals (carbohydrate, fat, protein, mixed) as well as water and mannitol. The peak increase in SMA blood flow was most rapid (20 minutes) after the carbohydrate meal and occured 30 minutes after the other foods. The response was greatest after mixed (164 ± 30%) and fat (118 ± 23%) meals, suggesting that long chain fatty acids are potent stimulators of intestinal blood flow. The postprandial hyperaemia persisted for over 90 minutes. Although water produced no change, mannitol increased blood flow suggesting that osmolarity of intestinal content might have some hyperaemic effect, contrary to experimental evidence [58].

Intestinal blood flow in dumping syndrome

A significant increase in postprandial but not resting superior mesenteric blood flow occurs in patients with dumping syndrome compared with normal and non-dumping post-gastrectomy controls [43]. The peak increase was at 10 minutes after the end of the meal and was 42–76% greater but did not occur earlier than the maximal response in the controls. Norryd *et al.* had measured a massive increase in superior mesenteric artery flow in normal subjects in response to hypertonic glusose within the jejunal lumen [39]. Experimental studies had shown an increase in superior mesenteric blood flow accompanied by a parallel decrease in carotid, renal and femoral artery flow in reponse to injection of 50% glucose solution into the proximal jejunum of dogs [59].

A reduction in plasma volume associated with peripheral vasodilatation is a feature of dumping syndrome [60], and may be the cause of the commonly associated dizziness, hypotension (or need to lie down), weakness or palpitations. The mechanism by which these changes occur is still unclear. Perhaps an inflow of extracellular fluid into the bowel occurs in response to the hyperosmolar load; the resulting fall in plasma volume might trigger the release of vasoactive substances such as serotonin [61], kinins [62] or vasoactive intestinal peptide [63].

The effect of exercise on intestinal blood flow

Bradley [2] simultaneously measured cardiac output (direct Fick method), and estimated renal blood flow (PAH clearance) and total splanchnic, blood flow using bromsulphalein (BSP) clearance before and during exercise in the form of cycling in the recumbent position. He demonstrated a doubling in cardiac output associated with a fall in splanchnic blood flow of about 30% and in renal blood flow of 16%, with no change in systemic blood pressure. Again using BSP extraction to estimate changes in splanchnic blood flow and radio-iodine 131 to measure changes in splanchnic blood volume in normal subects in response to light, supine exercise, Wade *et al.* [1] demonstrated a fall in splanchnic blood flow by 20–25%, a simultaneous fall in splanchnic oxygen uptake and a fall in splanchnic blood volume from 1100 to 800 ml.

Qamar [47] confirmed these observations by demonstrating a 43% fall in SMA blood flow after moderately severe treadmill exercise. Exercise significantly reduced the postprandial hyperaemic response to a liquid meal when this was taken simultaneously.

Blood pressure changes little during exercise, so the fall in splanchnic blood flow must be due to increased splanchnic vascular resistance, presumably due to increased sympathetic tone. The decrease in splanchnic blood volume has been conceived in terms of an autotransfusion that primes the cardiac pump and makes possible the rapid increase in cardiac output that occurs in the first 90 seconds of exercise [64]. When the exercising cardiac output may reach 30–35 l/min, it is difficult to believe that in healthy humans the splachnic effects are sufficiently great to be of importance, but those with a reduced cardiac reserve are more likely to benefit from such a relatively small circulatory redistribution [65].

Mesenteric ischaemia

The intestine is very vulnerable to ischaemia; whenever there is a lack of tissue viability, bacterial invasion from the bowel contents will occur. In other words, infarction inevitably leads to gangrene.

Acute intestinal failure due to mesenteric ischaemia

Despite all advances in management, the very high mortality of this disorder 80–90% [66–68] has remained unchanged over 20 years. The condition increasingly affects old and seriously ill patients and the diagnosis is often delayed resulting in a high mortality. Even with apparently successful revascularisation or adequate bowel resection, the continuing high mortality suggests the involvement of many other factors in the usual fatal outcome. A favourable outcome depends upon early diagnosis, but a reliable diagnostic test is unfortunately lacking.

Sudden occlusion of the superior mesenteric artery usually results in intestinal infarction. In most cases occlusion is due to atherosclerotic occlusion or thrombosis. The large size and oblique origin of the superior mesenteric artery make it a preferential route for systemic emboli, but this an uncommon cause of mesenteric artery occlusion nowadays, because rheumatic valve disease is less common. Those emboli that do occur generally complicate myocardial infarction.

Bowel infarction due to primary venous thrombosis carries a favourable prognosis when treated with bowel resection and correction of the hypercoagulable state [67, 69], but when due to secondary venous thrombosis the outlook is bad.

Fifty per cent of fatal cases of acute intestinal failure due to ischaemia have nonocclusive thrombosis of the superior mesenteric artery or entirely patent vessels [70]. Such cases are usually old and very ill with severe cardiogenic shock. Acute changes in blood pressure or cardiac output lead to a reduction in splanchnic flow and a redistribution of blood within the bowel wall at the expense of perfusion of the mucosa, the cells of which suffer ischaemic damage [71]. Moreover, reperfusion of hypoxic intestinal mucosal cells results in release of oxygen-derived free-radicals which inflict further cell damage [72, 73].

Experimental prevention of intestinal tissue damage due to ischaemia, vasoconstriction or reperfusion has been studied widely. In rats, intravenous glucagon, methylprednisolone and PGI_2 all improved survival after superior mesenteric artery ligation [74]. Glucagon has been considered suitable for clinical use, but the prevention of intestinal damage *in vitro* depended upon minimal delay in administration. All forms of infarction seem to be associated with persistent vasoconstriction, and vasodilators have produced favourable results both experimentally [75] and clinically [76–78]. The importance of the release of oxygen-derived free-radicals in the pathogenesis of tissue damage has recently emerged, and suggestions have been made that this might be prevented this by using competitive inhibitors of purine metabolism such as allopurinol [67], dimethyl sulphoxide [79], superoxide dismutase [80] or xanthine oxidase inhibitors [73].

Clinical aspects

Whatever the aetiology of superior mesenteric artery occusion, the result is a sudden intense spasm of the small intestine, so the earliest clue to diagnosis is of colic in a patient with generalised arterial disease in the presence of circulatory failure or pre-existing cardiovascular disease. The pain becomes dull and generalised, the mucosa ulcerates and blood or mucus may be passed. Ileus supervenes followed by peritonitis, intestinal perforation and death. By the time florid signs have appeared no recovery is possible. The classical history is not very typical, however, and late diagnosis is the norm.

A good prognosis is associated with younger patients with a short history, early dianosis and a short length of involved intestine. Conversely, a bad prognosis can be expected in patients with peritonitis, cardiac failure, a high leucocytosis or greater than 1.5 metres of infarcted intestine [67].

The traditional approach of surgery alone in the treatment of acute intestinal ischaemia is associated with poor results and should probably be accompanied by pharmacological measures to prevent mesenteric vasoconstriction and reperfusion tissue damage, if a high rate of recurrent ischaemia is to be avoided. Increased survival with injection into the superior mesenteric artery of papaverine [76], phenoxybenzamine [81] and PGE_1 [77] suggest these agents may be of use in preventing persistent vasoconstriction in nonocclusive infarction.

The continuing effects of tissue damage after reperfusion makes a policy of a 'second look' operation advisable on the day following resection with or without revascularisation [70, 82].

Towards earlier diagnosis

A favourable outcome depends upon early diagnosis, but a good diagnostic test is unfortunately lacking. Raised serum inorganic phosphate, especially if accompanied by high white cell count and a metabolic acidosis which remains after shock has been corrected [83]. Less useful laboratory tests are raised serum amylase, lactate dehydrogenase, creatinine phosphokinase or ammonia.

The role of early angiography is not clearly defined. It enables diagnosis to be made in cases with mesenteric artery occlusion and offers the option of selectively perfusing the superior mesenteric artery with vasodilators [76, 77]. A further option made available is percutaneous transluminal angioplasty, which has been used with success [84]. Apart from invasiveness and possibly delaying other treatments, obvious disadvantages of relying on an aggressive arteriographic policy of diagnosis arise from a lack of correlation between the clinical picture, the degree of ischaemic visceral damage and the state of the superior mesenteric artery as assessed angiographically. Visceral artery occlusion without intestinal ischaemia is not uncommon [4], and would lead to a false positive diagnosis. More importantly are false negatives, because many fatal cases are associated with nonocclusive thrombus.

A highly attractive method of obtaining haemodynamic information about blood flow in the superior mesenteric artery is, of course, duplex Doppler ultrasound [6, 49, 85]. By contrast with arteriography, the method is entirely noninvasive; it should be rapid, specific and offer dynamic information about the blood flow. In an occluded artery, blood flow will not be detectable and reduced flow in a diseased vessel will alter the velocity waveform. Unfortunately, both the abdominal tenderness and the gaseous distension of the small bowel ileus associated with acute ischaemia make duplex scanning of the superior mesenteric artery difficult. Moreover, the condition is not common and the few published data [86] suggest none of the major vascular laboratories have much experience of duplex scanning in acute mesenteric ischaemia.

Chronic intestinal ischaemia

The classical clinical picture of an emaciated patient who will not eat because he fears the severe abdominal pain which is brought on by eating, the "intestinal angina" described by Mikkelsen [87], is rarely seen. The condition is in any case very rare [4].

Other causes of abdominal pain should be excluded, and arteriography in two planes may demonstrate the responsible superior mesenteric artery stenosis. But arteriography can only document anatomical abnormalities; it cannot give information about their functional significance. Once again, duplex Doppler ultrasonic techniques are very attractive for the investigation of chronic mesenteric ischaemia. In the case of chronic superior mesenteric ischaemia, or intestinal angina, distorted flow signals may be detected in the fasting and postprandial states. Doppler ultrasound signals show high peak blood flow velocity and spectral broadening due to turbulent flow at the site of narrowing in the superior mesenteric or any other diseased artery [49]. High diastolic flow is present, always an abnormal finding in the fasting superior mesenteric artery, and the elevated end-diastolic blood flow velocity is a parameter more easily measured than the volume blood flow [50]. An intestinal stress test, comparable to treadmill exercise in the assessment of lower limb peripheral vascular disease has been proposed to unmask chronic visceral ischaemia. This may take the form of a test meal or intravenous injection of glucagon [51]. In severe case, a stress test may not be required for diagnosis, however [88], but as with acute intestinal ischaemia, diagnostic criteria are as yet poorly defined.

Doppler flow studies in the visceral arteries of neonates

Blood flow after the first feed

For the measurement of blood flow velocity in neonates duplex Doppler ultrasonic techniques have been a great advance; when only invasive techniques were available, the study of visceral blood flow in human neonates was not feasible. Unlike the adult, diastolic flow in the superior mesenteric artery is a normal finding even at rest, and Van Bel *et al.* [89] estimate this vessel receives 17–20% of the cardiac output. The effects of the first feed of life on coeliac and superior mesenteric blood flow have been studied in premature neonates [90, 91]. Time averaged mean blood flow velocity in the superior mesenteric artery (and, therefore, blood flow) rose by 15 minutes after starting the feed and peaked at 45 minutes with a doubling of the resting flow value. Gladman [90] also observed an almost immediate rise in the coeliac artery blood flow, and found the blood flow changes were unrelated to the babies' gestational ages or weights. The abruptness of the rise in coeliac blood flow suggests that a local regulatory mechanism operates in the stomach whereby mechanical stimulation of the mucosa causes increased blood flow.

Effect of congenital heart disease and risk of necrotising enterocolitis

In preterm babies with patent ducti arteriosi, superior mesenteric blood flow shows an abnormal waveform, with retrograde or absent flow in diastole. This profound disturbance in mid-gut perfusion is exacerbated by parenteral indomethacin [89] especially if infused rapidly. This seems to be a direct action of indomethacin on the splanchnic bed, and not due to its effect on the ductus arteriosus; similar changes have been observed in an infant with

Fallot's tetralogy given indomethacin [92]. Preterm infants with such congenital heart problems are at increased risk of developing necrotising enterocolitis. Although there is no direct evidence that abnormal intestinal blood flow is responsible for necrotising enterocolitis in man, studies on animals and on severely growth-retarded fetuses suggest it may be [93].

Liver blood flow

The liver receives arterial and partially deoxygenated portal venous blood. The fasting portal venous oxygen saturation may be 85% or more, and although this falls postprandially as more oxygen is extracted by the intestinal mucosa, the portal flow contributes about 70% of the total liver oxygen supply [3]. This predominantly nourishes the hepatocytes, for the cells of the bile ducts and canaliculi require arterial blood for survival [94]. The arterial supply is via the common hepatic artery which usually arises from the coeliac trunk; in neonates it is the largest coeliac branch. There are common variations in the pattern of arterial anatomy, and some or all of the supply may be via the superior mesenteric artery [95]. Branches of the hepatic artery are distributed with those of the portal vein in the portal tracts; once within the liver they are functionally end arteries. The portal veins arborise into extensive venous sinusoids which perfuse the hepatocytes. Venous drainage is via central veins and the three hepatic veins to the inferior vena cava.

The hepatic blood volume is 10–15% of total blood volume [96], but in cardiac failure the liver may contain twice the normal volume of blood, mostly in venous capacitance vessels. After moderate blood loss in experimental animals, the liver capacitance vessels may expel blood to make good up to 25% of the loss. This reflex uses afferents from atrial stretch receptors and sympathetic efferents to the large capacitance veins of the liver; although probably important in animals, it is of doubtful importance even in young fit humans [97].

The total liver blood flow at rest is about 25% of the cardiac output [2]. Since this is also the total splanchnic blood flow, factors which alter intestinal blood flow will also alter portal venous flow and hence liver blood flow. So total liver blood flow increases postprandially [2, 16, 98] and decreases during exercise [1, 2]. Hepatic blood flow does not rise and fall according to the oxygen requirements of the liver cells. At rest, the liver only extracts up to 40% of the oxygen supplied; when the liver blood flow or oxygen supply falls the liver compensates by increasing oxygen extraction, rather than by attempting to increase its blood flow.

Control of hepatic blood flow

Autoregulation occurs in the liver, as in all tissues. A reduction in hepatic artery pressure leads to a reduction in resistance in an attempt to keep blood flow constant. In the portal system, however, autoregulation does not occur; if portal pressure falls the peripheral resistance increases to help sustain it [99].

If portal inflow is diverted or temporarily occluded, arterial blood flow shows a compensatory increase, but hepatic artery occlusion produces no change in portal haemodynamics [100].

Effect of hormones and vasoactive substances

Catecholamines

Intravenous adrenaline causes a transient rise in hepatic artery flow, and a more sustained rise in portal flow due to splanchnic vasodilatation. This effect is reversed by β-adrenergic blockers, which, by increasing splanchnic vascular resistance and reducing mesenteric blood flow, lower portal venous pressure in portal hypertension.

Noradrenaline produces a fall in portal flow as a result of mesenteric vasoconstriction. This effect is short-lived, as the intestinal blood flow is restored by autoregulatory escape.

Angiotensin and vasopressin

Infusion of angiotensin was found to produce a 17.5% fall in cardiac output and a 26% fall in total hepatic blood flow measured by Indocyanine Green clearance. The peripheral resistance in the splanchnic bed increased by 100%, but portal pressure did not fall [101]. Vasopressin is a yet more potent splanchnic vasoconstrictor [30], causing a sustained fall in portal pressure and hepatic blood flow. When infused directly into the canine hepatic artery or portal vein, vasopressin produces a transient fall in hepatic artery blood flow which is restored rapidly by autoregulatory escape, but systemic infusion does not alter hepatic artery flow. Vasopressin reduces portal pressure by profoundly reducing mesenteric blood flow; this effect is not influenced by the route of administration, local or systemic [102]. Moreover, the superior mesenteric artery does not exhibit autoregulatory escape from vasopressin-induced vasoconstriction.

Somatostatin reduces portal pressure by splanchnic vasoconstriction; it appears to be as effective as vasopressin for arresting acute variceal hae-morrhage in portal hypertension, but is associated with less serious complications [103].

The measurement of hepatic blood flow

In 1974, Bradley [104] classified the then available methods of measuring hepatic blood flow clinically:

1. those depending upon hepatic clearance of an infused substance;
2. indicator dilution techniques;
3. other methods, such as inert gas diffusion and electromagnetic flowmetry.

The principal advance since then has been the study of portal venous and, to a much lesser extent, hepatic arterial haemodynamics using Doppler ultrasound.

Hepatic clearance

Bromsulphalein (BSP) is cleared from circulating blood almost exclusively by the liver. Bradley estimated total hepatic blood flow in 50 normal conscious human subiects using BSP clearance as 1490 (950–1840) ml/min [2]. Calculation of total liver blood flow was made according to the indirect Fick principle and required continuous infusion of BSP and sampling of peripheral arterial and hepatic venous blood. Bolus infusion of BSP allows sequential measurements of flow to be made, but with considerably less accuracy. Hepatic clearance of indocyanine green (ICG) is preferred by some to BSP in that it is cleared solely by the liver, whereas some renal clearance of BSP occurs [105]. Even this technique is limited by hepatic function, being a measurement of hepatic extraction of ICG, and did not correlate well when compared with electromagnetic flowmetry [106].

Indicator dilution

The advantage of indicator dilution methods over hepatic clearance is that the former do not depend upon hepatic function and may be used to measure blood flow in disease states. A bolus of a tracer (for example ^{131}I-labelled albumin) is injected upstream of the liver (into the superior mesenteric or splenic artery, or intrasplenic injection) and samples taken from the hepatic vein [107].

Doppler ultrasonic techniques

The portal vein was one of the first blood vessels in which volume blood flow was measured noninvasively using ultrasonic techniques [108], and several studies have been reported since [98, 109–114]; (Table 33.2). Its large size and relative accessibility make error of measurement small, and flow is relatively constant, without marked variation due to cardiac or respiratory cycles. Moreover, the information provided is likely to be of clinical value, enabling monitoring of portal haemodynamics and liver disease. Unfortu-

Table 33.2. Resting blood flow in the portal vein of normal and cirrhotic subjets.

Blood flow (ml/min)		Method	Author
Normal	Cirrhotic		
447	359	electromagnetic	Moreno, 1967 [120]
889 ± 284[a]		duplex Doppler	Moriyasu, 1986 [111]
966 ± 344[a]	579 ± 252[a]	duplex Doppler	Okazaki, 1986 [98]
694 ± 23[a]	736 ± 46[a]	duplex Doppler	Zoli, 1986 [110]
632 ± 203[a]	1218 ± 394[b]	duplex Doppler	Oshnishi, 1987 [109]
	640 ± 108[b]		
874 ± 207[a]	450 ± 85[a]	duplex Doppler	Ozaki, 1988 [112]

[a] Mean ± standard deviation.
[b] Early and advanced disease; see text.

nately, there is a lack of agreement in studies of the effects of cirrhosis on portal and hepatic arterial volume flow (see below), and a good case can be made for relying on Doppler-derived blood flow velocity patterns, rather than volume flow calculations in studying the portal vein. These are more simply calculated, since measurement of the portal vein cross-sectional area is not required. This is often wrongly assumed to be circular, and its measurement is considered a major source of error. A directional Doppler flow detector can provide important information about the quality of blood flow; for example, whether hepatofugal flow occurs, and if so during what phases of the cardiac cycle. Duplex Doppler also provides the ideal method of observing the postoperative effects of portal-systemic shunts [114] and checking for continued patency [115].

Portal vein blood flow velocity

Doppler signals from the portal vein in a normal fasted adult show continuous forward flow with a time averaged mean velocity of 10–15 cm/sec. After a meal the flow increases within minutes; the vein distends and the time averaged mean velocity increases to 20–25 cm/sec.

In most patients with mild to moderate liver disease the portal flow is normal. In more advanced cirrhosis the time averaged mean velocity is reduced at rest as well as postprandially. Eventually increased pressure within the portal vein is insufficient to compensate for hepatic resistance and retrograde diastolic flow occurs. In more advanced cases, established continuous flow reversal develops.

In the acute phase of Budd-Chiari syndrome, reversed flow will occur in the portal vein and flow in the hepatic veins will be undetectable. In portal vein occlusion no flow is detectable, unless the thrombosis occured early in life, when cavernous transformation takes places as a means of recanalisation.

Hepatic artery blood flow measurement

The volume of blood flow in the common hepatic artery at rest has been measured using Doppler ultrasound as 254 ± 131 ml/min; less, that is, than resting flow in the splenic (370 ± 181 ml/min) and superior mesenteric (478 ± 166) arteries [54]. Visualisation of an adequate length of common hepatic artery for flow measurement is difficult, however, and the frequency of hepatic arterial anomalies makes a flow value difficult to interpret. Flow measurements in a single arterial or portal branch are more easily performed, and may be used sequentially to monitor the effects of drugs on liver blood flow [116].

Cirrhosis and portal hypertension

Portal venous pressure is normally 6–10 mm Hg and sinusoidal vein pressure 2–4 mm Hg above vena caval pressure. The portal pressure depends primarily on the degree of constriction or dilatation of splanchnic arterioles and on the intrahepatic resistance. Normal hepatic artery pressure has no effect on portal pressure.

All forms of cirrhosis may lead to intrahepatic portal hypertension. Fibrous contraction leads to distortion and reduction of the portal vascular bed, producing mechanical obstruction. The sinusoids and hepatic venous radicals are also compressed. Blood is diverted away from the liver into the major collateral channels and up to 30% of the liver blood flow bypasses functioning hepatocytes being shunted through abnormal portal-hepatic anastamoses. The proportion of blood shunted in this way has been calculated by measuring the distribution of degradeable $^{99}Tc^m$ albumin labelled microspheres [117]. The regenerating nodules, divorced from portal blood, become dependent upon the hepatic artery for oxygen supply, and arterial oxygen extraction increases.

In advanced cases the systemic circulation is hyperdynamic, as systemic and pulmonary arteriovenous fistulae open up; this is not a feature of prehepatic and other non-cirrhotic causes of portal hypertension [118]. The cause of the hyperaemia is uncertain; vasoactive false transmitters of intestinal origin which the diseased liver fails to metabolise have been incriminated but not identified. There is considerable evidence that an increase in the volume of blood entering the portal system by way of increased flow through the splenic and, perhaps, mesenteric circulations is an important factor in the development of portal hypertension [119], even in non-cirrhotic patients [109, 119].

Bradley [2] found the total splanchnic blood flow was reduced in cirrhotics and the oxygen extraction was increased. Moreover, since BSP uptake by the cirrhotic liver is impaired, the estimate of blood flow is likely to be falsely high. Okazaki *et al.* [98] and Ozaki *et al.* [112] both demonstrated reduced portal blood flow in cirrhotics with portal hypertension. Portal hyperaemia, both postprandially and induced by glucagon and secretin, were found to be significantly less in the cirrhotics, but the reduction in portal blood flow by vasopressin was not impaired. These observations confirm that the volume of portal blood flow depends primarily upon mesenteric flow, and suggest that the latter is reduced in cirrhotics with portal hypertension. Other workers, however, found no reduction in portal flow in cirrhotic patients with portal hypertension [109, 110, 113], and some have found that it was considerably increased [114].

Zoli and colleagues [110] found that the portal flow volume was not altered in cirrhotic patients, but that flow patterns were, the mean velocity of the portal flow in cirrhotics 10.5 ± 0.6 cm/sec) being significantly less than in controls 16.0 ± 0.5. Ohinishi and associates [109] found two distinct patterns in patients with benign intrahepatic portal hypertension. One group had markedly increased portal vein volume blood flow (measured by duplex ultrasound) and total hepatic flow (measured by IGG clearance), associated with moderate elevation of the portal blood pressure. The other group had more advanced disease, with higher pressures and hepatic resistance, but portal and total hepatic blood flow not significantly different from normal. Sato *et al.* [53] measured increased blood flow in the superior mesenteric and splenic arteries of patients with cirrhosis but not those with chronic hepatitis, reflecting the hyperdynamic state found in cirrhotics; they propose that increased flow into the portal vein is an important aetiological factor in the development of portal hypertension. There are many inconsistencies in these data. Perhaps these are due to a difference in technique; it is not always clear where in the portal vein the measurement were made or even whether flow was hepatofugal or hepatopetal (Table 33.2). The changes in the mesenteric and splenic circulations in portal hypertension are still poorly understood, and clearly this an area begging for further study.

Splenic blood flow

Anatomical considerations

The splenic artery is the largest of the coeliac branches in adults. It branches at the splenic hilum and further ramifies within the splenic substance into *central arteries* which enter the trabeculae and acquire coats of lymphatic tissue. On emerging from the lymphatic layer the vessels divide further in the splenic pulp, losing their muscular coats; here they are called *penicillar arteries*. Blood drains into venous sinuses, occupying the red pulp, which are capable of containing considerable quanttties of blood under low pressure. These drain via pulp veins into trabecular veins, accompanying the arteries, and thence to the splenic vein and portal vein. The smooth muscle of the arteries, arterioles and veins has a sympathetic but not a parasympathetic innervation.

The microcirculation of the spleen, perhaps the most complex of any organ [121], is adapted to its filtrative function. The delivery of blood from the arteries into the unique splenic sinuses shows considerable species variation. Two pathways exist, each serving a separate function. In the "closed" system, an endothelialised communication exists between artery and vein providing a rapid circuit of low resistance. In the red pulp the arteriolar terminations have no endothelial continuity with venous structures, and the circulation is predominantly "open" in form with the blood crossing a connective tissue lined space. It is in this open anatomical system that filtration takes place.

Functional considerations

Radial branches of the central arteries have the effect of skimming off the more slowly-moving outer layers of the streaming blood and leaving the central axial elements of the flow, containing most of the red blood cells, to flow onwards into the red pulp. In this way the plasma is directed into the white pulp in low resistance closed pathways bypassing the filtration system, and the remaining red cell concentrated blood doubles its haematocrit and passes into the filtration system. The plasma flow through the spleen is thus as rapid as in active skeletal muscle, and 90% of the splenic flow passes through the closed system. But the time taken for a red blood cell to pass through the splenic filtration system may be a thousand times greater. The result is a highly efficient filtration system; a very high proportion of abnormal red cells is retained on a single passage through the spleen [122].

In some animals, such as dogs, cats, horses and seals, the spleen functions as a red cell reservoir; in the cat 40–50% of the total volme of the relaxed spleen consists of red cells. The relatively large spleen of these creatures has much smooth muscle within its trabeculae and capsule. Contraction of this splenic smooth muscle, which occurs in response to symathetic stimulation and to adrenergic sympathomimetics, contracts the filtration beds and releases the cells held there into the circulation. It also has the effect of closing the open pathways and speeding up blood flow through the red pulp.

In portal hypertensive patients, increased splenic vein pressure leads to congestive splenomegaly as the venous reservoir becomes progressively engorged, and the volume and mass of the spleen increase considerably.

Splenic blood flow

Although the relatively small human spleen does not not seem to have an important function as a circulatory reservoir, regulation of the volume and distribution of blood flow by intrinsic and extrinsic sympathetic control of vascular muscular tone is critically important if it is to function effectively.

Unfortunately, the splenic blood flow and its measurement in man have received relatively little attention.

Normal splenic artery flow has been estimated as 100–200 ml/min by William *et al.* using an inert gas washout technique [119]. They found an increase in total splenic flow in 13 patients with congenital haemolytic disorders. These patients also had increased portal venous pressure, suggesting that increased flow through the splenic artery must be considered an aetiological factor in portal hypertension. Cirrhotic patients were found to have significantly reduced flow per unit mass of spleen, but since the spleen was enlarged in all these portal hypertensive patients, *total* splenic blood flow was increased. In those with significant natural or surgical portal systemic shunts the splenic flow was grossly elevated.

Using duplex Doppler ultrasound, Nakamura [54] obtained values of 370 ± 181, 478 ± 166 and 254 ± 131 ml/min for blood flow in the splenic, superior mesenteric and common hepatic arteries respectively. Sato *et al.* [53] measured blood flow in the splenic and superior mesenteric arteries as 179 ± 37 and 383 ± 90 ml/min respectively; flow in both arteries was significantly increased in portal hypertensive patients. Zoli and colleagues [110] also found significantly increased blood flow in cirrhotic patients compared with normal controls (372 ± 43 *versus* 231 ± 19 ml/min), although they found no increase in portal venous flow.

References

1. Wade OL, Combes B, Childs AW *et al.* The effect of exercise on the splanchnic blood flow and splanchnic blood volume in normal man. Clin Science 1956;13:457–68.
2. Bradley SE. Variations in hepatic blood flow in man during health and disease. N Eng J Med 1949;240:456–61.
3. Sherlock S. Portal venous system and portal hypertension. In: Diseases of the liver and biliary system. 7th ed. Oxford: Blackwell, 1985:135–81.
4. Marston A, Clarke JFM, Garcia JC *et al.* Intestinal function and intestinal blood supply: a 20 year surgical study. Gut 1985;260:656–66.
5. Grainger DN, Richardson PDI, Kvietys PR *et al.* Intestinal blood flow. Gastroenterology 1980;78:837–63.
6. Qamar MI, Read AE. Intestinal blood flow. Q J Med 1985;56:417.
7. Taylor G. Blood flow measurement in the superior mesenteric artery: estimation with Doppler ultrasound [editorial]. Radiology 1990;174:15–6.
8. Hallback DA, Hulten J, Jodal M *et al.* Evidence for the existence of a countercurrent exchanger in the small intestine in man. Gastroenterology 1978;74:683–90.
9. Parks DA, Jacobson ED. Mesenteric circulation. In: Johnson LR (ed), Physiology of the gastrointestinal tract. 2nd ed. New York: Raven Press, 1987:1649–70.
10. Gallavan RH, Chou CC, Kvietys *et sl.* Regional blood flow during digestion in the conscious dog. Am J Physiol 1980;238:G131–4.
11. Bond JH, Prentiss RA, Levitt MD. The effects of feeding on blood flow to the stomach, small bowel and colon of the conscious dog. J Lab Clin Med 1979;93:594–9,
12. Biber B, Lundgren O, Svanvik J. Studies on the intestinal vasodilatation observed after mechanical stimulation of the mucosa of the gut. Acta Physiol Scand 1971;82:177–92.

13. Chou CC, Kvietys P, Post J *et al.* Constituents of chyme responsible for postprandial intestinal hyperaemia. Am J Physiol 1978;235:H677–82.
14. Siregar H, Chou G. Relative contribution of fat, protein, carbohydrate, and ethanol to intestinal hyperemia. *Am J Physiol* 1982;242:G27–31.
15. Moneta GL, Taylor DC, Helton WS *et al.* Duplex ultrasound measurement of postprandial intestinal blood flow: effect of meal composition. Gastroenterology 1988;95:1294–301.
16. Brandt JL, Castleman L, Ruskin HD *et al.* The effect of oral protein and glucose feeding on splanchnic blood flow and oxygen utilisation in normal and cirrhotic subjects. J Clin Invest 1955;34:1017–25.
17. Qamar MI, Read AE. Effects of ingestion of carbohydrate, fat, protein and water on the mesenteric blood flow in man. Scand J Gastroenterol 1988;23:26–30.
18. Chou CC, Burns TD, Hsieh CP *et al.* Mechanisms of local vasodilation with hypertonic glucose in the jejunum. Surgery 1972;71:380.
19. Fara JW, Rubenstein EH, Sonnenshein RR. Intestinal hormones in mesenteric dilatation after intraduodenal agents. Am J Physiol 1972;223:1058–67.
20. Biber B, Fara J, Lundgren O. A pharmacological study of intestinal vasodilation mechanisms in the cat. *Acta Physiol Scand* 1974;90:673–83.
21. Cobbold A, Folkow B, Lundren *et al.* Blood flow capillary filtration coefficient and regional blood volume responses in the intestines of the cat during stimulation of the hypothalamic 'defence' area. Acta Physiol Scand 1964;61;467.
22. Folkow B, Rubenstein EH. Behavioral and autonomic patterns evoked by stimulation of the lateral hypothalamic area in the cat. Acta Physiol Scand 1965;65:292–9.
23. Mancia G, Adams DB, Baccelli G *et al.* Regional blood flow during desynchronised sleep in the cat. Experimentia 1969;25:48
24. Greenway CV, Scott GD, Zink J. Sites of autoregulatory escape in the mesenteric vascular bed. J Physiol (Lond) 1976;259:1–12.
25. Shepherd AP, Mailman D, Burks TF *et al.* Effects of norepinephrine and sympathetic stimulation on the extraction of oxygen and ^{86}Rb in perfused canine small bowel. Circ Res 1981;33:166,
26. Kerr JC, Reynold DG, Swan KG. Adrenergic stimulation and blockade in the mesenteric circulation of the baboon. Am J Physiol 1978;234:E452–62.
27. Pawlik WW, Xailman D, Shanbour LL *et al.* Dopamine effects on the intestinal circulation. Am Heart J 1976;91:325.
28. Bowen JC, Pawlik W, Fang W-F *et al.* Pharmacological effects of gastrointestinal hormones on intestinal oxygen consumption and blood flow. Surgery 1975;78:515–9.
29. Gallavan RH, Chen MH, Joffe SN *et al.* Vasoactive intestinal peptide, cholecystokinin, glucagon, and bile-oleate-induced jejunal hyperaemia. Am J Physiol 1985;248:G208.
30. Norryd C, Dencker H, Lunderquist A *et al.* Superior mesenteric blood flow in man following injection of bradykinin and vasopressin into the superior mesenteric artery. Acta Chir Scand 1975;141:119–28.
31. McNeill JR, Stark RD, Greenway CV. Intestinal vasoconstriction after haemorrhage; roles of vasopressin and angiotensin. Am J Physiol 1970;219:1342.
32. Pawlik W, Tague LL, Tepperman BL *et al.* Histamine H-1 and H-2 receptor vasodilatation of the canine intestinal circulation. Am J Physiol 1977;233:E219.
33. Banks RO, Jacobson ED. Renal vasodilation with ureteric occlusion and prostaglandins: attenuation by histamine H-1 antagonists. Am J Physiol 1985;249:F851.
34. Blumberg AL, Denny SE, Marshall GR *et al.* Blood vessel hormone interactions: angiotensin, bradykinin and prostaglandins. Am J Physiol 1977;232:H305.
35. Biber B, Fara J, Lundgren O. A pharmacological study of intestinal vasodilator mechanisms in the cat. Acta Physiol Scand 1974;90:673.
36. Lantz M, Link D, Holcroft J *et al.* Video dilution technique. Angiographic determination of splanchnic blood flow. In: Grainger D, Buckley G (eds) Measurement of blood flow in applications to the splanchnic circulation. Baltimore: Williams and Wilkins, 1981:425–35.

37. Norryd C, Dencker H, Lunderquist A *et al*. Superior mesenteric blood flow in man studied with a dye-dilution technique. Acta Chir Scand 1974;141:109–18.
38. Norryd C, Dencker H, Lunderquist A *et al*. Superior mesenteric blood flow during digestion in man. Acta Chir Scand 1975;141:197–202.
39. Norryd C, Dencker H, Lunderquist A *et al*. Superior mesenteric blood flow during expeimentally induced dumping in man. Acta Chir Scand 1975;141:187–96.
40. Clark R, Colley D, Jacobson E *et al*. Superior mesenteric angiography and blood flow measurement following intra-arterial injection of prostaglandin E_1. Radiology 1980;134:327–38.
41. Hulten L, Jodal M, Lindhagen J *et al*. Blood flow in the small intestine of cat and man as analysed by an inert gas washout technique. Gastroenterology 1976;70:45.
42. Qamar MI, Read AE, Skidmore R *et al*. Pulsatility index of superior mesenteric artery blood velocity waveforms. Ultrasound Med Biol 1986;12:773–7.
43. Aldoori MI, Qamar MI, Read AE *et al*. Increased flow in the superior mesenteric artery in dumping syndrome. Br J Surg 1985;72:389.
44. Qamar MI, Read AE, Skidmore R *et al*. Transcutaneous Doppler ultrasonic measurement of coeliac axis blood flow in man. Br J Surg 1985;72:391.
45. Qamar MI, Read AE, Skidmore R *et al*. Transcutaneous Doppler ultrasonic measurement of superior mesenteric blood flow in man. Gut 1986;27:100.
46. Qamar MI, Read AE, Mountford R. Increased superior mesenteric artery blood flow after glucose but not lactose ingestion. Q J Med 1986;60:893,
47. Qamar MI, Read AE. Effects of exercise on mesenteric blood flow in man. Gut 1987;27:583.
48. Gill RW. Measurement of blood flow by ultrasound: accuracy and sources of error. Ultrasound Med Biol 1985;11:625.
49. Nichols SG, Kohler TR, Martin RS *et al*. Use of hemodynamic parameters in the diagnosis of mesenteric insufficiency. J Vasc Surg 1986;3:507.
50. Jager K, Bollinger A, Valli C *et al*. Measurement of mesenteric blood flow by duplex scanning. J Vasc Surg 1986;3:462.
51. Lilly MP, Harward TRS, Flinn WR *et al*. Duplex ultrasound measurement of changes in mesenteric blood velocity with pharmacologic and physiologic alteration of intestinal blood flow in man. J Vasc Surg 1989;9:18.
52. Qamar MI, Beard J, Evans JM *et al*. Accuracy and errors of non-invasive measurenents of blood flow by Doppler ultrasound. Br J Radiol 1986;59:838.
53. Sato S, Ohnishi K, Sugita OK *et al*. Splenic artery and superior mesenteric artery blood flow: nonsurgical Doppler ultrasound measurement in healthy subject and patients with chronic liver disease. Radiology 1987;164:347.
54. Nakamura T, Moriyasu F, Ban N *et al*. Quantitative measurement of abdominal arterial blood flow using image-directed Doppler ultrasonography: superior mesenteric, splenic and common hepatic arterial blood flow in normal adults. J Clin Ultrasound 1989;17:261.
55. Fara JW. Postprandial mesenteric hyperemia. In: Shepherd AP, Grainger DN (eds), Physiology of the intestinal circulation. New York: Raven Press, 1984;99–106.
56. Chou CC, Burns TD, Hsieh CP *et al*. Mechanisms of local vasodilatation with hypertonic glucose in the jejunum. Surgery 1972;71:380–7.
57. Sit SP, Nyhof R, Gallavan R *et al*. Mechanisms of glucose-induced hyperemia in the jejunum. Proc Soc Exp Biol Med 1980:163:273.
58. Kveitys P, Pittman R, Chou C. Contribution of the luminal concentration of nutrients and osmolality to postprandial intestinal hyperaemia in dogs. Proc Soc Exp Biol ed 1976;152:659.
59. Hues WM, Hinshaw DB. Blood flow studies in the experimental dumping syndrome. Surg Forum 1961;11:316.
60. Hinshaw DB, Joergenson EJ, Davis HA *et al*. Peripheral blood flow and blood volume in the dumping syndrome. Arch Surg 1957;74:686.

61. Drapanas T, McDonald JC, Stewart JD. Serotinin release following instillation of hypertonic glucose into the proximal intestine. Ann Surg 1962,156:528.
62. Wong PY, Talamo RC, Babior BM *et al*. Kallikrein-kinin system in post-gastrectomy dumping syndrome. Ann Int Med 1980;80:577.
63. Sagor GR, Bryant MG, Ghatei MA *et al*. Release of vasoactive intestinal peptide in the dumping syndrome. Br Med J 1981;282:507.
64. Donald KW, Bishop J, Cumming G *et al*. The effect of exercise on the cardiac output and circulatory dynamics of normal subjects. Clin Sci 1955;14:37.
65. Bishop JM, Donald KW, Wade OL. Changes in the oxygen content of hepatic venous blood during exercise in patients wlth rhematic heart disease. J Clin Invest 1955;34:1115.
66. Williams LF. Mesenteric ischemia. Surg Clin Am 9168;68(ii):331.
67. Clavien PA, Muller C, Harder F. Treatment of mesenteric infarction. Br J Surg 1987;74:500.
68. Wilson C, Gupta R, Gilmore DG *et al*. Acute superior mesenteric ischaemia. Br J Surg 1987;74:279.
69. Grendell GH, Ockner RK. Mesenteric venous thrombosis. Gastroenterology,1982;82:358.
70. Ottinger LW. The surgical management of acute occlusion of the superior mesenteric artery. Ann Surg 1978;188:721.
71. Gottlieb JE, Menashe PI, Cruz E. Gastrointestinal complications in critically ill patients: the intensivist's overview. Am J Gastroenterol 1986;81:227.
72. Bounous G. Pancreatic proteases and oxygen-derived free radicals in acute ischemic enteropathy. Surgery 1986;199:92.
73. Grainger DN, McCord JM, Parks DA *et al*. Xanthine oxidase inhibitors attenuate ischemia-induced vascular permiability changes in the cat intestine. Gastroenterology 1986;90:80.
74. Kasmers A, Zwolak R, Appleman H *et al*. Pharmacologic interventions in acute mesenteric ischemia: improved survival with intravenous glucagon, methyl prednisolone and prostacyclin. J Vasc Surg 1984;1:472.
75. MacCannell KL. Comparison of an intravenous selective mesenteric vasodilator with intra-arterial papaverine in experimental nonocclusive mesenteric ischemia. Gastroenterology 1986;91:79.
76. Boley SJ, Feinstein FR, Sammartano R *et al*. New concepts in the management of emboli of the superior mesenteric artery. Surg Gynecol Ostet 1981;153:561.
77. Clark RA, Gallant TE. Acute mesenteric ischemia: angiographic spectrum. A J R 184;42:555.
78. Athanasoulis CA, Wittenberg J, Bernstein R *et al*. Vasodilatory drugs in the management of nonocclusive bowel ischemia. Gastroenterology 1975;68:146.
79. Demetriou AA, Kagoma PK, Kaiser S *et al*. Effect of dimethyl sulfoxide and glycerol on acute bowel ischemia in the rat. Am J Surg 1985;149:91.
80. Bulkley GB. The role of oxygen free radicals in human disease proceses. Surg 1983;94:407.
81. Bailey RW, Bulkley GB, Hamilton SR *et al*. Protection of the small intestine from nonocclusive mesenteric ischemic injury due to cardiogenic shock. Am J Surg 1987;153:108–16.
82. Glotzer DJ, Glotzer P. Superior mesenteric embolectomy. Report of two successful cases using the Fogarty catheter. Arch Surg 1966;93:421.
83. Jamieson WG, Marchuk S, Rowsom J *et al*. The early diagnosis of massive acute intestinal ischaemia. Br J Surg 1982;96(Suppl): S52.
84. Van Deinse WH, Zawacki J, Phillips D. Treatment of acute mesenteric ischemia by percutaneous transluminal angioplasty. Gastroenterology 1986;91:475.
85. Flinn R, Rizzo RJ, Park JS *et al*. Duplex scanning for assessment of mesenteric ischemia. Surg Clin N Am 1990;70(i):99.
86. Takahashi H, Takezawa J, Okada T *et al*. Portal blood flow measured by duplex scanning during mesenteric infarction. Crit Care Med 1986;14:253–4.
87. Mikkelsen WP. Intestinal angina: its surgical significance. Am J Surg 1957;194:262.
88. Strandness DE. Comment. J Vasc Surg 1989;9:24–5.
89. Van Bel F, Van Zweiten PHT, Guit GL *et al*. Superior mesenteric artery blood flow

velocity and estimated volume flow: duplex Doppler ultrasound study of preterm and term neonates. Radiology, 1990;74:165.

90. Leidig E. Doppler analysis of superior mesenteric artery blood flow in preterm infants. Arch Dis Child 1989;64:476.

91. Gladman G, Sims DG, Chiswick ML. Gastrointestinal blood flow velocity after the first feed. Arch Dis Child 1991;6:17.

92. Coombs RC, Morgan MEI, Durbin GM *et al.* Gut blood flow velocities in the newborn; effects of patent ductus arteriosus and parenteral indomethacin. Arch Dis child 1990;65:1067.

93. Hackett GA, Campbell S, Gam SU *et al.* Doppler studies in the growth retarded fetus and prediction of neonatal necrotising enterocolitis, haemorrhage and neonatal morbidity. Br Med J 1987;294:13.

94. Northover JMA, Terblanche J. The importance of the blood supply to the bile duct in human liver transplantation. Transplantation 1978;26:67-73.

95. Michels NA. Newer anatomy of the liver and its variant blood supply and collateral circulation. Am J Surg 1966;112:337.

96. Lautt WW. Hepatic vasculature: A conceptual review. Gastroenterology 1977;73:1163-9.

98. Okazaki K, Miyazaki M, Onishi S *et al.* Effects of food intake and various extrinsic hormones on portal blood flow in patients with liver cirrhosis demonstrated by pulsed Doppler with the Octoson. Scand J Gastroenterol 1986;21:1029-38.

99. Campra JL, Reynolds TB. The hepatic circulation. In: Arias IM Jacoby WB, Poppr H *et al.* (eds), The liver: biology and pathobiology. 2nd ed. New York: Raven Press, 1988:911.

100. Schenk WG, McDonald JC, McDonald K *et al.* Direct measurement of hepatic blood flow in surgical patients; with related observations on hepatic flow dynamics in experimental animals. Ann Surg 1962;156:463.

101. Chiandussi L, Vaccarino A, Greco F *et al.* Effect of drug infusion on the splanchnic circulation. I. Angiotensin infusion in normal and cirrhotic subjects. Proc Soc Exp Biol Med 1963;112:324-6.

102. Kerr JC, Hobson RW, Seelig RF *et al.* Vasopressin: route of administration and effects on canine hepatic and superior mesenteric blood flow. Ann Surg 1978;187:137.

103. Jenkins SA, Baxter JN, Corbett W *et al.* A prospective randomised controlled clinical trial comparing somatostatin and vasopressin in controlling acute variceal haemorrhage. Br Med J 1985;290:275.

104. Bradley SE. Measurement of hepatic blood flow in man. Surgery 1974;75:783-9.

105. Leevy CM, Mendenhall CL, Lesko W *et al.* Estimation of hepatic blood flow with indocyanine green. J Clin Invest 1962;41:1169.

106. Daeman MJAP, Thijssen HHW, Van Essen H *et al.* Liver blood flow measurement in the rat. The electromagnetic versus the microsphere and the clearance methods. J Pharmacol Methods 1989;21:287.

107. Reichmann S, Davis WD, Storaasli JP *et al.* Measurement of hepatic blood flow by indicator dilution techniques. J Clin Invest 1958;137:1848.

108. Nimura Y, Miyatake K, Kinoshita *et al.* New approach to noninvasive assessment of blood flow in the major arteries in the abdomen by two-dimensional Doppler echography. In: Lerski RA, Morley P (eds) Ultrasound '82. Proceedings of the third Meeting of the World Federation for Ultrasound in Medicine and Biology, Oxford: Pergamon Press, 1983:477.

109. Ohnishi K, Saito M, Sato S *et al.* Portal hemodynamics in idiopathic portal hypertension (Banti's syndrome): comparison with chronic persistent hepatitis and normal subjects. Gastroenterology 1987;92:751.

110. Zoli M, Marchesini G, Cordiani MR *et al.* Echo Doppler measurement of splachnic blood flow in control and cirrhotic subjects. J Clin Ultrasound 1986;14:429.

111. Moriyasu F, Ban N, Nishida O *et al.* Clinical application of an ultrasonic duplex system in the quantitative measurement of portal blood flow. J Clin Ultrasound 1986;14:579.

112. Ozaki CF, Anderson JC, Lieberman RP *et al.* Duplex ultrasonography as a noninvasive technique for assessing portal hemodynamics. Amer J Surg 1988;155:70-5.

113. Burns P, Taylor K, Blei AT. Doppler flowmetry and portal hypertension. Gastroenterology, 1987;92:824–6.
114. Moriyasu F, Nishida O, Ban N *et al*. Ultrasonic Doppler duplex study of hemodynamic changes from portasystemic shunt operations. Ann Surg 1987;205:151.
115. Berger LA, Sagar G, George P. The ultrasonic demonstration of portacaval shunts. Br J Surg 1979;66:166.
116. Horn JR, Zierler B, Bauer LA *et al*. Estimation of hepatic blood flow in branches of hepatic vessels utilizing a noninasive, duplex Doppler method. J Clin Pharmacol 1990;30:922.
117. Syrota A, Vinot JM, Paraf A *et al*. Scintillation splenoportagraphy: haemodynamic and morphologic study of the portal circulation. Gastroenterology 1976;71:652.
118. Murray JF, Dawson AM, Sherlock S. Circulatory changes in chronic liver disease. Am J Med, 24:358.
119. Williams R, Condon RE, Williams HS *et al*. Splenic blood flow in cirrhosis and portal hypertension. Clin Sci 1968;34:441.
120. Moreno AH, Burchell AR, Rousselot EM *et al*. Portal blood flow in cirrhosis of the liver. J Clin Invest 1967;46:436.
121. Chamberlain JK. The microanatomy of the spleen in man. In: The spleen. Structure, function and clinical significance. London: Chapman and Hill Medical, 1990:9.
122. Weiss L. Mechanisms of splenic clearance of the blood. In: The spleen. Structure, function and clinical significance. London: Chapman and Hill Medical, 1990:23–45.

34. Blood flow to the limbs

RICHARD E. LEE, JONATHAN D. BEARD and
MUNTHER I. ALDOORI

The blood flowing into the limbs supplies skin, subcutaneous tissue, muscle
and bone. While blood flow to the bone, nerve and connective tissue of the
limb is relatively constant, that to skin and muscle show a great range. The
circulation to the skin, and especially that of the extremities, is determined
by the need for temperature regulation so that any change in the blood flow
in the resting limb occurs as a result of change in the local or ambient
temperature. Enormous changes in blood flow to skeletal muscle occur during
exercise in response to the workload, and continue afterwards in repayment
of the flow debt incurred during exercise. Thus, the resting blood flow is
determined by temperature, and exercising blood flow by the degree of
muscle activity.

Cutaneous and digital blood flow

The ratio of muscle to skin and bone decreases from the upper arm and
thigh distally in each limb, so that there is no muscle blood flow in the
terminal phalanges. Thus, whereas the volume of blood supplying the calf and
thigh is determined by muscular activity, the digital blood flow is essentially
cutaneous blood flow. Changes in the blood flow of the digits may be measured using plethysmometry, pulse volume recording or laser Doppler; in
response to temperature challenges or vasoactive drugs, for example, such
measurements may be used as an index of cutaneous blood flow.

The blood supply to the fingers is extraordinarily rich; much greater on a
volume basis than the toe circulation. Warming the hand from 20°C to 35°C
increases the blood flow at least threefold [1]; of the total hand blood flow
at 35°C, 30% perfuses the distal phalanges, which comprise only 5% of the
hand volume [2]. Fingertip flow may vary 150–fold depending upon local
and body temperatures and autonomic vasomotor tone. This enormous range
of flow is a function of the great density of temperature-regulating arteriovenous shunts in the skin of the fingertips, and in high cutaneous flow states it
is through these channels that most of the hyperaemia takes place. Nutrient
blood flow contributes only a small proportion of total cutaneous flow except
at low temperatures.

Hyperaemia through cutaneous arteriovenous shunts occurs very rapidly

A.-M. Salmasi and A.S. Iskandrian (eds): Cardiac output and regional flow in health and disease, 505–522.
© 1993 *Kluwer Academic Publishers. Printed in the Netherlands.*

in response to temperature changes, and in normal subjects rewarming occurs rapidly after the removal of a mild cold stimulus. In patients with *Raynaud's disease* there is a latent period before rewarming takes place, and even then this is slow. Rather than an exaggerated autonomic response to cold stimulation, Raynaud's disease is characterised by a failure to recover from the cold stimulus.

Reactive hyperaemia

The augmented blood flow which follows the restoration of arterial inflow to a limb after a period of circulatory exclusion is almost exclusively confined to the skin. This response, which is unaffected by sympathetic and somatic denervation [3], is probably mediated by local mechanisms [4]. It is likely that myogenic and chemical mechanisms are involved. The concept of a repayment of a flow debt lends weight to control by a chemical mechanism, and pH, osmolality, and the concentration of magnesium ions, potassium ions, histamine and bradykinin have all been proposed as vasoactive metabolites. Hypoxia is probably not a factor *per se*, but the removal of vasoactive substances does seem to depend upon a critical level of oxygen and blood flow.

The reactive hyperaemic response in patients with peripheral vascular disease is highly abnormal, and offers a relatively straightforward method of revealing abnormalities in an arteriopathic patient who has normal resting femoral blood flow or ankle pressure measurements [5–8].

In the normal reactive hyperaemic response, a *peak flow* several times the resting level occurs within about five seconds of releasing the circulatory occlusion; thereafter, the flow returns to resting levels over a variable period, generally of a few minutes (Figure 34.1). The magnitude of the peak flow which is a measure of the capacity of the resistance vessels in the ischaemic tissues to dilate, increases in a linear fashion with increasing periods of occlusion up to about five minutes [5]. The *total excess flow* increases progressively as the period of ischaemia is increased, but for circulatory arrest up to five minutes, nearly 80% occurs during the the first minute of circulatory release. There is a linear correlation between flow debt and hyperaemic flow, but as resting flow far exceeds need in the normal limb, the volume of blood flow debited and repaid are seldom equal.

In patients with peripheral vascular disease, the total vascular resistance is greatly increased and is invariable as a result of occlusive disease involving the main limb arteries. The resistance vessels in the microcirculation of the skin and muscles of such patients are already dilated to reduce the vascular resistance, in an attempt to promote normal blood flow at rest. Thus, when circulatory occlusion is released, even maximal dilatation of the resistance vessels cannot substantially alter the total vascular resistance, and the hyperemic response is very different from that in which blood at systemic arterial pressure is suddenly allowed to flow into a circulation with minimal peripheral

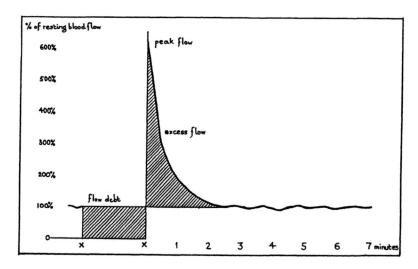

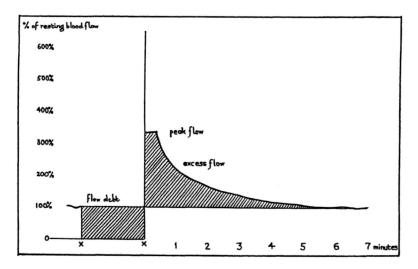

Figure 34.1. Reactive hyperaemic blood flow measured ultrasonically following a two-minute circulatory arrest (X – X) with a pneumatic cuff applied to the thigh in a normal subject (above) and in a patient with occlusive disease of the iliac artery (below). Note effect of the diseased inflow vessel reducing peak flow on release of the cuff and prolonging the hyperaemia. (After: Lee, RE, An evaluation of ultrasonic flowmetry in vascular surgery.)

resistance. In the presence of occlusive arterial disease the magnitude of the peak is decreased and its onset delayed beyond five seconds occasionally as long as two minutes [5]. As a result, a much smaller proportion of the excess flow takes place within the first minute, and although the hyperaemia may last for twenty minutes or more, the flow debt is usually substantially under-paid [9].

Muscle blood flow

Most of the blood supplying the limbs enters by way of the subclavian-axillary and external iliac-common femoral arterial systems. The proportion of limb blood flow contributed by the scapular/pelvic anastamoses and subcu-taneous collaterals is usually very small, but in the presence of occlusive disease of the main arterial channels these alternative pathways must supply all the blood reaching the limb. In the healthy lower limb, for example, common femoral artery flow approximates to total limb flow, but in the presence of an occlusion of the external iliac artery most of the blood supplying the limb must travel by way of gluteal and other pelvic collaterals, and common femoral flow will be markedly reduced. Similarly, if the superfi-cial femoral artery is occluded the calf muscles are supplied by collaterals arising from the profunda femoris system.

At 20°C, muscle flow accounts for about half the total calf blood flow at rest [5, 10], but the hyperaemia of exercising muscle may be over 20 times the resting flow level, increasing up to 90% of the cardiac output [11]. The increased limb blood flow is compensated for by an increase in the cardiac output [12] and oxygen consumption may rise ten- or twenty-fold with severe exercise [13]. Redistribution of blood flow from the splanchnic circulation may be an important mechanism in some animals, but is relatively unimpor-tant in man (this is discussed more fully in the chapter *The splanchnic circulation*).

Blood flow only occurs during muscle relaxation. This seems to be due to local compression of arteries and veins rather than to an effect on the microcirculation [14]. Passive stretching and sustained isometric contractions produce a decrease in blood flow proportionate to the degree of muscle tension, but isotonic contraction has a much less pronounced effect. Sus-tained isometric contraction, as produced by standing on tip toe for example, results in almost complete cessation of blood flow in the contracted muscles.

During muscular contraction, blood pressure rises equally in arteries and in veins, so that arterial inflow is decreased and venous outflow is increased. When muscular relaxation occurs the void in the venous channels results in a decrease in venous pressure which encourages a rapid inflow of blood [15]. During rhythmic exercise with the limbs dependent, as in a running man, a perpetual decrease in intramuscular venous pressure results, provided the venous system has competent valves. The increased hydrostatic pressure produced by upright position thus encourages blood flow, up to 60% more than resulting from supine exercise.

Although sympathetic efferent nerves seem to mediate in the earliest phase of muscle hyperaemia in cats and other lower mammals, in humans changes in blood flow with exercise occur independently of innervation [16]. It is likely that both myogenic and chemical mechanisms for local control are involved in regulating the muscle flow. The disappearance of accumulated metabolites after exercise would show an exponential decay in concentrations as they are 'washed out' of the muscle; this corresponds to the exponential fall in excess blood flow which occurs in the post-exercise period. Metabolic changes which occur during muscular contraction include venous oxygen desaturation, increased venous osmolality, regional hyperosmolality, increased extracellular concentration of potassium ions, protons and ATP, and a raised pCO_2. All of these have been proposed as vasoactive metabolites; it is likely that hypoxia, regional osmolality and potassium ion concentration are of greatest importance, and that a complex interrelationship amongst them contributes to muscular hyperaemia [17, 18].

The effects of training

Athletes have a greater capacity to increase cardiac output and blood flow than sedentary subjects [10] and require lower blood flows than untrained subjects to perform a given workload [19]. The post-exercise responses in untrained subjects resemble those recorded in athletes after performing ischaemic exercise, suggesting that untrained individuals have a relative ischaemia during exercise. Exercising and postexercise excess blood flow can be reduced in normal individuals following a course of training [20], and it has long been recognised that exercise training has a beneficial effect upon the symptoms and exercise tolerance of patients with intermittent claudication [21]. This is likely to arise as a combination of improved mechanical efficiency, increased capillary ingrowth, increased blood flow and increased oxygen extraction; there is little evidence that exercise promotes a significant growth of collateral blood vessels or that any major changes occur in muscle metabolism.

Peripheral vascular disease

Atherosclerosis is the commonest cause of chronic arterial insufficiency of the lower limbs. The superficial femoral and external iliac arteries are most commonly affected. Patients affected are most usually men over 50 years old, and almost all are cigarette smokers. Diabetes, hypertension, a family history of peripheral vascular disease and certain hyperlipidaemias constitute other risk factors. Provided occlusive disease is confined to one or two main arteries compensatory dilatation of collateral arteries and the peripheral vascular bed will allow an adequate supply of blood at rest. When the limb is exercised, however, the capacity of the collateral circulation to supply blood is easily exceeded, and the relative ischaemia of the muscles gives rise to intermittent claudication.

Intermittent claudication is the characteristic symptom of chronic arterial occlusive disease of the lower limb. A cramp like pain develops in one or more muscle groups after a relatively constant amount of exertion. The pain is relieved by a few seconds of rest. The muscle group most distal to the arterial occlusion is rendered most ischaemic by exercise. An external iliac artery occlusion produces calf muscle pain before thigh pain for example. Claudication is caused by an inadequate flow of blood to supply nutrients and remove metabolite sufficiently quickly to meet the needs of the exercising muscles. Despite maximal dilatation of the microvasculature of the muscles in response to exercise, occlusion of a major artery increases the total vascular resistance beyond the level at which sufficient flow can occur. Blood has to flow through collateral channels of high resistance, reducing the pressure of blood perfusing tissue distal to each arterial occlusion.

Ischaemic rest pain

Where a functional end artery is occluded, where chronic arterial disease has produced multiple occlusions at different levels, or where collateral inflow or outflow vessels are diseased in addition to main vessels, the proximal resistance to blood flow may be high enough to make peripheral vasodilatation insufficient to compensate and tissue ischaemia at rest will result. Ischaemic rest pain is unusual where the resting ankle systolic pressure exceeds 40–50 mm Hg. The pressure drop increases with each collateral bed through which the blood must pass, so distal structures, usually the toes, are involved first.

Ischaemic rest pain results from a disparity between blood supplied and tissue requirement for nutrition and removal of waste metabolites. True ischaemic rest pain is relieved by adequate restoration of the circulation. It is characteristically also relieved by walking a few steps and by holding the foot dependent. Muscular effort reduces venous pressure, improving blood flow by increasing the pressure gradient across the capillary bed [22]. Although it does not improve the arteriovenous pressure gradient alone, dependency produces an rise in arterial hydrostatic pressure increasing transmural pressure across the microvasculature, distending the resistance vessels and increases tissue perfusion by reducing peripheral resistance. Similarly, elevation reduces tissue perfusion by increasing vascular resistance. Gaskell and Baker [23] found that a change from supine to seated posture caused a decrease in pedal blood flow in normal subjects, but a 44% *increase* in patients with occlusion of the superficial femoral artery.

In the normal limb circulation, reflex vasoconstriction and local myogenic responses prevent an increase in blood flow on standing up; within ischaemic tissues, a state of vasomotor paralysis exists where arterioles become maximally dilated and insensitive to the stimuli which would normally result in vasoconstriction. This is the basis of *Buerger's test*. When the foot of a patient with severe occlusive arterial disease is elevated blood flow ceases and the foot becomes pale and waxy; when placed in dependency it becomes suffused with blood and flushes a deep red.

Assessment of the limb circulation

Assessment of the circulation rests upon evaluation of the pulses and their characteristics, measurement of the blood pressure and measurement of blood flow.

The arterial pulse pressure

A palpable pulse provides the most readily available information for the assessment of the circulation. A palpable pulse of normal character and volume is a taken as a reassuring sign of an adequate circulation. Below a stenosis or occlusion the pulse may be decreased or impossible to detect by the examining finger. Blood flowing through a stenosis increases its velocity and energy losses occur. These affect peak systolic more than diastolic flow. Beyond the stenosis the mean blood flow velocity returns to its previous value but the character of the pulse wave is altered, with a decreased pulse pressure and a rounded pulse contour. A reduction in the luminal diameter of at least 75% is required before a pulse is diminished clinically; a 99% stenosis may be required before a pulse is clinically absent [24]. In the presence of haemodynamically significant arterial disease, a previously palpable pulse may disappear during and after exercise as a result of steal of blood by working muscles.

The arterial pulse volume

With the arrival of each arterial pulse wave the limb, digit or organ increases in volume. The shape of the volume-time curve is largely determined by the rate at which blood enters and at which it flows out. Initially, arterial blood flow in more rapidly than venous blood flows out, thereafter blood leaves more rapidly than it enters. The volume rises rapidly to a peak (upstroke time), and falls more slowly with a dicrotic notch on the downslope (Figure 34.2).

The pulse volume changes can be recorded by segmental plethysmography using pneumatic cuffs, and qualitative information about the state of the circulation may be inferred. For example, distal to an arterial stenosis or

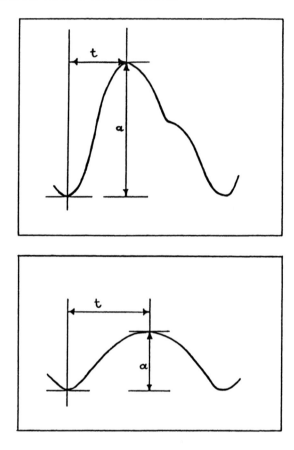

Figure 34.2. Pulse volume recordings from the calf of a normal subject (above) and a patient with occlusive disease of the iliac artery (below). The inflow arterial disease prolongs the upstroke time (**t**) and reduces the amplitude (**a**) of the pulse volume.

occlusion, the pulse volume contour is rounded, with a delay in the upstroke time, a reduction in the upstroke angle and a loss of the dicrotic notch [25]. Similarly, venous insufficiency produces measurable changes in the rate of blood emptying from the limb. Although pulse volume recordings are easily made, the information yielded is qualitative and, in our hands, insensitive for the detection of venous problems.

Although pulse volume varies directly with blood flow, the degree of volume change per unit change in blood flow varies greatly from one individual to another and from one organ to another. Thus, the percentage change in volume with each pulse cannot be used to measure blood flow. If the venous outflow to a limb is occluded, however, and provided venous occlusion is not maintained so long as to impede capillary filling, volume changes can be used to measure regional blood flow. This is the basis of the plethysmographic techniques mentioned below.

Arterial blood pressure

Changes in blood pressure are far more easily measured than changes in blood flow, and have proved an accurate and sensitive indicator of functional disability.

In the normal circulation, the mean arterial pressure falls slightly (up to 10 mm Hg) as the pulse wave travels from heart to toes. The fall is predominantly in diastole so the pulse pressure widens as blood flows distally; the systolic pressure rises slightly.

The systolic blood pressure is easily measured at the ankle using a sphygmomanometer and a Doppler ultrasonic blood flow detector. The ankle arteries are easily compressed and this is an accurate method of estimating true pressure when compared with invasive direct pressure measurements. The ankle systolic pressure is most usefully expressed as a ratio of brachial arterial pressure, as an approximation to aortic pressure (ankle systolic pressure index, or A.S.P.I.) [26]. In undiseased limbs the normal A.S.P.I. is 1.11 ± 0.10, and usually falls to less than 1.0 in patients with lower limb arterial occlusions. The A.S.P.I. correlates well with the patients' degree of functional disability [27]. Segmental blood pressure measurement may be made at thigh and below knee levels using a similar technique. In these locations the systolic pressure measurement is likely to be an overestimate, since a pneumatic cuff is not wide enough to transmit its pressure accurately deep inside a very muscular or fat limb. For example, a normal thigh pressure measurement may be 150% of the brachial pressure. A pressure gradient of over 20 mm Hg between any two adjacent points of measurement indicates occlusive disease within that segment [28].

Changes in arterial blood pressure with exercise

The increased flow during exercise leads to a drop in pressure across the major arterial channel of the lower limb. Since the total arterial resistance in a healthy subject is very small, the pressure drop following mild or moderate effort is generally undetectable. However, increasingly strenuous effort may be associated with a progressive fall in ankle systolic pressure and an increasing time to recovery [29]. In the presence of occlusive arterial disease, exercise produces a marked fall in A.S.P.I. and a delayed return to normal [30]. This is most marked in those with iliac and combined segment disease. Even a short period of exercise will unmask asymptomatic arterial insufficiency in patients in whom this is not severe enough to affect the A.S.P.I. at rest [31], and can be used to identify femoropopliteal reconstructions in danger of occlusion [32]. Increasing the workload results in an increased fall in the initial post-exercise pressure and progressive prolongation of the recovery time.

The A.S.P.I. and post-exercise calf muscle blood flow are inversely related because both depend upon the conductance of inflow vessels. If the main arterial channels are free from disease then the inflow resistance (R_o) is negligible, the drop between distal artery pressure (P_D) and aortic pressure (P_A) is small, and A.S.P.I. does not alter appreciably with exercise. In the presence of narrowing or occlusion of the major arterial channel upstream, R_o is high as blood has to travel by way of high resistance collaterals. The increased blood flow through the exercising muscles (Q_{CM}) resulting from a fall in resistance of the muscle vascular bed (R_{CM}) produces a profound fall in the pressure distally (P_D); the greater the muscle blood flow (Q_{CM}), the greater the fall in ankle pressure [33].

$$P_A - P_D = Q_{CM} \cdot (R_o + R_{CM})$$

Where occlusive disease is present at combined levels, for example when iliac and superficial femoral arteries are both occluded, the ankle pressure falls abruptly with exercise. The intramuscular arteriolar bed widely dilates in response to exercise as in a normal subject. This decreases the total hemodynamic resistance of the limb, and blood from the pelvic collateral circulation is diverted to supply the augmented flow through the thigh muscles. The effect of this is to reduce the pressure in the common femoral artery and thus the filling pressure of the calf muscles, which would depend for their blood supply upon collaterals via the profunda femoris artery. The blood passing distally is diverted into the low resistance circulation of the exercising calf muscles, reducing the popliteal artery pressure even further. After exercise, the flow debt is relatively rapidly paid as a result of the preferential supply of blood to the thigh muscle mass during exercise; so as the arteriolar bed of the thigh muscle constricts and imposes resistance again, the femoral pressure rises and calf muscle flow increases. Ultimately, the ankle pressure returns to normal.

Blood flow measurement

Regional blood flow to the whole or part of a limb may be measured, and is expressed as flow per unit mass or volume of tissue supplied (usually ml/100 ml/min or ml/100 mg/min). Indicator dilution, isotope clearance and plethysmographic techniques have all been used to measure regional blood flow in the lower limb.

Volume blood flow in a given artery of conscious subjects may be measured using indicator dilution techniques and by duplex Doppler ultrasound, or if the vessel is isolated as at surgical operation, by electromagnetic flowmetry. This is usually expressed as ml/min.

Regional blood flow

If venous outflow is occluded then limb blood flow can be measured plethys-mographically [34], and modifications of the *mercury strain gauge plethysmo-meter* introduced by Whitney [35] have been used to measure upper and lower limb blood flow at rest and to quantify the response to reactive hyperae-mia and exercise. The technique has the advantage of being reproducible, noninvasive, and of providing continuous measurement so that changes with exercise or other stimuli can be monitored. The normal resting calf blood flow is 1.5–6.5 ml/100 ml/min [5–7, 9, 20, 30, 36, 37], varying with the ambient temperature and physical fitness. Changes in blood flow with reactive hyperaemia [5, 6] and exercise [6, 37] have been measured in normal subjects and patients with peripheral vascular disease. The technique has been used to provide criteria for the diagnosis of peripheral vascular disease [7, 38] and for assessing the results of surgical reconstruction [9].

Limb blood flow measurement using ^{99m}Tc clearance is currently used as a screening test for vascular insufficiency. Its use in conjunction with reactive hyperaemia improves its diagnostic accuracy [39].

Volume blood flow

Common femoral artery flow has been measured using indicator dilution techniques. Although this entails sampling blood from the femoral or external iliac vein, measurements have been made at rest and during exercise [40, 41, 43, 44]. For example, using a dye-dilution technique sampling blood from a cannula in the external iliac vein Pentecost demonstrated a five-fold rise in blood flow during bicycling exercise (from 473 to 2523 ml/min) which was associated with a ten-fold rise in oxygen consumption [40]. Values for resting flow measurements in the femoral arteries are set out In Table 34.1.

The use of electromagnetic flowmetry in human studies is limited to intra-operative measurements, but these have proved of value in predicting the outcome of vascular reconstructions [49].

Doppler ultrasonic techniques enable blood flow measurements to be made noninvasively. Ultrasound reflected by moving blood undergoes a frequency modulation according to the Doppler effect, producing an audible signal proportionate in frequency to the velocity of the moving blood. Although the signal may be accurately assessed by a practiced ear, more useful information is available if the signals are analysed mathematically.

The Doppler shift signal from a normal limb artery at rest has three phases. During systole, blood flows rapidly forwards producing a high fre-quency signal of short duration. After systole, the blood flow velocity falls dramatically and a reversed flow phase occurs, followed by another phase of forward flow. These two phases produce softer low-pitched sounds in diastole. Beyond an arterial stenosis or occlusion, the systolic sound is re-duced in frequency and prolonged, and the reversed flow phase disappears.

Table 34.1. Resting blood flow in the common femoral artery.

Using indicator dilution		
Agrifoglio *et al.* 1961 [42]	635 [450–886] ml/min	n = 12
Pentecost *et al.* 1964 [40]	440 [334–605] ml/min	n = 6
Folse, 1965 [43]	301 [196–484] ml/min	n = 48
Cobb *et al.* 1969 [41]	345 ± 126 ml/min	n = 19
Wahren *et al.* 1973 [44]	390 ± 20 ml/min	
Using thermodilution		
Ganz *et al.* 1964 [45]	636 [384–1114] ml/min	
Using electromagnetic flowmetry		
Vanttinen, 1975 [46]	239 [150–420] ml/min	n = 20
	134 [80–250] ml/min (S.F.A.)	n = 20
	104 [50–210] ml/min (P.F.A.)	n = 20
Using continuous wave Doppler ultrasound		
Regan *et al.* 1971 [47]	376 [93–627] ml/min	n = 18
Using pulsed wave Doppler ultrasound		
Lee, 1987 [8]	347 [161–463] ml/min	n = 58
	198 [110–316] ml/min (S.F.A.)	n = 58
	120 [53–183] ml/min (P.F.A.)	n = 21
Lewis, 1990 [48]	344 [109–714] ml/min	n = 109

Published values for resting flow in the normal common, superficial (S.F.A) and deep (P.F.A.) femoral arteries.

Blood flowing through a stenosis does so with increased velocity, and this may be detected by a localised high frequency signal.

The peak or mean flow velocity can be computed from Doppler shift signals. If the spacial mean flow velocity, averaged over several cardiac cycles, is multiplied by cross-sectional area of the artery under study, the volume of blood flow is obtained. This measurement is most conveniently carried out using a duplex scanner and has been used to provide data in the carotid, splachnic, fetal and limb circulations. The technique relies upon accurate measurement of the blood vessel cross section and of the angle subtended by the ultrasound beam with the moving blood, which should not be allowed to exceed 60° [50]. A pulsed wave Doppler beam with a sample volume just large enough to encompass the blood vessel cross section will ensure even reflection of ultrasound from all parts of the vessel cross section.

A Doppler ultrasonic flowmeter has been developed by one of us for intra-operative use on isolated arteries [51]. This instrument is free from many of the problems associated with the use of electromagnetic flowmeters, and overcomes sources of error in Doppler flowmetry by a fixed angle of inson-ation and by imposing a strict diameter upon the vessel under study.

Blood flow measurements In peripheral vascular disease

In patients with intermittent claudication, the total limb blood flow at rest is usually not significantly different from normal [6, 30]. The volume of blood flow in a given artery just proximal or distal to stenosis will certainly be reduced, however, as collateral circulations contribute more to the total limb flow. In the presence of occlusive disease of the iliac or superficial femoral arteries, the volume of blood flowing in the common femoral artery is reduced significantly below the normal range [8]. But the wide range of normal resting blood flow in any artery makes the interpretation of isolated flow measurements difficult to interpret, and the measurement of resting blood flow is of limited value in the assessment of peripheral vascular disease. A stenosis or occlusion proximal or distal to the site of measurement will alter the pattern of blood flow, and Doppler flow velocity curves mathematically modelled using fast Fourier or laPlace transform techniques enable the computation of parameters which correlate with upstream stenosis disease or the state of the distal circulation [52, 53]. As with segmental pressure studies, the value of measurements made in a state of hyperaemia is far greater than those made at rest.

Measurement of hyperaemic blood flow

Measurement of blood flow during exercise is difficult because the movement of exercise interferes with the measurement technique. Despite this, measurements of flow during exercise have been made using dye dilution and venous occlusion plethysmography, and form the basis of our understanding of the haemodynamic changes which take place with exercise and reactive hyperaemia in humans.

It is much easier to measure post exercise hyperaemia, of course. This bears a linear relationship with work performed provided this exceeds a minimum quantity. Below this critical level, increased flow during exercise meets increased needs adequately; any flow debt remaining at the end of the period of exercise may be discharged without any post-exercise hyperaemia since the resting flow rate is much greater than necessary for basal metabolic needs. The maximum post-exercise flow rate is broadly the same as the flow during exercise [10]; it may even be slightly greater, because of the effects of sustained isometric muscular contraction. The total excess postexercise blood flow is directly proportional to the excess blood flow during exercise [40] up to a work load of 50–70% of maximum capacity. Above this level, exercise blood flow plateaus at a critical value but post exercise excess flow is increased by prolongation of the period of hyperaemia [10, 54]. When ischaemic exercise has been performed, for example with a pneumatic thigh cuff inflated to arrest the circulation, both peak post exercise flow and total excess blood flow are markedly increased [5].

A problem with the measurement of post-exercise hyperaemia using duplex

TREADMILL EXERCISE TESTING

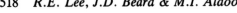

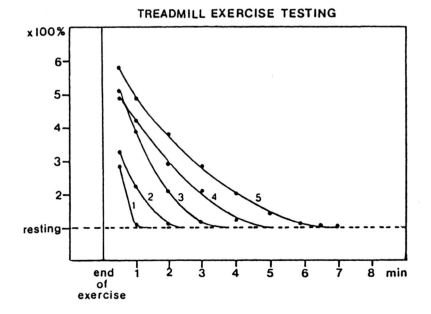

POST-OCCLUSION HYPERÆMIA

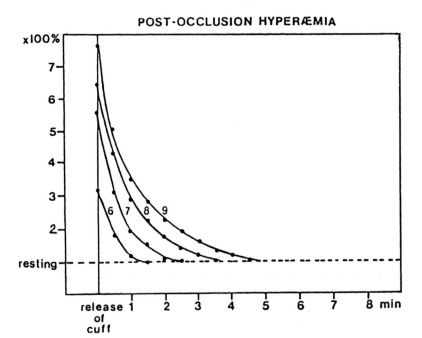

Doppler ultrasound is that the duration of hyperaemia must be of at least two minutes duration. Even then, in patients with intermittent claudication this may be too short a time to move them to the examination couch and perform a flow measurement. As post exercise flow decays exponentially, the flow measurement should be made as early as possible. On the other hand, measurement of post-occlusion reactive hyperemia can be made without moving the patient from the examination couch. We compared common femoral blood flow in normal young adults following five treadmill exercise tests of graded severity and of reactive hyperemia following four periods of thigh cuff arterial occlusion (Figure 34.3). The hyperaemia following one minute of exercise and one minute of occlusion were shortlived; flow returned to resting values within one minute. Longer periods of exercise and occlusion than five minutes increased the duration of excess flow proportionately more than the peak flow. Three minutes of occlusion produced a hyperaemia which lasted for over two minutes, and which was comparable to that following two minutes of exercise. On the basis of these findings, we evaluated a hyperaemic index (the ratio of peak hyperaemic flow following three minutes of occlusion to resting blood flow) as a standard clinical test to stress the circulation and to accentuate the haemodynamic effect of occlusive arterial lesions. This enabled us to separate normal subjects from patients with superficial femoral arterial occlusions and those with combined level occlusions. Hyperaemic flow ratios less than 1.5 and post exercise A.S.P.I. less than 0.8 were accurate in identifying occult haemodynamic problems in femoro-popliteal reconstructions and predicting graft failure, whereas mea-

Figure 34.3. Increased blood flow in six normal subjects each subjected to five treadmill exercise tests of increasing severity (1–5) and reactive hyperaemia following four periods of circulatory arrest using a thigh occlusion cuff (6–9). Measurements were made using duplex Doppler ultrasound following release of the occluding cuff and as soon as possible after completing each exercise test, and were repeated every 30 seconds until resting flow values were reached (median of flow values expressed as percentage of resting flow). (After: Lee RE, An evaluation of ultrasonic flowmetry in vascular surgery.)
Treadmill exercise tests:
   1: minute at 4 km/hr on a 10° gradient.
   2: 2 minutes at 4 km/hr on a 10° gradient.
   3: 5 minute, at 4 km/hr on a 10° gradient.
   4: 5 minutes at 6.5 km/hr on a 20° gradient.
   5: 10 minutes at 6.5 km/hr on a 20° gradient.
Reactive hyperaemia tests:
   6: 1 minute of circulatory arrest.
   7: 3 minutes of circulatory arrest.
   8: 6 minutes of circulatory arrest.
   9: 10 minutes of circulatory arrest.

surements made in resting limbs proved no more accurate than pulse palpation [32].

References

1. Ludbrook J, Collins GM. Venous occlusion pressure plethysmography in the human upper limb. Circ Res 1967;21:139–47.
2. Price WH. Measurement of blood flow in the vasodilated fingers. Clin Sci 1966;30:13–8.
3. Lewis T, Grant R. Observations upon reactive hyperaemia in man. Heart 1925;12:73.
4. Shepherd JT. Reactive hyperaemia in human extremities. Circ Res 1964;14–15(Suppl 1):76–9.
5. Hillestad LK. The peripheral blood flow in intermittent claudication. Acta Med Scand 1963;174:23–41, 671–700.
6. Strandell T, Wahren J. Circulation in the calf at rest, after arterial occlusion and after exercise in normal subjects and in patients with intermittent claudication. Acta Med Scand 1963;173:99–105.
7. Myers K. The investigation of peripheral arterial disease by strain gauge pleythysmography. Angiology, 1964;15:293–304.
8. Lee RE. An evaluation of ultrasonic flowmetry in vascular surgery. Master of Surgery Thesis, University of Edinburgh, 1987.
9. Snell ES, Eastcott HHG. Circulation in the lower limb before and after reconstruction of obstructed main artery. Lancet, 1960;i:242–8.
10. Lassen NA, Kampp M. Calf muscle blood flow during walking studies by the Xenon[133] method in normals and in patients with intermittent claudication. Scand J Clin Lab Invest 1965;17:447–53.
11. Wade OL, Bishop JM. Cardfac output and regional blood flow. Oxford: Blackwell Scientific Publications, 1962;99.
12. Ekblom B, Hermans L. Cardiac output in athletes. J Applied Physiol 1968;25:619–25.
13. Jorfeldt L, Wahren J. Leg blood flow during exercise in man. Clin Sci 1971;41:459.
14. Gray SD, Carlsson E, Snaub NC. Site of increased vascular resistance during isometric muscle contraction. Am J Physiol 1967;213:683–9.
15. Folkow B, Gaskell P, Waaler BA. Blood flow through limb muscles during heavy rhythmic exercise. Acta Physiol Scand 1970;81:157–63.
16. Hilton SM. Experiments upon the postcontraction hyperaemia of skeletal muscles. J Physiol (Lond) 1953;120:230–45.
17. Mellander S, Lundvall J. Role of tissue hyperosmolality in exercise hyperaemia. Circ Res 1971;28–29(Suppl 1):139–45.
18. Skinner NS, Costin JC. Interactions between oxygen, potassium and osmolality in regulation of skeletal muscle flow. Circ Res (Suppl 1) 1971;28:9173–9.
19. Grimby G, Haggendal E, Saltin B. Local Xenon[133] clearance from the quadriceps muscle during exercise in man. J Applied Physiol 1967;22:305–10.
20. Elsner RW, Carlson LD. Postexercise hyperemia in trained and untrained subjects. J Applied physiol 1962;17:436–40.
21. Skinner JS, Strandness DE. Exercise and intermittent claudication. I. Effect of repetition and intensity of exercise. II. Effect of physical training. Circulation 1967;36:15–29.
22. Folkow B, Gaskell P, Waaler BA. Pathophysiological aspects of blood flow distal to an obliterated main artery with special regard to the possibilities of affecting the collateral resistance and the arterioles in the distal low pressure system. Scan J Clin Lab Invest 1967;19(Suppl 93):211–8.
23. Gaskell P, Becker WJ. The erect posture as an aid to the circulation in the feet in the presence of arterial obstruction. Can Med Assoc J 1971;105:930–4.

24. Weese JA, Van de Berg L, May AC. *et al.* Stenoses of arteries of the lower extremity. Arch Surg 1964;89:806–16.
25. Strandness DE, Bell JW. Peripheral vascular disease. Diagnosis and critical evaluation using a mercury strain gauge. Ann Surg 1965;161(suppl):1.
26. Yao ST, Hobbs JT, Irvine WT. Ankle systolic pressure measurements in arterial disease affecting the lower extremities. Br J Surg 1969;56:676–9.
27. Yao ST. Haemodynamic studies in peripheral arterial disease. Br J Surg 1970;57:761–8.
28. Strandness DE, Bell JW. An evaluation of the hemodynamic response of the claudicating extremity to exercise. Surg Gynecol Obstet 1964;119:1237–42.
29. Stadler C, Strandness DE. Ankle blood pressure response to graduated treadmill exercise. Angiology 1967;18:237–41.
30. Sumner DS, Strandness DE. The relationship between calf blood flow and ankle blood pressure in patients with intermittent claudication. Surgery 1969;65:763–71.
31. Laing S, Greenhalgh RM. The detection and progression of asymptomatic peripheral arterial disease. Br J Surg 1983;70:628–30.
32. Lee RE, Baird RN. Predicting failure of femoropopliteal bypasses using ultrasonic flowmetry. Br J Surg 1987;74:328.
33. Strandness DE. Blood flow to the limbs. In: Standness DE, Sumner DS (eds.), Hemodynamics for surgeons. New York: Grune and Strutton, 1975.
34. Brodie T G, Russell AE. On the determination of the rate of blood flow through an organ. J Physiol (Lond.) 1905;32:xlvii.
35. Whitney RJ. The measurement of volume changes in human limbs. J Physiol (Lond.) 1953;121:1–187.
36. Halliday JA. Blood flow in the human calf after prolonged walking. Am Heart J 1960;60:100.
37. Livingstone RA. Blood flow in the calf of the leg after running. Am Heart J 1961;61:219–24.
38. Strandness DE, Gibbons GE, Bell JW. Use of a new simplified plethysmometer in the clinical evaluation of patients with arteriosclerosis obliterans. Surg Gynecol Obstet 1961;112:751–6.
39. Parkin A, Wiggins PA, Robinson PJ *et al.* Use of a gamma camera for measuring limb blood flow in peripheral vascular disease. Br J Surg 1987;74:271–4.
40. Pentecost BL. The effect of exercise on the external iliac vein blood flow and local oxygen consumption in normal subjects and in those with occlusive arterial disease. Clin Sci 1964;27:437–45.
41. Cobb LA, Smith PH, Lwai S. *et al.* External iliac flow: its response to exercise and relation to lactate production. J Applied Physiol 1969;26:606–10.
42. Agrifoglio G, Thorburn GD, Edwards EA. Measurement of blood flow in the human lower extremity by indicator dilution method. Surg Gynecol & Obstet 1961;113:1641–5.
43. Folse R. Alterations in femoral blood flow and resistance during rhythmic exercise and sustained muscular contractions in patients with arteriosclerosis. Surg Gynecol & Obstet 1965;121:767–76.
44. Wahren J, Torfeldt L. Determination of leg blood flow during exercise in man: an indicator-dilution technique based on femoral venous dye infusion. Clin Sci Mol Med 1973;45:135–46.
45. Ganz V, Hlavavá A, Fronèk A. *et al.* Measurement of blood flow in the femoral artery in man at rest and during exercise by local thermodilution. Circulation 1964;30:86–9.
46. Vanttinen E. Electromagnetic measurement of the arterial blood flow in the femoro-popliteal region. Acta Chir Scand 1975;141:353.
47. Reagan TR, Miller CW, Strandness DE. Transcutaneous measurement of femoral flow. J Surg Res 1971;11:477–82.
48. Lewis P, Psaila.JV, Morgan RH. *et al.* Common femoral artery volume flow in peripheral vascular disease. Br J Surg 1990;77:183–7.
49. Cappelan C, Hall KV. Electromagnetic flowmetry in clinical surgery. Acta Chir Scand 1967;368(Suppl):3.

50. Gill RW. Measurement of blood flow by ultrasound: accuracy and sources of error. Ultrasound Med Biol 1985;11:625–41.
51. Beard JD, Evan,.JM, Skidmore R. *et al*. A Doppler flowmeter for use in theatre. Ultrasound Med Biol 1986;12:883–9.
52. Gosling RG, Dunbar G, King DH *et al*. The quantitative analysis of peripheral arterial disease by a nonintrusive ultrasonic technique. Angiology 1971;22:52–5.
53. Skidmore R, Woodcock JP, Well:, PNT. *et al*. Physiological interpretation of Doppler shift waveforms. III. Clinical results. Ultrasound Med Biol 1980;6:227.
54. Tønessen KH. Blood flow through muscle during rhythmic contraction measured by [133]xenon. Scand J Clin Lab Invest 1964;16:646–53.

35. Carotid blood flow and pathogenesis of cerebral ischaemia

MUNTHER I. ALDOORI and RICHARD E. LEE

The carotid bifurcation is the most frequent site for the development of cerebrovascular atherosclerosis [1]. Preferential development of atherosclerotic plaque along the outer wall of carotid sinus has been observed on carotid angiograms [2], in post mortem [3] and in plaque morphology studies following carotid endarterectomies [4]. The carotid artery has one of the most complex bifurcations in the arterial system. The internal and external carotid arteries supply vascular beds of different resistance, and therefore they have different flow patterns. While flow in the external carotid artery is more or less similar to other peripheral arteries, flow in the internal carotid artery is almost steady due to high diastolic flow which is a reflection of low intra-cerebral resistance. The presence of the carotid sinus produces an unusual geometry which results in flow disturbances [5], which play a role in plaque formation. Therefore, knowledge of flow behaviour in the carotid bifurcation is of great importance in understanding of plaque initiation and promotion.

In vitro haemodynamic studies of human carotid bifurcation

Bharadvaj and associates (1982) [6,7] developed glass models of the human carotid bifurcation based upon 124 biplanar arteriograms, and used a laser-Doppler anemometer to study the flow field under steady flow conditions in which the Reynolds numbers and flow division ratios were physiological. They identified the region of flow separation along the outer wall of the carotid sinus with reverse and helical flow associated with low wall shear stress, in contrast to the inner wall region (flow divider) which contains zones of quite high velocity and areas of relatively high wall shear stress.

Ku and Giddens (1987) [8] extended the work of Bharadvaj et al. using a pulsatile pump which could be programmed to provide the desired carotid flow wave form, while using an identical carotid bifurcation glass model, flow system and laser Doppler anemometer. They confirmed the complexity of flow in the carotid sinus and its variation during the cycle. Forward flow was found throughout the branches during early systole, followed by separation and flow reversal near the outer wall of the sinus during late systole. This results in an oscillatory shear stress at the outer wall during systole with an

A.-M. Salmasi and A.S. Iskandrian (eds): Cardiac output and regional flow in health and disease, 523–547.

average mean value of -0.5 dyn cm^{-2}, in contrast to flow divider wall shear stress of an average mean of 26 dyn cm^{-2}. They also noticed that the flow accelerates as it moves from the sinus into the internal carotid branch due to the decrease in cross sectional area which results in forward flow during the entire cycle. This is associated with an abrupt increase in the sheer stress value towards the distal portion of the sinus and internal carotid branch. Motomiya and Karin (1984) [9] reported the same observation of flow separation in an isolated transparent natural post-mortem carotid bifurcation.

These studies support Caro's [10] low sheer stress hypothesis in contrast to Fry's [11] high sheer stress experiment and hypothesis in which he showed, using a mechanical device placed in the canine aorta, that sudden elevations in sheer stress to levels of about 400 dyn cm^{-2} may cause endothelial damage. This, he postulated, enhanced lipid transport from the blood to the intima resulting in the development of atheroma. However, the sheer stress required is far beyond that found in the human carotid artery under physiological conditions.

Caro et al. [10], in 1971, observed in post mortem studies that early atherosclerotic lesions tend to develop in the areas of low wall sheer stress, like the inner walls of curved vessels and at the hips of a bifurcation. They suggested that low wall sheer stress may retard the transport of circulating particles away from the wall, resulting in increased intimal accumulation of lipids.

LoGerefo et al. [12], in 1985, elegantly demonstrated the region of flow separation by using a dye flow visualization technique in a plastic model of the human carotid bifurcation during steady and pulsatile flow. They suggested that although flow separation itself is a site of low sheer, it is possible that low and high sheer may act independently or synergistically to explain the link between flow separation and atherogenesis. They suggested that platelet activation may occur at a flow divider due to high sheer stress [13]. The same platelets can cause damage when they enter and retained in the separation zone and then have the opportunity for prolonged wall contact. Kartino and Goldsmith [14], in 1979, showed that adhesion of platelets to the vessel wall was significantly enhanced in the region of disturbed flow. If endothelial injury occurred as a result of the metabolic effects of low sheer, the activated platelets could adhere to the subendothelial surface and stimulate smooth muscle proliferation [15].

These in vitro haemodynamic studies are supported by the clinical observation of boundary layer separation in the normal human carotid bulb using ultrasound techniques, especially duplex scanning (Figure 35.1).

In vivo haemodynamic studies of human carotid bifurcation

Duplex ultrasonic scanners, which combine a real time, B-mode imager and a pulsed/continuous wave Doppler flowmeter with an on-board wave form

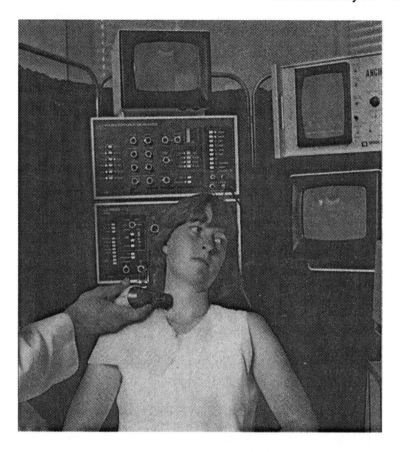

Figure 35.1. Carotid duplex scanning.

spectral analyzer, are used extensively in the evaluation of carotid bifurcation in health and disease (Figure 35.2). The first system was developed and Christened "duplex" by Baber *et al.*, in 1974 [16]. When duplex scanning was first used to evaluate the carotid arteries, the specificity of the tests (or the ability to identify normal vessels) was very low (37%) [17]. This was due to false interpretation of the normal flow disturbance in the carotid bulb as abnormal. Wood *et al.*, in 1982 [18], were the first to demonstrate the phenomena of flow separation in the healthy normal carotid bulb. Soon afterwards, Phillips *et al.*, in 1983 [5], confirmed the presence of an area of boundary layer separation near the outer wall of the normal carotid bulb using duplex scanning. Recognition of the complexity of carotid flow helped to increase the specificity of duplex scanning to 84% [19] by the same group of investigators. Aldoori and Baird, in 1987 [20], correlated duplex scanning

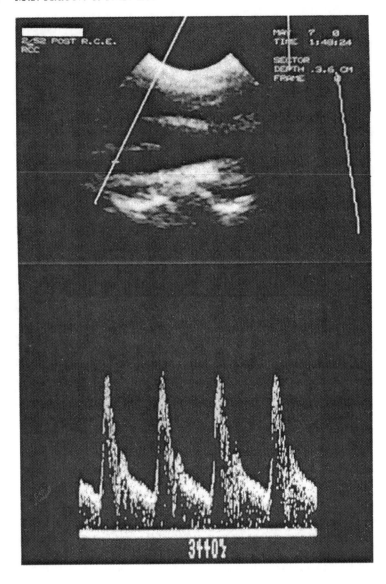

Figure 35.2. Normal carotid duplex scanning. Top: B-Mode image of carotid bifurcation. Bottom: pulsed Doppler signals. Laminar flow (systolic frequency <4000 Hz).

with triplanar angiography in 109 patients. They reported a sensitivity of 98.8%, and specificity of 90% ($\kappa = 0.854 \pm 0.026$).

With the introduction of colour-flow ultrasound scanners our understanding of the complexity of the flow in carotids bulb is more fully appreciated. Zierler *et al.*, in 1982 [21], studied the flow in ten normal volunteers using a colour-flow Doppler duplex scanner. They confirm the presence of a zone of boundary layer separation along the outer wall of the bulb. The length and width of the zone fluctuated during the cardic cycle, with maximum appearances around peak systole. These zones of flow separation were limited to the proximal internal carotid and bulb and were not observed in the distal internal carotid artery. This finding corresponds to the observation by vascular surgeons that the atheroma usually does not extend very far into the internal carotid artery.

Middleton and his associates, in 1988 [22], were able to detect flow reversal in 99% of their 50 normal, young volunteers. They suggested that the absence of flow reversal should be considered abnormal, while Hennerici's [23] group attributed the absence of flow separation and reversal to the anatomical absence of a carotid bulb in 6.4% of their presumed normal volunteers (23 men and 33 women; mean age 46 years, range 17–81 years). Comparison of colour flow and 3D images using computer graphics showed that wall configuration, bulb dilatation and curvature play an important role in flow reversal and stagnation in the carotid bulb [24]. A minor degree of flow separation has been shown to occur simultaneously at the origin of the external carotid artery [24].

In summary, it may be said that atherosclerosis tends to occur in the area of flow reversal and stagnation, but the precise reason is still unknown.

Carotid volume blood flow

The first measurement of cerebral blood volume flow in healthy men using nitrous oxide washout technique was reported by Kety and Schmit in 1945 [25]. Their mean value was 54 ml/100 gram/min, which corresponds with an internal carotid blood flow of 200–300 mil/min (assuming the mean brain weight is 1400 grams and that each internal carotid artery carries one third of cerebral blood flow). A wide range of values has been reported using electromagnetic flowmetry (201–364 ml/min) [26, 27]. We used duplex scanner to measure volume flow in both common and internal carotid arteries in 59 subjects, and correlated flow with the degree of stenosis measured using ultrasound (Figure 35.3) and triplanar angiography (Figure 35.4). Resting blood flow in undiseased arteries was 420 (258–697) ml/min (median range) for common arotid and 276 (172–411) ml/min for the internal carotid. In 37 diseased internal carotid arteries a stenosis of at least 75% was found to be needed to reduce the blood flow significantly from normal [28].

These findings are in agreement with Archie and Feldtman's [29] sugges-

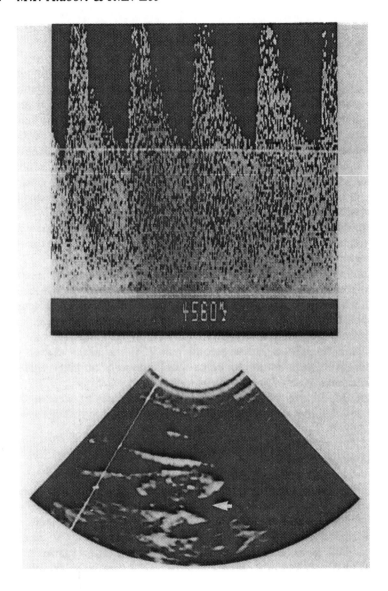

Figure 35.3. Duplex scanning of abnormal internal carotid artery with a stenosis of at least 75% luminal narrowing. Top: Real time Doppler shift wave form of blood flow velocity showing turbulent flow. Systolic and diastolic frequencies are both abnormally high (diastolic frequency >4000 Hz). Bottom: B mode ultrasonic image showing (arrowed) a large heterogeneous echolucent plaque filling the bulb and origin of the internal carotid artery.

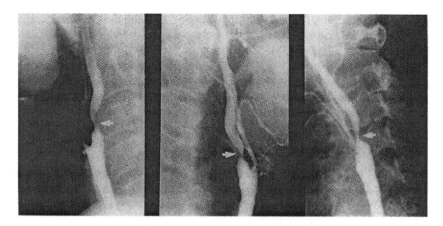

Figure 35.4. Triplanar carotid angiogram. >75% stenosis seen in all three views. Arrows.

tion that a reduction in luminal diameter of at least 75% (94 % area stenosis) is required to produce critical stenosis. Wada *et al.*, in 1990 [30], correlated the degree of stenosis measured at autopsy with the common carotid volume flow measurement obtained previously while the patients were alive. Volume flow of 384 ml/min or less was associated with >50% stenosis and 45% of the patients had >75% stenosis.

We observed in the presence of >75% stenosis there is enhancement of the flow in the patent contralateral internal carotid artery. In the literature there are contradictory reports, some have observed the same phenomenon [31, 32], others have not [33].

Pathogenesis of cerebral ischaemia

The atherosclerotic plaque may progress to a severe stenotic lesion, or even to complete occlusion without producing symptoms. This is due to the remarkable adaptive facility of the brain through the collateral circulation provided by the circle of Willis. Eklof and Schwartz, in 1969 [33], demonstrated this ability in baboons' brains by producing gradual stenosis of the major vessels in the neck. Bilateral occlusion of vertebral arteries increased carotid flow by 15%. When occlusion of one carotid artery was carried out, the flow in the contralateral vessel increased by 88% of normal value. The anatomy of the circle of Willis in the baboon differs from that of humans in one regard, namely that the anterior cerebral arteries arise independently from the internal carotid arteries and fuse in the midline to form single anterior cerebral artery.

Anomalies of the vessels forming the circle of Willis which are likely to be functionally significant are present in up to one third of normal human brains. A normal configuration of the polygon occurred in only 52% of 350 brains studied at autopsy [35].

The question as to what events convert asymptomatic atheromatous plaques into initiators of acute ischaemic symptoms remains unresolved. Both haemodynamic and thrombo-embolic theories have been put forward in an attempt to answer the mechanism of transient ischaemic attacks.

Haemodynamic theory

The mechanism by which a constant stenosis produces transient ischaemic attacks (TIAs) and temporary monocular blindness is difficult to postulate with certainty. One explanation is that the blood pressure and cardiac output are reduced by hypotension and dysrhythmia. However, Kendall and Marshall, in 1963 [36], were unable to reproduce TIAs with deliberately induced hypotension in 37 patients who had presented with frequent attacks of TIAs. Furthermore, several authors have noted that TIAs disappear at the time of carotid occlusion [37, 38] (Figure 35.5). Similarly, temporary occlusion of common carotid artery with a vascular clamp during endartectomy under local anaesthesia is usually well tolerated. Hafiner and Evans, in 1988 [39], reported 1200 carotid endarterectomies performed under local anaesthesia. Only 9% required intraoperative shunting for brain protection as determined by neurological signs and symptoms. Patients with a contralateral severe stenosis or occlusion required shunting six times more frequently than those with a unilateral lesion. Mann and associates in 1938 [40], defined critical stenosis as the level at which small increases in the degree of stenosis cause a significant reduction in blood flow and pressure distal to the construction. Crawford and colleagues in 1960 [41], stated that the criterion for carotid endarterectomy should be relevant symptoms in the presence of pressure gradient across a stenosis involving the internal carotid artery. They performed simultaneous measurement of mean intra-arterial pressure immediately proximal and distal to a carotid stenosis in 22 patients and correlated the pressure gradient with the degree of stenosis, estimated both at operation and from lateral view arteriograms. Eleven of the twelve patients who had >55% reduction in luminal diameter had a pressure gradient of more than 20 mm Hg. All but three had insignificant contralateral stenoses. It was assumed the presence of pressure gradient associated with reduction in blood flow. May *et al.*, in 1963 [42], confirmed Crawford's findings using electromagnetic flowmetry. Archie and Feldtman, in 1981 [29], suggested that a >75% reduction in luminal diameter (94% area stenosis) is required to produce critical stenosis. They measured pressure and flow in 47 patients in whom carotid endarterectomies were performed. All had normal or near normal contralateral internal carotid arteries diagnosed by biplaner arteriograms. In addition to the adequacy of the collateral circulation, other variables include the length of the stenosis, as well as the viscosity and velocity

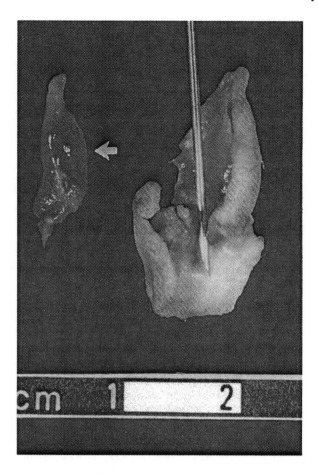

Figure 35.5. Endarterectomy specimen showing very severe stenosis. TIAs disappeared when the artery become occluded. Needle – indicates very tight stenosis. Arrow – fresh thrombus occluded the origin of the artery.

of the blood flow which are important in determining when a stenosis becomes critical [43].

Thrombo-embolic theory

The hypothesis of embolization of thrombotic or atheromatous material is widely accepted [37, 44, 45]. The fact that atheromatous plaques can be a source of emboli was first suggested by Panum in 1862 [46], highlighted by

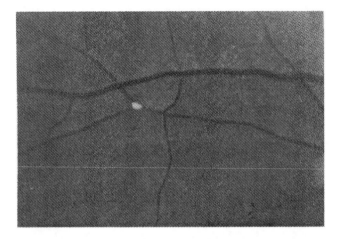

Figure 35.6. "Hollenhorst plaque" golden yellow cholestrol embolus obstructing the branches of the retinal artery.

Chiari, in 1905 [47], and conclusively documented by Meyer in 1947 [48]. Disappearance of TIA's following anti-coagulant therapy was noted by Fisher in 1958 [49]. A year later he reported white platelet-fibrin microemboli in a patient undergoing a transient episode of monocular blindness [44]. Hollenhorst, in 1961 [50], described bright yellow plaques from cholesterol emboli in the retinal arterioles of 9.4% of 235 patients with occlusive extracranial disease of the carotid system (Figure 35.6). McBrien, Bradley and Ashton, in 1963 [51], histologically confirmed the nature of the microemboli in the retinal vessels of a patient who had temporary monocular blindness. In the same year Julian *et al.* [52] reported the presence of ulcerated atheroma in 17 of 231 carotid endarterectomies they had performed (Figure 35.7). This evidence encouraged Moore and Hall [37] to operate successfully on symptomatic patients with non-stenotic ulcerative lesions. Thiele and Strandness, in 1982 [53], studied 104 carotid arteriograms and found that irregularity and ulceration occurred with almost equal frequency whether the degree of stenosis was considered haemodynamically significant or not. Eikelboom *et al.*, in 1983 [54], studied the morphology of surgical specimens and found that ulceration was present to a similar extent in all categories of stenosis.

We studied plaque morphology and ulceration in 78 symptomatic patients presenting with TIAs and monocular temporary blindness. All had non-stenotic carotid lesions (<50% reduction in luminal diameter) in the ipsilateral sides diagnosed by ultrasound (Figure 35.8) and confirmed by triplanar angiography in 46% (Figure 35.9) All except 10 had non-stenotic lesions in the contralateral arteries (10 were normal), which were used as controls. Echolucent "soft" plaques (Figure 35.10) were more commonly found in the

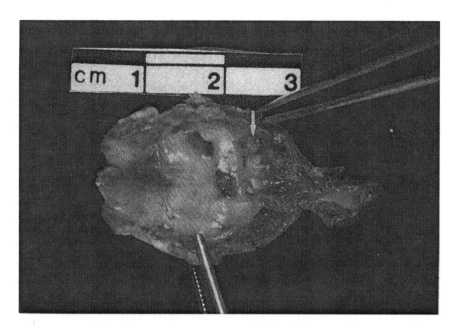

Figure 35.7. Endarterectomy specimen showing ulcerated atheroma. Arrow – inded the site of ulcer.

symptomatic sides (63% versus 23%; $p < 0.005$, $\chi^2 = 12.4$). The occurrence of echogenic "dense" Fibrous plaques was reversed (Figure 35.11) (30% versus 70%), while calcified plaques were equally distributed (6.4% versus 5.8%). Ulceration (Figure 35.12), like soft plaques, were predominant in the symptomatic sides (25.6% versus 7.3%; $p < 0.5$, $\chi^2 = 5.64$) [55].

Stereotype TIAs pose a problem for the embolic theory. However, in more than one study, artificial emboli injected in the carotid circulation tended to gather in the same vessel, because of laminar flow [56, 57]. It seems that the pathogenesis of TIAs is more likely to be due to embolization irrespective of whether there is a haemodynamically significant stenosis or not (Figure 35.13).

Intraplaque haemorrhage

The casual relation between plaque disruption [58–60], intra-plaque haemorrhage [61, 62] and coronary artery thrombosis in acute myocardial infarction has long been recognised. Although Fisher, in 1954 [63], drew attention to the presence of intraplaque haemorrhage in carotid atheroma, no serious study was performed until 1979, when Imparato *et al.*, [4] published a review of histology versus gross morphology in 69 carotid plaque specimens from

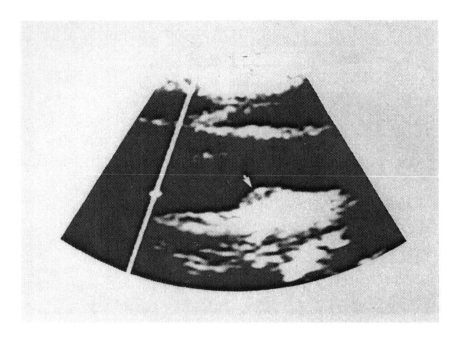

Figure 35.8. B-mode image showing <50% stenosis at the bulb – arrow.

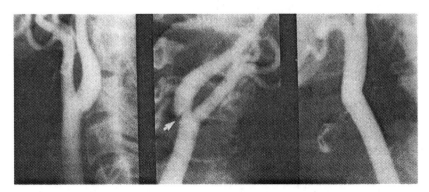

Figure 35.9. Triplanar carotid angiogram. The arrow indicates <50% stenosis in the middle view. Other views appeared normal.

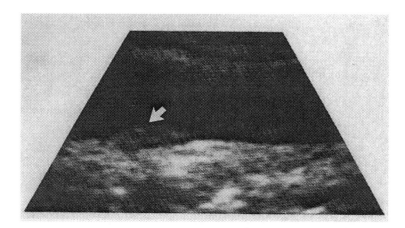

Figure 35.10. Echolucent "soft" plaque. Arrow – the black areas within the plaque represent soft atheroma or lipid. Blood can give similar appearance. B-mode image indicates <50% stenosis.

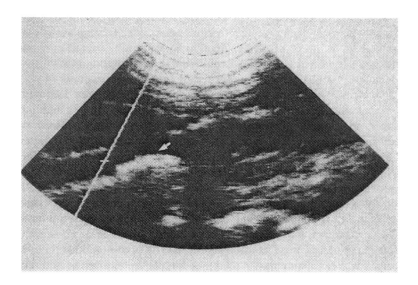

Figure 35.11. Echogenic homogeneous "dense" fibrous plaque. Arrow – B-mode image indicates <50% stenosis.

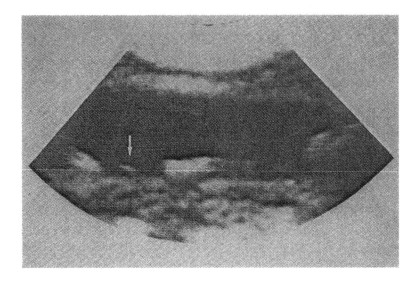

Figure 35.12. Long plaque in the posterior wall of the bulb. Arrow indicates large ulcer in the plaque. B-Mode image indicates <50% stenosis.

50 patients. They noted some degree of intraplaque haemorrhage was present in 65% of the specimens examined. They concluded that "significant" intramural haemorrhage was the single most important factor in carotid atheromatous plaques responsible for focal neurological deficits. Imparato *et al.*,1983 [64], conducted further study on 376 carotid plaques harvested at endarterectomy (275 symptomatic and 101 asymptomatic). They found that intraplaque haemorrhage was significantly more common in symptomatic (46%) compared with asymptomatic (31%) plaques and correlated well with increasing severity of plaque stenosis (Figure 35.14). Lusby *et al.*, in 1982 [65], emphasized the importance of the age of the haemorrhage. They showed a significantly higher incidence of recent haemorrhage among symptomatic patients (92%) than amongst asymptomatic patients (27%). However, Ammer *et al.*, 1984 [66], failed to confirm it, in spite of the high incidence of intraplaque haemorrhage they reported in their symptomatic patients (82%). In a further study 1986, they found repeated episodes of haemorrhage were associated more with laterilising symptoms than non-laterilising or no symptoms [67].

The mechanism of cerebral ischaemia caused by intraplaque haemorrhage can be explained by both haemodynamic and thrombo-embolic theories [68]. Blood inside the plaque may lead to sudden plaque expansion and reduction in blood flow, i.e. "closed haemorrhage" (Figure 35.15) [68]. Alternatively, an acute plaque haemorrhage might rupture the overlying intimal surface and connection may develop with the arterial lumen, i.e. "open haemor-

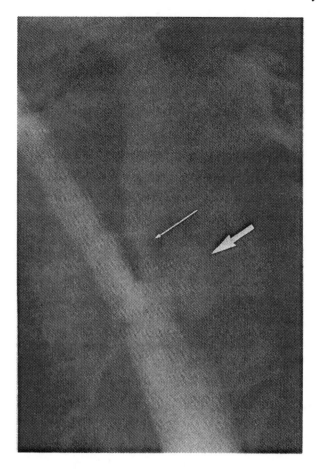

Figure 35.13. Carotid angiogram. Large arrow – large ulcer. Small arrow – tight stenosis.

rhage" (Figure 35.16) [68]. Open haemorrhage might obstruct the flow or cause thrombo-embolisation due to plaque eruption or act as a nidus on which blood constituents, platelets and clotting proteins could cause thrombosis and intra-luminal clot [69] (Figure 35.16).

The mechanism of carotid intraplaque haemorrhage is not well understood. It is most probably due to mechanical stress due to differences in vessel wall compliance [68], but the source of the blood is not clear. Imparato [64] believes it results from breaks in the intimal surface and dissection of blood into the plaque. Others postulated its origin as rupture of newly formed fragile vessels [65]. Neovascularity has been reported with equal frequency

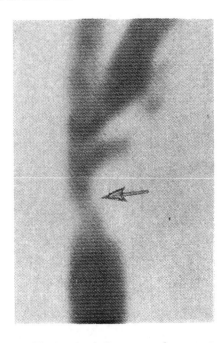

Figure 35.14. Intra-arterial DSA. Arrow – indicates smooth severe stenosis due to intraplaque haemorrhage. Rare diagnosis by X-ray.

in symptomatic and asymptomatic plaques as well as in the superficial and deep parts of the plaques [69]. They are predominantly thin walled and poorly supported by a stroma of cholesterol debris and foam cells [69]. There is still controversy whether plaque haemorrhage is a primary process or secondary to plaque disruption [70]. Fisher and Ojemann [71] showed plaque disruption (ulceration) and haemorrhage did occur in the same frequency and they were associated more frequently with symptoms. A more recent study by Avril *et al.*, in 1991 [72], showed intraplaque haemorrhage was closely associated with presence of symptoms but was encountered less frequently (16.7%), while ulceration was commoner (72.2%). These findings may suggest that intraplaque haemorrhage is sequence rather than primary event.

Carotid endarterectomy

Every 5 minutes someone in Britain suffers a stroke [73]. It is the cause of one in eight deaths [73]. Stroke from cerebral infarction is a devastating human illness because of its high initial mortality (up to 30%) [74] and its high incidence of serious and incapacitating permanent neurological deficits

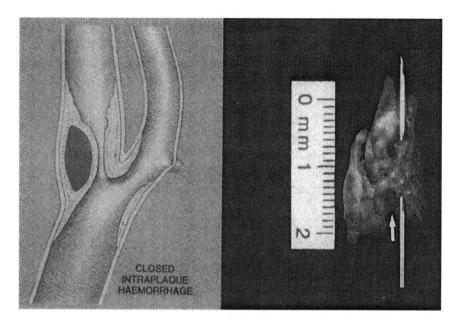

Figure 35.15. "Closed" intraplaque haemorrhage. Endarterectomy specimen showing very tight stenosis – needle. The arrow indicates the site of haemorrhage.

(up to 30%) [75]. Although the overall mortality from stoke in the United Kingdom fell by about 20% between 1976 and 1986, it is still double that in the United States [76]. A large proportion of strokes should be preventable by controlling blood pressure and stopping smoking [77, 78]. Secondary prevention can be achieved by improvement in medical [79] and surgical management [80, 81].

Fortunately not all strokes come without warning. 10–79% of ischaemic strokes are preceded by TIAs [82]. It is very difficult to determine the exact incidence and prevalence of TIAs, as they can be unheeded by physicians and unreported by patients, particularly by those who later develop a stroke [83]. In the Harvard Stroke Registry, approximately 50% of atherothrombotic stroke presented with preliminary TIAs [82]. At present much of what is known about the prognosis of TIAs has been obtained from series which have considered TIAs as a whole and have not allowed for the separate identifications of their aetiology. Millikan and McDowell in 1978 reported the natural history of TIAs based on a retrospective review of 13 published TIA studies. They found that 35–40% of patients with TIAs would eventually have cerebral infarction if followed for as long as 5 years, giving a cumulative annual risk of 5–8% [74]. Recently the results of Oxfordshire Community Stroke Project showed 11.6% was the actual risk of stroke during the first

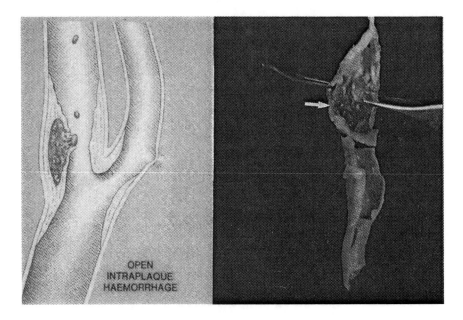

Figure 35.16. "Open" intraplaque haemorrhage – arrow.

year following TIAs and approximately 5.9% per annum over the first 5 years [84]. Several angiographic studies in patients with hemispheric TIAs have shown that about half are associated with >50% reduction in luminal diameter of the ipsilateral extracranial internal carotid artery [85].

For asymptomatic patients, antiplatelet agents have no proven benefit in stroke prevention [86]. Aldoori *et al.*, in 1987 [87], have reported 50% stroke rate at 3 years in asymptomatic patients with >75% carotid stenosis treated conservatively (43% were taking aspirin, dose range 300–1200 mg daily). Carotid endarterectomy can be justified only if it is clearly superior to optimal medical therapy in offering stroke prevention to patients suffering from carotid bifurcation atherosclerosis [86].

Carotid endarterectomy for symptomatic carotid stenosis

Many published uncontrolled series showed that carotid endarterectomy can be performed with very low peri-operative stroke and mortality (1–3% and around 1% respectively) [86, 88–91]. Nonetheless, some authors [92–94] have reported very high rates of morbidity and mortality, which make 100,000 operations performed per annum difficult to justify [95]. Therefore, three symptomatic carotid endarterectomy trials were launched in the 1980s: the

MRC European Carotid Surgery Trial (ESCT) [80]; the North American Symptomatic Carotid Endarterectomy Trial (NASCET) [81]; and the Symptomatic Carotid Stenosis Veterans Administration Trial [96]. All three trials have demonstrated that surgery confers a significant benefit in patients with severe (70–99%) stenosis.

The ESCT trial [80] included 2518 randomized patients; 778 were in the category of 70–99% stenosis and 455 were treated surgically. 7.5% had a stroke or died within 30 days of surgery, but during the next 3 years only another 2.8% had strokes, compared to 16.8% of the control group (sixfold reduction). Surgery conferred no benefit on patients with mild (0–29%) stenosis, so the trial has been stopped for both mild and severe stenosis, and continues to assess those with moderate (30–69%) stenosis. The incidence of stroke or death during the first 30 days following randomization was 7.5% after carotid endarterectomy group and 5% for controls in the group with moderate stenoses.

The NASCET trial [81] results are remarkably similar to those of the European trial. There were 595 patients; 300 underwent carotid endarterectomy and 295 were controls. Between the time of randomization and 30 days later, 5% of the surgical group and 3% of the control died or suffered stroke. The incidence of death and stroke in the surgical group was 2%, compared to 21% in the control group (tenfold reduction), with a mean follow up of 18 months. For moderate (30–69%) stenosis the interim analysis was inconclusive, so the study continues recruiting more patients.

The Veterans Administration Trial [96] showed a significant reduction in stroke and crescendo TIAs in patients who received carotid endarterectomy (7.7%) compared with control group (19.4%). The benefit of surgery was more profound in patients with severe (>70%) stenosis.

Carotid endarterectomy for asymptomatic carotid stenosis

Carotid surgery for asymptomatic patients remains controversial. However, patients with asymptomatic diffuse or localized carotid murmur are approximately three times more likely to suffer ischaemic stroke than an age and sex match population sample known to have a carotid murmur [97].

The substantial variation in published results suggests that sub-groups may exist amongst the asymptomatic patients [87]. Chambers and Norris, 1986 [98], studied 500 asymptomatic patients with cervical murmurs followed prospectively by clinical and Doppler examination for up to 4 years. An increased risk of stroke was noted with increasing severity of carotid stenosis. Patients who had a >75% carotid stenosis had an incidence of either TIAs or stroke of 22% at 2 years. Roderer *et al.*, in 1984 [99], found that patients with >80% stenosis had a higher risk of TIAs, stroke and occlusion, than patients with <80% stenosis. Aldoori *et al.*, in 1987 [87], suggested that patients with >75% stenosis are at an increased risk of stroke in comparison to those with <75% stenosis (Figures 35.17, 37.18).

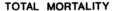

TOTAL MORTALITY

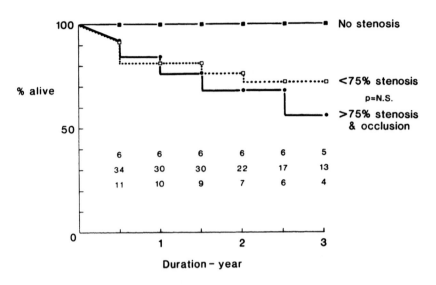

Figure 35.17. Life table analysis of survival by severity of carotid stenosis showing numbers of patients entering each follow up interval: ■, no stenosis: □, <75% stenosis: ●, >75% stenosis. For □ versus ● p = 11.3.

Two recent reports [100, 101] comparing the operative and non-operative outcome of patients with high grade asymptomatic stenosis support the use of prophylactic carotid endarterectomy. Moneta *et al.* (1987) [100] studied 115 patients with >80% stenoses, 56 of whom underwent prophylactic carotid endarterectomy. Life-table analysis of 24 months showed a higher incidence of stroke, TIAs and occlusion in the non-operative group. Though this study was prospective, treatment was not randomized. Caracci *et al.* (1989) [101] found in retrospective study that surgery gave better results, although follow-up was unavailable for 25% of the population group. The management of asymptomatic patients will remain controversial until the result of two currently conducted multicenteric studies [102, 103] are available.

The Veterans Administration Asymptomatic Carotid Stenosis Trial [102]. Four hundred and forty-four patients were randomized between aspirin treatment (233 patients) and carotid endarterectomy plus aspirin (211 patients). The recruitment was carried out between 1983 and 1987. The final report should be published in 1992. The interim report published in 1990 showed a 2.4% stroke rate in the surgical group with 1.9% mortality, all due to cardiac disease.

The asymptomatic Carotid Atherosclerosis Study (ACAS) [103] was started in 1988, and 810 patients have so far been randomized. The overall

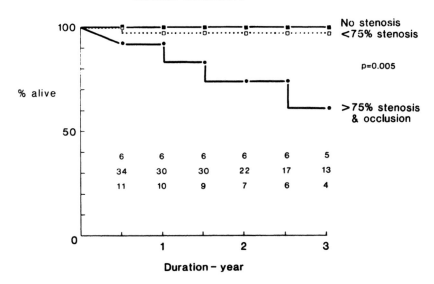

Figure 35.18. Stroke mortality related to severity of carotid stenosis. Life table analysis showing number entering each following interval: ■, no stenosis: □, <75% stenosis: ●, >75% stenosis. For □ versus ● p = 10.005.

surgical mortality and stroke rate of the surgeons involved in the study is expected to be <3%. If it rises above this figure the trial will be stopped. When the 117 participating surgeons' results before the study were analysed, their combined mortality and stroke rates after 1511 carotid endarterectomies for symptomatic stenosis were 0.8% and 0.9% respectively. The results of this study are unlikely to be published before 1994–1995.

References

1. Hass WK, Fields WS, North RR *et al.* Joint study of extracranial arterial occlusion. JAMA 1968;203:159–66.
2. Jeans WD, Mackenziel S, Baird RN. Angiography in transient cerebral ischaemia using three views of the carotid bifurcation. Br J Radiol 1986;59:135–42.
3. Heath D, Smita P, Harris P *et al.* The atherosclrotic human carotid sinus. J Pathol 1973;110:49–58.
4. Imparato AM, Riles TS, Gorstein F. Carotid bufurcation plaque: pathologic findings associated with cerebral ischaemia. Stroke 1979;10:238–45.
5. Phillips DJ, Greene FM, Langlois Y *et al.* Flow velocity patterns in the carotid bifurcations of young presumed normal subjects. Ultrasound Med Biol 1983;9:39–49.
6. Bharadvaj BK, Mabon RF, Giddens DP. Steady flow in a model of the human carotid bifurcation. Part 1 – flow visualization. J Biomechanics 1982;15:349–62.

7. Bharadvaj BK, Mabon RF, Giddens DP. Steady flow in a model of the human carotid bifurcation. Part II - laser–Doppler anomometer measurement. J Biomechanics 1982;15:363–78.
8. Ku, DN, Giddens DP. Laser Doppler anomometer measurement of pulsatile flow in a model carotid bifurcation. J Biomechanics 1987;20:407–21.
9. Motomiya M. Flow patterns in the human carotid artery bifurcation. Stroke 1984;15:50–6.
10. Caro CG, Fitz-Gerald JM, Shorter RC. Observation, correlation and proposal of a sheer dependent mass transfer mechanism for atherogenesis. Proc Roy Soc Lond [Biol] 1971;177:109–59.
11. Fry DL. Acute vascular endothelial changes associated with increased blood velocity gradients. Circ Res 1968;22:165–7.
12. Lo Gerfo FW, Nowak MD, Quist WC. Structural details of boundary layer separation in a model human carotid bifurcation under steady and pulsatile flow conditions. J. Vasc Surg 1985;2:263–9.
13. Brown CH, Leverette LB, Lewis CW et al. Morphological, biochemical and functional changes in human platelets subjected to sheer stress. J Lab Clin Med 1975;86:462–71.
14. Karino T, Goldsmith HL. Adhesion of human platelets in an annular vortex distal to a tubular expansion. Microvasc Res 1979;17:238–62.
15. Ross R, Glomset J, Kanyla B et al. Platelet-dependent serum factor that stimulates proliferation of arterial smooth muscle cells in vitro. Proc Natl Acad Sci USA 1974;71:1207–10.
16. Baber FE, Baker DW, Nation AWC et al. Ultrasonic duplex echo-Doppler scanner. IEEE Trans Biomed Eng 1974;109.
17. Fell G, Phillips DJ, Chikos PM et al. Ultrasonic duplex scanning for disease of the carotid artery. Circulation 1981;64:1191–5.
18. Wood CPL, Smith BT, Nunn CL et al. Noninvasive detection of boundary layer separation in the normal carotid artery bifurcation [abstract]. Stroke 1982;13:11.
19. Roederer GO, Langlois YE, Chan A et al. Ultrasonic duplex scanning of extracranial carotid arteries. Improved accuracy using new features from the common carotid artery. J Cardiovasc Ultrasound 1982;1:373–9.
20. Aldoori MI, Baird RN. Prospective assessment of carotid endarterectomy by clinical and ultrasonic methods. Br J Surg 1987;74:926–9.
21. Zierler RE, Phillips DJ, Beach KW et al. Noninvasive assessment of normal carotid bifurcation haemodynamics with colour-flow ultrasound imaging. Ultrasound Med Biol 1987;13:471–6.
22. Middleton WD, Foley WD, Lawson TL. Flow reversal in the normal carotid bifurcation: colour Doppler flow imaging analysis. Neuroradiol 1988;167:207–10.
23. Steinke W, Kloetzsch C, Hennerici M. Variability of flow patterns in the normal carotid bifurcation. Atherosclerosis 1990;84:121–7.
24. Houi K, Mochio S, Isogai Y et al. Comparison of colour flow and 3D imaging by computer graphics for the evaluation of carotid disease. Angiology 1990; April:305–12.
25. Kety SS, Schmidt CF. The determination of cerebral blood flow in man by the use of nitrous oxide in low concentrations. Am Phys 1945;143:53–66.
26. Greenfield JC, Tindall GT. Effect of acute increase in intracranial pressure on blood flow in the internal carotid artery of man. J Clint Invest 1965;44:1343–51.
27. Hardesty WH, Roberts VB, Toole JF et al. Studies on carotid artery-flow. Surgery 1960;49:251–6.
28. Lee RE. An evaluation of ultrasonic flowmetry in vascular surgery. University of Edinburgh Ch.M. thesis, 1987.
29. Archie JP. Critical stenosis of the internal carotid artery. Surgery 1981;89:67–72.
30. Wada T, Kodaira K, Fujishiro K et al. Correlation of common carotid flow volume measured by ultrasonic quantitative flowmeter with pathological findings. Stroke 1991;22:319–23.

31. Zwiebel WJ. Spectrum analysis of carotid sonography. Ultrasound Med Biol 1987;13:625–36.
32. Roberts R, Hardesty WH, Holling HE *et al.* Studies on extracranial blood flow. Surgery 1964;56:826–33.
33. Benetos A, Simon A, Levenson J *et al.* Pulsed Doppler: an evaluation of diameter, blood velocity and blood flow of the common carotid artery in patients with unilateral stenosis of the internal carotid artery. Stroke 1985;16:969–72.
34. Eklof B, Schwartz SI. Effect of critical stenosis of the carotid artery and compromised cephalic blood flow. Arch Surg 1969;99:695701.
35. Alpers BJ, Berry RG, Paddison RM. Anatomical studies of the circle of Willis in normal brain. A.M.A. Arch Neurol Psych 1959;81:409–18.
36. Kendall RE, Marshall J. Role of hypertension in the genesis of transient local cerebral ischaemic attacks. Br Med J 1963;2:344.
37. Moore WS, Hall AD. Importance of emboli from carotid bifurcation in pathogenesis of cerebral ischaemic attacks. Arch Surg 1970;101:708–16.
38. Russell RWR. Observations on the retinal blood-vessels in monocular blindness. Lancet 1961;2:1422.
39. Hafner CD, Evans WE. Carotid endarterectomy with local anaesthesia. Results and advantages. J, Vasc Surg 1988;7:232–9.
40. Mann FC, Herrick JF, Essex HE *et al.* The Effect on the blood flow of decreasing the lumen of a blood vessel. Surgery 1938;4:249–52.
41. Crawford ES, DeBakey ME, Frank WB *et al.* Haemodynamic alterations in patients with cerebral arterial insufficiency before and after operation. Surgery 1960;48:76–94.
42. May AG, Van de Berg L, DeWeese JA *et al.* Critical stenosis. Surgery 1963;54:250–9.
43. Moher JP, Pessin MS. Extracranial carotid artery disease. In: Barnett HJM, Stein BM, Moher JP *et al.* (eds.), Stroke: pathophysiology, disgnosis and management. New York: Churchill Livingstone, 1986:293–336.
44. Fisher CM. Observation of the fundus oculi in transient monocular blindness. Neurology 1959;9:333–47.
45. Zukowski AJ, Nicolaides AN, Lewis RT *et al.* The correlation between carotid plaque ulceration and cerebral infarction seen on CT scan. J Vasc Surg 1984;1:782–6.
46. Pancum PL. Experimentelle Beitrage zur Lehre von der Embolie. Virchows Arch (Pathol Anat) 1862;25:308.
47. Chiari H. Über das Verhalten des Teilungswinkels der carotid Communis bei der Endarteriitis Chronica Deformans. Verh Dtsch Ges Pathol 1905;9:326.
48. Meyer WW. Cholesterinkrystallembolie kleiner Organarterien und ihre Folgen. Virchows Arch (Pathol Anat) 1947;314:616.
49. Fisher CM. The use of anticoagulants in cerebral trombosis. Neurology 1958;8:311.
50. Hollenhorst RW. Significance of bright plaques in the retinal arterioles. JAMA 1961;178:23–9.
51. McBrien DJ, Bradley RD, Ashton N. The nature of retinal emboli in stenosis of the internal carotid artery. Lancet 1963;1:697.
52. Julian OC, Dye WS, Javid H *et al.* Ulcerative lesions of the carotid artery bifurcation. Arch Surg 1963;86:803–9.
53. Theile BL, Strandness IE. Distribution of intracranial and extracranial arterial lesions in patients with symptomatic cerebrovascular disease. In: Bernstein EF (ed.), Noninvasive diagnostic techniques in vascular disease. St Louis: The C V Mosby Company, 1982:193.
54. Eikelboom BC, Ackerstaff RGA, Ludwig JW *et al.* Digital video subtraction angiography and duplex scanning in assessment of carotid disease: comparison with conventional angiography. Surgery 1983;94:821–5.
55. Aldoori MI. Ultrasound and related studies in carotid disease. University of Bristol. Ph.D. thesis, 1986.
56. Millikan CH. The pathogenesis of transient focal cerebral ischaemia. Circulation 1965;32:438–50.

57. Whisnant JP. Multiple particles injected may all to to the same cerebral branch. Stroke. 1982;13:720.
58. Benson RL. The present status of coronary arterial disease. Arch Pathol Lab Med 1926;2:876–916.
59. Saphir D, Priest WS, Hamburger WW *et al.* Coronary atherosclerosis, coronary thrombosis and the resulting myocardial changes. Am Heart J 1935;10:567–95.
60. Clarke E, Graef I, Chasis H. Thrombosis of the aorta and coronary arteries. Arch Pathol Lab Med 1936;22:183–212.
61. Paterson JC. Capillary rupture with intimal haemorrhage as a causative factor in coronary thrombosis. Arch.Pathol 1938;25:474–84.
62. Geiringer E. Intimal vascularisation and atherosclerosis. J. Pathol. Bacteriol 1951;63:201–11.
63. Fisher CM. Occlusion of the internal carotid artery. Arch Neurol Psychiatr 1954; 72:187–203.
64. Imparato AM, Riles TS, Mintzer RM *et al.* The importance of haemorrhage in the relationship between gross morphological characteristics and cerebral symptoms in 379 carotid artery plaques. Ann Surg 1983;197:195–203.
65. Lusby RJ, Ferrell LD, Ehrenfield WK *et al.* Carotid plaque haemorrhage. Its role in production of cerebral ischaemia. Arch Surg 1982;117:1479–88.
66. Ammer AD, Wilson RL, Travers H *et al.* Intraplaque haemorrhage: its significance in cerebrovascular disease. Am J Surg 1984;148:840–3.
67. Ammer AD, Ernst RL, Lin JJ *et al.* The influence of repeated carotid plaque haemorrhages on the production of cerebrovascular symptoms. J Vasc Sur 1986;3:857–9.
68. Aldoori MI, Baird RN, Al-Sam SZ *et al.* Duplex scanning and plaque histology in cerebral ischaemia. Eur J Vasc Surg 1987;1:159–64.
69. Fryer JA, Myers PC, Appleberg MA. Carotid intraplaque haemorrhage: the significance of neovascularity. J Vasc Surg 1987;6:341–9.
70. Fisher M, Blumenfeld AM, Smith TW. The importance of carotid artery plaque disruption and haemorrhage. Arch Neurol 1987;44:1086–9.
71. Fisher CM, Ojemann RG. A clinicopathologic study of carotid endarterectomy plaques. Rev Neurol 1986;42:573–89.
72. Avril G, Batt M Guidoin R *et al.* Carotid endarterectomy plaques: correlation of clinical and anatomic findings. Ann Vasc Surg 1991;5:50–4.
73. Panel of Kings Fund Forum. Treatment of Stroke. 1988;297:126–8.
74. Millikan CH, McDowell FH. Treatment of transient ischaemic attacks. Stroke 1978;9:299–300.
75. Marqursden J. Epidemiology of strokes in Europe. In: Barnett HJM, Bennett MS, Mohr JP *et al.* (eds.), Stroke: pathophysiology, diagnosis and management. New York: Churchill Livingston, 1986: 31–44.
76. Dale S. Stroke. London: Office of Health Economics, 1988 ((No 89).
77. Shaper AG, Phillips AN, Pocock SJ *et al.* Risk factors for stroke in middle aged British men 1991;302:1111–5.
78. Wolf PA, D'Agostino, Kannel WB *et al.* Cigarette smoking as a risk factor for stroke. The Framingham study. JAMA 1988;259:1025–9.
79. Bousser MD, Eschwege R, Haguenau M *et al.* "A ICLA" controlled trial of aspirin and dsrpyridamole in the secondary prevention of atherothrombotic cerebral ischaemia. Stroke 1983;14:5–14.
80. European Carotid Surgery Trialists Conaborative Group. MRC European carotid surgery trial, interim results for symptomatic patients with severe (70–90%) or with mild (0–29%) carotid stenosis. Lancet 1991;337:235–43.
81. Barnett HJM, MASCET. North American symptomatic carotid endarterectomy trial. May 1991 (personal communication).
82. Barnett HJM. Progress towards stroke prevention: Robert Wartenberg lecture. Neurology 1980;30:1212–24.

83. Warlow C. Medical management. In: Warlow C, Morris PJ (eds.), Transient ischaemic attack. New York: Marcel Dekker, 1982:221–50.
84. Dennis M, Bamford J, Sandercock P *et al.* Prognosis of transient ischaemic attacks in the Oxfordshire community stroke project. Stroke 1990;21:848–53.
85. Harrison MJG, Marshall J. Indications for angiography and surgery in carotid artery disease. Br Med J 1975;1:616–7.
86. Callow AD, Mackey WC. Optimum results of the surgical treatment of carotid territory ischaemia. circulation 1991;83(Suppl 1):1-190–5.
87. Aldoori MI, Beneveniste GL, Baird RN *et al.* Asymptomatic carotid murmur: ultrasonic factors influencing outcome. Br J Surg 1987;74:496.
88. Hertzer NR, Flanagan RA, O'Hara PJ *et al.* Surgical versus nonoperative treatment of symptomatic carotid stenosis. 211 patients documented by intravenous angiography. Ann Surg 1986;20:154–62.
89. Healy DA, Clowes AW, Zierler RE *et al.* Immediate and long-term results of carotid endarterectomy. Stroke 1989;20:1138–42.
90. Hafner CD. Minimizing the risks of carotid endarterectomy. J Vasc Surg 1984;1:329–7.
91. Browse NL, Roos-Russel R. Carotid endarterectomy and the Javid shunt. The early results of 215 consecutive operations for transient ischaemic attacks. Br J Surg 1984;71:53–7.
92. Cafferata HT, Gainey MD. Carotid endarterectomy in the community hospital. A continuing controversy. J Cardiovasc Surg 1986;27:557–6.
93. Brott T, Thalinger K. The practice of carotid endarterectomy in a large metropolitan area. Stroke 1984;15:950–4.
94. Easton JD, Sherman DG. Stroke and mortality rate in carotid endarterectomy. 228 consecutive operations. 197;8:565–8.
95. Pokras R, Dyken ML. Dramatic changes in the performance of endarterectomy for diseases of the extracranial arteries of the head. Stroke 1988;19:1289– 90.
96. Mayberg MR, Wilson E, Yatsu F *et al.* Carotid endarterectomy and prevention of cerebral ischaemia in symptomatic carotid stenosis. JAMA 1991;266:3289–94.
97. Wiebers DO, Whisnaut JP, Sandok BA *et al.* Prospective comparison of a cohort with asymptomatic carotid bruit and a population-based cohort without carotid bruit. Stroke 1990;21:984–8.
98. Chambers BR, Morris JW. Outcome in patients with asymptomatic neck bruits. N Engl J Med 1986;315:860–5.
99. Reoederer GO, Langlois YE, Jager KA *et al.* The natural history of carotid arterial disease in asymptomatic patients with cervical bruits. Stroke 1984;15:605–13.
100. Moneta GL, Taylor DC, Nicholls SC *et al.* Operative versus nonoperative management of asymptomatic high-grade internal carotid artery stenosis. Improved results with endarterectomy. Stroke 1987;18:1005–10.
101. Caracci BF, Zukocoski AJ, Hurley JJ *et al.* Asymptomatic severe carotid stenosis. J Vasc Surg 1989;9:361.
102. Towne JB, Weiss DG, Hobson RW. First phase reports of co-operative VA Asymptomatic Carotid Stenosis Study – operative morbidity and mortality J Vasc Surg 1990;11:252–8.
103. Asymptomatic Carotid Atherosclerosis Study Group. Study design for randomised prospective trials of carotid endarterectomy for asymptomatic atherosclerosis. Stroke 1989;20:844–9.

Index of Subjects

Developments in Cardiovascular Medicine

50. J. Meyer, R. Erbel and H.J. Rupprecht (eds.): *Improvement of Myocardial Perfusion.* Thrombolysis, Angioplasty, Bypass Surgery. Proceedings of a Symposium, held in Mainz, F.R.G. (1984). 1985　　　　　　　　　　　ISBN 0-89838-748-5
51. J.H.C. Reiber, P.W. Serruys and C.J. Slager (eds.): *Quantitative Coronary and Left Ventricular Cineangiography.* Methodology and Clinical Applications. 1986
　　　　　　　　　　　　　　　　　　　　　　　　　　ISBN 0-89838-760-4
52. R.H. Fagard and I.E. Bekaert (eds.): *Sports Cardiology.* Exercise in Health and Cardiovascular Disease. Proceedings from an International Conference, held in Knokke, Belgium (1985). 1986　　　　　　　　　　ISBN 0-89838-782-5
53. J.H.C. Reiber and P.W. Serruys (eds.): *State of the Art in Quantitative Cornary Arteriography.* 1986　　　　　　　　　　　　　ISBN 0-89838-804-X
54. J. Roelandt (ed.): *Color Doppler Flow Imaging and Other Advances in Doppler Echocardiography.* 1986　　　　　　　　　　　　　ISBN 0-89838-806-6
55. E.E. van der Wall (ed.): *Noninvasive Imaging of Cardiac Metabolism.* Single Photon Scintigraphy, Positron Emission Tomography and Nuclear Magnetic Resonance. 1987
　　　　　　　　　　　　　　　　　　　　　　　　　　ISBN 0-89838-812-0
56. J. Liebman, R. Plonsey and Y. Rudy (eds.): *Pediatric and Fundamental Electrocardiography.* 1987　　　　　　　　　　　　　ISBN 0-89838-815-5
57. H.H. Hilger, V. Hombach and W.J. Rashkind (eds.), *Invasive Cardiovascular Therapy.* Proceedings of an International Symposium, held in Cologne, F.R.G. (1985). 1987　　　　　　　　　　　　　　　　　　ISBN 0-89838-818-X
58. P.W. Serruys and G.T. Meester (eds.): *Coronary Angioplasty.* A Controlled Model for Ischemia. 1986　　　　　　　　　　　　　　ISBN 0-89838-819-8
59. J.E. Tooke and L.H. Smaje (eds.): *Clinical Investigation of the Microcirculation.* Proceedings of an International Meeting, held in London, U.K. (1985). 1987
　　　　　　　　　　　　　　　　　　　　　　　　　　ISBN 0-89838-833-3
60. R.Th. van Dam and A. van Oosterom (eds.): *Electrocardiographic Body Surface Mapping.* Proceedings of the 3rd International Symposium on B.S.M., held in Nijmegen, The Netherlands (1985). 1986　　　　　　ISBN 0-89838-834-1
61. M.P. Spencer (ed.): *Ultrasonic Diagnosis of Cerebrovascular Disease.* Doppler Techniques and Pulse Echo Imaging. 1987　　　　　ISBN 0-89838-836-8
62. M.J. Legato (ed.): *The Stressed Heart.* 1987　　　　　ISBN 0-89838-849-X
63. M.E. Safar (ed.): *Arterial and Venous Systems in Essential Hypertension.* With Assistance of G.M. London, A.Ch. Simon and Y.A. Weiss. 1987
　　　　　　　　　　　　　　　　　　　　　　　　　　ISBN 0-89838-857-0
64. J. Roelandt (ed.): *Digital Techniques in Echocardiography.* 1987
　　　　　　　　　　　　　　　　　　　　　　　　　　ISBN 0-89838-861-9
65. N.S. Dhalla, P.K. Singal and R.E. Beamish (eds.): *Pathology of Heart Disease.* Proceedings of the 8th Annual Meeting of the American Section of the I.S.H.R., held in Winnipeg, Canada, 1986 (Vol. 1). 1987　　　　　ISBN 0-89838-864-3
66. N.S. Dhalla, G.N. Pierce and R.E. Beamish (eds.): *Heart Function and Metabolism.* Proceedings of the 8th Annual Meeting of the American Section of the I.S.H.R., held in Winnipeg, Canada, 1986 (Vol. 2). 1987　　　　　ISBN 0-89838-865-1
67. N.S. Dhalla, I.R. Innes and R.E. Beamish (eds.): *Myocardial Ischemia.* Proceedings of a Satellite Symposium of the 30th International Physiological Congress, held in Winnipeg, Canada (1986). 1987　　　　　　ISBN 0-89838-866-X
68. R.E. Beamish, V. Panagia and N.S. Dhalla (eds.): *Pharmacological Aspects of Heart Disease.* Proceedings of an International Symposium, held in Winnipeg, Canada (1986). 1987　　　　　　　　　　　　　　ISBN 0-89838-867-8
69. H.E.D.J. ter Keurs and J.V. Tyberg (eds.): *Mechanics of the Circulation.* Proceedings of a Satellite Symposium of the 30th International Physiological Congress, held in Banff, Alberta, Canada (1986). 1987　　　　　ISBN 0-89838-870-8
70. S. Sideman and R. Beyar (eds.): *Activation, Metabolism and Perfusion of the Heart.* Simulation and Experimental Models. Proceedings of the 3rd Henry Goldberg Workshop, held in Piscataway, N.J., U.S.A. (1986). 1987　ISBN 0-89838-871-6

Developments in Cardiovascular Medicine

71. E. Aliot and R. Lazzara (eds.): *Ventricular Tachycardias. From Mechanism to Therapy.* 1987 ISBN 0-89838-881-3
72. A. Schneeweiss and G. Schettler: *Cardiovascular Drug Therapoy in the Elderly.* 1988 ISBN 0-89838-883-X
73. J.V. Chapman and A. Sgalambro (eds.): *Basic Concepts in Doppler Echocardiography.* Methods of Clinical Applications based on a Multi-modality Doppler Approach. 1987 ISBN 0-89838-888-0
74. S. Chien, J. Dormandy, E. Ernst and A. Matrai (eds.): *Clinical Hemorheology.* Applications in Cardiovascular and Hematological Disease, Diabetes, Surgery and Gynecology. 1987 ISBN 0-89838-807-4
75. J. Morganroth and E.N. Moore (eds.): *Congestive Heart Failure.* Proceedings of the 7th Annual Symposium on New Drugs and Devices, held in Philadelphia, Pa., U.S.A. (1986). 1987 ISBN 0-89838-955-0
76. F.H. Messerli (ed.): *Cardiovascular Disease in the Elderly.* 2nd ed. 1988 ISBN 0-89838-962-3
77. P.H. Heintzen and J.H. Bürsch (eds.): *Progress in Digital Angiocardiography.* 1988 ISBN 0-89838-965-8
78. M.M. Scheinman (ed.): *Catheter Ablation of Cardiac Arrhythmias.* Basic Bioelectrical Effects and Clinical Indications. 1988 ISBN 0-89838-967-4
79. J.A.E. Spaan, A.V.G. Bruschke and A.C. Gittenberger-De Groot (eds.): *Coronary Circulation.* From Basic Mechanisms to Clinical Implications. 1987 ISBN 0-89838-978-X
80. C. Visser, G. Kan and R.S. Meltzer (eds.): *Echocardiography in Coronary Artery Disease.* 1988 ISBN 0-89838-979-8
81. A. Bayés de Luna, A. Betriu and G. Permanyer (eds.): *Therapeutics in Cardiology.* 1988 ISBN 0-89838-981-X
82. D.M. Mirvis (ed.): *Body Surface Electrocardiographic Mapping.* 1988 ISBN 0-89838-983-6
83. M.A. Konstam and J.M. Isner (eds.): *The Right Ventricle.* 1988 ISBN 0-89838-987-9
84. C.T. Kappagoda and P.V. Greenwood (eds.): *Long-term Management of Patients after Myocardial Infarction.* 1988 ISBN 0-89838-352-8
85. W.H. Gaasch and H.J. Levine (eds.): *Chronic Aortic Regurgitation.* 1988 ISBN 0-89838-364-1
86. P.K. Singal (ed.): *Oxygen Radicals in the Pathophysiology of Heart Disease.* 1988 ISBN 0-89838-375-7
87. J.H.C. Reiber and P.W. Serruys (eds.): *New Developments in Quantitative Coronary Arteriography.* 1988 ISBN 0-89838-377-3
88. J. Morganroth and E.N. Moore (eds.): *Silent Myocardial Ischemia.* Proceedings of the 8th Annual Symposium on New Drugs and Devices (1987). 1988 ISBN 0-89838-380-3
89. H.E.D.J. ter Keurs and M.I.M. Noble (eds.): *Starling's Law of the Heart Revisited.* 1988 ISBN 0-89838-382-X
90. N. Sperelakis (ed.): *Physiology and Pathophysiology of the Heart.* (Rev. ed.) 1988 ISBN 0-89838-388-9
91. J.W. de Jong (ed.): *Myocardial Energy Metabolism.* 1988 ISBN 0-89838-394-3
92. V. Hombach, H.H. Hilger and H.L. Kennedy (eds.): *Electrocardiography and Cardiac Drug Therapy.* Proceedings of an International Symposium, held in Cologne, F.R.G. (1987). 1988 ISBN 0-89838-395-1
93. H. Iwata, J.B. Lombardini and T. Segawa (eds.): *Taurine and the Heart.* 1988 ISBN 0-89838-396-X
94. M.R. Rosen and Y. Palti (eds.): *Lethal Arrhythmias Resulting from Myocardial Ischemia and Infarction.* Proceedings of the 2nd Rappaport Symposium, held in Haifa, Israel (1988). 1988 ISBN 0-89838-401-X
95. M. Iwase and I. Sotobata: *Clinical Echocardiography.* With a Foreword by M.P. Spencer. 1989 ISBN 0-7923-0004-1

Developments in Cardiovascular Medicine

Developments in Cardiovascular Medicine

Previous volumes are still available

KLUWER ACADEMIC PUBLISHERS – DORDRECHT / BOSTON / LONDON

CPSIA information can be obtained
at www.ICGtesting.com
Printed in the USA
LVOW10*1725120617
537835LV00010B/185/P